Visit our website

to find out about other books from W.B. Saunders and our sister companies in Harcourt Health Sciences

Register free at
www.harcourt-international.com

and you will get

- the latest information on new books, journals and electronic products in your chosen subject areas

- the choice of e-mail or post alerts or both, when there are any new books in your chosen areas

- news of special offers and promotions

- information about products from all Harcourt Health Sciences' companies including W. B. Saunders, Churchill Livingstone, and Mosby

You will also find an easily searchable catalogue, online ordering, information on our extensive list of journals...and much more!

Visit the Harcourt Health Sciences' website today!

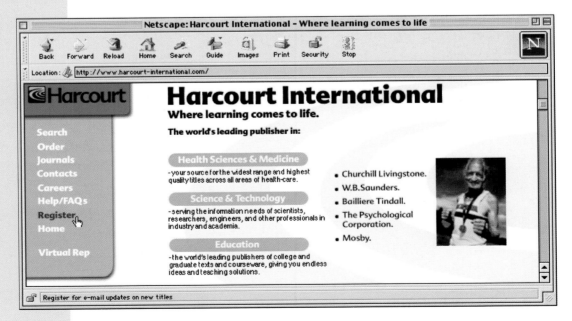

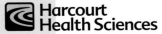

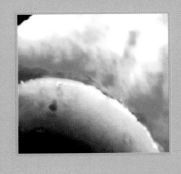

PRACTICE OF THERAPEUTIC ENDOSCOPY
second edition

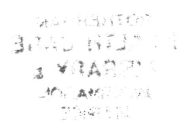

Commissioning Editor: **Sue Hodgson**
Project Development Manager: **Paul Fam**
Project Manager: **Cheryl Brant**
Senior Production Controller: **Helen Sofio**
Designer: **Greg Smith**

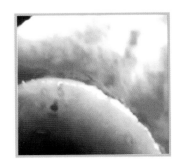

PRACTICE OF THERAPEUTIC ENDOSCOPY
second edition

G.N.J. Tytgat MD PhD FRCP
Professor of Gastroenterology, Academic Medical Centre,
University of Amsterdam, Amsterdam, The Netherlands

Meinhard Classen MD MDhc
Professor and Head of the Department of Internal Medicine II,
Technical University, Munich, Germany

Jerome D. Waye MD
Clinical Professor of Medicine, The Mount Sinai Medical Center,
City University of New York; Chief Gastrointestinal Endoscopy
Unit, Mount Sinai Hospital; Chief, Gastrointestinal Endoscopy
Unit, Lennox Hill Hospital, New York, New York, USA

Saburo Nakazawa MD
Professor of Medicine, Second Teaching Hospital, Fujita Health
University School of Medicine, Nagoya, Japan

 London Edinburgh New York Philadelphia St Louis Sydney Toronto 2000

WB Saunders
An imprint of Harcourt Publishers Limited

First edition published in 1994

ISBN 0 7020 2561 5

British Library Cataloguing in Publication Data
A catalogue record for this book is available from the British Library

Library of Congress Cataloging in Publication Data
A catalog record for this book is available from the Library of Congress

Note

Medical knowledge is constantly changing. As new information becomes available, changes in treatment, procedures, equipment and the use of drugs become necessary. The editors/authors/contributors and the publishers have taken care to ensure that the information given in this text is accurate and up to date. However, readers are strongly advised to confirm that the information, especially with regard to drug usage, complies with the latest legislation and standards of practice.

Printed in Spain

The
Publisher's
policy is **to use**
paper manufactured
from sustainable forests

CONTENTS

Preface to First Edition   viii
Preface to Second Edition   ix
Contributors   xi

1. **Practical management of non-variceal upper gastrointestinal bleeding**
   James Y.W. Lau & Sydney Sheong-Chee Chung   1

2. **Endoscopic treatment of variceal bleeding**
   Tilman Sauerbruch, Christian Scheurlen & Michael Neubrand   13

3. **Dilation procedures**
   Jacques Deviere   29

4. **Bridging intestinal narrowing with prostheses**
   Richard A. Kozarek   39

5.1 **Modalities for tissue coagulation or ablation: electrocoagulation**
   Louis-Michel Wong Kee Song & Norman E. Marcon   59

5.2 **Modalities for tissue coagulation or ablation: laser application**
   Rainer R. Sander   75

5.3 **Clinical application of argon plasma coagulation in flexible endoscopy**
   Karl E. Grund & Gunter Farin   87

6. **Photodynamic therapy in gastroenterology**
   L. Gossner & C. Ell   101

7. **Endoscopic mucosal resection for entire gastrointestinal mucosal cancers**
   Haruhiro Inoue   117

8. **Endoscopic sphincterotomy**
   Meinhard Classen & Peter Born   129

9.1 **Biliary tract stone disease: transpapillary endoscopic management**
   Gregory B. Haber & Alessandro Repici   147

9.2 **Biliary tract stone disease: transhepatic therapy**
   Horst Neuhaus   165

10. **Endoscopic management of benign pancreatic diseases**
    Michael J. Levy & Joseph E. Geenen   177

11. **Biliary stenting**
    Kees Huibregtse & Vinod Dhir   199

12. **Colonoscopic polypectomy**
    Jerome D. Waye   213

13. **Endoscopic treatment of lower intestinal bleeding**
    Christopher B. Williams   235

14. **Proctologic intervention**
    John Hartley & Peter Lee   245

15. **Endosonography-guided interventions**
    Manoop S. Bhutani   265

16. **Gastrostomy and enterostomy**
    E.M.H. Mathus-Vliegen   277

Index   301

The contribution of diagnostic endoscopy to medicine has been tremendous. Perhaps of even greater impact is the development of therapeutic endoscopy, which now attracts the interest of many physicians and surgeons in training.This atlas and textbook presents the current state of knowledge in the practice of therapeutic endoscopy. Obviously, this is not a surrogate for hands-on training. Rather, it is intended to teach the essentials of the various techniques in a systematic and straightforward way and to provide the background information which is necessary before practical training begin.

All the chapters have been written by experts who have had substantial clinical experience. The editors believe that these outstanding contributions from North American and European leaders on the field cover the relevant recent advances in an accessible but comprehensive way. Some minor items have been omitted because their applicability to routine practice has not yet been established. We have deliberately avoided including glamorous novel techniques which are still at the experimental stage and are not ready to be applied in clinical practice.

The editors would like to thank Churchill Livingstone for their support in preparing the book for the 1994 World Congress in Los Angeles.

We hope that *The Practice of Therapeutic Endoscopy* will meet the needs of gastroenterologists and surgeons in training and in practice. may this book help improve the care we provide to our patients.

G N J Tytgat
Meinhard Classen

PREFACE TO THE SECOND EDITION

Few discoveries in medicine have contributed so much to the development of gastroenterology and hepatology than the development of diagnostic and therapeutic endoscopy. Spectacular advances in other imaging modalities such as spiral computer tomography or magnetic resonance imaging undoubtedly compete with diagnostic endoscopy. Yet the possibility for targeted mucosal sampling remains unique for flexible endoscopy. Of even more importance is the realization that no other technology can rival endoscopy with respect to its therapeutic potential. Developments in therapeutic endoscopy have evolved so rapidly over the past few years that it was more than justified to produce and launch a new edition of this 'classic' book on therapeutic endoscopy. Just consider the developments in the endoscopic therapy of bleeding, stenting, biliary-pancreatic interventions, endosonographically guided therapy, and so on.

In line with the first edition, the aim of the editors was to produce a highly practical up-to-date textbook and atlas on all aspects of therapeutic endoscopy. A team of world renowned endoscopic interventionists has been willing to contribute to this second edition. They have provided superbly illustrated chapters which truly reflect the international coverage of therapeutic endoscopy. Clearly illustrated with colour line drawings and photographs, this practical and accessible book explains all steps involved in different endoscopic procedures and illustrates potential pitfalls, complications and results. Throughout this volume the reader will notice a 'personal touch' of the expert, reflecting their vast experience in practice. The editors are convinced that this issue will be well received by the practising gastroenterologist, both the novice and the experienced clinician. We are confident that this edition will become the genuine reflection of the global standard for endoscopic intervention.

On behalf of the editors, Professors Classen, Waye and Nakazawa,

G N J Tytgat
2000

CONTRIBUTORS

Manoop S. Bhutani MD FACG FACP
Director, Center for Endoscopic Ultrasound, Director, Center for Experimental Endoscopy, Associate Professor of Medicine, University of Florida, Gainesville, Florida, USA

Peter Born MD
Associate Professor Department of Internal Medicine II, Technical University, Munich, Germany

Sydney S. C. Chung MD
Professor, Department of Surgery, Faculty of Medicine, Prince of Wales Hospital, Shatin, New Territories, Hong Kong

Meinhard Classen MD MDhc
Professor and Head of the Department of Internal Medicine II, Technical University, Munich, Germany

Jacques Deviere MD PhD
Professor and Head of the Department of Gastroenterology and Hepatopancreatology, Hôspital Erasme, Bruselles, Belgium

Vinod Dhir MD
Department of Gastroenterology and Hepatology, Academic Medical Center, Amsterdam, The Netherlands

Christian Ell MD PhD
Professor of Medicine, Second Medical Department, Wiesbaden Hospital, Wiesbaden, Germany

Gunter Farin Dipl Ing
Center for Medical Research, Eberhard – Karls University, Tuebingen, Germany

Joseph E. Geenen MD
Professor of Medicine, Medical College of Wisconsin, Milwaukee, Wisconsin, USA

L. Gossner MD PhD
Professor of Medicine, Second Medical Department, Wiesbaden Hospital, Wiesbaden, Germany

Karl E. Grund MD
Professor of Surgery, Department of Surgical Endoscopy, Center for Medical Research, Eberhard – Karls University, University Hospital, Tuebingen, Germany

Gregory B. Haber MD, FRCP (C)
Assistant Professor, The Centre for Advanced Therapeutic Endoscopy and Endoscopic Oncology, The Wellesley Hospital, The University of Toronto, Toronto, Ontario, Canada

John Hartley MD FRCS
Lecturer and Honorary Registrar, Hull and East Yorkshire Hospital Trusts, Academic Surgical Unit, University of Hull Medical School, Hull, UK

Kees Huibregtse MD PhD
Professor of Gastrointestinal Endoscopy, Department of Gastroenterology and Hepatology, Academic Medical Center, Amsterdam, The Netherlands

Haruhiro Inoue MD
Chief of Endoscopic Surgery, First Department of Surgery, Tokyo Medical and Dental University, Tokyo, Japan

Richard A. Kozarek MD
Chief of Gastroenterology, Section of Gastroenterology, Virginia Mason Medical Center, Seattle, Washington, USA

James Y.W. Lau MD
Professor and Chairman, Department of Surgery, The Chinese University of Hong Kong, Prince of Wales Hospital, Ngan Shing Hospital, Shatin, Hong Kong

Peter Lee MD FRCS
Consultant Colon and Rectal Surgeon, Hull and East Yorkshire Hospital Trusts, Honorary Senior Lecturer, Academic Surgical Unit, University of Hull Medical School, Hull, UK

Michael J. Levy MD
Assistant Professor of Medicine, Emory University, Atlanta, Georgia, USA

Norman E. Marcon MD FRCP (C)
Associate Professor of Medicine, Division of Gastroenterology, The Wellesley Hospital, Toronto, Ontario, Canada

E.M.H. Mathus-Vliegen MD PhD
Professor of Clinical Nutrition, Department of Gastroenterology, Academic Medical Center University of Amsterdam, Amsterdam, The Netherlands

Michael Neubrand MD
Professor, Department of General Internal Medicine, University of Bonn, Bonn, Germany

Horst Neuhaus MD
Professor and Head of Department of Internal Medicine, Evangelisches Krankenhaus, Dusseldorf, Germany

Alessandro Repici MD, FRCP (C)
Fellow in Gastroenterology The Centre for Advanced Therapeutic Endoscopy and Endoscopic Oncology, The Wellesley Hospital, The University of Toronto, Toronto, Ontario, Canada

Rainer R. Sander MD
Internist, Gastroenterology, F.A.C.G., Stadtisches Krankenhaus Munchen-Harlaching, Akademisches Lehrkrrankenhaus Munchen, Germany

Tilman Sauerbruch MD
Professor, Department of General Internal Medicine, University of Bonn, Bonn, Germany

Christian Scheurlen MD
Professor, Department of General Internal Medicine, University of Bonn, Bonn, Germany

Jerome D. Waye MD
Clinical Professor of Medicine, The Mount Sinai Medical Center, City University of New York; Chief Gastrointestinal Endoscopy Unit, Mount Sinai Hospital; Chief, Gastrointestinal Endoscopy Unit, Lennox Hill Hospital, New York, New York, USA

Christopher B. Williams BM FRCP FRCS
Consultant Physician (Endoscopy), St. Mark's Hospital, London, UK

Louis-Michel Wong Kee Song MD FRCP (C)
Fellow in Therapeutic Endoscopy, Division of Gastroenterology, The Wellesley Hospital, Toronto, Ontario, Canada

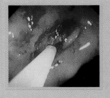

1.
PRACTICAL MANAGEMENT OF NON-VARICEAL UPPER GASTROINTESTINAL BLEEDING

JAMES YW LAU

SYDNEY SHEONG-CHEE CHUNG

OVERVIEW

Upper gastrointestinal bleeding continues to be a common cause of emergency hospital admission. Bleeding peptic ulcer is the commonest cause of an acute upper gastrointestinal bleed. In spite of a general decline in the incidence of peptic ulcer disease, the incidence of ulcer bleeding has paradoxically increased in recent years. In a recent national audit in the UK, the overall incidence of acute upper gastrointestinal bleeding was 103/100 000 adults per year.[1] Over the last few decades, patients presenting with bleeding are increasingly older. The proportion of patients aged over 60 was 33% in the 1940s compared to 68% in the 1990s. During this time major advances have been made in the practical management of gastrointestinal bleeding. Endoscopic hemostasis has become the first-line treatment for upper gastrointestinal bleeding in many hospitals. Endoscopy can often be performed within a few hours of admission. Many endoscopic hemostatic methods have been shown to be effective.[2,3] From specialized centers, very low mortality rates from 2 to 6% were reported. However, despite these advances, overall mortality of gastrointestinal bleeding has changed little in larger, population-based series. An aging population has appeared to offset advances made in the management of gastrointestinal bleeding.

THE ANATOMY OF A BLEEDING ULCER

Peptic ulcers bleed because an artery in the ulcer base is eroded by acid–peptic digestion. In most cases, the eroded artery is a medium-sized vessel in the submucosal plexus. Swain et al found 26 eroded arteries in 27 gastrectomy specimens in patients who required emergency surgery for bleeding.[4] The artery was plugged by a blood clot in 17 cases. Twenty of these arteries were below 1 mm in size.

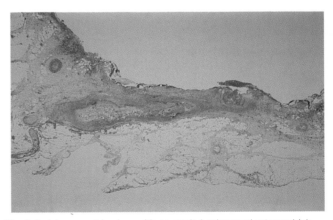

Fig. 1.1 A large gastric ulcer with an eroded subserosal artery which measures 1 mm in diameter.

Currently popular endoscopic devices such as electrocoagulation or heat probe can seal vessels of up to 1 mm in size. In the majority of bleeding ulcers, bleeding can be stopped by endoscopic treatment. In the event where larger serosal vessels are eroded, endoscopic therapy is less likely to succeed (Fig. 1.1). Examples are posterior duodenal ulcers eroding into the gastroduodenal artery, and lesser curve gastric ulcers eroding into the left gastric artery. In units that pursue an aggressive policy of endoscopic hemostasis, most of the patients who need surgical intervention fall into this category.

BASICS

Timing of endoscopy
Patients presenting with an acute gastrointestinal bleed should be endoscoped within 12 hours of admission. Most units would endoscope stable patients on the next day's list.

Urgent endoscopy should be performed after an initial period of resuscitation in those who are hemodynamically unstable, have vomited fresh blood, or when variceal bleeding is suspected. Rarely, patients with torrential bleeding cannot be stabilized before the bleeding is controlled. In these patients, endoscopy should be performed in the operating room with the patient intubated. If bleeding cannot be controlled endoscopically, surgery can be carried out without delay. The value of intubation is that the cuffed endotracheal tube protects against aspiration of blood.

CHOICE OF ENDOSCOPES

A standard endoscope with a 2.8 mm channel is more flexible and easier to manipulate than a wide therapeutic instrument. Unfortunately, the channel size limits the ability to suction blood and clots and the size of therapeutic devices. We prefer to use a therapeutic twin-channel endoscope (Fig. 1.2). The larger channel permits the use of 3.2 mm thermal devices. A twin-channel endoscope also permits suction and irrigation while therapy is being delivered via the other channel. If injection treatment is carried out, a twin-channel scope allows the needle to be inserted via either channel and therefore directed at different angles, allowing better targeting. In rare instances, the use of a side viewing scope allows en face access when an ulcer is in an awkward place, e.g. at the junction of the first and second part of the duodenum.

MONITORING

The condition of a bleeding patient may change rapidly. Pulse oximetry and automatic blood pressure monitoring should always be used. Supplemental oxygen by nasal cannula is useful to prevent desaturation during the procedure. Facilities for rapid blood transfusion such as pressurized infusion bags should be readily accessible. Resuscitation equipment including endotracheal tubes, life-support drugs and defibrillators should all be close by. As the endoscopist is likely to be preoccupied with the procedure, the condition of the patient must be monitored by other competent staff such as an anesthetist, a gastrointestinal assistant or a nurse.

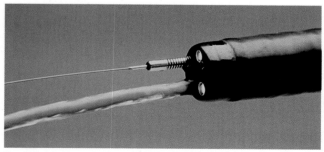

Fig. 1.2 A twin-channel therapeutic endoscope (2T-10, Olympus, Tokyo) allowing therapy and irrigation to be carried out at the same time.

PATIENT PREPARATION

Position of the patient

In the left lateral position adopted for routine endoscopy, blood in the stomach tends to gravitate towards the fundus and body of the stomach. Most bleeding lesions are located in the esophagus, along the lesser curvature, the antrum, or the duodenum. By avoiding the pool of blood in the fundus, adequate viewing is often possible, even in a stomach that is full of blood. If a red-out is encountered, the scope should be pulled back into the esophagogastric junction and then the stomach re-entered by following the lesser curvature into the antrum. Occasionally, rolling the patient over to the right side (the roll-over technique) can help expose the fundus and the greater curvature. Sitting the patient up at an angle may sometimes be useful to shift blood away from the cardia, e.g. in a patient with bleeding varices.

PROCEDURE

Gastric lavage and irrigation

We do not use gastric lavage routinely before endoscopy. When gastric lavage is required, an overtube is passed over the scope (Fig. 1.3). This protects against aspiration and facilitates repeated passage of the lavage tube. For washing blood and clots away from the bleeding lesion, the Water-pik device is useful (Fig. 1.4). This consists of a modified tooth-cleaning device with pulsed water jet fitted with a foot switch. By connecting it to the instrument channel of the endoscope via a three-way tap, effective irrigation can be carried out. Alternatively the irrigation facilities of the heat probe or the multipolar probe can be used.

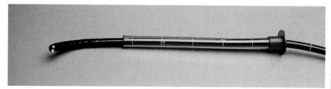

Fig. 1.3 An overtube passed over an endoscope.

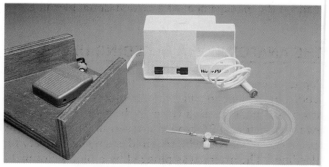

Fig. 1.4 A Water-pik device with a foot switch.

Who to treat

Bleeding stops spontaneously in 80% of bleeding peptic ulcers. In those who continue to bleed or develop recurrent bleeding, the mortality is substantially higher. It is therefore important to identify the latter group of patients for treatment. Before the days of endoscopic therapy, surgeons relied on clinical parameters such as shock at presentation, fresh hematemesis and age over 60 years to select patients for early surgical intervention.[5]

With emergency endoscopy, the appearance of the ulcer base also provides important clues to predict the likelihood of recurrent bleeding. In 1972, Forrest categorized bleeding peptic ulcers into those actively bleeding at endoscopy, those with stigmata of recent hemorrhage, and clean-based ulcers.[6] A modified version has been used widely in the literature to describe the appearance of the ulcer base. Actively bleeding ulcers (Forrest I) are further categorized into those with spurting or pulsatile bleeding (Ia) (Fig. 1.5) or those with oozing hemorrhage (Ib). Ulcers with stigmata of recent hemorrhage are subdivided into those with non-bleeding visible vessels (IIa), adherent clots (IIb), or flat pigmentation (IIc) (Figs 1.6 to 1.8). Essentially, these are eroded blood vessels plugged by a thrombus in different stages of evolution. Clean-based ulcers are designated as Forrest III.

Visual interpretation of stigmata of recent hemorrhage can be variable among endoscopists. Interobserver agreement studies on stigmata of hemorrhage revealed significant disparity in the visual interpretation of these stigmata, especially amongst endoscopists from different institutions.[7] The National Institute of Health Consensus Conference defined a non-bleeding visible vessel as 'protuberant' discoloration on the floor of an ulcer.[8] Adherent clots represent a heterogeneous group. Depending on the vigor of endoscopic washings, some of them may harbor an exposed vessel. Most endoscopists use targeted irrigation with a thermal probe with or without pre-injection around the clot with epinephrine, while others use mechanical methods such as a mini-snare to cheese-wire the clot off. In at least one-third of the cases, the adherent clot hides an eroded blood vessel. Both non-bleeding visible vessels and adherent clots are considered major stigmata and carry a rebleeding risk of 30 to 45% if left untreated. Flat spots (IIc), however, carry a much lower risk of rebleeding and should be left untreated. Clean-based ulcers carry a minimal risk of recurrent bleeding.

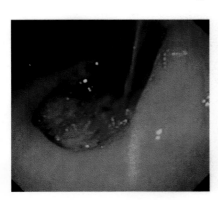

Fig. 1.5 A gastric ulcer with an arterial spurter.

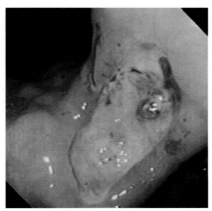

Fig. 1.6 A gastric ulcer at the angular notch with a protuberant discoloration or a non-bleeding visible vessel.

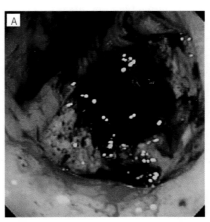

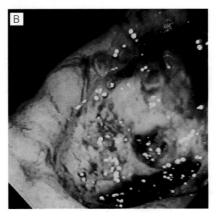

Fig. 1.7A and B An adherent clot in a gastric ulcer; a 'vessel' is noted after lifting the clot.

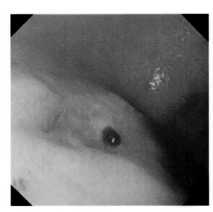

Fig. 1.8 A duodenal-ulcer with a flat pigmentation or a 'dot'.

Table 1.1 Prevalence and rebleeding risks of bleeding ulcers according to ulcer appearance at endoscopy (modified from Laine L, Peterson W. N Engl J Med 1994).[42]

Prevalence and rebleeding risks of bleeding ulcers			
Endoscopic appearance	Forrest class	Prevalence % (range)	Further bleeding % (range)
Clean base	III	42 (19–52)	5 (0–10)
Flat spot	II c	20 (0–42)	10 (0–13)
Adherent clot	II b	17 (0–49)	22 (14–36)
Non-bleeding visible vessel	II a	17 (4–35)	43 (0–81)
Active bleeding	I	18 (4–26)	55 (17–100)

Despite discrepancies in the reported prevalence and rebleeding risks of stigmata of recent hemorrhage, they are of prognostic significance (Table 1.1). These stigmata should be interpreted in the context of the clinical setting. Endoscopic treatment of an active bleeding ulcer is clearly warranted. The National Institute of Health Consensus Conference recommended that treatment also be applied to the non-bleeding visible vessel. There is currently no consensus in the case of adherent clots. Some endoscopists are wary to disturb an adherent clot for fear of provoking bleeding. Evidence is emerging, however, that a vigorous approach in removing the clot and treating the underlying vessel, if one is present, leads to a better clinical outcome. Patients with clean-based ulcers may be considered for early discharge if otherwise stable.

ENDOSCOPIC MODALITIES

Endoscopic therapy can be broadly divided into injection, thermal methods, and mechanical methods. Thermal methods can be further divided into non-contact methods such as laser photocoagulation or argon plasma coagulation and contact methods such as electrocoagulation and heater probes. The hemoclips are the only commercially available mechanical method at the current time.

Injection therapy
Because of wide availability and ease of use, injection therapy is the most widely practiced method of endoscopic therapy for ulcer bleeding. Soehendra first used the technique in 1976 when he injected 1% polidocanol to stop bleeding from a gastric ulcer.[9] Later, the technique was modified to use epinephrine injection to stop the bleeding followed by targeted injection of a sclerosant.[10]

Diluted epinephrine
Submucosal injection of epinephrine causes local tissue tamponade, vasoconstriction, and platelet aggregation. Unlike sclerosants, epinephrine does not cause tissue damage and large volumes (up to 20 mL) can be safely injected. The liver rapidly metabolizes epinephrine injected into the stomach or duodenum (1st pass effect) and adverse cardiovascular effects are rarely seen.[11] Caution should be exercised in patients with limited hepatic reserve, or if epinephrine injection is used outside the drainage area of the portal vein, e.g. in injecting a Mallory–Weiss tear. We favor the use of a 23 gauge sclerotherapy needle (Marcon–Haber

Injector, Wilson–Cook, Winston–Salem, USA). The needle should have a short bevel and protrude for about 5 mm beyond the plastic sheath. In chronic ulcers with a fibrotic base, more force is needed to push the fluid into the tissues and a metallic needle (NM-1K, Olympus Optical Co., Tokyo, Japan) is preferred.

Before use, the needle should be checked for patency and the ability to extend and retract. It is then primed with the injection solution. Aliquots of 0.5–1 mL are injected into and around the bleeding point. During epinephrine injection, accurate targeting is not necessary. Injection close to the bleeding vessel is sufficient to control the bleeding. During injection, the nurse-assistant will feel considerable resistance as the solution is injected, especially in a chronic ulcer with a fibrotic base. Submucosal injection will result in blanching around the ulcer. In actively bleeding ulcers, cessation of bleeding constitutes the therapeutic endpoint (Fig. 1.9A and B). In non-bleeding visible vessels, the

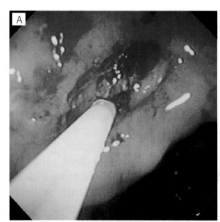
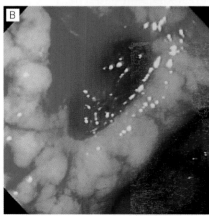

Fig. 1.9A and B Submucosal injection of a bleeding gastric ulcer stops bleeding and causes mucosal blanching.

endpoint is more difficult to define. Most endoscopists will inject at four quadrants up to a total of about 10 mL. The most commonly used dilution of epinephrine is 1/10 000. More dilute solutions (1/100 000) have also been used successfully; indeed, other authors have reported equally good results with dextrose water or even water, suggesting that tissue tamponade may be the main mechanism of hemostasis.

Epinephrine injection is highly effective in stopping active bleeding. The major drawback is that it does not induce permanent thrombosis of the bleeding artery. Recurrent bleeding occurs in about 15 to 20% of patients after epinephrine injection. Our opinion is that epinephrine should be used as the initial agent for stopping the bleeding and gaining a clear view of the vessel. A second agent should then be targeted to the artery to obliterate the vessel and reduce the chance of rebleeding.

Sclerosants

Agents used for variceal sclerotherapy such as polidocanol, sodium tetradecyl sulfate and ethanolamine have been used successfully to control ulcer bleeding. When injected into the gastric mucosa, they cause tissue necrosis and ulcer extension in a dose-dependent manner. Because of the dangers of stomach wall necrosis and perforation, the maximum volume that can be injected is limited. Most endoscopists would use epinephrine to control the active bleeding and to gain a good view before injecting the sclerosant.

Absolute alcohol causes rapid tissue dehydration and is the most potent agent in causing thrombosis. Because of the potent tissue-damaging effect, alcohol should be injected in 0.2–0.4 mL aliquots using a tuberculin syringe. The maximum permissible volume is 2 mL.

Several trials have examined the value of adding a sclerosant after epinephrine injection. We studied 200 patients with actively bleeding ulcers and randomly assigned them to epinephrine injection alone or epinephrine injection plus 3% sodium tetradecyl sulfate.[12] Initial hemostasis was comparable in either group (94 vs 97%). No difference was noted between the two groups in their requirement for emergency surgery, blood transfusion, and death. A group from Edinburgh compared injection of epinephrine to epinephrine plus 5% ethanolamine in 107 patients.[13] Permanent hemostasis was achieved in 85% of patients in either group. In another trial with 63 patients, Villanueva was unable to demonstrate any difference in outcome following the addition of polidocanol.[14] The addition of alcohol after epinephrine injection was studied in two randomized trials. In a trial with 160 patients with active bleeding, our group was unable to show any difference in rebleeding, surgery, or death.[15] Lin et al randomized 64 patients and also found that rebleeding was similar in either group.[16]

There have been case reports of gastric necrosis following sclerosant injection, some of which were fatal (Fig. 1.10).[17,18] In view of the lack of evidence showing any added benefit, and the potential for serious complications,

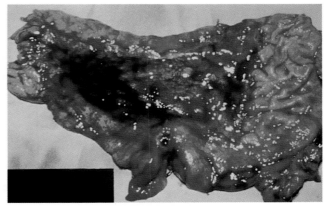

Fig. 1.10 Gastrectomy specimen from a patient with extensive gastric necrosis after endoscopic injection of a sclerosant.

we do not recommend adding a sclerosant after epinephrine injection.

Thrombogenic substances

Thrombin initiates the clotting cascade and is arguably the most physiological agent used in injection therapy. Thrombin injection does not cause local tissue damage and has even been claimed to promote ulcer healing. To limit the amount of thrombin used, it is usual to pre-inject with epinephrine in actively bleeding ulcers. There are theoretical concerns of intravascular injection leading to systemic thrombosis and anaphylaxis but none of these postulated complications has been reported. Initially, bovine thrombin was used, but the current product is human thrombin derived from pooled plasma. The preparation is solvent treated and the risk of viral transmission should be minimal. Kubba et al compared epinephrine injection alone with epinephrine followed by human thrombin in high concentration. A significant reduction in recurrent bleeding, transfusion, and mortality was observed in the dual treatment group.[19]

Fibrin sealant (Figs 1.11A, B and C)

Fibrin sealant is a two-component product. It consists of (1) thrombin constituted in aprotonin solution and (2) fibrinogen in calcium chloride solution. When these two components are mixed, a fibrin sealant forms. Injection of fibrin glue requires a dual-channel injection needle. Mixing of the two components of the glue occurs at the needle tip. The needle has a wider channel for the more viscous fibrinogen and a narrower channel for the thrombin. The injector is color-coded to ensure that the respective solutions are injected through the correct channel.

The technique of injection is referred to as the plug technique (Fig. 1.12). Considerable force is needed to advance the needle deep into the submucosa. The aim is to surround the bleeding point in four quadrants with submucosal blebs before injecting the vessel itself. The needle is placed about 5 mm from the bleeding point and 0.5 mL of fibrinogen and 0.5 mL of thrombin (1 mL of fibrin sealant) is injected into each quadrant. With the needle

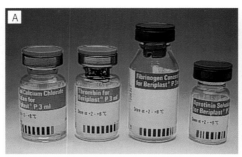
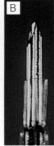
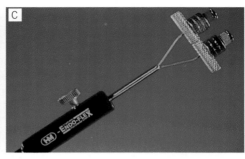

Fig. 1.11A, B and C The fibrin sealant is a two-component adhesive mixed by reconstituted thrombin in calcium chloride solution and fibrinogen in aprotonin solution (Beriplast P). Injection of fibrin sealant requires a twin-channel needle. One of the channels is larger, allowing for injection of the more viscous fibrinogen. Both the injector and the solutions are color-coded so that the two solutions are injected into respective channels. Mixing occurs submucosally at the tip of the needle.

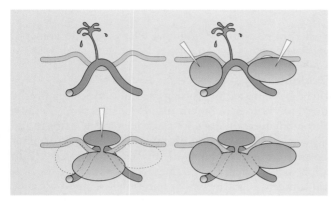

Fig. 1.12 The plug technique with four-quadrant injection followed by injection into the bleeding point. The needle is slowly withdrawn, allowing a central fibrin plug.

still in the tissue, 1–1.5 mL of normal saline is injected to drive the glue submucosally. Consequently the volume injected at a single site adds up to approximately 2.5 mL. Following four-quadrant injection, the bleeding point is then injected. As the glue is being injected, the needle is slowly withdrawn leaving a central fibrin plug.

Many European centers recommend repeated fibrin glue injection at scheduled daily endoscopy until bleeding stigmata disappear from the ulcer floor. In a large multicenter trial, patients with actively bleeding ulcers, visible vessels and clots were randomized into three groups: polidocanol alone, single injection with epinephrine and fibrin sealant, and repeated daily injections of epinephrine and fibrin sealant until complete fading of stigmata from the ulcer floor.[20] The repeated fibrin sealant group had the lowest rebleeding rate (15.2%), compared to 19.2% for once-only fibrin sealant and 22.8% for once-only polidocanol. Statistically, the rebleeding rates for polidocanol and repeated fibrin sealant were significantly different. Unfortunately, it was not possible to ascertain whether the difference resulted from the repeated treatment or the use of fibrin sealant.

Thermal methods
Thermal methods can be divided into contact and non-contact methods.

Non-contact thermal probes. Non-contact methods include laser treatment and, more recently, argon plasma coagulation (APC). These methods depend on the heating of tissue protein, contraction of the arterial wall, and vessel shrinkage. One drawback of non-contact thermal methods is the 'heat sink effect' where flowing arterial blood leads to dissipation of the thermal energy. Because of the higher tissue penetration, the neodymium: yttrium aluminum garnet (Nd:YAG) laser is superior to the argon laser for ulcer hemostasis. Laser units are expensive, bulky and generally not portable. They are also difficult to use as an en face view of the bleeding ulcer is required. For these reasons, laser photocoagulation has fallen out of favor for ulcer bleeding. The argon plasma coagulator uses a flowing stream of argon gas as the conductor for electrocoagulation. This method is excellent for mucosal bleeding but may not be effective in coagulating the eroded artery in a bleeding ulcer. As flowing argon gas is needed, care must be taken to avoid overdistention of the stomach during treatment.

Contact thermal probes. Multipolar electrocoagulation and the heat probe device fall into this group. Unipolar electrocoagulation results in unpredictable tissue damage and cannot be recommended.

Contact thermal probes utilize the principle of 'coaptive coagulation' (Fig. 1.13); firm tamponade of the blood vessel brings the two walls of the blood vessel together. Heat is then applied to seal the two walls together. Compression of the blood vessel also stops the blood flow and reduces the heat sink effect. In experimental settings, contact thermal probes consistently seal bleeding vessels of up to 2 mm in diameter.[21] Both electrocoagulation and the heat probe have been shown to be effective in randomized controlled clinical trials (RCTs).[22–24]

The BICAP probe has three pairs of electrodes at its tip. The electrical circuit is completed when two adjacent electrodes of different polarity are in contact with the tissues. The Gold probe (Microvasive) has alternating electrodes arranged in a spiral manner. The Injector-Gold probe (Microvasive) also incorporates an injection needle for pre-injection with epinephrine (Fig. 1.14). Effective electrocoagulation requires:

2.
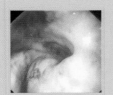
ENDOSCOPIC TREATMENT OF VARICEAL BLEEDING

TILMAN SAUERBRUCH

CHRISTIAN SCHEURLEN

MICHAEL NEUBRAND

Esophageal varices are caused either by portal hypertension or by an increased outflow resistance above the level of the azygos vein. In the latter situation, varices that have developed in the esophagus are also called 'downhill varices'. The vast majority of esophageal varices are caused by portal hypertension where the varices constitute a collateral system to bypass an outflow obstruction of the splenic or portal vein. The elevated pressure in the portal system is due to liver cirrhosis in most patients, in whom not only outflow obstruction but also increased portal inflow contributes to portal hypertension.[1] The prevalence of esophageal varices in patients with liver cirrhosis ranges between 40% and 80%.[2] Nine out of 10 patients in whom cirrhosis has been known for 10 or more years eventually develop esophageal varices (Fig. 2.1A–E).[3] Ten percent of these patients will have

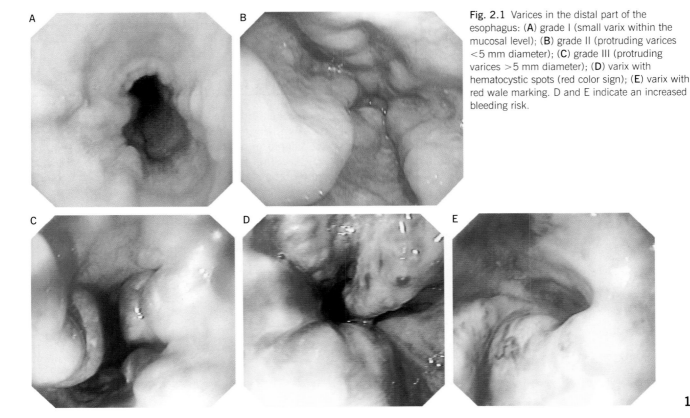

Fig. 2.1 Varices in the distal part of the esophagus: (**A**) grade I (small varix within the mucosal level); (**B**) grade II (protruding varices <5 mm diameter); (**C**) grade III (protruding varices >5 mm diameter); (**D**) varix with hematocystic spots (red color sign); (**E**) varix with red wale marking. D and E indicate an increased bleeding risk.

Calculation of the risk of bleeding in esophageal varies[†]	
Variable	Points
Size of varices	
Small	8.7
Medium	13.0
Large	17.4
Red wale markings	
Absent	3.2
Mild	6.4
Moderate	9.6
Severe	12.8
Child's grade	
A	6.5
B	13.0
C	19.5

*The score is computed by adding the corresponding three points.
Probability of first bleeding within 1 year:

< 20 points	< 10%
20–40 points	10–40%
> 40 points	around 70%

† Modified from The North Italian Endoscopic Club for the Study and Treatment of Esophageal Varices. Prediction of the first variceal hemorrhage in patients with cirrhosis of the liver and esophageal varices. N Engl J Med 1988; 319:983–989.

Table 2.1 Score* for calculation of the risk of bleeding in esophageal varices[†]

concomitant varices in the fundal region of the stomach.[4,5] Furthermore, 50 to 100% of patients with varices and liver cirrhosis have been reported to have congestive or hypertensive gastropathy defined as cherry red spots on a finely granular mucosa.[6–8]

Esophageal varices may rupture and bleed. This occurs in about 30 to 40% of patients with varices. Several risk scores, mainly based on endoscopic findings, have been published (Tables 2.1 and 2.2; Fig. 2.1A–E).[5,9] These scores may help to decide whether measures for prophylaxis of bleeding are mandatory.

Measurements of the variceal radius by endosonography together with the transmural pressure may also be used to estimate the tension of the variceal wall and therewith the bleeding risk.[10]

ENDOSCOPIC THERAPY OF ESOPHAGEAL VARICES

Injection sclerotherapy was first described more than 50 years ago.[11] It required a rigid endoscope as well as general anesthesia, and the procedure failed to gain a significant place in the treatment of varices. Thus, variceal hemorrhage was mainly managed by balloon tamponade with the Linton or Sengstaken–Blakemore tube,[12] vasopressin and/or shunt surgery.[13] This situation changed when the first negative results of controlled trials on portacaval anastomoses appeared.[13] Together with the development of flexible endoscopes, the technique of sclerotherapy was revitalized by several pioneers in Europe between the mid-1950s and the early 1970s.[14–16] It has now to a large extent been replaced by endoscopic variceal band ligation.

Sclerotherapy and ligation are applied to achieve three major goals: hemostasis of active hemorrhage, prophylaxis of first hemorrhage, or prophylaxis of recurrent variceal bleeding. The technique of sclerotherapy varies from center to center with regard to sclerosants, needles, endoscopes, injection sites, time schedules, and adjuvant measures, although the results may be quite similar.

Two major new developments have been added to the armamentarium of variceal treatment within recent years, namely variceal ligation[17,18] and the transjugular intrahepatic portosystemic shunt (TIPS).[19] TIPS is of special value in patients with recurrent bleeding who are refractory to local measures – such as sclerotherapy or ligation – or who exhibit concomitant ascites that is poorly managed with diuretics. Ligation has become the initial treatment of choice to prevent rebleeding.[20] Some trials suggest a combination of ligation and sclerotherapy[21–23] although its superior effect compared to ligation alone is not proven by all authors.[24–27]

INDICATIONS AND CONTRAINDICATIONS

Elective local endoscopic treatment of esophageal varices, whether by injection sclerotherapy or ligation, is principally indicated in all patients with proven or suspected variceal bleeding. However, it must be remembered that reduction of the bleeding risk is not achieved prior to oblit-

Clinical, serological and endoscopic parameters indicating an increased bleeding risk					
					P-value
Gastric varices	Absent	24%	Present	69%	<0.0001
Red color sign	Absent	25%	Present	46%	0.002
Ascites	Absent	28%	Severe	43%	0.01
Alcoholic liver disease	Absent	17%	Present	25%	0.02
Child's grade	A	23%	B or C	33%	0.03
Size of largest varix	<5 mm	12%	>5 mm	33%	0.08

Encephalopathy, age, number of varices, bilirubin and albumin levels, prothrombin time and platelets had no influence on bleeding risk.[5]

Table 2.2 Clinical, serological and endoscopic parameters indicating an increased bleeding risk within a mean follow-up of 21 ± 15 months in 109 patients with gastric and/or esophageal varices and without history of bleeding

eration of most of the varices, which takes at least 1 to 2 months. Endoscopic treatment should not be continued in those patients who suffer from recurrent bleeding despite repeated procedures. Local endoscopic therapy requires a compliant and cooperative patient. Otherwise, less time-consuming procedures (e.g. a shunt) or those which are less invasive (e.g. drugs, i.e. propranolol) should be applied depending on the circumstances.

Emergency treatment of intestinal bleeding requires endoscopy as soon as possible. In these patients, localization of variceal hemorrhage should always be followed by immediate local treatment for hemostasis. It is effective in up to 90% of patients, be it injection or ligation.[18,20,28,29]

The indication for endoscopic therapy for prophylaxis of first variceal hemorrhage is controversial. A possible benefit of prevention of bleeding in patients with large varices and a high bleeding risk may be outweighed by complications of sclerotherapy.[30,31] It is debatable whether ligation may overcome some of the drawbacks and gain a place in the prophylaxis of first bleeding.[32]

EQUIPMENT

Endoscopes

Injection of varices is now generally performed with normal forward-viewing endoscopes (diameter 9.8 mm). Oblique-viewing endoscopes (e.g. $GIFK_{10}$, Olympus) may have some advantages but are no longer available. In cases of heavy bleeding, glass fiber endoscopes may permit better vision, but many endoscopists use videoendoscopes in this situation.

Ligation is performed with standard endoscopes onto which the hollow plastic cylinders carrying the rubber bands are placed.

Overtubes

Overtubes with a distal slot,[33,34] formerly used as a working channel for sclerotherapy, have been abandoned in favor of the free hand technique. The overtube with bite block which initially was obligatory for rubber band ligation[29,35–37] is now rarely used after the advent of multiple-shooter systems, especially since it carries a small risk of additional complications.[38,39] The plastic overtube (length 25 cm, diameter 20 mm) is sometimes of value in the situation of heavy bleeding, allowing rapid suction of blood clots. In this case, patients should be intubated and care has to be taken not to lacerate the esophageal wall. A tear of the pharyngeal mucosa may be minimized by introducing a tapered dilator (which some endoscopists prefer to place over a guidewire) through the overtube.

Needles and agents used for injection sclerotherapy

A number of different needles are available for injection sclerotherapy. Normally a 23 or 25 gauge needle is used with a length of 6 or 7 mm.

> **BOX 2.1 Sclerosants generally used for injection sclerotherapy of esophageal varices**
>
> - 5% Ethanolamine oleate
> - 0.5–2% Polidocanol (e.g. Aethoxysclerol)
> - 0.75–3% Sodium tetradecyl sulfate
> - 1.6% or 5% Sodium morrhuate
> - N-butyl-2-cyanoacrylate
> - Fibrin glue

A variety of sclerosants available for injection of esophageal varices is shown in Box 2.1. In the UK, Japan, North America and South Africa, sodium tetradecyl sulfate and ethanolamine oleate are widely employed, whereas a mixture of 5–20 mg/mL of polidocanol with 0.05 mL of ethanol is used most frequently in continental Europe. The effect, i.e. thrombosis, inflammation, and fibrosis, is similar with all sclerosants.[40,41] However, there are only a few studies in which a systematic comparison was carried out. In the clinical setting, ethanolamine oleate was more effective than sodium tetradecyl sulfate[42] with respect to rebleeding and complications (esophageal ulcers).

Two trials[43,44] (one of them controlled[44]) showed that fibrin glue was as effective as polidocanol, but may prevent the development of post-sclerotherapy ulcers. However, injection of fibrin requires more sessions to achieve obliteration of varices and is expensive. Conventional sclerosants are not effective for the treatment of bleeding fundal varices. Butyl-cyanoacrylate, a 'glue' which hardens on contact with blood, has been shown to be superior.[15] One group favors administration of butyl-cyanoacrylate for first-line injection of esophageal varices in cases of heavy bleeding.[45]

Ligation device

The chamber of all ligation devices consists of an outer cylinder which is affixed to the tip of a standard flexible endoscope and an inner cylinder mounted with one or several rubber rings (Fig. 2.2A). This latter cylinder is connected with a trip wire running through the biopsy channel of the endoscope. Pulling the wire moves the inner cylinder towards the endoscope and releases the rubber ring which contracts onto the base of the mucosa and varix which were pulled into the cylinder device by suction/aspiration. The more recent devices are constructed of a transparent hollow plastic cylinder which several rubber bands are stretched. The p rim of this device consists of stretchable e polyvinyl allowing adaption to different end trigger unit (Fig. 2.2B) pulls a braided draw is led through the biopsy channel and relea rings one after another (Fig. 2.2A).[46]

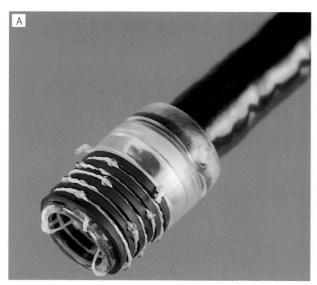

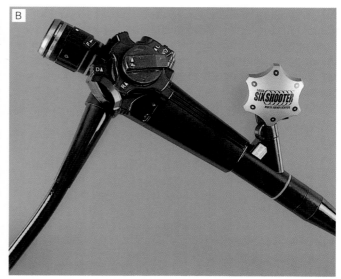

Fig. 2.2 Multiligator tip with six elastic rubber bands (**A**) which are released by a trigger unit at the entrance of the working channel (**B**).

PATIENT PREPARATION

Emergency treatment

A large-bore intravenous (IV) catheter is inserted into a peripheral vein. In an acute emergency when peripheral veins are not available, access may be via a jugular, subclavian, or femoral vein. Blood can be drawn at this time for initial studies which should include a complete blood count, electrolytes, blood urea nitrogen, creatinine, glucose, coagulation parameters, and blood for typing and cross-matching.

Sedatives should be administered with care because of the danger of aspiration. Systemic injection of vasoactive drugs (e.g. glycylpressin, 1–2 mg initially, then 1 mg every 4–6 h, or the somatostatin analog, octreotide, 50 µg/h with an initial 50 µg bolus)[47] should be started even prior to emergency endoscopy if bleeding associated with portal hypertension is suspected.[48,49] If possible, the emergency procedure should be performed in a critical care facility. Prophylactic intubation with mechanical ventilation prevents aspiration, but is not generally recommended. High-risk patients, e.g. patients with pre-existing severe pulmonary disease or severe encephalopathy, should be ventilated. Prophylactic administration of antibiotics is mandatory in patients with known valvular heart disease. Several studies showed that routine treatment with peri-operative antibiotics reduces bacteremia and infection of ascites.[50]

Elective treatment

For elective treatment, the patient is endoscoped after an overnight fast. Sedatives and scopolamine should be given depending on the patient's condition (e.g. 5 mg midazolam or 20–40 mg propofol initially), considering the altered bioavailability of these drugs in cirrhotic patients. Patients with considerable impairment of coagulation (e.g. pro-hrombin time less 30%) may receive coagulation factors frozen plasma) or vitamin K prior to endoscopy.

PROCEDURE

Technique of sclerotherapy

Variceal bleeding mostly occurs in the distal part of the esophagus and at the gastroesophageal junction. In this region, varices are only covered by a thin layer of squamous cell epithelium and are thus particularly prone to bleed.[51] Therefore most of the injection treatment is directed to the varices in the distal third of the esophagus up to 3–6 cm above the squamocolumnar junction. There are three different techniques for injection sclerotherapy: intravariceal injection, paravariceal injection or the combined technique (Figs 2.3 and 2.4), using mostly 23 gauge needles with a length of 4–8 mm. Some authors doubt whether the distinction between the different techniques is valid since nearly 50% of attempted intravariceal injections result in paravariceal accumulation of the injected material.[52] The injection of sclerosants (see Box 2.1) directly into the lumen of the vessel may lead to more systemic side effects, especially in the lungs. However, thrombosis of the vessel is probably achieved more rapidly. Some authors favor the combined technique.[4,53] The sclerosant is first injected into the vessel and then the needle is withdrawn to apply a deposit to the variceal wall and the adjacent mucosa (Figs 2.3 and 2.4). This may reduce bleeding after

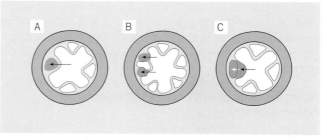

Fig. 2.3 Scheme of different injection techniques: (**A**) intravariceal; (**B**) paravariceal; (**C**) combined.

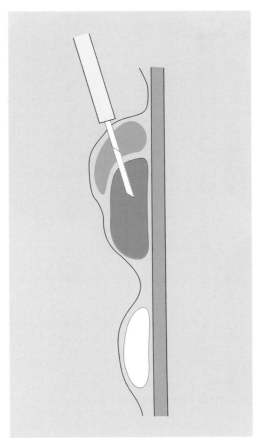

Fig. 2.4 Scheme of combined injection technique.

injection. We start injection precisely at the gastroesophageal junction and then proceed stepwise orally. Each varix is injected beginning at 6 o'clock if the patient is in the left lateral position, because the blood pools in the deepest point and prevents precise targeting of the varices at the site when injection is started elsewhere. The injections are performed at about three levels with a distance of 2–3 cm between sites.

The volume applied per session and per injection depends on the chosen sclerosant. While a large amount of sclerosant may lead to a more rapid obliteration of varices, it carries a higher risk of complications such as bleeding ulcers or perforations. At present, there is a tendency to use smaller amounts of sclerosant to avoid these complications. When using polidocanol 1%, 15–20 mL per session, and 0.5–5 mL per injection, appear to be most appropriate. Similar volumes have been used for ethanolamine oleate and sodium tetradecyl sulfate. In cases of more pronounced bleeding from the injection site, two manoeuvers can be performed: the endoscope may be passed into the stomach to tamponade the varix for several minutes or, if bleeding has not stopped, a second injection of fibrin glue or butyl-cyanoacrylate may be given.

Butyl-cyanoacrylate is often mixed with a fat-soluble dye (lipiodol 1/1 or 1/2 v/v) in order to allow radiologic visualization of the thrombus casts and to prevent the glue from hardening too rapidly; in most cases, 1–2 mL of this mixture are given per injection. A mixture of butyl-cyanoacrylate and dye is also used to treat gastric varices (Fig. 2.5A–C). Butyl-cyanoacrylate has to be injected as much as possible directly into the vessel. This may be tested by starting with saline. Prior to injection of butyl-cyanoacrylate, the endoscope must be prepared in order to prevent damage to the instrument. The tip of the scope and the biopsy channel are flushed with silicone oil which reduces the danger of the material sticking to exposed surfaces. In addition, the endoscope should be withdrawn with the needle in place after intravascular injection, otherwise the glue might drip into the channel if the needle is pulled back. Alternatively, the catheter and needle should be flushed with water to remove all glue before withdrawal.

Technique of ligation

The endoscope with the rubber-band ligating device can be introduced normally after topical oropharyngeal anesthesia and intravenous sedation. Ligation should be started as close to the gastroesophageal junction as possible. The target varix is approached (Fig. 2.6A) and suctioned to fill the inner chamber (with the rubber rings) (Fig. 2.6B). A ring is released by turning the trigger device

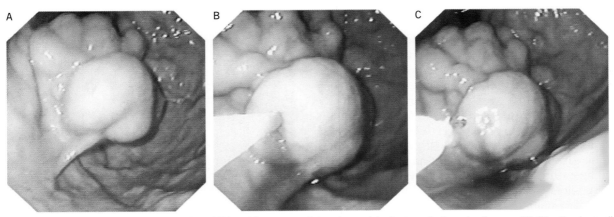

Fig. 2.5 (A) Gastric varix. (B) Varix during injection of N-butyl-2-cyanoacrylate using an injection needle for sclerotherapy. (C) Situation immediately after injection of the varix.

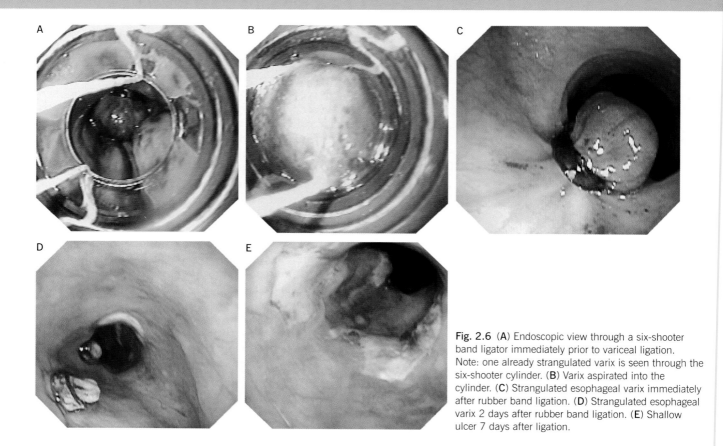

Fig. 2.6 (A) Endoscopic view through a six-shooter band ligator immediately prior to variceal ligation. Note: one already strangulated varix is seen through the six-shooter cylinder. (B) Varix aspirated into the cylinder. (C) Strangulated esophageal varix immediately after rubber band ligation. (D) Strangulated esophageal varix 2 days after rubber band ligation. (E) Shallow ulcer 7 days after ligation.

clockwise (Fig. 2.6C). Care must be taken to suck the varix as far as possible into the cylinder so that the varix can be completely ligated and blood flow interrupted at this site. Otherwise, the ring may fall off and cause heavy bleeding if the varix is not thrombosed. Other varices at the same level are then treated. Thereafter, the endoscope is drawn back 2–3 cm to treat varices at a more proximal level until the mid-esophagus is reached. On average 5 to 10 bands are placed per session. In cases of large varices up to 15 to 20 bands may be released at the first session. The value of ligation of gastric varices – despite anecdotal reports – is still debated, since it is questionable whether all feeding vessels can sufficiently be interrupted in one session.[54,55]

Treatment schedule

The intervals between endoscopic sessions vary in different reports. Most groups, however, leave an interval of 7 days during the initial phase of sclerotherapy and ligation as well. If the interval between sclerotherapy sessions is too short (less than a week), there is an increase in life-threatening complications, probably as a result of cumulative local tissue injury.[56] Longer intervals (3 weeks) between sclerotherapy sessions will prolong the total treatment time required for obliteration, with the risk of rebleeding events.[57] A comparative trial between 1- and 2-weekly sclerotherapy intervals found no relevant difference.[58] The number of sessions required for obliteration was similar in all trials. Most authors report that a total of 6 to 8 sessions during the initial treatment phase

was required to obliterate the majority of the varices (Fig. 2.7). Therefore, the bleeding risk is probably not reduced earlier than 2 or 3 months after initiation of sclerotherapy. Complete obliteration in most patients takes even longer (up to 1 year). On the other hand, there is some evidence[59] that total eradication of the varices may not be necessary to reduce the bleeding risk and that sclerotherapy can be stopped when reduction of the varices to small columns has been achieved. Varices may recur after obliteration in up to 60% of patients.[60] Therefore, control endoscopy every 6 months after the initial treatment period is advised by most authors.

Ligated parts of the varices are sloughed 3 to 10 days after the rubber bands have been set leaving shallow ulcers,

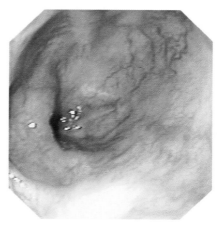

Fig. 2.7 Endoscopic aspect of the distal esophageal mucosa after five sessions of endoscopic treatment with injection of polidocanol. Note that former grade III varices are completely sclerosed with some remaining ectatic mucosal and submucosal vessels.

so that most endoscopists repeat the ligation after 1 week (Fig. 2.6D–E). On average it takes three to four sessions to achieve obliteration of the bulk of varices. However, smaller varices can persist and sometimes it is difficult to treat these vessels by banding because scarring decreases the compliance of the wall which will result in the inability to fully suction mucosa into the ligating cylinder. Therefore, several techniques have been developed to combine injection sclerotherapy with ligation. One technique injects the sclerosant immediately after ligation into the varix site proximal to the rubber band;[23] in another method, injection of the lower esophagus is followed by immediate ligation.[22] Still another technique uses sclerotherapy after most of the varices have been obliterated by ligation.[21] The technique of combination therapy is far from being standardized with respect to the time when sclerotherapy is started, injection volume of the sclerosant, and even site of injection.

Patients have to be carefully monitored after endoscopic therapy of varices for signs of rebleeding. After 2 hours, they may be given liquids and, if no rebleeding occurs, patients can advance to normal meals. They should, however, be told to chew adequately and drink sufficiently with meals.

COMPLICATIONS AND THEIR MANAGEMENT

The main complications of sclerotherapy and ligation are listed in Table 2.3. There is no significant difference between intravariceal or paravariceal injection with regard to adverse effects. Absolute alcohol more often leads to complications than polidocanol,[61,62] and there is some evidence that ethanolamine oleate may cause fewer complications than polidocanol or sodium tetradecyl sulfate.[42]

The reported cumulative rate of complications varies between 20% and 40%, with a procedure-related mortality of around 1 to 2%.[63,64] Most fatalities are caused by esophageal perforation, aspiration,[65] or bleeding ulcers. Perforation occurs more frequently after emergency sclerotherapy than after elective treatment. Esophageal wall

perforations or penetrations subsequent to sclerotherapy may induce serious damage to adjacent structures and organs, such as pleural and mediastinal alterations[66] or even pericarditis,[67,68] leading rarely to cardiac tamponade.[69] Complications and death are significantly associated with poor liver function.[70] Rarely, intramural hematoma may occur following injection sclerotherapy, mainly owing to coagulation disorders and insufficient injection.

Perforation normally can be managed conservatively.[59,71] Large pleural effusions may require drainage.

Ligation is easier to learn, requires less experience, and complications are less operator-dependent than sclerotherapy. The cumulative percentages of adverse effects range between 2% and 20%.[20,29,37] Shallow ulcers occur regularly, but only a minority are associated with bleeding. Less than 20% of patients may have chest pain and dysphagia within several days after the procedure. Endoscopy-related complications such as aspiration with bronchopneumonia are the main reason for fatal complications. Less often bleeding ulcers can cause fatalities. In a meta-analysis of controlled trials comparing ligation and sclerotherapy,[20] complications leading to death were seen in 1% of the ligation-patients and 3.3% of the patients who received sclerotherapy. Bleeding ulcers are managed by injection of epinephrine or fibrin glue.

Ulcers

Ulcers occur in most patients after sclerotherapy. They may be considerably deeper than after ligation where shallow ulcers are the rule, but deep ulcers are rare. Treatment-induced ulcer bleeding occurs in up to 12% of patients receiving sclerotherapy,[37] whereas the upper range of bleeding ulcers is around 8% in ligation patients.[18] According to a meta-analysis, bleeding ulcers are reduced by 40% when ligation is applied instead of sclerotherapy.[20]

Strictures

Post-sclerotherapy esophageal strictures are reported in up to 20% of patients. This rate, however, is considerably lower in more recent trials. The development of strictures is dependent on the total number of treatments and the cumulative amount of sclerosant required to obliterate the varices.[72] Severe strictures can be treated by bougienage. A small trial[73] postulates that a vigorous acid protection regimen (antacids, cimetidine, sucralfate) helps prevent stricture formation. However, this could not be confirmed in a larger double-blind randomized study.[74] Strictures do not occur after ligation.

Bacteremia

Sclerotherapy leads to bacteremia in up to 50% of patients,[75–79] although some studies showed no significant increase in bacteremia.[80,81] Emergency sclerotherapy has a higher risk of bacteremia than elective sclerotherapy.[82] The risk of bacteremia caused by upper endoscopy alone is probably higher in cirrhotic patients than in non-cirrhotic patients.[83] Most of the microorganisms isolated from the blood belong to the normal oropharyngeal flora (α-hemolytic streptococci and staphylococci spp).[77]

Main complications of sclerotherapy and ligation		
Complication	Percentage of patients (median from different controlled trials)	
	Sclerotherapy	Ligation
Complicated esophageal ulcers	15	3
Fever	14	5
Esophageal stenoses	12	0
Bronchopneumonia	6	4
Bacterial peritonitis	10	6
Esophageal perforation	2	<1
Fatal complication	1	<1

Table 2.3 Main complications of sclerotherapy and ligation

Although septic complications (e.g. bacterial peritonitis or brain abscess) occur rarely,[84–86] antibiotic prophylaxis may be advisable for high-risk patients, such as those prone to endocarditis (heart failure, prosthesis) or spontaneous peritonitis (patients with ascites and reduced liver function – Child's grade C – or ascites with low albumin content).

In cases of emergency treatment, patients should receive a prophylactic regimen of antibiotics which have been proven to reduce infectious complications in these patients.[50] When ligation is used, the risk of bacteremia is probably similar to sclerotherapy.[87]

Esophageal dysmotility

Since repeated injection sclerotherapy may lead to fibrosis and scarring of the esophageal wall, several authors have evaluated esophageal motor function in patients after repeated injection sessions. Peristalsis in the distal esophagus may be impaired,[88–90] although lower esophageal sphincter function was not affected in most studies.[89–90] The dysmotility, if present, is probably reversible.[90] These findings are in accordance with the observation that the transport and clearance function of the esophagus is only partially reduced after injection sclerotherapy[88] and that, on average, there is no increase in acid gastroesophageal reflux episodes in patients who have received repeated injections compared with controls with untreated esophageal varices.[91] In some patients, dependent on the total amount of sclerosant given, paravariceal injection sclerotherapy may cause pathologic gastroesophageal reflux.[92] Ligation does not seem to lead to major motility disorders.[17,18,93,94]

Systemic effects

The entry of sclerosant directly or through the azygos venous system into the systemic circulation following intravariceal injection has been documented radiologically,[95] and there are anecdotal reports of acute respiratory failure after application of sodium morrhuate.[96] In most cases, however, no more than 20% of the injected dose reaches the pulmonary circulation and a change in pulmonary diffusing capacity cannot be shown.[97] Furthermore, in a case control study with 11 patients, there was no difference in lung function tests and gas exchange before and after esophageal variceal sclerotherapy.[65] Some sclerosants may cause activation of the coagulation system.[98,99] This, however, rarely leads to thromboembolic or bleeding complications. Ligation, which needs no sclerosant, has no potential to produce pulmonary capillary injury. However, it may lead to decrease of cardiac output by unknown reasons with impairment of oxygen delivery.[100]

Thrombosis elsewhere

Portal vein thrombosis[101–104] and mesenteric vein thrombosis[105] have occasionally been seen following esophageal sclerotherapy. This may be due to communication between vessels of the lower esophagus and the short gastric veins, allowing dispersal of the sclerosant into the portal and mesenteric veins, especially in cases of caudal venous blood flow which has been documented in up to 50% of patients.[52,106] Activation of systemic blood coagulation in cirrhotic patients during and after sclerotherapy – demonstrated by an increase in plasma fibrinopeptide A,[107] fibrin degradation product E,[98] or elevated D-dimer levels[99] – especially together with vasopressin infusion,[101,105] is believed to promote venous thrombosis in the splanchnic bed after sclerotherapy. It may be inferred from these anecdotal findings that vasopressin infusion should not be combined with intravascular injection of sclerosant. On the other hand, no development of a portal or splanchnic vein thrombosis was found in an arteriographic study within an average of 2 years after sclerotherapy,[108] underlining the rarity of thrombosis elsewhere. Thrombosis in collaterals outside esophageal varices to date has not been reported after ligation to our knowledge.

Collaterals

It has been postulated that obliteration of esophageal varices could lead to the development of collaterals in the stomach, the duodenum,[109–111] or the large bowel. However, this is not the case in most patients,[112] probably because sufficient portal venous blood is drained along paraesophageal channels in the mediastinum to the azygos vein, even after complete obliteration of intramural esophageal collaterals.[113] Large paraesophageal varices as assessed by endoscopic ultrasound are postulated to be predictive for recurrent varices.[114] Furthermore, the portal venous fraction of the hepatic blood flow, which is significantly reduced in patients with liver cirrhosis, is not influenced by long-term sclerotherapy. A short-term study also found no difference in the hepatic venous pressure gradient and the azygos blood flow before and after sclerotherapy.[115] After ligation, a prompt decrease in left ventricular end-diastolic volume associated with a decline in the stroke volume and a rise of the systemic vascular resistance index is observed. This is probably caused by a sudden reduction of the cardiac preload.[116]

It has been postulated that sclerotherapy is associated with the development of spontaneous splenorenal shunts, which prevent reappearance of esophageal varices.[117] It has also been suggested that portal hypertensive gastropathy is seen more frequently in patients who have undergone endoscopic sclerotherapy and its frequency appears to increase with time as more sclerotherapy is performed. However, it is important to distinguish between transient changes occurring as a consequence of the procedure of variceal injection and longer-term abnormalities. It has been observed that injection of esophageal varices sometimes led to the earlier appearance of fundal gastropathy, but also resulted in its disappearance in a number of patients. Overall, there is still debate as to whether the frequency of congestive gastropathy and consequent bleeding are increased after sclerotherapy.[6,118] Portal hypertensive gastropathy has been reported to increase after ligation, especially if patients have no fundal varices, which may provide protection from mucosal congestion of the stomach.[119]

Adjuvant therapy

Adjuvant treatment has four major goals:

1. Interruption of active bleeding even before emergency endoscopy takes place so that the local treatment, be it sclerotherapy or ligation, is facilitated.
2. Prevention of rebleeding from ulcers or from untreated varices.
3. Prevention of septic complications.
4. Enhancement of healing of ulcers induced by endoscopic treatment.

These different therapeutic approaches are partly discussed in the above section dealing with complications and their management. They are also discussed in clinical results of endoscopic therapy of varices.

Chronic propranolol therapy decreases portal pressure and reduces the risk of variceal bleeding,[120] although studies on the value of propranolol adjuvant to sclerotherapy are somewhat conflicting. According to a meta-analysis, addition of propranolol to sclerotherapy further reduces the bleeding risk.[121] As stated above, terlipressin or octreotide adjuvant to endoscopic hemostasis is beneficial in the situation of acute bleeding.[48,49]

The prevention of post-sclerotherapy ulcers or strictures remains a problem. The data on the value of sucralfate administration are controversial. Ranitidine, although not decreasing the rate of ulcer occurrence, may hasten healing of post-injection ulcers,[122] and omeprazole in a dosage of 40 mg daily leads to healing of ulcers that had been resistant to conventional antacid treatment.[123]

Chemoprophylaxis for septic complications remains controversial. The incidence of pyrexia or elevated white blood cell count or erythrocyte sedimentation rate was not affected by 4×1 g ampicillin IV over 3 days in a randomized trial.[124] However, more recent trials support the concept of chemoprophylaxis, at least in an emergency situation.[50,125]

RESULTS

Efficacy of endoscopic treatment

Emergency studies showed that hemostasis of acute variceal hemorrhage can be achieved using injection sclerotherapy or ligation in about 90% of patients. Sclerotherapy is more effective than vasoactive treatment alone[126,127] and at least equally effective as,[128] or better than, balloon tamponade.[129]

However, rebleeding was found to occur in between 20% and 50% of these patients within the first year after initiation of sclerotherapy. The rebleeding rate depends to a considerable extent on the hepatic function as assessed by the Child's status.[130,131] Child's grade A patients receiving long-term sclerotherapy have an excellent prognosis after variceal hemorrhage with regard to both rebleeding and survival.[131] According to a meta-analysis, the rebleeding rate is reduced by 40 to 50% if ligation is used as first endoscopic treatment,[20] rather than sclerotherapy.

Some patients show a decrease in portal pressure following sclerotherapy, possibly because of spontaneous collaterals such as paraumbilical veins[103] or splenorenal shunts.[117] These patients may have a lower rebleeding risk.

Elevated portal pressure is observed in two-thirds of the patients after ligation, while one-third had decreased portal pressure. This might be an explanation why recurrence of varices occurs after complete variceal ligation therapy in some patients.[132]

Percutaneous portographic studies[133] showed that complete obliteration of varices and their feeding veins is important to reduce rebleeding, contrary to assumptions of other authors who believe that total eradication of the varices may not be necessary to reduce the bleeding risk.[59]

A considerable number of RCTs have now been published, comparing injection sclerotherapy with other therapeutic approaches to variceal hemorrhage. Sclerotherapy is more, or at least equally, effective for hemostasis of acute variceal bleeding than vasoactive drugs[47] or balloon tamponade.[129] Repeated injection sclerotherapy is also more effective for the prevention of rebleeding than conservative management alone (e.g. vasopressin or balloon tamponade). Furthermore, the use of sclerotherapy to initiate hemostasis followed by repeated sessions to prevent rebleeding may prolong survival compared with conservative management. This is in contrast to randomized portacaval shunt trials, in which survival was not significantly affected.[13] However, RCTs comparing sclerotherapy with open shunt operations did not reveal any difference in survival rates, although the portacaval shunt reduces the risk of recurrent gastrointestinal bleeding significantly compared to sclerotherapy.[134–137] It may well be that the higher risks of perioperative mortality, liver failure, and encephalopathy in the shunt group are outweighed by more rebleeding episodes in the sclerotherapy group. It should be kept in mind, however, that our conclusions are mainly based on elective trials and highly selected patients. In addition, combined or sequential treatment should be considered. For example, the trial from the Atlanta group[138] revealed that sclerotherapy as first-line treatment, with shunt rescue only in cases of recurrent hemorrhage, may prolong survival compared with shunt surgery as primary treatment.[134–136] Similar to shunt surgery, transection is more effective than sclerotherapy for the prevention of recurrent bleeding; however, it is not superior with respect to survival.[139–141]

All RCTs comparing the effect of sclerotherapy on rebleeding with medical portal decompressive therapy (mostly the β-adrenergic blocker propranolol) showed that death and recurrent gastrointestinal hemorrhage occur with about equal frequency in both groups.[142–146] Some authors found that the risk of rebleeding from esophageal varices is lower after repeated sclerotherapy compared with the chronic intake of propranolol.[144,147–149] However, propranolol probably has a positive effect on bleeding from a hypertensive gastropathy, which cannot be achieved by injection sclerotherapy.

When compared to sclerotherapy, rebleeding rates seem to be lower in the banding groups in all studies.[18,29,37,150–154]

Controlled trials exist comparing sclerotherapy with ligation. In all trials, ligation was at least equivalent to sclerotherapy. In eight trials, adverse effects (strictures, complicated ulcers) occurred less frequently in the ligation arm,[18,37,94,150-154] and in four trials ligation was even accompanied by slightly better survival.[18,151-153] These data suggest that ligation is the endoscopic therapy of choice for elective treatment. To date, it is unclear whether combination of both modalities offers an advantage (see above).

During the last 20 years, different treatment modalities for the arrest of acute variceal bleeding and prevention of recurrent bleeding have been developed. Endoscopic treatment plays the most important role in hemostasis of acute hemorrhage. Prevention of rebleeding remains more of an open question. The open surgical shunt or TIPS, repeated sclerotherapy, or ligation and β-blockers all have their place. Now the results of several RCTs comparing endoscopic therapy (sclerotherapy or ligation) with TIPS are available.[155-160] These outcomes are similar to the former trials comparing sclerotherapy and open shunts. TIPS patients had less rebleeding but a higher rate of encephalopathy, and survival was not influenced. There is some evidence to suggest that it is appropriate to begin with less invasive treatments, such as β-blockers or endoscopic treatment (preferably ligation) and to restrict portocaval surgery or TIPS to those patients with compensated liver function and recurrent bleeding. Liver function remains the most important prognostic indicator and appears to be independent of treatment or prophylaxis of bleeding. Thus some patients with advanced disease may qualify for transplantation after stabilization with endoscopic treatment of varices.[161]

Prophylactic endoscopic treatment

It has not been demonstrated convincingly that injection sclerotherapy for prophylaxis of first variceal hemorrhage is superior to a 'wait and see' policy. At present, prophylactic sclerotherapy should only be performed in controlled trials. It may be beneficial to patients with a very high bleeding risk[162] and to those with alcoholic liver cirrhosis. According to the available data, patients with a high bleeding risk are best classified by endoscopic criteria.[5,9,163] As far as prophylactic variceal banding therapy is concerned, studies are in progress. In three small RCTs, ligation was superior to 'wait and see'[164-166] or even propranolol.[167,168] However, this is debatable[32] and further trials are needed.

CHECKLIST OF PRACTICE POINTS

1. Assess the patient's general condition, including blood pressure and heart rate.
2. Review the results of prior laboratory data (coagulation parameters, red blood cell count, oxygen).
3. Obtain informed consent from the patient.
4. Insert a large-bore IV catheter into a peripheral vein.
5. Place the patient in the left lateral or prone position.
6. Check that all necessary equipment is available:
   Endoscopes
   Needles
   Ligation device
   Vacuum pump
   Light source
   Sengstaken–Blakemore or Linton–Nachlas balloon.
7. Ensure availability of appropriate drugs:
   Premedication and antagonists:
      benzodiazepines, pentazocine, flumazenil, naloxone
   Plasma expanders
   Sclerosing agents
   Butyl-cyanoacrylate
   Drugs for portal decompression (terlipressin, somatostatin).
8. Ensure immediate availability of cardiopulmonary resuscitation apparatus.
9. If possible, perform emergency procedure in a critical care facility. Monitor the patient with pulse oximetry.
10. Provide post-treatment instructions for nursing staff.
11. Provide patient with instructions and schedule for follow-up treatment before discharge.

REFERENCES

1. Genecin GE, Groszmann RJ. The biology of portal hypertension. In: Arias IM, Boyer JL, Fausto N, Jakoby WB, Schachter D, Shafritz DA, eds. The liver. Biology and pathobiology. 3rd ed. New York: Raven Press; 1994:1327–1341.

2. Calès P, Pascal JP. Histoire naturelle des varices oesophagiennes au cours de la cirrhose (de la naissance à la rupture). Gastroenterol Clin Biol 1988; 12:245–254.

3. Christensen E, Faverholdt L, Schlichting P, et al. Aspects of the natural history of gastrointestinal bleeding in cirrhosis and the effect of prednisone. Gastroenterology 1981; 81:944–952.

4. Sauerbruch T, Wotzka R, Köpcke W, et al. Prophylactic sclerotherapy before the first episode of variceal hemorrhage in patients with cirrhosis. N Engl J Med 1988; 319:8–15.

5. Kleber G, Sauerbruch T, Ansari H, Paumgartner G. Prediction of variceal hemorrhage in cirrhosis: a prospective follow-up study. Gastroenterology 1991; 100:1332–1337.

6. D'Amico G, Montalbano L, Traina M, et al. Natural history of congestive gastropathy in cirrhosis. Gastroenterology 1990; 99:1558–1564.

7. Papazian A, Braillon A, Dupas JL, et al. Portal hypertensive gastric mucosa: an endoscopic study. Gut 1986; 27:1199–1203.

8. Triger DR, Hosking SW. The gastric mucosa in portal hypertension. J Hepatol 1989; 8:267–272.

9. The North Italian Endoscopic Club for the Study and Treatment of Esophageal Varices. Prediction of the first variceal hemorrhage in patients with cirrhosis of the liver and esophageal varices. N Engl J Med 1988; 319:983–989.

10. Escorsell A, Bordas JM, Feu F, et al. Endoscopic assessment of variceal volume and wall tension in cirrhotic patients: effects of pharmacological therapy. Gastroenterology 1997; 113:1640–1646.

11. Crafoord C, Frenckner P. New surgical treatment of varicose veins of the oesophagus. Acta Otolaryngol 1939; 27:421–429.

12. Pitcher JL. Safety and effectiveness of the modified Sengstaken–Blakemore tube: a prospective study. Gastroenterology 1971; 61:291–298.

13. Conn HO. Ideal treatment of portal hypertension in 1985. Clin Gastroenterol 1985; 14:259–288.

14. Macbeth R. Treatment of oesophageal varices in portal hypertension by means of sclerosing injection. BMJ 1955; 2:877–880.

15. Binmoeller KF, Grimm H, Soehendra N. Treatment of esophageal varices. Endoscopy 1992; 24:52–57.

16. Paquet KJ, Oberhammer E. Sclerotherapy of bleeding oesophageal varices by means of endoscopy. Endoscopy 1978; 10:7–12.

17. Goff JJ, Reville RM, Van Stiegmann GV. Three years' experience of endoscopic ligation for treatment of bleeding varices. Endoscopy 1992; 24:401–404.

18. Van Stiegmann GV, Goff JS, Michaletz-Onody PA, et al. Endoscopic sclerotherapy as compared with endoscopic ligation for bleeding esophageal varices. N Engl J Med 1992; 326:1527–1532.

19. Zemel G, Katzen BT, Becker GJ, et al. Percutaneous transjugular portosystemic shunt. JAMA 1991; 266:390–393.

20. Laine L, Cook D. Endoscopic ligation compared with sclerotherapy for treatment of esophageal variceal bleeding. A meta-analysis. Ann Intern Med 1995; 123:280–287.

21. Bhargava DK, Pokharna R. Endoscopic variceal ligation versus endoscopic variceal ligation and endoscopic sclerotherapy. A prospective randomized study. Am J Gastroenterol 1997; 92:950–953.

22. Lo G-H, Lai K-H, Cheng J-S, et al. The additive effect of sclerotherapy to patients receiving repeated endoscopic variceal ligation: A prospective, randomized trial. Hepatology 1998; 28:391–395.

23. Umehara M, Onda M, Tajiri T, et al. Sclerotherapy plus ligation versus ligation for the treatment of esophageal varices: a prospective randomized study. Gastrointest Endosc 1999; 50:7–12.

24. Saeed ZA, Van Stiegmann GV, Ramirez FC, et al. Endoscopic variceal ligation is superior to combined ligation and sclerotherapy for esophageal varices: a multicenter prospective randomized trial. Hepatology 1997; 25:71–74.

25. Laine L, Stein C, Sharma V. Randomized comparison of ligation versus ligation plus sclerotherapy in patients with bleeding esophageal varices. Gastroenterology 1996; 110:529–533.

26. Traif IA, Fachartz FS, Jumah AA, et al. Randomized trial of ligation versus combined ligation and sclerotherapy for bleeding esophageal varices. Gastrointest Endosc 1999; 50:1–6.

27. Djurdjevic D, Janosevic S, Dapcevic B, et al. Combined ligation and sclerotherapy versus ligation alone for eradication of bleeding esophageal varices. A randomized and prospective trial. Endoscopy 1999; 31:286–290.

28. Lo G-H, Lai K-H, Cheng J-S, et al. Emergency banding ligation versus sclerotherapy for the control of active bleeding from esophageal varices. Hepatology 1997; 25:1101–1104.

29. Gimson AES, Ramage JK, Panos MZ, et al. Randomised trial of variceal banding ligation versus injection sclerotherapy for bleeding oesophageal varices. Lancet 1993; 342:391–394.

30. Pagliaro L, D'Amico G, Luca A, et al. Portal hypertension: Diagnosis and treatment. J Hepatol 1995; 23(Suppl 1):36–44.

31. D'Amico G, Pagliaro L, Bosch J. The treatment of portal hypertension: a meta-analysis review. Hepatology 1995; 22:332–354.

32. Burroughs AK, Patch D. Primary prevention of bleeding from esophageal varices (editorial). N Engl J Med 1999; 340:1033–1035.

33. Kawano T, Nakamura H, Inoue H, et al. Endoscopic injection sclerotherapy using a transparent overtube with intraluminal negative pressure for esophageal varices. Surg Endosc 1990; 4:15–17.

34. Williams KGD, Dawson JL. Fibreoptic injection of oesophageal varices. BMJ 1979; 2:766–767.

35. Van Stiegmann G, Cambre T, Sun JH. A new endoscopic elastic band ligating device. Gastrointest Endosc 1986; 32:230–232.

36. Van Stiegmann G, Goff JS, Sun JH, et al. Endoscopic ligation of esophageal varices. Am J Surg 1990; 159:21–26.

37. Laine L, El-Newihi HM, Migikovsky B, et al. Endoscopic ligation compared with sclerotherapy for treatment of bleeding esophageal varices. Ann Intern Med 1993; 119:1–7.

38. El-Newihi HM, Mihas AA. Endoscopic perforation as a complication of endoscopic overtube insertion. Am J Gastroenterol 1994; 89:953–954.

39. Hoepffner N, Foerster E, Menzel J, et al. Severe complications arising from esophageal varix ligation with the Stiegmann-Goff set. Endoscopy 1995; 27:345.

40. Helpap B, Bollweg L. Morphological changes in the terminal oesophagus with varices, following sclerosis of the wall. Endoscopy 1981; 13:229–233.

41. Soehendra N, De Heer K, Kempeneers I, et al. Morphological alterations of the esophagus after endoscopic sclerotherapy of varices. Endoscopy 1983; 15:291–296.

42. Kitano S, Iso Y, Yamaga H, et al. Trial of sclerosing agents in patients with oesophageal varices. Br J Surg 1988; 75:751–753.

43. Eimiller A, Berg P, Born P, et al. Fibrinkleber als Sklerotherapeuticum. Z Gastroenterol 1988; 26:458.

44. Zimmer T, Rucktaschel F, Stolzel U, et al. Endoscopic sclerotherapy with fibrin glue as compared with polidocanol to prevent early esophageal variceal rebleeding. J Hepatol 1988; 28:292–297.

45. Oho K, Iwao T, Sumino M, et al. Ethanolamine oleate versus butyl cyanoacrylate for bleeding gastric varices: A nonrandomized study. Endoscopy 1995; 27:349–354.

46. Saeed ZA. The Saeed six-shooter: a prospective study of a new endoscopic multiple rubber-band ligator for the treatment of varices. Endoscopy 1996; 28:559–564.

47. Sung JJY, Chung SCS, Lai CW, et al. Octreotide infusion or emergency sclerotherapy for variceal haemorrhage. Lancet 1993; 342:637–641.

48. Avgerinos A, Nevens F, Raptis S, et al. Early administration of somatostatin and efficacy of sclerotherapy in acute oesophageal variceal bleeds: the European acute bleeding oesophageal variceal episodes (ABOVE) randomised trial. Lancet 1997; 350:1495–1499.

49. Levacher S, Letroumelin P, Pateron D, et al. Early administration of terlipressin plus glyceryl trinitrate to control active upper gastrointestinal bleeding in cirrhotic patients. Lancet 1995; 246:865–868.

50. Soriano G, Guarner C, Tomás A, et al. Norfloxacin prevents bacterial infection in cirrhotics with gastrointestinal hemorrhage. Gastroenterology 1992; 103:1267–1272.

51. Noda T. Angioarchitectural study of esophageal varices. Virchows Arch A. Pathol Anat Histopathol 1984; 404:381–392.

52. Grobe JI, Kozarek RA, Sanowski RA, et al. Venography during endoscopic injection sclerotherapy of esophageal varices. Gastrointest Endosc 1984; 30:6–8.

53. Soehendra N, De Heer K, Kempeneers I, et al. Sclerotherapy of esophageal varices: acute arrest of gastrointestinal hemorrhage or long-term therapy? Endoscopy 1983; 15:136–140.

54. Shiha G, El-Sayed SS. Gastric variceal ligation: a new technique. Gastrointest Endosc 1999; 49:437–441.

55. Vitte RL, Eugene C, Fingerhut A, et al. Fatal outcome following endoscopic fundal variceal ligation (letter). Gastrointest Endosc 1996; 43:82.

56. Akriviadis E, Korula J, Gupta S, et al. Frequent endoscopic variceal sclerotherapy increases risk of complications. Prospective randomized controlled study of two treatment schedules. Dig Dis Sci 1989; 34:1068–1074.

57. Westaby D, Melia W, Macdougall BRD, et al. Injection sclerotherapy for oesophageal varices. A prospective randomized controlled trial of different treatment schedules. Gut 1984; 25:129–132.

58. Higashi H, Kitano S, Hashimoto M, et al. A prospective randomized trial of schedules for sclerosing esophageal varices. 1- versus 2-week intervals. Hepato-gastroenterol 1989; 36:337–340.

59. Burroughs AK, McCormick PA, Siringo S, et al. Prospective randomized trial of long term sclerotherapy for variceal rebleeding using the same protocol to treat rebleeding in all patients. Final report. J Hepatol 1989; 9(Suppl 1):12.

60. Terblanche J, Kahn D, Campbell JAH, et al. Failure of repeated injection sclerotherapy to improve long-term survival after oesophageal variceal bleeding. A five-year prospective controlled clinical trial. Lancet 1983; ii:1328–1332.

61. Atamkurj SP, Bhargava DK, Sharma MP. Endoscopic sclerotherapy for esophageal varices: a prospective, randomized trial of absolute alcohol versus polidocanol. Indian J Gastroenterol 1988; 7:87–89.

62. Paoluzi P, Pietroiusti A, Ferrari S, et al. Absolute alcohol in esophageal vein sclerosis. Gastrointest Endosc 1988; 34:400–402.

63. Schuman BM, Beckman JW, Tedesco FJ, et al. Complications of endoscopic injection sclerotherapy: a review. Am J Gastroenterol 1987; 82:823–830.

64. Sivak MV. Esophageal varices. In: Sivak MV, ed. Gastroenterologic endoscopy. Philadelphia: WB Saunders; 1987:342–372.

65. Korula J, Baydur A, Sassoon C, et al. Effect of esophageal variceal sclerotherapy (EVS) on lung function. A prospective controlled study. Arch Intern Med 1986; 146:1517–1520.

66. Saks BJ, Kilby AE, Dietrich PA, et al. Pleural and mediastinal changes following endoscopic injection sclerotherapy of esophageal varices. Radiology 1983; 149:639–642.

67. Knauer CM, Fogel MR. Pericarditis: complication of esophageal sclerotherapy. Gastroenterology 1987; 93:287–290.

68. Caletti GC, Brocchi E, Labriola E, et al. Pericarditis: a probably overlooked complication of endoscopic variceal sclerotherapy. Endoscopy 1990; 22:144–145.

69. Tabibian N, Schwartz JT, Smith JL, et al. Cardiac tamponade as a result of endoscopic sclerotherapy: report of a case. Surgery 1987; 102:546–547.

70. McKee RF, Garden OJ, Carter DC. Injection sclerotherapy for bleeding varices: risk factors and complications. Br J Surg 1991; 78:1098–1101.

71. Korula J, Pandya K, Yamada S. Perforation of esophagus after endoscopic variceal sclerotherapy. Incidence and clues to pathogenesis. Dig Dis Sci 1989; 34:324–329.

72. Guynn TP, Eckhauser FE, Knol JA, et al. Injection sclerotherapy-induced esophageal strictures. Am Surg 1991; 57:567–571.

73. Snady H, Rosman AS, Korsten MA. Prevention of stricture formation after endoscopic sclerotherapy of esophageal varices. Gastrointest Endosc 1989; 35:377–380.

74. Garg PK, Sidhu SS, Bhargava DK. Role of omeprazole in prevention and treatment of postendoscopic variceal sclerotherapy esophageal complications. Double-blind randomized study. Dig Dis Sci 1995; 40:1569–1574.

75. Camara DS, Gruber M, Barde CJ, et al. Transient bacteremia following endoscopic injection sclerotherapy of esophageal varices. Arch Intern Med 1983; 143:1350–1352.

ity for dilation of gastric, duodenal, or colonic stenoses. Another advantage is that the pressure is applied directly in a circumferential radial axis to the stricture while bougies or olives give a longitudinal shearing force downward to the tissues, with a risk of laceration. The third advantage is that the endoscope is only passed once through the oropharynx, while the TTS dilating balloons are introduced through the accessory channel, as opposed to the requirement for passing multiple instruments over a guidewire.

A possible disadvantage is that the dilation process with a balloon provides no tactile sensation for the endoscopist as to a 'feeling' for the resistance to dilation. Therefore, the balloon will reach its designated diameter without the operator's control over the degree of pressure applied to the stenosis. The first generation of TTS balloons had flexible tips without the possibility of guidewire insertion, which is now available with the latest generation balloons. All of these devices are inflated with mechanical syringe pumps (Boston Scientific Corp., USA; Wilson–Cook, USA; Cordis, USA) with continuous control of the pressure delivered.

Some TTS balloons can be reused several times after glutaraldehyde disinfection. Many of them are marketed as disposables and the latest models rapidly lose their mechanical properties, which happens after the first use of controlled radial expansion balloons.

Dilators for achalasia

These are used to forcefully stretch the lower esophageal sphincter and have diameters ranging from 30 to 40 mm. The older Reider–Moeller dilators have now been abandoned and the Rigiflex (Boston Scientific Corp., USA) dilators are those which are most widely used. These balloons are easy to insert, provide accurate control of their size during dilation without the risk of inadvertent overdilation. They are mounted over a guidewire and dilation is achieved under fluoroscopic control.

TECHNIQUE OF DILATION

Patient preparation

For any dilation performed in the upper gastrointestinal tract, the patient must fast for at least 12 hours before the examination. Special attention must be given to patients having distal esophageal or esophagogastric cancer, frequently associated with gastric stasis, and to patients with duodenal stenosis. In these cases, gastric stasis may be associated with an increased risk of aspiration during the procedure, especially if dilation is followed by stenting. Under these circumstances, dilation should be performed under general anesthesia with intubation in order to protect the airway.

The nature of the stricture should have been evaluated by endoscopy and other imaging techniques before making the decision as to the type of dilator required.

Antibiotic prophylaxis for prevention of endocarditis is justified by an incidence of bacteremia ranging from 11 to 25% in the published series.[4] It is recommended for patients with valvular heart disease although its efficacy has never been demonstrated in a prospective study.[5]

Equipment

All dilation performed with guided bougies and olives as well as duodenal dilations (where the introduction of the balloon through the stenosis is frequently difficult) should be performed in a room equipped with good quality fluoroscopy. For balloon dilation, a videoendoscope allows both the endoscopist and assistant to simultaneously observe the procedure.

Conscious sedation or general anesthesia

Peroral or transoral dilation can be performed under conscious sedation. It may however be painful for the patient and can take a long time with multiple passages through the oropharynx in the case of bougie or olive dilation. When the stenosis is tight or there is a consideration that it will be difficult, we prefer sedation with propofol (AstraZeneca, SW) under careful oxymetric monitoring and, when gastric stasis is suspected (in esophagogastric cancers or duodenal stenosis), general anesthesia may be considered to avoid the risk of aspiration. These recommendations are based on the author's experience since there are no data on the favorable or unfavorable role of deep sedation for these specific indications. This type of sedation has not been shown to increase the risk of the procedure but it permits the patient and the operator to work comfortably, spending enough time to properly perform the treatment. Although the presence of an anesthesiologist increases the cost of the procedure, treatment can be performed on an outpatient basis.

Techniques of endoscopic dilation

In every case, the stenosis must be evaluated with an endoscope. If the scope can be passed through the narrowed segment, its linear extent can be determined endoscopically. If the scope cannot traverse the stricture, an injection of contrast medium at the proximal end of the stenosis will permit fluoroscopic evaluation of its extent and its configuration (Fig. 3.4A). This is particularly useful in tortuous and tight stenoses as well as angulated duodenal compression. When using the wire-guided system with fluoroscopic control, an intramural injection of contrast medium[6] can be performed at the proximal part of the stenosis (Fig. 3.4B) or an external marker can be placed on the skin (this method is less precise if the procedure is performed under mild sedation and the patient moves during the procedure). The next step of the procedure is the introduction of a guidewire through the stricture under radiographic or endoscopic control depending on whether the endoscope can traverse the narrow segment. The flexible distal tip of the wire (Eder–Puestow stiff wire, Keymed, UK) is positioned and maintained in the antrum when withdrawing the endoscope (Fig. 3.4C). In difficult tortuous strictures, other guidewires (Stiff Terumo, Terumo Corp., Japan; Amplatz, Cook Co., Denmark) can be useful and may be maneuvered through a catheter in a fashion similar to that used

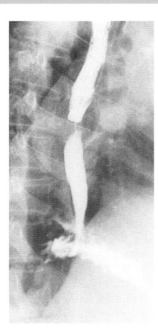

Fig. 3.4A Injection of contrast medium above the stenosis to delineate its extent and shape.

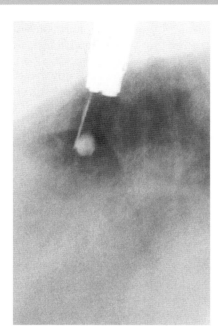

Fig. 3.4B Intramural injection of contrast medium at the upper level of the stenosis.

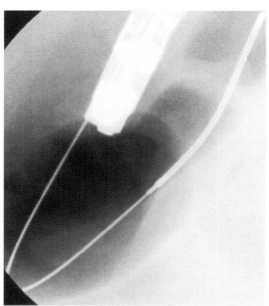

Fig. 3.4C Eder–Puestow guidewire advanced to the antrum.

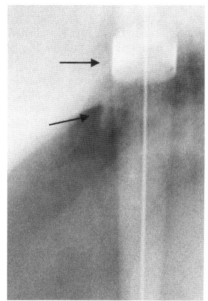

Fig. 3.4D Radiopaque marker on the bougie passed through the stricture.

for endoscopic retrograde cholangiopancreatography (ERCP). If a soft, flexible guidewire has to be used, it must be replaced by a stiffer one (Amplatz or similar) prior to the dilation. The exchange is performed through an ERCP injection catheter.

Dilation with polyvinyl dilators

Once the guidewire is in place, the endoscope is removed and an assistant holds the wire at the patient's mouth. The dilator is then advanced over the guidewire, ensuring that both the dilator and the guidewire do not move forward together. The operator pushes the dilator with the left hand while keeping the wire firmly fixed with the right hand. The size of the first dilator depends on the previous endoscopic evaluation. If an endoscope can pass the stenosis, dilation can be started with an 11 mm dilator. If the endoscope cannot intubate the stricture, the initial dilator size should be 8 or 9 mm. It is recommended to do the procedure step by step, performing dilation millimeter by millimeter, using bougies of increasing diameter. For very tight strictures, the procedure should be performed in two or more sessions, limiting the dilation instrument to 4 or 5 mm larger than the first dilator that meets resistance in each session. It must be kept in mind that, with polyvinyl bougies, dilation is performed with the distal flexible cone and is completely achieved when the largest diameter (at the radiopaque marker) of the bougie is passed through the stricture (Fig. 3.4D).

There are two recommendations to achieve dilation safely with polyvinyl bougies:

1. Be very careful during insertion of the cone through the stricture, exerting steady pressure on the bougie as it slides over the guidewire. Avoid too much pressure when resistance is felt. Instead of a rapid forceful dilation, it is better to apply moderate pressure for a longer time. The use of only two fingers of the left hand on the bougie will help to avoid too much pressure.

2. Once the full diameter of the bougie has passed the stricture, the dilation is finished and there is no reason to leave the dilator in place.

Dilation with through-the-scope balloons

The balloons are lubricated with liquid silicone before introduction into the endoscope's therapeutic channel which can also be lubricated with 1–2 mL of silicone. Those with an internal channel can be introduced over a guidewire previously inserted through the stricture. Once in place, the balloon is inflated with water or diluted contrast material, while the pressure is monitored with a manometer. Before inflation, it is important to be sure that the balloon covers symmetrically the full length of the stenosis. During dilation, there is a tendency for downward or upward migration of the balloon. Indeed, if the balloon is too proximal or too distal, there is a 'cone effect' which occurs during dilation and propels the balloon proximal or distal to the stenosis before effective dilation has been achieved.

For many stenoses, the dilation may be obtained at a pressure and therefore at a diameter lower than that recommended by the manufacturer but it should always be inflated up to the full pressure since a tight stricture, either fibrotic or malignant, may not permit the balloon to expand to its full diameter at less than the recommended pressure. Endoscopic control of dilation can be obtained during the procedure by pulling the inflated balloon up to the endoscope lens. This permits direct vision of the stricture through the balloon (Fig. 3.5). When the full diameter is reached, the stenosis can usually be passed using this balloon as an obturator, attached to the faceplate of the endoscope while both are pushed through the stricture.

The most frequently used balloons are 12, 15, 18, and 20 mm in diameter. For the larger sizes (18 and 20 mm), it may be safer to perform the dilation in two sessions, especially in malignant stenosis or in settings where the risk of perforation is high. Indeed, as the balloon reaches its full diameter in the absence of any 'tactile' control by the operator, the result of each successive dilation should be evaluated. Dilation with large size balloons is potentially hazardous and their use explains the high incidence of perforation, especially in malignant stenoses, that has been reported even in experienced centers.[7]

Choice between over-the-wire dilators and through-the-scope balloons

This choice arises only for esophageal or high gastric strictures. The currently available data have not demonstrated a definitive advantage of either technique in terms of safety and effectiveness.[8–10] TTS balloons have some practical advantages including the ability to be introduced during endoscopy without, in most instances, the need for fluoroscopy. They are undoubtedly the first and only choice for any stricture located beyond the cardia. Wire-guided bougies are still preferred by many experts since they allow a 'feel' of the stenosis and therefore the ability to monitor the dilation process on the basis of their experience. This is particularly true for malignant esophageal stenoses. The polyvinyl dilators are also more durable and cheaper than balloons.

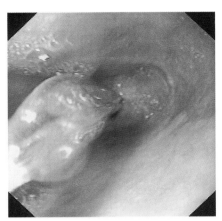

Fig. 3.5A Deflated 18 mm TTS balloon passed through an esophagogastric anastomotic stricture.

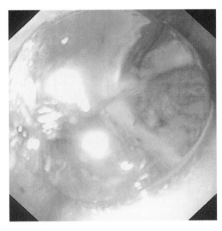

Fig. 3.5B Balloon inflated.

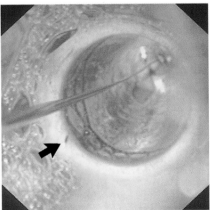

Fig. 3.5C The inflated balloon pulled back against the tip of the scope so that dilation of the stricture can be checked through the balloon. A metallic suture is visible (arrow).

Over-the-wire dilation for achalasia

Dilation for achalasia is unique in that it requires forceful disruption of the lower esophageal sphincter.[11] It is therefore critical to have the diagnosis confirmed beyond any doubt before dilation. Although manometry is the major diagnostic test, tumors or benign stenoses can mimic achalasia on clinical, radiographic, and manometric evaluation;[12] forceful dilation in these cases may result in major complications. Endoscopy is an important part of the overall evaluation to demonstrate the absence of mucosal disease at, or below, the cardia. The functional stenosis of achalasia can always be passed with an endoscope and, if endoscopic intubation is not possible, the diagnosis has to be reconsidered.

Forceful dilation of the sphincter is painful and we prefer to perform the procedure with sedation using propofol or general anesthesia. Achalasia balloons are available with diameters of 30, 35, and 40 mm. The first dilation is always performed with the smallest balloon, warning the patient that a repeat treatment with the larger size dilator will be necessary if symptoms persist or recur rapidly.

The balloon is threaded over a guidewire and positioned at the cardia under fluoroscopic control. Approximately two-thirds of the balloon length is placed above the cardia to minimize the 'cone' effect during inflation which tends to propel the balloon into the stomach. Should this occur, the balloon has to be repositioned to a higher level. The operator holding the flexible shaft of the balloon can feel this migration which renders the dilation ineffective. The balloon can be inflated with air or water. Some authors recommend that the balloon be inflated for 1 or 2 minutes but this is not sustained by clinical data. With the Rigiflex balloon, when the full pressure has been reached and the balloon is correctly sited, several seconds of dilation are as effective as prolonged dilation.[13]

Post-dilation procedures and recovery

In all stenoses where the balloon dilator is used, and the endoscope cannot be passed through prior to dilation, the stricture should be evaluated post-dilation. After balloon dilation, the endoscope may be pushed with the balloon through the stricture (as described above) and the endoscopic examination is performed when withdrawing the endoscope after balloon dilation. When the procedure is performed under fluoroscopy, we usually perform an injection of contrast medium with the endoscope placed proximal to the level of the dilation to rule out a perforation.

Dilation can be performed safely on an outpatient basis[14] but the patient should be kept under surveillance after the procedure and re-examined before discharge for any sign of perforation (pain, distress, subcutaneous emphysema, abdominal rebound, or tenderness). In case of a difficult esophageal dilation, a routine post-procedural esophagogram may be useful to detect intramural lacerations. These difficult cases require special attention; a soft diet is usually recommended for several days.

COMPLICATIONS AND THEIR MANAGEMENT

Endoscopic dilation should be a relatively safe method if performed carefully observing all the precautions described above. It is often erroneously considered as an easy procedure.

It is one of the most operator-dependent techniques in endoscopy, and esophageal dilation, for which the most data are available, carries a risk of complication which clearly varies with the experience of the operator and ranges from 0.5 to 9%.[15–18]

Perforation is the major complication and occurs with the same frequency when using balloons or bougies. It occurs with a greater incidence in tumors, in caustic stenosis, or after radiotherapy and is less frequent in benign stenoses where the risk in experienced hands is less than 5/1000 dilations.[10,16,19]

With bougies or olives, the most common site of perforation is proximal to or just above the stricture and may be related to a shearing effect. The risk of a perforation is reduced when dilation is performed gently and gradually as the tapered tip goes through the stricture. Perforation can also occur during guidewire manipulation through the stenosis and, when there is any cause for concern, the use of fluoroscopic guidance is mandatory.

Perforations must be recognized early, since the decision for conservative or surgical treatment must be made and therapy started as soon as possible.[20] Large perforations after dilation of a benign esophageal stricture, of achalasia in a fit patient, and free communication with the pleural cavity or peritoneal leakage, are solid indications for rapid surgical management, especially if the clinical status worsens during the first 24 hours. The majority of patients with post-dilation perforations can be treated conservatively. An early diagnosis and immediate action are required for a successful outcome. Treatment consists of stopping oral intake, starting parenteral nutrition, antibiotics, analgesics, and continuous aspiration at the site of the injury (with suction holes placed above and below it) until the perforation closes. An absolute requirement for conservative treatment is daily medical–surgical evaluation. If the perforation occurs during dilation of a malignant stenosis, immediate treatment entails placement of an expandable covered stent[21] and intravenous antibiotics.

GENERAL COMMENTS ON SELECTED INDICATIONS

Benign esophageal stenoses

The two most common causes for benign esophageal stenosis are acid reflux and surgical anastomoses.

Peptic stenoses can be located at the level of the gastroesophageal sphincter or higher (in this latter case, it is often associated with a Barrett's esophagus). Endoscopy is essential for evaluation but a subtle stricture can be missed even though it is symptomatic;[22] a barium esophagogram completes the clinical evaluation. Esophagitis above a peptic stricture is seen in about 50% of the cases but biopsy must be taken in every stricture. The first dilation should not exceed 15 mm and can be repeated shortly up to 18 mm, using balloons or bougies. This effectively relieves dysphagia with a response rate >80%.[23] The long-term outcome is that 45% of patients will develop a recurrent stricture within 1 year. Adequate acid control is mandatory with full-dose proton pump inhibitors after dilation to reduce the recurrence rate.[24]

Surgical anastomotic strictures may be very tight and tortuous, especially when they appear after a postoperative leak. They occur in up to 40% of gastroesophageal anastomoses[25] and develop more frequently after an anastomotic leakage or with stapled rather than hand-sewn anastomoses. Endoscopic bougie or balloon dilation is successful in 75–92% of the cases[25,26] but have to be repeated a median of three to five times. The number of dilations required is even higher when the stenosis occurs after healing of an anastomatic leakage. To minimize the risk of recurrence, dilation up to 18–20 mm must always be performed. Some very tight anastomotic strictures require bougie dilation since the balloon may fail to inflate to its predetermined diameter. If the anastomotic strictures recur, it is better to repeat dilation than to place a stent, the long-term complications of which are unacceptable for patients with a prolonged life expectancy.

Upper esophageal webs and Schatzki rings are usually dilated up to 20 mm during a single session. Long caustic strictures are usually very difficult to dilate, have a higher rate of recurrence than those of any other etiology,[17,27] and are associated with a greater risk of perforation, ranging between 1% and 2% per procedure. Extreme caution must be taken even during dilation with relatively small caliber bougies or balloons.

Achalasia

Achalasia is a unique indication for dilation since the purpose is to physically disrupt the lower esophageal sphincter and thereby relieve the functional obstruction. Dilation is not operator-dependent and only the rule of starting with a 30 mm balloon after clear confirmation of the diagnosis may limit the complications.[28] Perforation occurs in 2–8% of achalasia dilations and is the major limitation of this technique although it can be treated conservatively in the majority of the cases if recognized early.[29] This complication is less frequent with a single 30 mm balloon dilation which results in a short-term benefit of 70–85% and long-term relief of symptoms in 50–65% of cases.[30] It is logical to propose pneumatic dilation as an initial procedure and to consider laparoscopic Heller esophagomyotomy[31] in case of failure or relapse after the first pneumatic dilation attempt in fit patients.

Esophageal tumors

Endoscopic dilation of esophageal tumors will reduce dysphagia in more than 90% of cases. The duration of improvement is often very short, ranging from a few days to 2–4 weeks. Dilation is therefore frequently combined with stenting or thermal ablative treatment. Because the compliance of the tumor may vary widely from one case to another, we prefer Savary–Gilliard bougies over balloon dilation in order to better judge the degree of force necessary to effect a successful outcome. During the last decade, perforation caused by the pre-stent insertion stricture dilation was the major complication related to stenting. Indeed, placement of a plastic stent required prior dilation to a diameter of 17–19 mm. The availability of self-expandable stents[7] has dramatically reduced this complication since a dilation of only 14 mm is required.

Stenoses located into the stomach

With the development of gastroplasty for treating morbid obesity, stenosis of the outlet of the gastric pouch has become the most frequent indication for gastric dilation. Stenosis may occur in up to 25% of patients and is usually manifested as vomiting, gastroesophageal reflux, or pain.[32] Food impaction may also occur causing complete dysphagia. Balloon dilation is usually effective but may have to be repeated several times. The size of the balloon for dilation is usually equal to or 1–2 mm larger than the diameter of the stenosis. In relapsing stenoses, our practice is to leave the balloon inflated for several minutes in hopes of inducing a degree of necrosis of the inflammatory tissue in the stenotic segment.

Anastomotic gastrointestinal stenoses are dilated similarly to esophagogastric anastomoses, using a TTS balloon.[33,34]

The incidence of peptic stenoses at the pylorus is becoming infrequent in parallel with the reduced incidence of peptic ulcers. Balloon dilation is very effective in this circumstance. Stenoses in the distal stomach or duodenum are often associated with gastric stasis and caution has to be taken to avoid aspiration of gastric contents especially in older patients.

Duodenal stenoses

These include peptic stenoses and those related to Crohn's disease: they are both good candidates for balloon dilation. In duodenal stenoses associated with chronic pancreatitis, dilation may only give temporary benefit when symptoms occur during an acute exacerbation of the disease. In malignant stenosis, dilation is performed before stent placement[35] in patients who are not candidates for surgery.

Colorectal stricture

A TTS balloon is the usual dilator, introduced after colonic preparation when possible or lavage enema in case of tight stenosis. Anastomotic colorectal stenoses benefit from dilation with a similar outcome as for other anastomotic locations. Interestingly, two to three dilations are usually required to achieve long-term dilation.[36,37]

Endoscopic dilation of ileocolonic stenoses occurring in the setting of Crohn's disease has been reported in limited series.[38,39] It seems that satisfactory results can be expected when dilation is performed in non-active disease.

CONCLUSION

There are only a few instruments available for dilation of stenoses in the gastrointestinal tract. The major advance in this field occurred with the development of the TTS balloon which has made dilation accessible to any lesion that can be reached with an endoscope. Inspite of the limited armamentarium, this apparently simple technique is associated with a significant morbidity. Precise knowledge of the rules for each indication as well as experience in each technique are mandatory to prevent complications.

CHECKLIST OF PRACTICE POINTS

Before dilation
1. Precise diagnosis is available.
2. Overall management of the patient has been discussed.
3. Patient has fasted.
4. Antibiotic prophylaxis has been planned (if necessary).
5. Conscious sedation or general anesthesia.
6. The material is ready and available. Both the gastroenterologist and the GI assistant know what they will be doing during the procedure.

During dilation
1. Evaluate the stenosis endoscopically and, if possible, fluoroscopically.
2. Put a marker at the proximal part.
3. Know about the length, the shape and the tightness of the stenosis.
4. Introduce a guide wire deeply in the antrum. Avoid the traumatic and/or hydrophilic guide wire.
5. If bougies are used, start dilation progressively. Do not increase pressure when you feel more resistance (two fingers).
6. Always check the absence of leakage at the end of the procedure, endoscopically and with contrast injection level to the stenosis.
7. Watch the patient for 4 hours before feeding and/or discharge.

REFERENCES

1. Puestow KL. Conservative treatment of stenosing diseases of the esophagus. Postgrad Med 1955; 18:6–14.

2. Monnier PH, Hsieh V, Savary M. Endoscopic treatment of esophageal stenosis using Savary–Gilliard bougies: technical innovations. Acta Endoscop 1985; 15:119–124.

3. McGovern R, Barkin JS. Short tipped Savary dilators. Gastrointest Endosc 1990; 36:593–594.

4. Zuccaro GJR, Richter JE, Rice TW, et al. Viridans streptococcal bacteremia after esophageal stricture dilation. Gastrointest Endosc 1998; 48:568–573.

5. Meyer GW. Endocarditis prophylaxis for esophageal dilation: a confusing issue? Gastrointest Endosc 1998; 48:641–643.

6. Ismael AE, Leong HT, Sung JJ, et al. Submucosal injection of contrast medium as a radiologic marker for insertion of esophageal prosthesis. Gastrointest Endosc 1993; 39:470–471.

7. Knyrim K, Wagner HJ, Bethge N, et al. A controlled trial of an expansile metal stent for palliation of esophageal obstruction due to inoperable cancer. N Engl J Med 1993; 329:1302–1307.

8. Cox JGC, Winter RK, Maslin SC, et al. Balloon or bougie for dilation of benign esophageal stricture? Dig Dis Sci 1994; 39:776–781.

9. Saeed ZA, Winchester CB, Ferro PS, et al. Prospective randomized comparison of polyvinyl bougies and through the scope balloons for dilation of peptic strictures of the esophagus. Gastrointest Endosc 1994; 41:189–195.

10. Scolapio JS, Pasha TM, Gostout CJ, et al. A randomized prospective study comparing rigid to balloon dilators for benign esophageal strictures and rings. Gastrointest Endosc 1999; 50:13–17.

11. Van Trappen G, Hellemans J. Treatment of achalasia and related motor disorders. Gastroenterology 1980; 79:144–154.

12. Tucker HJ, Snape WJ, Cohen S. Achalasia secondary to carcinoma: manometric and clinical features. Ann Intern Med 1978; 89:315–318.

13. Khan AA, Shah SW, Alam A, et al. Pneumatic balloon dilation in achalasia: a prospective comparison of balloon distension time. Am J Gastroenterol 1998; 93:1064–1067.

14. Bradpiece HA, Galland RB, Spencer J. Esophageal dilation as an outpatient procedure. Surg Gynecol Obstet 1988; 167:45–48.

15. Tulman AB, Boyce HW. Complications of esophageal dilation and guidelines for their prevention. Gastrointest Endosc 1981; 27:229–234.

16. Tytgat GNJ. Dilation therapy of benign esophageal stenoses. World J Surg 1989; 13:142–148.

17. Pereira-Lima JC, Ramires RP, Zamin I. Endoscopic dilation of benign esophageal strictures: report on 1043 procedures. Am J Gastroenterol 1999; 94:1497–1501.

18. Silvis SE, Nebel O, Rogers G, et al. Endoscopic complications. Results of the 1974 American Society of Gastrointestinal Endoscopy survey. JAMA 1976; 235:928–930.

19. Kozarek RA. Hydrostatic balloon dilation of gastrointestinal stenoses: a national survey. Gastrointest Endosc 1986; 32:15–19.

20. Wesdorp ICE, Bartelsman JFWM, Huibregtse K, et al. Treatment of esophageal perforation. Gut 1984; 25:398–404.

21. Dumonceau JM, Cremer M, Lalmand B, et al. Esophageal fistula sealing: choice of stent, practical management and cost. Gastrointest Endosc 1999; 49:70–78.

22. Ott DJ, Gelfand DW, Lane TJ, et al. Radiologic detection and spectrum of appearances of peptic esophageal strictures. J Clin Gastroenterol 1982; 4:11–15.

23. Marks RD, Richter JE. Peptic strictures of the esophagus. Am J Gastroenterol 1993; 88:1160–1173.

24. Smith PL, Kerr GD, Cockel R, et al. A comparison of omeprazole and ranitidine in the prevention of recurrence of benign esophageal stricture. Gastroenterology 1994; 107:1312–1318.

25. Honkoop P, Siersema PD, Tilanus HW, et al. Benign anastomotic strictures after transhiatal esophagectomy and cervical esophagogastrostomy: risk factors and management. J Thorac Cardiovasc Surg 1996; 111:1141–1146.

26. Ikeya T, Ohwada S, Ogawa T, et al. Endoscopic balloon dilation for benign esophageal anastomotic stricture: factors influencing its effectiveness. Hepatogastroenterology 1999; 46:959–966.

27. Broor SL, Lahoti D, Bose PP, et al. Benign esophageal strictures in children and adolescents: etiology, clinical profile and results of endoscopic dilation. Gastrointest Endosc 1996; 43:474–477.

28. Kadakia SC, Wong RKH. Graded pneumatic dilation using Rigiflex achalasia dilators in patients with primary achalasia. Am J Gastroenterol 1993; 88:34–38.

29. Swedlund A, Traube M, Siskind BN, et al. Non surgical management of esophageal perforation from pneumatic dilation in achalasia. Dig Dis Sci 1989; 34:379–384.

30. Parkman HP, Reynolds JC, Ouyang A, et al. Pneumatic dilation and esophagomyotomy for idiopathic achalasia: clinical outcomes and cost analysis. Dig Dis Sci 1993; 37:75–85.

31. Spiess AE, Kahrilas PJ. Treating achalasia. From whalebone to laparoscope. JAMA 1998; 280:638–642.

32. Verset D, Houben JJ, Gay F, et al. The place of upper gastrointestinal tract endoscopy before and after vertical banded gastroplasty for morbid obesity. Dig Dis Sci 1997; 42:2333–2337.

33. Holt PD, de Lange EE, Shaffer HA Jr. Strictures after gastric surgery: treatment with fluoroscopically guided balloon dilation. Am J Roentgenol 1995; 164:895–899.

34. Kozarek RA, Botoman VA, Paterson DJ. Long term follow up of patients who have undergone balloon dilation for gastric outlet obstruction. Gastrointest Endosc 1990; 36:558–561.

35. Venu RP, Pastika BJ, Kini M, et al. Self expandable metal stents for malignant gastric outlet obstruction: a modified technique. Endoscopy 1998; 30:553–558.

36. Pietropaolo V, Masoni L, Ferrera M, et al. Endoscopic dilation of colonic postoperative strictures. Surg Endosc 1990; 4:26–38.

37. Dinneen MD, Motson RW. Treatment of colonic anastomosis with 'through the scope' balloon dilators. J R Soc Med 1991; 84:264–266.

38. Williams AJK, Palmer KR. Endoscopic balloon dilation as a therapeutic in the management of intestinal strictures resulting from Crohn's disease. Br J Surg 1991; 78:453–454.

39. Breysem Y, Janssens JF, Coremans G, et al. Endoscopic balloon dilatation of colonic and ileocolonic Crohn's strictures: long term results. Gastrointest Endosc 1992; 38:142–147.

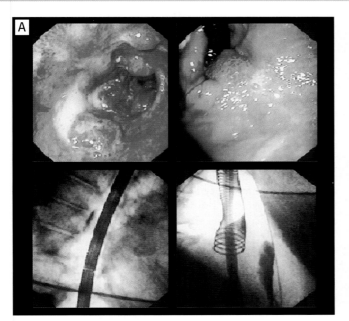

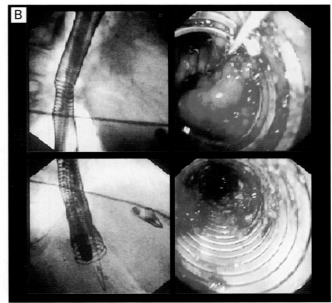

Fig. 4.6 (A) Bulky, exophytic esophageal neoplasm stented with Esophacoil (B).

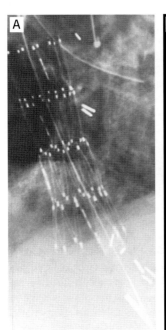

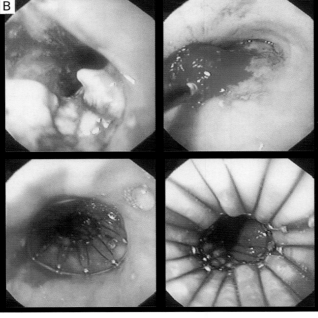

Fig. 4.7 (A and B) Exophytic tumor localized fluoroscopically with contrast injection and bypassed with 8 cm Z stent.

5. **Miscellaneous.** Recently, a woven, self-expandable, plastic stent has been tested in Germany. Consisting of a compressed polyethylene polymer, the advantage of this prosthesis is purported to be comparable palliation at lesser cost ($450 vs $1500–2000 for expandable metallic stents).[55] Data regarding efficacy are limited to a single center and at the time of writing, this particular prosthesis has not been commercially marketed.

PROCEDURE

Expandable stent placement is a palliative maneuver, should be considered as permanent unless a completely covered stent is used, and must be considered in the context of other complementary and competing therapies. In the esophagus, for instance, not only does stent placement compete with available ablative modalities (Nd:YAG laser, caustic injection, multipolar cautery, photodynamic therapy, PEG placement) but also with chemoirradiation.[56–61] In malignant gastric outlet and colon obstruction, palliative bypass or resection are the historic therapies by which placement of an expandable prosthesis must be compared.[27] The informed consent given by patients should include treatment options, risks of both the dilation and insertion procedures (bleeding, perforation, drug reaction), and subsequent complications (migration, tumor ingrowth/overgrowth, erosion with elicitation of bleeding or perforation, or occlusion by luminal contents).

Conscious sedation with an intravenous narcotic and/or benzodiazepine is sufficient for prosthesis insertion in the vast majority of individuals. Tumor localization is best defined using a combination of endoscopic and fluoroscopic techniques. As such, both the stricture length and angulation are important considerations when selecting the type of prosthesis. Assuming that an endoscope can be passed through the malignancy, its proximal and distal margins can be marked by either injecting contrast, preferably lipid soluble to preclude rapid absorption, with a sclerotherapy needle (Figs 4.5 and 4.7) or placement of clips. The alternative is to place external markers on the patient although even slight patient movement may be associated with maldeployment if only fluoroscopic monitoring is used during the placement. If scope passage through the stricture proves impossible, delineation of the tumor length, tightness, and angulation can be defined by luminal injection of contrast through an endoscopic retrograde cholangiopancreatography (ERCP) catheter or by pre-stent bougienage.

Dilation

Stricture dilation is mandatory for the insertion of conventional esophageal prostheses and may be advisable for inserting expandable stents into some patients.[1,47,48] This latter circumstance may arise in patients with significant mediastinal tumor or primary lung carcinoma who may develop acute stridor after stent insertion by virtue of airway compression by the prosthesis. This is perhaps less of a problem in patients in whom a conventional stent can be rapidly removed but may be life-threatening after Wallstent placement in which the exposed proximal wires often preclude safe retrieval. Such patients, therefore, either should have pre-stent bronchoscopy with placement of an airway stent, if indicated, or insertion of a dilator prior to stent insertion to assure that stridor and oxygen desaturation do not occur.[57] This is the sole setting in which I use balloon dilation in the esophagus.

In the vast majority of patients with esophageal malignancy, I use Savary-type dilators (American Endoscopy, Mentor, OH) under fluoroscopic control as I consider balloons an unnecessary expense, mercury-filled dilators to be dangerous in this setting, and Eder–Peustow metal olives to be of historical interest only.[1] Occasionally, with acutely angulated or extremely tight stenoses, finding the lumen is best accomplished with an 0.35 inch or hydrophilic guidewire. Once this is placed, a semi-rigid, piano-style wire can be inserted alongside the smaller wire which is removed.

Bougienage can usually be accomplished in a single session when placing an expandable, esophageal prosthesis (current delivery systems 18–28 Fr), usually dilating to 3–6 Fr larger than the delivery system, particularly if initial scope passage was significantly impaired. In patients in whom a conventional plastic stent is to be inserted, dilation diameters of 48–54 Fr are usually required to insert a commercial prosthesis. In this circumstance, it is often unsafe to dilate a luminal diameter of 3 mm up to 16–17 mm in a single session. Accordingly, a dilation schedule should be considered which increases luminal diameter 2–3 mm every other day or so, although tumor length and resistance, prior experience, and common sense all play significant roles in defining how rapidly to dilate.

Patients with gastric outlet or colonic obstruction are usually dilated with TTS balloon technology (Fig. 4.8). This is a consequence of both the acute angulation of many of these strictures as well as the distance from the mouth and anus, respectively, precluding Savary dilator passage. Balloon application should be used under fluoroscopic control not only because fluoroscopy helps with positioning and assessment of a false passage through necrotic neoplasms, but also because it is impossible to ascertain from visualizing the back end of a balloon whether the balloon's waist has been effaced during the attempted dilation. Waist effacement is critical for stricture fracture and effective dilation. There are no data to support increased efficacy with increased inflation time, although various endoscopists use insufflation times ranging from a few seconds up to 3 minutes.[1] I usually reposition the balloon after an initial dilation as occasionally balloons will be pulled beyond or pushed back from the stricture if the balloon is relatively short or not centered well. Balloon reposition also allows dilation of strictures that are longer than the balloon utilized (usually 3–8 cm).

Stent placement presupposes adequate dilation of the malignant stenosis (48–54 Fr for conventional prostheses; 3–6 Fr larger than the insertion system for expandable stents), measurement of malignancy length and angulation, and in the esophagus, delineation of presence or absence of an associated esophago-airway fistula. Prostheses are chosen for their physical characteristics within both an anatomical and clinical context. For instance, fully covered prostheses that bridge esophagogastric neoplasms have a penchant for migration. Uncovered metal mesh stents have no place in the treatment of fistulous disease, and use of rigid stents in acutely angulated strictures predisposes to proximal and distal pressure necrosis from the vector forces that occur with straightening of the prostheses.[2,3] Acutely angled esophageal strictures may be better treated with stents that angle without kinking (i.e. Ultraflex or Esophacoil), whereas more central stenoses, particularly those beyond the length of currently marketed delivery systems, require TTS technology using an Enteral Wallstent.

Esophageal stents

Rigid prostheses Most rigid stents are passed over a well-lubricated 30–33 Fr Savary-type dilator (insertion tube) using a pushing tube to permit forceful passage through

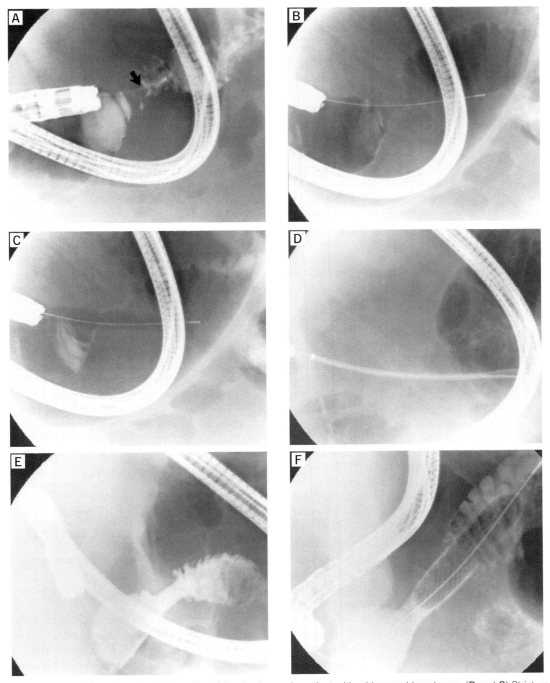

Fig. 4.8 (**A**) Arrow delineates tight stricture in third portion of the duodenum in patient with widespread lymphoma. (**B** and **C**) Stricture is balloon dilated, and (**D** and **E**) stented with through-the-scope Wallstent. (**F**) Incompletely expanded distal end subsequently dilated with 18 mm through-the-scope balloon.

the neoplastic stenosis.[1,47] Assuming that a stent has been chosen which is 5–6 cm longer than the neoplasm and that this tumor has been localized by injecting contrast proximally and distally, fluoroscopic monitoring of stent and insertion tube position is more important than measurements from the tumor to the incisors. Using fluoroscopic control, the insertion tube, stent, and pushing tube are advanced as a unit until 2–3 cm of prosthesis projects beyond the distal injection mark which will leave an addi-

tional 2–3 cm of prosthesis above the proximal injection site. After ascertaining that stent position is correct, the insertion tube is withdrawn keeping the pushing tube within the stent's proximal funnel. The latter is removed using a rotational movement and stent position subsequently checked endoscopically (Fig. 4.2). If the prosthesis has been malplaced, stent reposition can be attempted using a foreign body retrieval device (Shark's tooth, alligator or stent retrieval forceps) but reposition is usually easier inserting an 18 mm balloon with a 34 Fr shaft marketed by Wilson–Cook for this purpose. Occasionally, stents that have been inserted too far need to be pushed into the stomach and retrieved with a polyp snare trailing the proximal funnel to ease its passage through the malignant stenosis.

Expandable prostheses As noted, many patients in whom expandable stents are placed require no dilation or dilation only 1–2 mm larger than the introduction system.[1–3] Tumor measurement and marking, however, remain as important as during insertion of a conventional prosthesis. Moreover, knowledge regarding the characteristics of the various insertion systems as well as the types of stent dysfunction that can occur with individual prosthesis design is crucial for successful palliation. For instance, most of these stents shorten from 20 to 50% during delivery (the exception is the Z stent). Knowledge regarding the length of shortening and whether shortening occurs from the distal end (Ultraflex) or equally from both ends (Endocoil, Wallstent) is crucial to assure proper placement. Also important is familiarity with the delivery systems, many of which are deployed differently – use of an introducer catheter: all systems; withdrawal of compression catheter: Z and Wallstents; pulling back a single suture: Ultraflex; and turning a knob that releases sequential restraining wires: Endocoil. Some stents are introduced through an endoscope in a tightly wrapped small caliber system, while others are passed over a guidewire and positioned with fluoroscopy and by an endoscope passed alongside the insertion catheter. As important as experience with stent release is knowledge about what is required if the stent fails to adequately expand or subsequent retrieval of the introducer catheter threatens to displace the stent proximally. Balloon dilation (15–18 mm) may be required alongside the insertion catheter in order to permit its withdrawal. Retrieval of the insertion catheter may also be facilitated by its rotation and the position of the stent is best evaluated fluoroscopically. Stent position is better evaluated endoscopically as far as its relation to the proximal edge of the tumor. On the other hand, it may be wise to use contrast injection through a catheter to assure that the distal stent end does not abut against the contralateral wall in esophagogastric junction tumors because scope passage through a partially expanded prosthesis (most will completely expand spontaneously within 24 to 48 hours) may displace it.

Whether a conventional or expandable prosthesis has been placed, I personally monitor all patients in an overnight observation unit. This allows me to obtain a chest X-ray and barium swallow later in the day of placement to detect possible perforation and assure adequate stent function. It allows a dietary consultant to reinforce eating in an upright position, taking copious liquids with meals, the need to chew food well, and the restriction of heavy breads and steak. The period of overnight hospitalization allows reinforcement of elevation of the bed head and need for proton pump inhibitors and prokinetic agents for most patients in whom the stent bridges the esophagogastric junction.

Non-esophageal stents
Obstructing distal colonic tumors and some malignant pyloric obstructions can be stented with the expandable prostheses currently marketed for the esophagus (Figs 4.8–4.13).[18,38] This is particularly true of the Esophacoil and Ultraflex stents that adapt readily to acutely angulated anatomy. However, many of the delivery systems are either too short or have a tendency to stretch the stomach or rectosigmoid rather than advance through the neoplasm. For non-esophageal locations, the Enteral Wallstent is used most often, being introduced through an endoscope although the insertion shaft tends to buckle if there is significant angulation or channel resistance, even when using a large channel endoscope. Copious lubrication is required and occasionally a duodenoscope with its added advantage of the elevator may facilitate placement in a patient subset. As with esophageal neoplasms, a stent 5–6 cm longer than the neoplasm length is selected and delivered by pulling back the restraining membrane. Position is ascertained endoscopically immediately after delivery, although incomplete expansion may require TTS balloon dilation. Alternatively, contrast injection through a catheter may be needed to visualize the distal end. Once placed, the sharp wires proximally and distally usually preclude repositioning and occasionally a second stent placed through the first is required for effective palliation. Follow-up may include an upper gastrointestinal tract series or barium enema in patients with enteral or colonic Wallstent placement, respectively. More often, however, follow-up is only expectant.

COMPLICATIONS AND THEIR MANAGEMENT

Complications of prosthesis placement can be divided into acute, subacute, or chronic.[41]

Acute complications
Acute complications, regardless of stent type or location, include prosthesis misplacement or perforation. Inadequate expansion of metallic stents (Fig. 4.14) may also occur as can many of the more standard complications of endoscopic procedures (drug reaction, aspiration, medication-related phlebitis). Perforation may be asymptomatic and be manifested as mediastinal air or neck crepitation and is treatable simply with insertion of a covered stent (Fig. 4.15). Alternatively, large tears, particularly those below the diaphragm or associated with contamination from colonic flora, may be life-threatening. Perforation may occur with preplacement dilation alone or the dilation that occurs in conjunction with stent insertion. In the esophagus, data are clear that perforation rates approximate 6 to 8% with rigid prostheses and usually 1 to 2% with expandable ones.[2,3,47,48] This appears to be a consequence of the need for greater dilation when inserting rigid prostheses and possibly local tears as a consequence of rigid stent design.

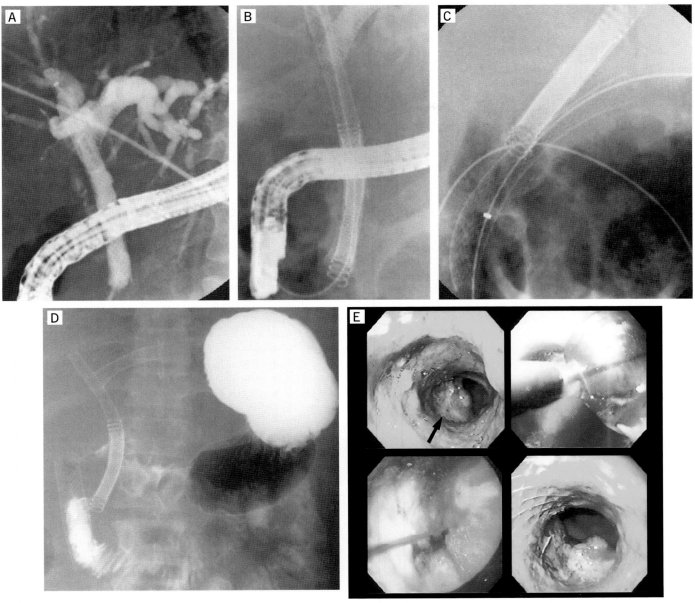

Fig. 4.9 A 39-year-old patient with bilateral biliary Wallstents, metastatic colorectal cancer, presents with distal Wallstent (**A**) and partial gastric outlet obstruction. (**B**) The former is treated with biliary Endocoil and the latter with an enteral Wallstent (**C** and **D**). (**E**) Note tumor ingrowth/overgrowth (arrow) at 3 months treated with balloon dilation, and subsequently with laser.

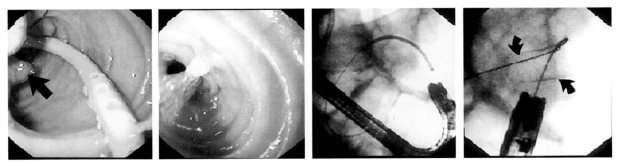

Fig. 4.10 Arrow (upper left) depicts invasive pancreatic cancer causing biliary and duodenal obstruction treated with enteral Wallstent (arrows). Note percutaneous transhepatic biliary drainage catheter upper left.

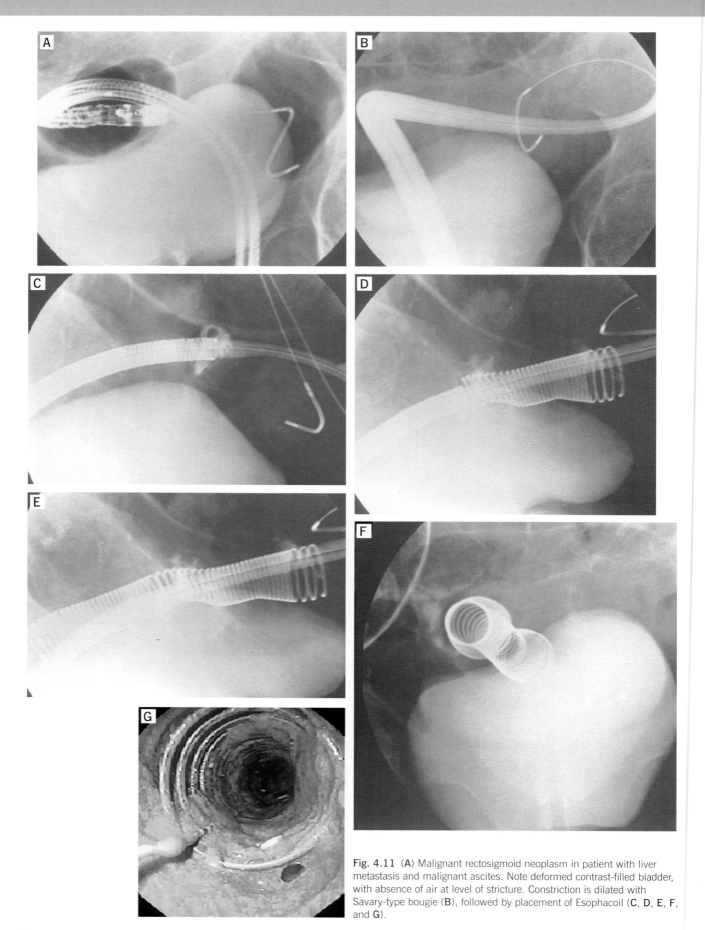

Fig. 4.11 (**A**) Malignant rectosigmoid neoplasm in patient with liver metastasis and malignant ascites. Note deformed contrast-filled bladder, with absence of air at level of stricture. Constriction is dilated with Savary-type bougie (**B**), followed by placement of Esophacoil (**C**, **D**, **E**, **F**, and **G**).

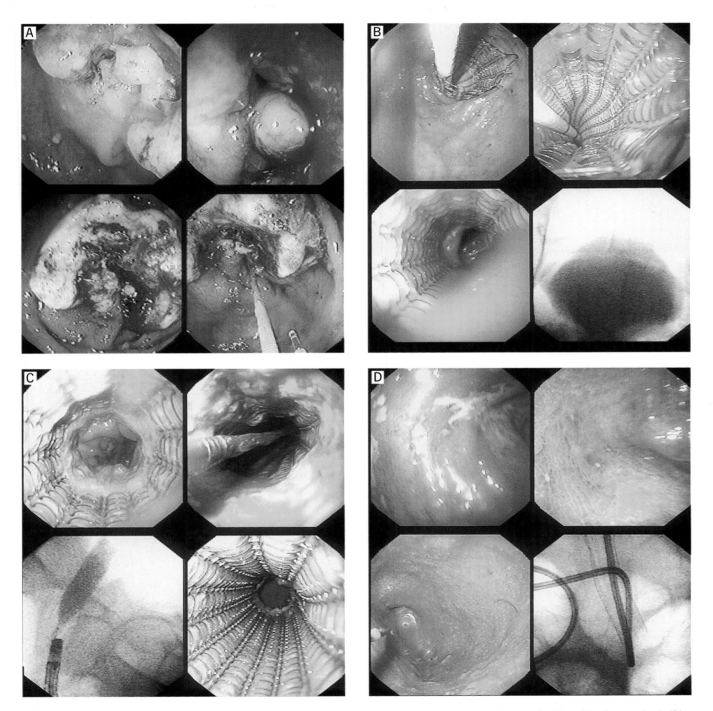

Fig. 4.12 (**A**) Bulky rectal carcinoma causing obstruction in patient with Duke's D colon carcinoma. Latter is stented with an Ultraflex prosthesis (**B**) followed by balloon dilation (**C**) and placement of decompressive tube into more proximal ischemic bowel (**D**).

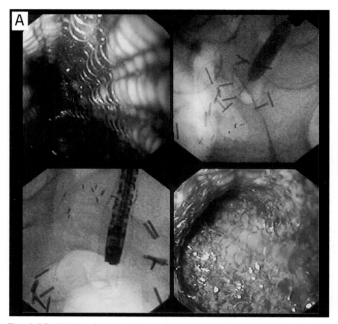

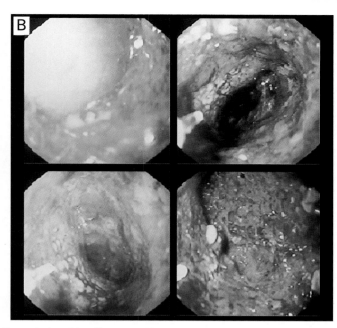

Fig. 4.13 (A) Ultraflex insertion and balloon dilation in patient with obstructing rectosigmoid malignancy, widespread metastatic disease. (B) Tumor ingrowth, mucosal hyperplasia subsequently treated with Nd:YAG photoablation.

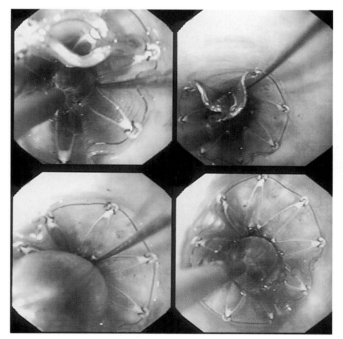

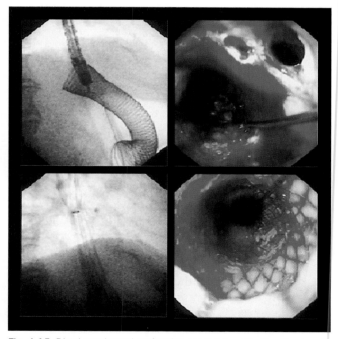

Fig. 4.14 Inadequate expansion of proximal Z stent treated with balloon dilation.

Fig. 4.15 Distal esophageal perforation caused by migrating Esophacoil treated by Esophacoil retrieval and Wallstent I placement.

A perforation may be observed at time of endoscopic visualization of the esophagus post-dilation or stent insertion. Alternatively, it may be noted at the time of post-procedure, contrast swallow (water soluble, if suspected). Eighty to 90% of esophageal leaks will respond to stent insertion, broad-spectrum antibiotics, nasogastric suction, and acid suppression with intravenous proton pump inhibitors or H$_2$-receptor antagonists. In contrast, perforations associated with enteral or colonic stents usually require surgical intervention that may include attempts at oversew, diverting gastrostomy, or diverting colostomy/ileostomy for duodenal and colonic leaks, respectively.

Malplacement, in turn, may simply require retrieval (conventional/Z stent) and replacement or the addition of another expandable stent (Figs 4.15 and 4.16). However, Esophacoils may maldeploy with significant tissue captured within the coils and require retrieval by grasping the proximal end with a snare and pulling the prosthesis through

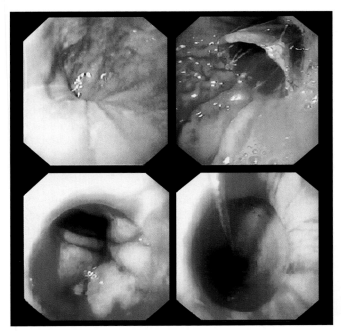

Fig. 4.16 Migrated Z stent treated with retrieval and conventional stent placement (lower right).

an overtube to prevent additional tissue damage. A maldeployed Wallstent may be a particular problem as the exposed wire barbs may be associated with both tissue and scope sheath laceration during attempted retrieval. Use of an overtube in conjunction with a polyp snare for retrieval is occasionally useful although placement of a conventional or additional type of expandable prosthesis may be required to achieve a functional result.

Subacute complications

Subacute complications are most commonly the consequence of stent design or tumor location.[41,52,53] One multicenter trial of Z stents noted an inordinate migration rate when 21 mm-flanged Z stents were placed across the esophagogastric junction, a problem partly solved by addition of shaft barbs, changing the proximal flange to a diameter of 25 mm, or uncovering a portion of the proximal flange. Tumors located at the esophagogastric junction are predisposed to both reflux and the potential for aspiration once a stent, open at both ends, obliterates the normal antireflux mechanisms. Occasionally, patients who have enteral or colonic Wallstents will be found to have widespread neoplastic implants with additional levels of obstruction beyond the stent. This is most often manifest in the first 24 to 48 hours after stent placement following contrast studies or an attempt at refeeding.

Chronic complications

Chronic complications include food impaction in patients who may ignore dietary advice, have long or acutely angulated stents, or tumor ingrowth or overgrowth with mucosal hyperplasia at the proximal or distal stent margins.[52,53] Although carbonated beverages may help the passage of a minor esophageal food impaction, some patients require

ablative therapy of recurrent tumor (Nd:YAG laser [Fig. 4.13], argon plasma coagulation), dilation through the prosthesis (Fig. 4.17), or insertion of an additional stent (Fig. 4.18).

Pressure necrosis, in turn, is usually a consequence of an acutely angulated stricture with proximal or distal erosion by the edge of the stent. In the esophagus, this may result in mediastinal erosion with a contained perforation, formation of an esophago-airway fistula, or exsanguination if the erosion occurs into the aorta, atrium, or a bronchial artery. Erosion into the peritoneal cavity for more distal prostheses may be catastrophic and associated with acute peritonitis. Alternatively, local abscess

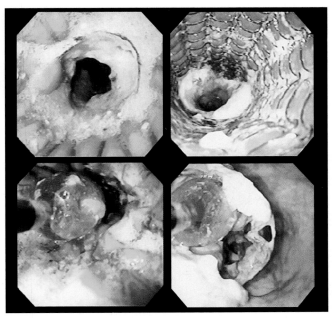

Fig. 4.17 Food impaction with Ultraflex prosthesis treated with disimpaction and balloon dilation.

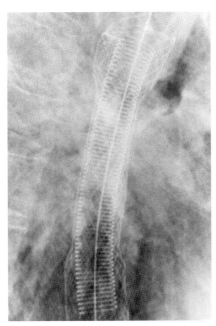

Fig. 4.18 Conventional prosthesis placed through Wallstent in patient with tumor ingrowth.

formation may require percutaneous drainage or surgical decompression and drainage.

In addition to the above, stent placement across the esophagogastric junction may be associated with a reflux stenosis above the prosthesis. This may be treated with dilation, insertion of a longer prosthesis, or potentially with a stent that incorporates an antireflux valve.[54] All patients with stents that straddle the esophagogastric junction require acid suppression as well as elevation of the bed head and prokinetic agents to minimize reflux.

RESULTS

Dilation therapy

Although relatively simple, dilation alone is not sufficient for most malignant obstructions of the esophagus,

stomach, or colon.[1] More often, it is used in conjunction with chemoirradiation, application of various ablative modalities, or stent insertion.

Stent placement
Esophagus

Although RCTs have confirmed lesser procedural morbidity when comparing expandable esophageal stents with conventional ones,[5,6] ultimate survival appears identical and approximates 2 to 6 months. Patients with a successfully palliated esophago-airway fistula have even shorter survival times.

Studies summarizing some of the recently published clinical series using expandable prostheses are included in Tables 4.1 to 4.4. RCTs have compared conventional stents with Z stents and Wallstents,[5,6] and an additional prospective study has demonstrated that there are fewer subse-

	Esophageal endoprosthesis – early clinical experience with the Wallstent						
Author	No. of pts	Design	Stent covered	Technical success	Early complications	Late complications	Follow-up
Bethge 1992	8	p	No	100%	0%	25%	12 weeks[1]
Neuhaus 1992	10	r (?)	No	100%	10%	40%	7 days[1]
Wagner 1992	17	p	No	100%	0%	29%	15 days[2]
Knyrim 1993	21	p	No	100%	0%	30%	167 days[2]
Ell 1994	23	p	No	100%	17%	48%	89 days[2]
Vermeijden 1995	32	p	No	97%	25%	47%	73 days[1]
Watkinson 1995	32	p	Yes	100%	34%	16%	78 days[1]
Bethge 1996	17	p	No	100%	6%	35%	124 days[2]
Dorta 1997	46	r	No	100%	13%	30%	84 days[1]
Nelson 1997	21	p	Yes	100%	33%	43%	53 days[1]
Total number	192						
Average	23			100%	14%	34%	

pts=patients; p=prospective; r=retrospective.
[1] Median.
[2] Mean.
Source: Ell & May.[69] Endoscopy 1997;29:392–398.

Table 4.1 Esophageal endoprosthesis – early clinical experience with the Wallstent

	Esophageal endoprosthesis – clinical experience with the Gianturco-Z/Song stent						
Author	No. of pts	Design	Stent	Technical success	Early complications	Late complications	Follow-up
Schaer 1992	6	r	American	100%	0%	67%	4 months[1]
Song 1994	119	p	Song	100%	34% (total)		16 weeks[1]
Wu 1994	32	p	American	100%	3%	28%	3 months[1]
Ell 1995	20	p	European	100%	5%	20%	69 days[2]
Kozarek 1996	56	p	American	96%	28%	41%	56 days[1]
Kinsman 1996	59	r	American	100%	10%	37%	–
Bartelsman 1998	153	r	Song	100%	30%	28%	78 days[1]
Total number	288						
Average	64			99%	13%	37%	

pts=patients; p=prospective; r=retrospective.
[1]Mean.
[2]Median.
Source: Ell & May.[69] Endoscopy 1997;29:392–398.

Table 4.2 Esophageal endoprosthesis – clinical experience with the Gianturco-Z/Song stent

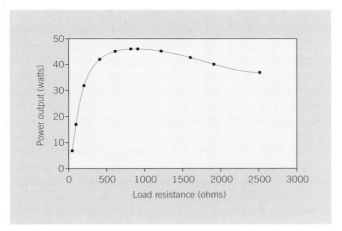

Fig. 5.1.3 The power output versus load resistance for a bipolar generator (Everest Medical, Minneapolis, MN) designed for bipolar cutting and coagulating electrodes. (Reproduced with permission from Tucker RD, Sievert CE, Kramolowsky EV, et al. The interaction between electrosurgical generators, endoscopic electrodes, and tissue. Gastrointest Endosc 1992; 38:118–122.)

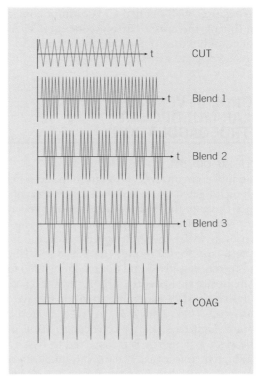

Fig. 5.1.4 Electrosurgical waveforms (not to scale). The CUT waveform is a high-current, low peak-to-peak voltage continuous waveform. The COAG waveform is a higher voltage, intermittent waveform. A BLEND current is a mixture of both cutting and coagulating waveforms. BLEND 1 cuts tissue with minimal coagulation. BLEND 3 produces more coagulation but cutting is less efficient.

injury. Electrocoagulation is a dynamic process with non-uniform changes occurring in tissue as treatment progresses. For instance, resistance increases heterogeneously within tissue during electrocoagulation. The current will select the path of least resistance towards the return electrode, which may change the intended direction of current flow and heat deposition. Similarly, the cooling effect of surrounding blood flow (heat sink effect) can reduce the intended amount of energy delivered to the target site. Lastly, the power output of the generator may also vary (Fig. 5.1.2) with tissue resistance, which changes the amount of power deposited over time.

Most generators allow selection of a particular current waveform depending on the effect desired. They display waveform settings such as CUT or COAG (coagulation), as well as a mixture (BLEND) of these waveforms (Fig. 5.1.4). The difference between these waveforms relates to the percentage of time that the current is on during the activation period (duty cycle).

The CUT mode uses a high-current, low peak-to-peak voltage, continuous (100% duty cycle) sinusoidal waveform that raises the tissue temperature rapidly (>100°C) at the point of contact, producing vaporization of tissue while minimizing lateral thermal spread (coagulation) to the walls of the incision. Because of low-peak voltage (force required to push current through tissue), the cutting current is less able to traverse dessicated tissue and to heat deeply. An increase in voltage, however, will result in an increase in the depth and width of thermal injury.

The COAG mode produces a waveform that gives off current intermittently. Coagulation waveforms have duty cycles varying between 5% and 50%. As noted in Figure 5.1.4, since current is intermittent, a higher peak-to-peak voltage is required to keep power constant (Power = Voltage × Current). The higher voltage permits deeper spread of current across tissue with deeper heating, but the current-off periods reduce air ionization, sparking,

and tissue ablation. Fulguration is a higher-voltage, low-current, non-continuous waveform designed to coagulate by spraying long electrical sparks to tissue. The benefit of fulguration is its ability to efficiently stop oozing emanating from a large area. The depth of necrosis is limited owing to the low duty cycle and lack of tissue contact, and is most effective for capillary/oozing bleeding. However, for hemostasis of larger vessels as in bleeding peptic ulcers, contact electrocoagulation is preferred because of the added advantage of coaptive coagulation.

The BLEND mode corresponds to a mix between cutting and coagulation waveforms. The duty cycle typically varies between 50% and 80% depending on the effect wanted. The lower the duty cycle, the higher the voltage, and the greater the hemostatic effect.[2] Likewise, the higher the duty cycle, the more of a cutting characteristic obtained.

During endoscopic electrocoagulation, power output may be more important than current waveform because high-power settings of COAG current on some generators can achieve reasonable cutting and, likewise, a low-power output of CUT current may provide adequate coagulation. Modern generators (e.g. ERBE, Tübingen, Germany) are available that offer automatic voltage or electric arc regulation to permit automatically fractionated cutting (Endocut) and control of the cutting speed so as to ensure a well-defined and constant zone of coagulation during the entire cutting process. Experience is being accumulated to determine the safety and efficacy of these newer generators.

MONOPOLAR VERSUS BIPOLAR/MULTIPOLAR ELECTROCOAGULATION

Monopolar circuit

In a monopolar circuit, RFC flows from the active electrode through the targeted tissue and then follows a path of least resistance through the body to return to the generator via a distant return electrode. Controlled monopolar electrocoagulation is widely used for specific indications such as polypectomy or sphincterotomy (see Chs 8 and 12). In contrast, it is rarely employed and not recommended for endoscopic hemostasis. Recently, argon plasma coagulation (APC) has received considerable attention in gastrointestinal endoscopy (see Ch. 5.3). APC is a non-contact, monopolar, high-frequency electrocoagulation modality whereby electrical energy is transferred to tissue via ionized conductive argon gas. The maximum depth of injury is about 2–3 mm. However, the probe has to be moved sufficiently close to the target to ignite the plasma without touching the mucosa. For discrete lesions, this proves to be difficult in practice since maintaining a distance of 1–2 mm from tissue amidst respiratory movement and heartbeats is challenging. Contact electrocoagulation may thus be advantageous in 'anchoring' the probe to the target site while providing the added benefit of coaptive coagulation, especially for larger arterial vessels.

Bipolar circuit

In a bipolar circuit, the passage of current is limited to the small volume of tissue that is in contact and confined within the closely spaced electrodes. The bipolar mode is essentially used for tissue coagulation or hemostasis. A typical bipolar hemostasis probe is really *multipolar*, consisting of multiple alternating active and return electrodes aligned next to each other at the end of the probe. Because current flows through only a small volume of tissue from one electrode to its adjacent partner, a bipolar unit requires lower power settings than its monopolar counterpart. Tissue injury is also limited, and placement of the return electrode (grounding pad) and the possibility of skin burns are a non-issue.

ELECTRICAL HAZARDS

Burn injury

For older, ground-referenced monopolar generators, unintended burn sites could occur as a result of current division to alternate ground points. With any misconnections between the return electrode and the generator, current seeking the path of least resistance could travel through electrically conductive grounded materials such as cardiac monitoring leads, causing alternate-site burns. Newer safety features in generators include *isolated generator outputs* where any break in the return circuit will effectively shut off the system and eliminate alternate-site burns through other ground paths, and *contact quality monitors* to prevent burns at the patient-return electrode site. Proper placement of the grounding pad is nevertheless important (usually across the upper thigh), and high-resistance areas such as bony prominences and prosthetic joints should be avoided. The phenomenon by which high-frequency current appears to leak across insulation and out of wires is related to the process of capacitive coupling.[1] The escape of secondary currents can thus cause inadvertent burns away from the target site. Insulation failure occurs when the instrument's shaft is compromised due to wear and tear or poor handling. Small cracks are more hazardous than easily detectable ones because they concentrate current and are more likely to cause burns. Similarly, stray currents can occur with frayed or broken cutting wires. Therefore, careful inspection of all devices prior to use is mandatory and damaged ones should be discarded.

Implanted electronic devices

Caution is warranted when the patient has implanted electronic devices such as a pacemaker, internal cardiac defibrillator, or medication pumps. Pacemaker malfunction and conduction disturbances have rarely been reported but defibrillator activation causing unnecessary shocks may occur.[3,4] Nevertheless, endoscopic electrocoagulation can be performed in such patients following a few precautionary measures:

- knowledge of the manufacturer's instructions and patient's cardiologist consultation before the procedure
- cardiac monitoring during the procedure and resuscitation equipment availability
- defibrillator inactivation prior to the procedure
- return electrode placement away from heart or medication pump
- use of low-power, low-voltage electrocoagulation if feasible
- use of bipolar mode instead of monopolar if possible.[5]

Intestinal gas explosion

Bowel gas explosion has occurred in unprepped colons exposed to electrocoagulation therapy.[6] Polyethylene glycol electrolyte lavage solutions safely prepare the bowel for electrocoagulation by decreasing the concentrations of combustible gases, mainly hydrogen and methane. Carbohydrate alcohols such as mannitol or sorbitol are contraindicated when using electrocautery in the colon because of hydrogen gas production from these sugars by colonic bacterial fermentation. Electrocoagulation should not be performed during flexible sigmoidoscopy following a standard phosphosoda enema preparation since an enema is insufficient at reducing combustible gas levels.[7]

EQUIPMENT

Many generators are now available and marketed for specific accessories although most are adaptable with other devices. Multipurpose generators such as the Valleylab SSE2L offer both monopolar and bipolar modes but there are bipolar generators specifically conceived for endoscopic electrocoagulation (e.g. CIRCON/ACMI, Stamford, CT) and others designed for optimal bipolar cutting (e.g. Everest Medical, Minneapolis, MN). Regardless, it is the endoscopist's responsibility to be familiar with a particular generator and its output characteristics. Generators with dial settings from 0 to 10 are still in use and each setting may correspond to a different power output from one model to the next. Newer versions such as the Valleylab Force generator allow selection of a specific power level in watts. Of note, if bipolar cutting is desired, the use of a bipolar mode of a standard multipurpose generator or a bipolar coagulation generator is inadequate owing to suboptimal power output.[8] For cutting, the bipolar electrodes should be used with a monopolar generator at $\frac{1}{3}$ to $\frac{1}{2}$ the power required for standard monopolar electrodes or a generator specifically designed for this purpose (e.g. Everest Medical, Minneapolis, MN).

A variety of monopolar and bipolar/multipolar electrocoagulation devices are available for hemostasis, tumor ablation, biopsy, polypectomy, and sphincterotomy. Monopolar accessories including sphincterotomes, snares, and hot biopsy forceps are traditionally used for sphincterotomy or polypectomy as described in Chapters 8 and 12, respectively. Bipolar polypectomy snares, where each half of the wire loop serves as an electrode with current flowing across the polyp, were developed to reduce or eliminate complications such as contralateral wall burns and perforations. Although seemingly effective and safe,[9] clinical application has been limited and larger comparative studies with their monopolar counterparts are required. The bipolar biopsy forceps has also received limited interest in view of the denaturation and histologic compromise of tissue caught between the forceps' jaws. A bipolar sphincterotome has been developed to reduce monopolar sphincterotomy complications. The device performed smooth, controlled, hemostatic sphincter cuts via open surgical access on dogs at reduced power.[10] In a prospective randomized control trial (RCT), the bipolar sphincterotome appeared to reduce the frequency of pancreatitis when compared to monopolar technology.[11] Overall, however, bipolar cutting devices have not yet enjoyed widespread use and further studies to determine efficacy, safety, and cost benefits are required before firm recommendations can be made.

Dry and liquid (electrohydrothermal – EHT) monopolar hemostasis probes have been available but are no longer recommended because of safer bipolar/multipolar alternatives. Two commonly used multipolar hemostasis probes are the BICAP (Circon-ACMI, Stamford, CT) and Gold probes (Microvasive, Boston Scientific Corp., Natick, MA). They come in small 2.3 mm (7 Fr) or large 3.2 mm (10 Fr) sizes and allow omnidirectional applications. The Gold probe allows firmer tamponade owing to its greater rigidity.[12] The probes contain a central irrigation channel to improve field visualization and recent versions also contain a retractable injection needle permitting combination therapy (Figs 5.1.5A and B). Other thermal probes such as the heater probe are available for treatment of bleeding lesions. However, the heater probe is a direct thermal device and not an electrosurgical device per se because there is a heating element, but no flow of current from the probe to tissue.

The distinctive multipolar hemorrhoid probe is a rigid probe that fits into a reusable handle connected to a standard bipolar generator. The electrodes are aligned and distributed over 180° of the surface of the probe tip. There is no water irrigation channel and treatment is applied through a slotted anoscope.[13] A multipolar tumor probe is available, similar in shape to an Eder–Puestow dilator with six pairs of bipolar electrodes oriented longitudinally on the surface of the olive, the latter available in diameters of 6, 9, 12, and 15 mm. These tumor probes have been used primarily for palliation of circumferential esophageal cancers.[14,15]

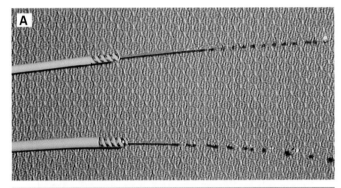

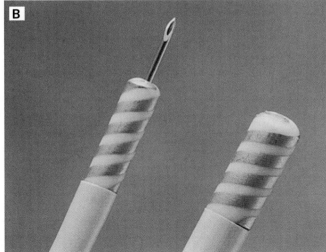

Fig. 5.1.5 (A) Small (2.3 mm) and large (3.2 mm) Gold probes with central irrigation channel. (B) Injection-Gold probes allowing combination therapy (injection and electrocoagulation) with the same probe. (Courtesy of Microvasive, Boston Scientific Corp., Natick, MA.)

CLINICAL APPLICATIONS

Hemostasis

The general approach to the management of non-variceal upper and lower gastrointestinal bleeding is addressed in Chapters 1 and 13 respectively. Electrocoagulation, in particular bipolar/multipolar, is primarily used for tissue coagulation or hemostasis. Patients should be appropriately resuscitated, coagulopathy corrected as best possible, and surgical back-up available for severe bleeding before attempting electrocoagulation. For emergent endoscopy of severe upper gastrointestinal hemorrhage, a therapeutic endoscope with two working channels is recommended; one channel for the introduction of a large 3.2 mm hemostatic probe if required and the other channel for washing and suctioning excess air, fluid, or blood. For significant lower gastrointestinal bleeding, a colonoscope with a large working channel (~3.7 mm) is recommended to allow passage of a large hemostasis probe if required and to permit simultaneous suctioning. The ESU in bipolar coagulation mode should be tested prior to clinical use. The multipolar probe can be checked by depressing the COAG pedal and placing the tip in several drops of saline with the power output adjusted to 10 W. A crackling sound should be heard from the discharge of energy. Thereafter, the power setting can be increased as appropriate.

Peptic ulcers

Peptic ulcer bleeding with high-risk stigmata can benefit from endoscopic electrocoagulation. These stigmata are active bleeding, non-bleeding visible vessels, and possibly adherent clots.

Monopolar electrocoagulation

Techniques. In expert hands, monopolar electrocoagulation using either the dry or liquid (EHT) probes is an effective modality in arresting peptic ulcer bleeding with major stigmata. Papp applied the dry monopolar probe within 2–3 mm of the vessel in the ulcer base as it is moved circumferentially around the vessel.[16] An arterial vessel should not be directly coagulated with the dry monopolar probe owing to thermal adherence of coagulum to the probe, which may be avulsed as the probe is withdrawn with increased bleeding. To minimize sticking, the dry technique has been modified by simultaneously instilling water (or saline) via holes drilled in the probe so as to produce a liquid interface between tissue and probe.[16] With the liquid probe, the bleeding site can be directly targeted. Jensen proposed direct tamponade of the bleeding point, en face if possible, and coagulation with 50–100 W/pulse and multiple short (0.5 seconds) coagulation pulses.[17] With the EHT probe, a two-channel endoscope is necessary so that blood or lavage solution can simultaneously be suctioned.

Results. Three RCTs using either dry[18] or liquid[19,20] monopolar electrocoagulation have demonstrated effective hemostasis of bleeding peptic ulcers with major stigmata (Table 5.1.2). Although no significant complications were reported in these trials, perforations have been reported in uncontrolled studies.[16] Despite some improvement with the EHT probes, the coagulation of briskly bleeding or tangentially-oriented ulcers is challenging, and the depth and extent of tissue injury remain unpredictable. Safer methods such as injection therapy, multipolar electrocoagulation (MPEC), or heater probe have essentially replaced monopolar electrocoagulation for ulcer hemostasis. Similarly, monopolar electrocoagulation is not recommended as a primary hemostatic modality for other lesions such as angioectasias.

Bipolar/multipolar electrocoagulation

The bleeding artery in recurrently bleeding gastric ulcers averages 0.7 mm in diameter with a range of 0.1–1.8 mm.[21] MPEC can effectively coagulate arteries ≤ 2 mm and has proven superior to non-contact modalities such as Nd:YAG laser or monopolar electrofulguration in a canine model.[22] The added benefit of contact electrocoagulation results from compression of the target artery with the MPEC probe before heat delivery (coaptive coagulation). Vessel compression significantly reduces the heat sink effect (where flowing blood rapidly dissipates the heat applied) and facilitates welding of the closely apposited vessel

Randomized controlled trials of monopolar electrocoagulation for peptic ulcer bleeding											
Author	Lesion	No.		1° Hemostasis (%)		Rebleeding (%)		Surgery (%)		Death (%)		Complications of ME
		Control	ME	Control	ME	Control	ME	Control	ME	Control	ME	
Papp[18]	NBVV	16	16			13 (81)	1 (6)*	9 (56)	1 (6)*	1 (6)	0 (0)	Nil
Freitas et al[19]	AB	10	11	4 (40)	9 (82)	6 (60)	4 (36)	4 (40)	4 (36)	2 (20)	1 (9)	Nil
	NBVV	17	14	–	–	9 (53)	3 (21)*	8 (47)	2 (14)*	3 (18)	1 (7)	
	Spots	15	11	–	–	2 (13)	0 (0)	1 (7)	0 (0)	1 (7)	0 (0)	
Moreto et al[20]	AB	6	6	6 (100)	0 (0)	6 (100)	0 (0)	8 (38)	0 (0)	2 (33)	1 (17)	Nil
	NBVV	15	10	–	–	5 (33)	1 (10)		0 (0)	1 (7)	0 (0)	

AB = active bleeding, oozing or spurting; ME = monopolar electrocoagulation; NBVV = non-bleeding visible vessel.
*P <0.05 versus control group.

Table 5.1.2 Randomized controlled trials of monopolar electrocoagulation for peptic ulcer bleeding

walls. The maximum temperature achieved with MPEC is 100°C and tissue erosion is also avoided. Other advantages include the ability to irrigate with the probe, gain access to ulcers obscured by folds, and treat lesions that can be approached only tangentially. Additionally, the newer Injection-Gold probe (IGP) allows combination therapy with the same probe. Disadvantages include sporadic difficulty passing the stiffer Gold probe out of the working channel of the endoscope when retroflexed, and occasional tissue adhesion. Indications for MPEC include a well-visualized ulcer with high-risk stigmata (active bleeding or a non-bleeding visible vessel), and perhaps an ulcer with overlying adherent clot. Absolute contraindications include inadequate visualization of the bleeding site to massive bleeding or inopportune location of the ulcer, and free intraperitoneal air. Although perforation using MPEC has been reported,[23,24] this complication is quite uncommon. When properly used, MPEC is a safe hemostatic modality for bleeding peptic ulcers with major stigmata.

Techniques. The correct application and power settings are critical in achieving successful permanent ulcer hemostasis. Although we tend to directly apply the MPEC probe to the bleeding point, circumferential application around the bleeding site prior to direct application is also used. Based on laboratory and clinical studies,[12,25–29] the recommended MPEC parameters for ulcer hemostasis are:

a. selection of a large 3.2 mm (10 Fr) hemostasis probe
b. forceful tamponade of the bleeding lesion with an en face approach if possible

c. coagulation with low power settings (15–25 W) at 10–14 seconds pulse duration per tamponade station before moving the probe
d. probe repositioning and repeat coagulation treatments if necessary.

Greater stiffness of the Gold probe, compared to the BICAP probe, provides greater application force, particularly when the probe is extended some distance from the tip of the endoscope and tangential coagulation is required.

Results. A few RCTs have shown MPEC to be effective in achieving hemostasis of ulcers with high-risk stigmata (Table 5.1.3). In general, these studies have demonstrated a reduction in the risk of rebleeding, blood transfusion requirements, emergency surgery, or hospital costs.[17,28–30] Although an effect on mortality is not apparent in individual trials, meta-analyses do show an improvement in survival compared to controls for the subgroups with active bleeding or non-bleeding visible vessels.[31] Three RCTs from the UK have not shown a significant difference in outcomes between MPEC-treated and medically-treated patients.[23,32,33] These discordant results may be explained by differences in patient selection and techniques in the UK studies, including the use of small bipolar probes, higher power settings, short pulse duration, and inclusion of patients with low-risk stigmata such as flat spots, with a low likelihood of rebleeding.

The management of the *adherent clot* has not been clearly defined. In a prospective study, adherent clots were subjected to vigorous washing, defined by irrigation using a 3.2 mm multipolar probe for up to 5 minutes. For persistently adherent clots, no endoscopic treatment was given.

Randomized controlled trials of bipolar/multipolar electrocoagulation for peptic ulcer bleeding													
Author	Lesion	No.		1° Hemostasis (%)		Rebleeding (%)		Surgery (%)		Death (%)		Complications of MPEC	
		Control	MPEC	Control	MPEC	Control	MPEC	Control	MPEC	Control	MPEC		
Goudie et al[32]	Any stigma	25	21	NA	NA	5 (20)	7 (33)	2 (8)	2 (10)	0 (0)	0 (0)	1 uncontrolled bleed	
Kernohan et al[33]	Overall	24	21	NA	NA	7 (29)	9 (43)	5 (21)	3 (14)	1 (4)	0 (0)	Nil	
	VV	2	5										
	Spots	22	16										
Brearley et al[23]	NBVV	21	20	–	–	8 (38)	6 (30)	4 (19)	5 (25)	0 (0)	0 (0)	1 duodenal perforation	
O'Brien et al[30]	AB	21	40	NA	NA	13 (62)	6 (15)*	NA	NA	NA	NA	Nil	
	NBVV	43	43	–	–	16 (37)	7 (16)*	NA	NA	NA	NA		
	Clots	39	18	–	–	5 (13)	4 (22)	NA	NA	NA	NA		
Laine[28]	AB	14	10	2 (14)	8 (80)	9 (64)	3 (30)	9 (64)	3 (30)	2 (14)	0 (0)	Nil	
Laine[29]	NBVV	37	38	–	–	15 (41)	7 (18)*	11 (30)	3 (8)*	0 (0)	1 (3)	1 uncontrolled bleed	
Jensen[17]	AB	14	14	13 (93)	2 (14)*	13 (93)	7 (47)*	8 (57)	4 (29)	1 (5)	1 (7)	NA	
	NBVV	27	27	–	–	14 (52)	9 (35)	9 (33)	8 (28)	0 (0)	1 (5)		

AB = active bleeding; MPEC = bipolar/multipolar electrocoagulation; NA = not available or reported; NBVV = non-bleeding visible vessel; Spots = bleeding or non-bleeding; VV = visible vessel, bleeding or non-bleeding.
*P <0.05 versus control group.

Table 5.1.3 Randomized controlled trials of bipolar/multipolar electrocoagulation for peptic ulcer bleeding

Out of 26 patients with persistently adherent clots, only 2 (8%) patients subsequently developed rebleeding which was successfully controlled with MPEC. This small study suggests that observation of patients with adherent clots resistant to 'vigorous' irrigation results in an excellent outcome.[34] More recently, a prospective RCT comparing endoscopic therapy with medical therapy for adherent clots in bleeding ulcers demonstrated a statistically significant reduction in rebleeding rates in the endoscopically-treated group (1/21 patients; 4.8%) versus the medically-treated group (12/35 patients; 34%) ($P = 0.02$). In this study, all clots were forcefully irrigated with 200 mL of syringe water prior to randomization. Those randomized to endoscopic therapy received four-quadrant 1:10 000 epinephrine injection of the base of the clot, followed by clot removal with suction, forceps manipulation, or the endoscope tip, and then heat probe coagulation.[35] Our approach is to first attempt clot removal with aggressive irrigation. If the clot is dislodged and reveals high-risk stigmata, our preferred thermal modality is MPEC with the treatment parameters described previously. If the clot remains adherent despite vigorous washing, epinephrine injection of the base is performed followed by attempted clot removal with the endoscope tip or by cold guillotine using a snare. MPEC is then applied only on ulcers with high-risk stigmata (Fig. 5.1.6).

MPEC has been compared to other endoscopic techniques for ulcer hemostasis. In a multicenter randomized prospective study, MPEC was comparable in safety and efficacy to heater probe for hemostasis of severe ulcer or Mallory–Weiss bleeding.[12] Hui et al performed an RCT on the efficacy of laser, heater probe, and BICAP for the treatment of actively bleeding ulcers. There was no significant difference among the three modalities with respect to rebleeding rate, hospital stay, or proportion of patients requiring emergency surgery. However, the cost per patient was higher with laser than heater probe or MPEC.[36] Likewise, in two trials, MPEC and injection sclerosis (absolute ethanol) were of comparable efficacy with respect to the major outcomes studied in the treatment of bleeding peptic ulcers.[24,37] Comparative trials may be difficult to interpret because of factors such as investigator's proficiency in one technique but not the other and suboptimal choice of treatment parameters. However, there does not seem to be a marked superiority of one modality over another in ulcer hemostasis and, in our opinion, these modalities are therapeutically equivalent with the use of proper techniques. The choice of a particular modality therefore rests on personal preference and expertise, instrument availability and costs, and lesion accessibility to a thermal contact probe.

In practice, many endoscopists use combination epinephrine injection followed by thermal coagulation for ulcer hemostasis although few clinical studies are available to support this approach. The vasoconstrictive properties of epinephrine may slow or halt bleeding and allow better visualization of the ulcer base, and the volume injected may act as a safety cushion prior to applying thermal therapy. For a non-bleeding visible vessel, epinephrine-induced vasoconstriction may also prevent bleeding precipitation upon manipulation of the vessel with the hemostasis probe. The need for separate injectors and thermal coagulation adds to the expense and duration of the procedure. However, the Injection-Gold Probe (IGP; Microvasive, Boston Scientific, Natick, MA) facilitates combination therapy by allowing irrigation, injection, and coagulation without probe removal (Fig. 5.1.5).

In a gastric ulcer canine model, the IGP was found to be safe, effective, and convenient.[38] Although protrusion of the needle may allow better anchoring of the probe for electrocoagulation, this technique is not recommended by the manufacturer because of the possibility of electrical current flowing between the probe and needle, causing deeper and more extensive tissue damage. This concern, however, was not substantiated in a porcine model,[39] although clinical studies are required to evaluate this method.

Lin et al prospectively randomized 96 ulcer patients with active bleeding or non-bleeding visible vessels to epinephrine alone, Gold probe alone, or combined treatment using the IGP. Rebleeding episodes were fewer in the IGP group (6.7%) than in the epinephrine (35.5%) and Gold probe (30%) group ($P < 0.05$). Transfusion requirements were also significantly less in the IGP group than in the other two. However, hospital stay, proportion of patients requiring urgent surgery, and death rate were not statistically different among the three groups. No treatment-related complications were reported.[40] Combination therapy is at least as effective as monotherapy and facilitated by accessories such as the IGP. Further studies are awaited to

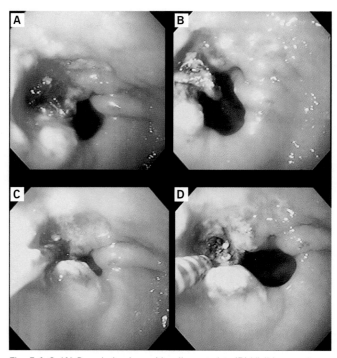

Fig. 5.1.6 (A) Prepyloric ulcer with adherent clot. (B) Visible vessel revealed following forceful irrigation. (C) Coaptive coagulation with firm tamponade directly on visible vessel using a large Gold probe. (D) Flattening of visible vessel.

demonstrate the superiority and safety of combined injection–MPEC therapy over single modalities.

Non-ulcer lesions

MPEC is an effective hemostatic modality for various non-peptic ulcer lesions including Mallory–Weiss tears, Dieulafoy's lesions, angioectasias, diverticular hemorrhage, post-polypectomy and post-sphinterotomy bleeding.

Techniques. For some of these conditions, general guidelines regarding the use of MPEC have been developed based on laboratory and clinical prospective studies, and are a useful tool to the endoscopist.[41–43] The MPEC guidelines for various gastrointestinal lesions put forth by the CURE Hemostasis Research Group are a good example (Tables 5.1.4 and 5.1.5), and suit current endoscopic practice reasonably well.

For a *Dieulafoy's lesion*, we commonly use epinephrine injection, especially in an actively bleeding lesion, followed by electrocoagulation. A large MPEC probe is placed directly and firmly on the bleeding point, preferably en face, and coagulated with a low power setting (~20 W) for 10 seconds pulse duration per tamponade station. Coagulation can be repeated and the probe repositioned, if need be, until bleeding ceases or the target vessel flattens and blanches. Alternative and equally effective methods, in our opinion, include rubber banding and hemostatic clips. A bleeding *Mallory–Weiss tear* is treated with moderate probe pressure applied on the bleeding point at a power setting of 15–20 W, 1 second pulse duration, and 2 to 4 pulses per tamponade station. *Watermelon stomach* and *upper gastrointestinal angioectasias* are approached with light pressure on the targeted sites at a power setting of 10–15 W, 1 second pulse duration, and 2 to 3 pulses per station with bleeding cessation or tissue blanching as an endpoint (Fig. 5.1.7). Multiple MPEC sessions and as many as 50 to 70 applications per session may be required for extensive disease. A non-contact modality such as APC may shorten treatment time but efficacy, in our experience, is similar.

Center for Ulcer Research and Education (CURE) Hemostasis Research Group's guidelines for endoscopic bipolar/multipolar electrocoagulation of upper gastrointestinal lesions

	Peptic ulcer		Dieulafoy's lesion		Mallory–Weiss tear
	Active bleeding	Non-bleeding visible vessel	Active bleeding	Non-bleeding visible vessel	Active bleeding
Probe size[a]	Large	Large	Large	Large	Large or small
Probe pressure[b]	Very firm	Very firm	Firm	Firm	Moderate
Power setting (W)	20	20	20	20	20
Pulse duration (s)[c]	10	10	10	10	4
Endpoint	Bleeding stops	Visible vessel flat and white	Bleeding stops	Visible vessel flat and white	Bleeding stops

*General standardized guidelines based on laboratory and randomized clinical endoscopic studies. Power, pressure, and power duration settings should be reduced for small, acute, or very deep upper gastrointestinal bleeding lesions.

[a]Large-diameter bipolar probes (3.2 mm diameter) are recommended for all non-variceal bleeding lesions or non-bleeding visible vessels except for small arteries (spurts) in Mallory–Weiss tears (<0.5 mm diameter) or small upper gastrointestinal angiomata (<3 mm diameter). Small bipolar probes (2.3 mm diameter) have less capability for tamponade, washing capacity, and volume of coagulation than large probes, and are recommended for coagulation via large-channel endoscopes only for small spurting arteries associated with Mallory–Weiss tears (<0.5 mm, stream) or small upper gastrointestinal angiomata (<3 mm diameter).

[b]Pressure is the tamponade pressure exerted en face or tangentially with the contact probe, directly on the bleeding lesion or non-bleeding visible vessel. For active bleeding, it is recommended that enough pressure is applied to stop the bleeding before initiating coagulation.

[c]Pulse duration refers to the duration of coagulation to the bleeding point, after tamponade, before changing the position of the probe.

Table 5.1.4 Center for Ulcer Research and Education (CURE) Hemostasis Research Group's guidelines for endoscopic bipolar/multipolar electrocoagulation of upper gastrointestinal lesions.* (Courtesy of Dennis Jensen, MD, CURE Hemostasis Research Group.)

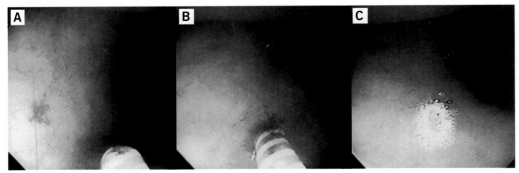

Fig. 5.1.7 (A) Vascular malformation of the duodenum. (B) Multipolar hemostasis probe placed directly on the lesion with light pressure and treated using a low-power setting and short pulse duration. (C) White coagulum formation.

	Angiomata or radiation telangiectasia		Polyp stalk	Focal ulcer	Diverticulosis		Cancer
	Active bleeding	Non-bleeding	Active bleeding	Active bleeding	Non-vessel active bleeding	Bleeding visible vessel	Active bleeding
Probe size[a]	Large	Large or small	Large	Large	Large	Large	Large
Probe pressure[b]	Light	Light	Moderate	Moderate	Moderate	Moderate	Moderate
Power setting (W)	10–15	10–15	15–20	15–20	15–20	15–20	20–25
Pulse duration (s)	1	1	1–2	1–2	1–2	1–2	1–2
Endpoint[c]	Bleeding stops	White coagulum	Bleeding stops	Bleeding stops	Bleeding stops	Vessel flattens	Bleeding stops

Center for Ulcer Research and Education (CURE) Hemostasis Research Group's guidelines for endoscopic bipolar/multipolar electrocoagulation of lower gastrointestinal lesions

*General standardized guidelines developed from laboratory and clinical prospective studies. Power, pressure, and pulse duration should be reduced for small or deep colonic lesions. Repeated coagulation on the same point of flat lesions such as angiomata will cause transmural coagulation and increase the risk of perforation.
[a]Large bipolar probes (3.2 mm) are recommended for treatment of all actively bleeding lesions and for treatment of angiomata or radiation telangiectasias >3 mm in diameter. Small diameter probes (2.3 mm) have less washing capacity, less volume of coagulation, and are more likely to bend with passage through a colonoscope. They are recommended for coagulation of small angiomata or radiation telangiectasias.
[b]Pressure can be exerted en face or tangentially directly on the bleeding or non-bleeding lesion. In the colon, firm tamponade with the probe and colonic distention should be avoided because of increased risks of transmural injury and perforation.
[c]The endpoint for actively bleeding lesions is acute hemostasis. However, repeated coagulation to the same point to control oozing from angiomata and to achieve a totally dry field may be unnecessary and will increase the risk of transmural injury.

Table 5.1.5 Center for Ulcer Research and Education (CURE) Hemostasis Research Group's guidelines for endoscopic bipolar/multipolar electrocoagulation of lower gastrointestinal lesions.* (Courtesy of Dennis Jensen, MD, CURE Hemostasis Research Group.)

Unlike electrocoagulation of bleeding peptic ulcers, upper gastrointestinal and *colonic angioectasias* require a lower power setting, shorter pulse duration, and lighter probe pressure to avoid transmural injury and perforation owing to the relatively thinner gastrointestinal wall associated with these lesions (Table 5.1.5). In particular, angioectasias involving the right colon should receive surface electrocoagulation to limit depth of injury. Additionally, for larger angioectatic lesions, it is preferable to apply point coagulation around the lesion followed by one or more applications in the middle to avoid excessive electrocoagulation in one area alone.

Colonic distension should also be avoided so as not to thin out the wall. Monopolar electrocoagulation using the 'hot biopsy' forceps has been reported for the treatment of colonic angioectasias.[44,45] A small but significant incidence of serious complications including bleeding and perforation exists because of a greater frequency of transmural colonic injury.[46] With the availability of safer techniques, we do not recommend the 'hot biopsy' forceps for ablation of angioectasias.

Radiation-induced telangiectasias are usually approached by non-contact methods such as lasers or APC. MPEC is likely to be as safe and effective as laser therapy, and is more economical. The contact nature of the technique, however, makes therapy slower and is more likely to induce bleeding from these friable lesions, obscuring the treatment field. The suggested MPEC parameters for radiation-induced proctopathy are given in Table 5.1.5.

For *diverticular hemorrhage*, thermal means of hemostasis are not suitable for bleeding emanating from *within* a diverticulum, because of the risk of perforation of the thin-walled diverticular dome. Epinephrine injection or use of hemoclips are safer alternatives in this situation and unassociated with tissue damage. MPEC is feasible for visible vessels on the *edge* of the diverticula.[47] A large MPEC probe, preceded by injection, can be applied with moderate pressure on the bleeding point with power settings of 15–20 W and 1–2 seconds pulse duration. Coagulation is repeated until bleeding stops or the visible vessel is flattened and blanched.

The use of coagulation current at low power settings has been advocated by some to reduce the risk of post-snare polypectomy bleeding. Nevertheless, *post-polypectomy hemorrhage* does occur and may be immediate or delayed. The control of *immediate* bleeding usually involves ensnaring the residual pedicle for a further 5 to 10 minutes. Further application of current carries the risk of shortening the residual stalk to a point where it can no longer be grasped and should be avoided. Subsequently, either epinephrine injection or MPEC may be used. Alternatively, an endoloop or endoclip may also be employed. Few studies are available regarding endoscopic hemostasis of *delayed* and persistent hemorrhage.[48] Tamponade of the bleeding site should be moderate in the colon and we would recommend a lower power setting (~15 W) and a shorter pulse duration (~3 seconds). If there is concern about the wall thickness underneath the excision site, endoclips should be used. *Post-sphincterotomy hemorrhage* can be managed using a large probe with firm tamponade at a power setting of ~20 W and 2–5 seconds pulse duration. MPEC has been shown to be an effective therapy for sphincterotomy-induced bleeding not responding to conservative or other endoscopic measures.[49]

Results. Unlike peptic ulcers, RCTs of MPEC for the above-mentioned conditions are scant. Multiple endoscopic modalities have also been used for these various lesions but comparative trials are few. For bleeding *Mallory–Weiss tears*, MPEC as compared with sham treatment was associated with significantly greater hemostatic efficacy (9/9 vs 1/8 patients), fewer emergency interventions (0/9 vs 4/8 patients), and a trend toward decreased transfusion requirements.[28] MPEC and heater probe controlled active bleeding more often than epinephrine/alcohol injection (100% vs 60%) in another small study, and without treatment-related complications.[50]

A prospective randomized study of 83 patients with *upper gastrointestinal angiomas* or *watermelon stomach* treated with either bipolar or heater probe demonstrated a reduction in rebleeding rates and transfusion requirements for the 2 years or more while on endoscopic treatment versus the 2 years prior while on medical therapy.[43] In patients with recurrent hemorrhage from *colonic angioectasias*, both MPEC and heater probe were associated with significantly fewer bleeding episodes, transfusions, and hospitalizations for gastrointestinal hemorrhage for the 2 years post-therapy versus the 2 years prior to endoscopic therapy.[51] Complications including post-coagulation syndrome and delayed gastrointestinal bleeding were somewhat higher in heater probe-treated patients (8.7%) compared to MPEC-treated patients (4.5%). MPEC and heater probe were equally safe and effective relative to medical therapy for palliation of patients with *radiation-induced bleeding*. Severe bleeding episodes and hematocrits improved significantly following endoscopic therapy.[52]

The effectiveness of MPEC for *diverticular bleeding* is based on anecdotal reports.[47] Prospective and comparative studies are not available. In a small descriptive study, MPEC in conjunction with epinephrine injection arrested *delayed post-polypectomy hemorrhage*.[48] In one prospective study, 8/9 patients with moderate or severe *sphincterotomy-induced hemorrhage* treated with MPEC, following epinephrine injection, achieved hemostasis. Rebleeding occurred in two patients, which was controlled by a second course of MPEC in one in whom it was attempted. No complications or death ensued and surgery was avoided in all cases.[49]

Hemorrhoid ablation

A variety of non-operative outpatient endoscopic and proctoscopic modalities for the management of internal hemorrhoids are available. These include injection sclerosis, rubber band ligation, cryotherapy, photocoagulation, electrocoagulation, and heater probe. Despite strong support for each of these modalities, few prospective RCTs are available.

Techniques. A disposable rigid bipolar hemorrhoid probe is available. Through a slotted anoscope, the tip of the probe is applied with moderate pressure at the base of the internal hemorrhoid. Jensen et al[13] set treatment parameters at 20 W and 1 second pulse duration, with 4 to 7 pulses delivered in a horseshoe pattern above the dentate line to each hemorrhoidal segment. Two to three non-contiguous hemorrhoidal segments are treated in this fashion at each treatment session.

A direct current (DC) hemorrhoid probe (Ultroid, Cabot Medical, Langhorne, PA) is also available and passes current between the double-pronged probe implanted at the base of the internal hemorrhoid, 1 cm or more proximal to the dentate line, with a grounding plate on the thigh or buttock. The current is gradually increased in 2 mA increments and typically 6–14 mA is used depending on patient tolerance. After 8 to 10 minutes, the current is gradually decreased to zero and the procedure repeated on another hemorrhoid segment.[53] This device is seldom used at present.

Results. Preliminary results of hemorrhoid electrocoagulation using the bipolar hemorrhoid probe compare favourably to injection sclerosis, rubber band ligation, or infrared photocoagulation.[54,55] The disadvantages of using DC electrocoagulation are the prolonged treatment times and patient discomfort.[53,56] In a prospective RCT of bipolar (50 patients) versus DC electrocoagulation (50 patients) for treatment of grade 1 to 3 bleeding internal hemorrhoids, both modalities were found to be effective with an overall success rate of 87% after 1-year follow-up. However, the mean treatment time per session was significantly less with multipolar (~25 seconds) than with DC coagulation (~16 min).[53]

Currently, we prefer traditional rubber band ligation for grade 2 to 3 internal hemorrhoids since it is simple, rapid, inexpensive, and painless when properly applied. The application of a multiligator banding device similar to variceal banding may be another option. For small, grade 1 hemorrhoids, the thermal devices, either the heater probe or the bipolar probe, seem favorable.

Tumor ablation

Tumor ingrowth or overgrowth

Cremer et al[57] initially described the use of electrocoagulation in diathermic cleaning of tumor ingrowth in *biliary metal stents*. An 8 Fr or 10 Fr sleeve with a diathermic tip is introduced into the stent and passed across the stricture by means of a hydrophilic, plastic-covered guidewire. With the wire in place to maintain the probe in the center of the stenosis, the probe is passed several times through the stenosis using cutting current. Successful recanalization was accomplished in two patients but short-lived, with repeated electrocoagulation necessary 1 to 2 months later. Ell et al[58] used the monopolar EHT probe in five cases of tumor ingrowth and biliary stent obstruction. One patient, however, demonstrated a broken biliary metal stent after repeated electrocoagulation. Based on these observations, *in vitro* studies were performed demonstrating melting of the metal filaments caused by local spark gap formation after 3–10 seconds of low-power monopolar electrocoagulation application. Electrocoagulation should be applied with great care in relieving obstructing cancerous tissue from a metal stent since contact of the probe with the steel filaments could result in melting and fracture of the stent. Other therapeutic means such as dragging an extraction balloon through the obstructed area, insertion of a polyethylene stent, or placement of a second metal expandable stent seem more appropriate.

Tumor overgrowth proximal or distal to an endoprosthesis may result in obstruction. Although electrocoagulation may be used, this problem is usually, and more effectively, corrected by insertion of a longer endoprosthesis after photoablation of the overgrowing cancerous tissue using Nd:YAG laser or after dilation of the narrowed segment.

Malignant strictures

For palliation of malignant *esophageal* tumors, the hemostasis probes such as the Gold probe do not usually provide an adequate degree of tumor coagulation and destruction for relief of dysphagia. Other drawbacks include the frequent need to clean the probe tip from charred tissue and the relatively longer treatment time required as compared to non-contact methods such as laser therapy or APC. The monopolar EHT probe may be more effective than the multipolar hemostasis probes because of greater depth of injury, but reports concerning therapy of malignant tumors using EHT probes are lacking. Moreover, the requirement for continuous liquid instillation while using the EHT probe predisposes the patient to a higher risk of aspiration as well as restricting visibility.

Olive-shaped BICAP tumor probes have been designed for the palliation of obstructing tumors.[14] The depth of injury is relatively superficial (~2 mm). Since energy is delivered in a 360° manner, these bipolar tumor probes are best suited for circumferential exophytic tumors but not recommended for non-circumferential tumors owing to the risks of perforation, stricture, or fistula formation from coagulation of adjacent normal tissue.

BICAP tumor probe technique.

Prior to BICAP therapy, the malignant esophageal stricture is topographically assessed using a small caliber endoscope. If the endoscope cannot pass through the stricture, a guidewire is placed under fluoroscopic guidance. Typically, standard tumor dilation to 15 mm or larger is performed if feasible and safe, followed by endoscopic inspection for tumor extent. The largest appropriate BICAP tumor probe usually approximates the diameter of the polyvinyl dilator used to dilate the stricture, and is passed over a guidewire under fluoroscopic guidance. The tumor probe can initially be placed at the proximal portion of the tumor where mild resistance is usually encountered. Alternatively, the probe can be introduced beyond the distal margin of the tumor and pulled back with a palpable impact felt as it engages the distal portion of the tumor. Appropriate position of the probe can be verified with a combination of previously placed endoscopic markers (injection of contrast material, application of clips, or markers placed on the skin at the proximal and distal tumor edges) and fluoroscopy.

Treatment to the proximal portion of the tumor can also be assessed by passing a small caliber endoscope alongside the probe shaft. Treatment can be rendered starting either at the proximal end or distal end of the tumor and moving the probe in an antegrade or retrograde fashion respectively. In some studies, both antegrade and retrograde coagulation were used at one treatment session.[59,60] The bipolar probe was positioned at overlapping stations throughout the tumor channel applying treatment with predetermined settings delivering energy in a 360°C manner. For example, five treatment stations will be required if the active electrode is 1 cm in length and the tumor is 5 cm in length. Fluoroscopic observations are made at each station. Typically, each station receives 40–50 W from a 50 W BICAP generator over a 10–20 second duration.[15,59] After therapy, endoscopic inspection of the treated tumor is performed, often revealing a circumferential white exudate over the entire area. If both antegrade and retrograde coagulation is performed at the same session, retreatment is rarely required but can be applied for any area that did not appear well coagulated.

Results.

Johnston et al[14] initially reported the use of a prototype BICAP tumor probe for palliation of obstructing circumferential esophageal cancer in 20 patients. In this multicenter pilot study, dysphagia and tumor channel diameter significantly improved after treatment. The mean number of initial treatment sessions was 1.7 and the mean treatment interval before repeat treatment was about 2 months. Major complications included delayed hemorrhage in two patients and tracheoesophageal fistula in another two. However, those complications are difficult to interpret since both bleeding and tracheoesophageal fistula may be part of the natural history of esophageal cancer.

Jensen et al[59] compared the efficacy and safety of the BICAP tumor probe to the Nd:YAG laser. Laser therapy required twice as much energy as the tumor probe but treatment results were similar during a median follow-up and survival of 16 weeks. Eighty-six percent of patients improved their intake from only liquids to soft or solid diet after initial therapy with the tumor probe or laser. The interval between treatments was similar for both groups, ranging from 6 to 10 weeks. Minor complications including pain or edema requiring dilation were more common in the laser-treated group than the electrocoagulation-treated group. A fistula developed in one patient with non-circumferential cancer treated with the BICAP probe whereas delayed strictures occurred in three patients treated with laser.

McIntyre et al[60] prospectively randomized patients with malignant esophageal strictures to either the bipolar tumor probe or silicone prosthetic tube insertion. Both therapies were comparable and resulted in good dysphagia relief in about 88% of patients. The median time interval between treatments was 28 days for the tumor probe group. A few patients had transient chest pains following electrocoagulation therapy and one patient suffered fistula formation 4 weeks after therapy. For the endoprosthesis-treated group, one esophageal perforation occurred during stent insertion, two had complications related to tube migration, and three had their tubes blocked by food.

The procedure of electrocoagulation with the tumor probe is usually accomplished within 30 minutes. It is portable, inexpensive, and can treat a large tumor area. Nevertheless, the rigid probe may not accommodate a very tortuous stricture, fluoroscopy is required, and it is a cumbersome technique as shown by the number of instrument passages required during each procedure: endoscope, guidewire, dilators, BICAP tumor probe, endoscope, BICAP probe removal, then endoscope again.[14] In our opinion, laser therapy is preferred for noncircumferential, short, exophytic, and distally located stenotic esophageal tumors. Additionally, the apparent longer lasting luminal patency provided by expandable metal stents limits usage of the tumor probe for palliation of esophageal cancers. Photodynamic therapy and APC are also other attractive alternatives for therapy of malignant esophageal strictures. However, one notable advantage of the tumor probe is in the treatment of high cervical strictures where stenting and laser applications are more challenging, undesirable, or associated with poor outcome.

Endoscopic palliation of *rectosigmoid cancers* can be achieved through a variety of modalities including balloon dilation, sclerosant injection, bipolar tumor probes or monopolar snare resection, laser photoablation, and stenting. Snare removal of portions of a malignant tumor has been used in addition to laser photoablation.[61] The use of the bipolar tumor probe has also been described for electrocoagulation of low-lying rectal cancers.[62] However, the efficacy and safety of electrocoagulation in this setting have not been established in large controlled trials. Laser photoablation is more commonly used and seems to be the preferred technique at this time.

Residual adenoma

Large sessile polyps are usually removed with conventional snare excision preceded by submucosal injection of saline or epinephrine and stained with methylene blue. Although no significant clinical studies are available, residual fragments at the edge of the polypectomy site can be coagulated or 'touched up' with either APC or the multipolar hemostasis probe (Fig. 5.1.8).

Barrett's esophagus ablation

For Barrett's esophagus, the goal of any endoscopic therapeutic modality is complete elimination of intestinal metaplasia with restoration of normal squamous epithelium. Compared to lasers or photodynamic therapy (PDT), MPEC is convenient, widely available, affordable, easy to apply, and has less severe side effects. However, MPEC usually requires multiple treatment sessions depending on the Barrett's length, and the depth of injury is limited. By endoscopic ultrasound, the average thickness of the Barrett's mucosa is 1.5 mm. In theory, MPEC should reach beyond this depth. In animal models, coagulation depths ranging from 1.7 mm to 4.8 mm were achieved depending on the power setting, application time, and force of tamponade.[25,63]

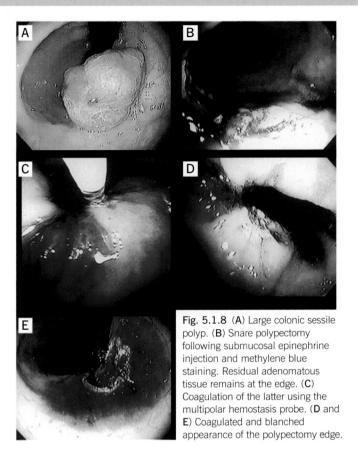

Fig. 5.1.8 (A) Large colonic sessile polyp. (B) Snare polypectomy following submucosal epinephrine injection and methylene blue staining. Residual adenomatous tissue remains at the edge. (C) Coagulation of the latter using the multipolar hemostasis probe. (D and E) Coagulated and blanched appearance of the polypectomy edge.

Techniques. The use of MPEC for Barrett's esophagus is not standardized and the optimal treatment parameters are unknown. In published reports, 2–3 cm Barrett's segment per session were treated using power outputs of 12–15 W (or dial setting of 3 on a 50 W generator), and applying either the small (2.3 mm) or large (3.2 mm) Gold probe to the mucosa until a white coagulum developed.[64,65]

Results. In a small study, 11 patients with a mean Barrett's length of 4.4 cm (range 2–9 cm) but without dysplasia demonstrated initial complete visual and histologic response to MPEC (mean 9.5 sessions/patient, range 2–19/patient). Mean follow-up was 39 months (range 28–53 months). However, three patients had intestinal metaplasia underlying the new squamous mucosa on follow-up biopsies.[66] This is of concern because of case reports of the development of adenocarcinoma after apparent squamous re-epithelization of Barrett's esophagus.[67] In another study, 27 patients with Barrett's esophagus but without dysplasia received a total of 67 MPEC sessions for a mean Barrett's length of 3.4 cm (range 2–10 cm). Sixteen patients demonstrated a normal endoscopic appearance at 18-week follow-up but one of these patients had specialized columnar epithelium on standard biopsy. The remaining 11 patients had apparent residual Barrett's mucosa at endoscopy although only four showed histologic evidence of specialized columnar epithelium.[65] Reported complications were minor and transient, including chest pain, odynophagia, and dysphagia. Unlike PDT, stricture formation requiring dilation is rare (0–5%). No perforations have yet been reported.[65,66]

As a contact point technique, MPEC may not be ideal for long-segment Barrett's esophagus but more appropriate for shorter segments or for 'touch-up' of residual islands of Barrett's mucosa treated by other means such as Photofrin-PDT. Although the stricture rate is minimal, the limited depth of injury achieved with MPEC may be problematic. As already mentioned, squamous re-epithelization overlying intestinal metaplasia following MPEC has been reported. Moreover, there is concern that the use of this technique may promote growth or malignant transformation of underlying surviving dysplastic cells. The endoscopic ablation of Barrett's mucosa with dysplasia or early carcinoma is of greater importance than treatment of Barrett's mucosa without premalignant histologic changes.

No data are currently available for the use of MPEC in dysplastic Barrett's esophagus. In a very small study, the combination of Nd:YAG laser and MPEC was successful in ablating intramucosal adenocarcinoma within Barrett's esophagus in five of six patients with a mean follow-up of 3.4 years (range 9–86 months).[68] The role of MPEC in the ablation of Barrett's esophagus remains unclear and its place among other therapeutic alternatives such as laser therapy, PDT, or surgery is undefined. Long-term follow-up is necessary. Furthermore, its impact on Barrett's epithelium with dysplasia and the risk of developing adenocarcinoma are unknown. Until these issues are resolved, the use of MPEC in Barrett's esophagus should be considered experimental and continued endoscopic surveillance is wise for those who are 'successfully' treated with this technique.

CHECKLIST OF PRACTICE POINTS

1. Be familiar with one ESU: check all connections and grounding pad placement (monopolar mode) before use, know the power output characteristics of the generator, and test the catheter or probe *ex vivo* prior to electrocoagulation.

2. For bipolar electrocoagulation, 25 W of power or less is usually sufficient. For monopolar cutting, 40–70 W usually suffices. If unusually high power settings are required, re-check the electrosurgical circuitry for misconnections and the electrode for damage or build-up of charred tissue. Power should be increased only after these correctable causes have been ruled out.

3. For patients with implanted electronic devices, consult the cardiologist and read the manufacturer's instructions prior to electrocoagulation. An implanted defibrillator should be inactivated prior to the procedure while the patient is kept under continuous electrocardiographic monitoring. Use low power electrocoagulation and bipolar mode if possible.

4. For hemostasis of bleeding ulcers, Dieulafoy's lesions, or upper gastrointestinal tumors, apply MPEC at a lower power setting (~20 W) for 10–14 seconds before moving the probe. Use a large hemostasis probe and apply firm pressure directly on the target lesion. The endpoint is bleeding cessation or flattening and whitening of the visible vessel. For hemostasis of gastrointestinal angioectasias, low power setting (10 W), short coagulation pulses (1–2 seconds), and light pressure are recommended. The endpoint is bleeding cessation or formation of a white coagulum.

5. Use of electrocoagulation for oncologic applications is limited. MPEC using the hemostasis probes for palliation of obstructing tumors is relatively inefficient. BICAP tumor probes are available for palliation of circumferential esophageal and rectal tumors, but are cumbersome in application and of limited clinical use. For cancer palliation, consider other more practical or more effective alternatives instead.

6. MPEC as a mucosal ablative technique (e.g. Barrett's ablation) is currently being investigated. Its role for this application is not yet defined and should be regarded as an investigational tool at present.

REFERENCES

1. Barlow DE. Endoscopic applications of electrosurgery: a review of basic principles. Gastrointest Endosc 1982; 28:73–76.

2. Tucker RD. Principles of electrosurgery. In: Sivak MV, ed. Gastroenterologic endoscopy. 2nd ed. Philadelphia: WB Saunders; 1999: ch 9.

3. Rubeiz GJ, Tobi M, Meisnner MD. Ventricular asystole during upper gastrointestinal endoscopic electrocoagulation. Gastrointest Endosc 1995; 41:261–263.

4. Veitch A, Fairclough P. Endoscopic diathermy in patients with cardiac pacemakers. Endoscopy 1998; 30:544–547.

5. Technology Assessment Status Evaluation. Electrocautery use in patients with implanted cardiac devices. Gastrointest Endosc 1994; 40:794–795.

6. Bigard MA, Gaucher P, Lassalle C. Fatal colonic explosion during colonoscopic polypectomy. Gastroenterology 1979; 77:1307–1310.

7. Monahan DW, Peluso FE, Goldner F. Combustible colonic gas levels during flexible sigmoidoscopy and colonoscopy. Gastrointest Endosc 1992; 38:40–43.

8. Tucker RD, Sievert CE, Kramolowsky EV, et al. The interaction between electrosurgical generators, endoscopic electrodes, and tissue. Gastrointest Endosc 1992; 38:118–122.

9. Forde KA, Treat MR, Tsai JL. Initial clinical experience with a bipolar snare for colon polypectomy. Surg Endosc 1993; 7:427–428.

10. Tucker RD, Sievert CE, Platz CE, et al. Bipolar electrosurgical sphincterotomy. Gastrointest Endosc 1992; 38:113–117.

11. Siegel JH, Veerappan A, Tucker R. Bipolar versus monopolar sphincterotomy: a prospective trial. Am J Gastroenterol 1994; 89:1827–1830.

12. Jensen DM, Kovacs TOG, Freeman M, et al. A multicenter randomized prospective study of Gold probe vs heater probe for hemostasis of very severe ulcer or Mallory–Weiss bleeding (abstract). Gastroenterology 1991; 100:A92.

13. Jensen DM, Jutabha R, Machicado GA, et al. Prospective randomized comparative study of bipolar electrocoagulation versus heater probe for treatment of chronically bleeding internal hemorrhoids. Gastrointest Endosc 1997; 46:435–443.

14. Johnston J, Quint R, Petruzzi C, et al. Development and experimental testing of a large BICAP probe for palliative treatment of obstructing esophageal and rectal malignancy. Gastrointest Endosc 1985; 31:156.

15. Johnston JH, Fleischer D, Petrini J, et al. Palliative bipolar electrocoagulation therapy of obstructing esophageal cancer. Gastrointest Endosc 1987; 33:349–353.

16. Papp JP. Monopolar and electrohydrothermal treatment of upper gastrointestinal bleeding. Gastrointest Endosc 1990; 36:S34–37.

17. Jensen DM. Thermal contact methods for endoscopic hemostasis. In: Sivak MV, ed. Gastroenterologic endoscopy, 2nd ed. Philadelphia: WB Saunders; 1999: ch 28.

18. Papp JP. Endoscopic electrocoagulation in the management of upper gastrointestinal tract bleeding. Surg Clin North Am 1982; 62:797–806.

19. Freitas D, Donato A, Monteiro JG. Controlled trial of liquid monopolar electrocoagulation in bleeding peptic ulcers. Am J Gastroenterol 1985; 80:853–857.

20. Moreto M, Zaballa M, Ibanez S, et al. Efficacy of monopolar electrocoagulation in the treatment of bleeding gastric ulcer: a controlled trial. Endoscopy 1987; 19:54–56.

21. Swain CP, Storey DW, Bown SG, et al. Nature of the bleeding vessel in recurrently bleeding gastric ulcers. Gastroenterology 1986; 90:595–608.

22. Johnston JH, Jensen DM, Auth D. Experimental comparison of endoscopic yttrium-aluminum-garnet laser, electrosurgery, and heater probe for canine gut arterial coagulation. Importance of compression and avoidance of erosion. Gastroenterology 1987; 92:1101–1108.

23. Brearley S, Hawker PC, Dykes PW et al. Per-endoscopic bipolar diathermy coagulation of visible vessels using a 3.2 mm probe – a randomised clinical trial. Endoscopy 1987; 19:160–163.

24. Laine L. Multipolar electrocoagulation versus injection therapy in the treatment of bleeding peptic ulcers. A prospective randomized trial. Gastroenterology 1990; 99:1303–1306.

25. Laine L. Determination of the optimal technique for bipolar electrocoagulation treatment. An experimental evaluation of the BICAP and Gold probes. Gastroenterology 1991; 100:107–112.

26. Dilley AV, Friend MAG, Morris DL. An experimental study of optimal parameters for bipolar electrocoagulation. Gastrointest Endosc 1995; 42:27–30.

27. Morris DL, Brearley S, Thompson H, et al. A comparison of the efficacy and depth of gastric wall injury with 3.2- and 2.3-mm bipolar probes in canine arterial hemorrhage. Gastrointest Endosc 1985; 31:361–363.

28. Laine L. Multipolar electrocoagulation in the treatment of active upper gastrointestinal hemorrhage: a prospective controlled trial. N Engl J Med 1987; 316:1613–1617.

29. Laine L. Multipolar electrocoagulation in the treatment of peptic ulcers with non-bleeding visible vessels: a prospective controlled trial. Ann Intern Med 1989; 110:510–514.

30. O'Brien JD, Day SJ, Burnham WR. Controlled trial of small bipolar probe in bleeding peptic ulcers. Lancet 1986; i:464–467.

31. Cook DJ, Guyatt GH, Saloma BJ, et al. Endoscopic therapy for acute non-variceal upper gastrointestinal hemorrhage – a meta-analysis. Gastroenterology 1992; 102:139–148.

32. Goudie BM, Mitchell KG, Birnie GG, et al. Controlled trial of endoscopic bipolar electrocoagulation in the treatment of bleeding peptic ulcers (abstract). Gut 1984; 25:A1185.

33. Kernohan RM, Anderson JR, McKelvey ST, et al. A controlled trial of bipolar electrocoagulation in patients with upper gastrointestinal bleeding. Br J Surg 1984; 71:889–891.

34. Laine L, Stein C, Sharma V. A prospective outcome study of patients with clot in an ulcer and the effect of irrigation. Gastrointest Endosc 1996; 43:107–110.

35. Bleu BF, Gostout CJ, Shaw MJ, et al. Final results: rebleeding from peptic ulcers associated with adherent clots: a prospective randomized controlled study comparing endoscopic therapy with medical therapy (abstract). Gastrointest Endosc 1997; 45:AB87.

36. Hui WM, Ng MMT, Lok ASF, et al. A randomized comparative study of laser photocoagulation, heater probe, and bipolar electrocoagulation in the treatment of actively bleeding ulcers. Gastrointest Endosc 1991; 37:299–304.

37. Waring JP, Sanowski RA, Sawyer RL, et al. A randomized comparison of multipolar electrocoagulation and injection sclerosis

for the treatment of bleeding peptic ulcer. Gastrointest Endosc 1991; 37:295–298.

38. Jutabha R, Jensen DM, Machicado G, et al. Randomized controlled studies of injection Gold probes compared with monotherapies for hemostasis of bleeding canine gastric ulcers. Gastrointest Endosc 1998; 48:598–605.

39. Chan LY, Sung JJY, Chan FKL, et al. Tissue injury of injection Gold probe. Gastrointest Endosc 1998; 48:291–295.

40. Lin HJ, Tseng GY, Perng CL, et al. Comparison of adrenaline injection and bipolar electrocoagulation for the arrest of peptic ulcer bleeding. Gut 1999; 44:715–719.

41. Kovacs TOG, Jensen DM. Endoscopic diagnosis and treatment of bleeding Mallory–Weiss tears. Gastrointest Endosc Clin North Am 1991; 1:387–400.

42. Narayan S, Jensen DM, Randall GA, et al. Gastric bleeding from Dieulafoy's lesion versus peptic ulcer (abstract). Gastrointest Endosc 1992; 38:1992.

43. Jensen DM, Kovacs TOG, Randall G, et al. Prospective randomised study of patients with bleeding watermelon stomach (WMS) vs other UGI angioma syndromes (UGAS) treated with bipolar or heater probe (abstract). Gastroenterology 1994; 106:A241.

44. Rogers BHG. Endoscopic diagnosis and therapy of mucosal vascular abnormalities of the gastrointestinal tract occurring in elderly patients and associated with cardiac, vascular, and pulmonary disease. Gastrointest Endosc 1980; 26:134–138.

45. Howard OM, Buchanan JD, Hunt RH. Angiodysplasia of the colon: experience of 26 cases. Lancet 1982; ii:16–19.

46. Wadas DD, Sanowski RA. Complications of the hot biopsy forceps technique. Gastrointest Endosc 1988; 34:32–37.

47. Savides TJ, Jensen DM, Machicado GA, et al. Colonoscopic hemostasis for recurrent diverticular hemorrhage associated with a visible vessel: a report of 3 cases. Gastrointest Endosc 1994; 40:70–73.

48. Rex DK, Lewis BS, Waye JD. Colonoscopy and endoscopic therapy for delayed post-polypectomy hemorrhage. Gastrointest Endosc 1992; 38:127–129.

49. Sherman S, Hawes RH, Nisi R, et al. Endoscopic sphincterotomy-induced hemorrhage: treatment with multipolar electrocoagulation. Gastrointest Endosc 1992; 38:123–126.

50. Jensen DM, Kovacs TOG, Machicado GA, et al. Prospective study of the stigmata of hemorrhage and endoscopic or medical treatment for bleeding Mallory–Weiss tears (abstract). Gastrointest Endosc 1992; 38:235.

51. Machicado GA, Jensen DM, Kovacs TG, et al. Patients with recurrent GI hemorrhage and colonic angiomas – a randomised study of endoscopic treatment with bipolar or heater probe coagulation (abstract). Gastrointest Endosc 1998; 47:AB100.

52. Jensen DM, Machicado GA, Cheng S, et al. A randomized prospective study of endoscopic bipolar electrocoagulation and heater probe treatment of chronic rectal bleeding from radiation telangiectasia. Gastrointest Endosc 1997; 45:20–25.

53. Randall GM, Jensen DM, Machicado GA, et al. Prospective randomized comparative study of bipolar versus direct current electrocoagulation for treatment of bleeding internal hemorrhoids. Gastrointest Endosc 1994; 40:403–410.

54. Dennison A, Whiston RJ, Ronney S, et al. A randomized study of infrared photocoagulation with bipolar diathermy for outpatient treatment of hemorrhoids. Dis Colon Rectum 1990; 33:32–34.

55. Griffith CDM, Morris DL, Wherry D, et al. Outpatient treatment of haemorrhoids: a randomized trial comparing contact bipolar diathermy with rubber band ligation. Coloproctology 1987; 6:322–334.

56. Hinton CP, Morris DL. A randomized trial comparing direct current therapy and bipolar diathermy in the outpatient treatment of third-degree hemorrhoids. Dis Colon Rectum 1990; 233:931–932.

57. Cremer M, Deviere J, Sugai B, et al. Expandable biliary metal stents for malignancies: endoscopic insertion and diathermic cleaning for tumor ingrowth. Gastrointest Endosc 1990; 36:451–457.

58. Ell C, Fleig WE, Hochberger J. Broken biliary metal stent after repeated electrocoagulation for tumor ingrowth. Gastrointest Endosc 1992; 38:197–198.

59. Jensen DM, Machicado G, Randall G, et al. Comparison of low-power YAG laser and BICAP tumor probe for palliation of esophageal cancer strictures. Gastroenterology 1988; 94:1263–1270.

60. McIntyre AS, Morris DL, Sloan RL, et al. Palliative therapy of malignant esophageal stricture with bipolar tumor probe and prosthetic tube. Gastrointest Endosc 1989; 35:531–535.

61. Aubert A, Meduri B, Fritsch J, et al. Endoscopic treatment by snare electrocoagulation prior to Nd:YAG laser photocoagulation in 85 voluminous colorectal villous adenomas. Dis Colon Rectum 1991; 34:372–377.

62. Paterlini A, Buffoli F, Cesari P, et al. Palliative treatment with the BICAP of recurrent neoplastic stenosis of the colon–rectum anastomosis. Endoscopy 1990; 22:96.

63. Jensen DM, Hirabayashi K. A comparative study of coagulation depths and efficacy of arterial coagulation for gold probe (abstract). Am J Gastroenterol 1989; 116:A89.

64. Sampliner RE, Fennerty B, Garewal HS. Reversal of Barrett's esophagus with acid suppression and multipolar electrocoagulation: preliminary results. Gastrointest Endosc 1996; 44:532–535.

65. Kovacs BJ, Chen YK, Lewis TD, et al. Successful reversal of Barrett's esophagus with multipolar electrocoagulation despite inadequate acid suppression. Gastrointest Endosc 1999; 49:547–553.

66. Sharma P, Camargo E, Garewal HS, et al. Long term reversal of patients with Barrett's esophagus with multipolar electrocoagulation (MPEC) and high dose omeprazole (abstract). Gastrointest Endosc 1998; 47:AB76.

67. Sampliner RE. Ablative therapies for the columnar-lined esophagus. Gastroenterol Clin North Am 1997; 26:685–694.

68. Sharma P, Jaffe PE, Bhattacharyya A, et al. Laser and multipolar electrocoagulation ablation of early Barrett's adenocarcinoma: long-term follow-up. Gastrointest Endosc 1999; 49:442–446.

5.2

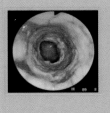

MODALITIES FOR TISSUE COAGULATION OR ABLATION: LASER APPLICATION

RAINER R. SANDER

INDICATIONS

Since the mid-1970s when Frühmorgen et al,[1] Dwyer et al,[2] and Kiefhaber et al[3] first applied laser light via a gastroscope in patients to achieve hemostasis, the therapeutic application of the laser beam has become standard practice in a wide range of medical specialties. In the field of gastroenterology, and especially in the framework of endoscopic-operative procedures, the indications for thermal laser treatment are:

- malignant tumors
- benign tumors
- non-neoplastic strictures
- actual and potential bleeding lesions.

Malignant tumors

The major use of endoscopic laser treatment in advanced malignant tumors of the gastrointestinal tract is to re-open a stenosis and keep the passage free for both liquid and solid food. Tumors suitable for treatment are exophytic lesions with tissue protruding into the lumen as well as intramural-spreading malignancies. Localized cancer can be cured in up to 81% of the cases[4] when surgical removal of the tumor is a contraindication because of the medical condition of the patient.[5,6]

Precursor lesions of cancer may be eradicated to prevent the subsequent development of malignancy.

Benign tumors

In inoperable or poor-risk patients, laser treatment is appropriate to debulk large benign tumors to relieve symptoms. When broad-based lesions cannot be completely removed endoscopically with a snare, complementary laser coagulation may be useful in eradicating the remaining tissue even in operable patients.

Non-neoplastic strictures

Stenoses induced by scars and inflammatory tissue may be amenable to laser treatment since the beam can be used as a cutting instrument to disrupt circumferential, cicatricial rings. This technique can be applied to symptomatic strictures where thickening of the wall causes the stenosis.

Actual and potential bleeding lesions

Although alternative methods offer similar results in hemostasis, thermal laser coagulation remains one of the classic and effective instruments in hemostasis for treatment of a broad variety of circumscribed potential and actual bleeding sources, including ulcers, erosions, tumors, and angiomas.

CONTRAINDICATIONS

There are no absolute contraindications for laser application in the gut except those cases where endoscopy should not be performed, i.e. in patients in a very poor and unstable general condition and those who cannot be properly prepared for treatment.

However, in every case alternative treatment regimens must be considered, which may result in a better outcome when applied alone or added to the laser therapy.

In several situations, the use of the laser may be associated with a high risk of complications, under which circumstances this modality should be employed with extreme caution. These circumstances are:

- esophageal and gastric varices
- deep penetrating ulcer of the posterior wall of the duodenal bulb with a visible non-bleeding vessel
- colonic lesions without proper bowel preparation
- lack of exact identification of the laser beam
- diffuse bleeding.

EQUIPMENT

Laser light is generated in an optically active medium which may be a gas, fluid, or solid material. It is amplified by external stimulation and reflection and emitted as a coherent, parallel, and monochromatic radiation.

Laser light is similar in properties to any light; when light shines on a material and is absorbed, it is converted into heat. The basic thermal effects of lasers with increasing temperatures are: reversible warming, denaturation of proteins, drying, carbonization, volatilization (or, in other words, hyperthermia, coagulation, shrinkage, and vaporization of tissue). The degree of the thermal effect depends on three parameters which are specific to the type of beam, the tissue, and the wavelength.

1. Beam-specific
   - spot diameter
   - power
   - time
2. Tissue-specific
   optical
   - absorption
   - scattering
   thermal
   - density
   - specific heat
   - thermal conductivity
   - blood circulation
3. Wavelength-specific
   - absorption in water.

For clinical use of thermal laser energy, medium-power, continuous wave lasers providing outputs of up to several hundred Watts per mm² are the most commonly employed. Of particular importance is the Nd:YAG laser, a solid-state laser, which operates at a wavelength of within the near infrared of 1064 nm and has an output of up to 100 W. The blue-green light of the argon laser (480–514 μm) and the frequency-doubled Nd:YAG laser (532 nm) show a more superficial effect. Advantages of these latter two lasers in gastrointestinal indications have not been demonstrated. This also applies to the Nd:YAG wavelength of 1318 nm.

Laser light is conducted through the endoscope via a Teflon-coated, quartz monofiber having a diameter of between 200 and 600 microns enclosed within an outer Teflon sheath, utilizing the principle of total internal reflection. The fiber is enclosed within a Teflon tube. The light guide system employed has an outer diameter of between 1.8 and 2.5 mm, and can be passed down the working channel of conventional endoscopes. At the tip of the laser light guide is a metal cap which envelops the end of the fiber and provides mechanical support to the system. A coaxial stream of a cooling medium which may be air, CO_2, nitrogen, or water keeps the tip free from contamination and prevents it from being destroyed by tissue contact. The invisible laser light emitted has a divergence of about 12°, so that the area of tissue exposed is dependent on the distance between the tip and the tissue. A red, heli-

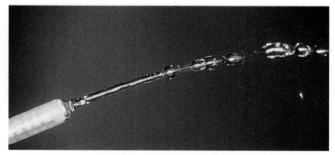

Fig. 5.2.1 The waterjet-guided laser beam, marked by the red dots of the helium-neon pilot laser.

um-neon pilot laser is an integral part of the system and is the visible source which identifies the direction and spot size of the therapeutic laser.

When water is used as the cooling medium (waterjet system),[7] the laser light follows the path of the waterjet and will deviate from a straight path (Fig. 5.2.1). The principle of transmission of laser light by the flexible conducting system is based on total internal reflection of the light at the interfaces between two materials having different refractive indices. The light is always reflected towards the medium with the higher refractive index. When gas is used to cool the light guide composed of quartz and Teflon, no energy is lost because of the total internal reflection, but once emitted from the fiber tip, the light is directed straight to the target of treatment. In the waterjet system, the water and air interface acts in a similar fashion to the quartz and Teflon but since the water flow extends beyond the tip of the fiber, the water stream will conduct the laser beam to the tissue in a gravity-dependent system.

In the gastrointestinal tract, the effect of laser application is dependent on the mode in which it is employed. In the non-contact mode, coagulation extends from the surface to a depth of up to 5 mm. Higher laser energies will result in tissue vaporization with progressively deeper tissue destruction, which can lead to an immediate perforation of the organ. The vaporization defect is surrounded by a coagulation zone and an area of edema (Fig. 5.2.2).

In contrast to the tissue effect of laser light in air is that produced by the waterjet system. Owing to the cooling effect of the water, the surface of the irradiated organ remains intact while deeper layers become coagulated and there is swelling and hyperemia of the surrounding area after several minutes (Fig. 5.2.3).

Modifications of transmission systems result in a wide range of other types of thermal injury: sapphire tips may induce a so-called popcorn effect with a slowly developing disruption of the wall of the organ related to smaller explosions of gas. The naked fiber shows unpredictable and delayed effects when used for interstitial application.

PATIENT PREPARATION

Basically laser treatment requires the same preparation as is used for the endoscopic procedure alone. As for any endoscopy, sedative and/or hypnotic medication (i.e.

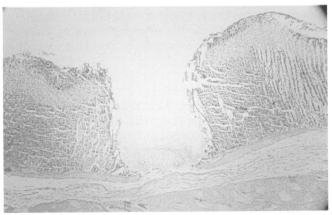

Fig. 5.2.2 Tissue-ablating effect of the non-contact system shown on a cross-section through the stomach of a rabbit with the tissue-ablating zone in the center, surrounded by coagulation and edema.

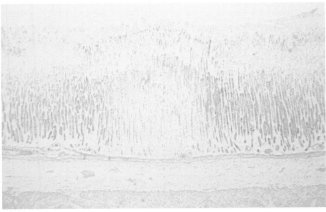

Fig. 5.2.3 In contrast, the tissue reaction after irradiation with the waterjet-guided laser beam. There is a deep-volume coagulation with coagulation of the deeper layers of the wall of the organ.

diazepam, midazolam/propofol, etomidat) is helpful to keep the patient calm and quiet. Although laser irradiation during gastrointestinal endoscopy generally is not painful, treatment in the proximal esophagus close to the pharynx or in the distal rectum in the neighborhood of the sphincter and the anal region may cause considerable discomfort.

Because of the risk of explosion related to flammable gases, laser therapy in the colon should be performed only after a complete bowel preparation.

PROCEDURE

Malignant tumors

Laser photodestruction is carried out through flexible endoscopes under visual control using the non-contact mode. When it is possible to traverse a malignant tumor, the laser is applied to the parts of the tumor located farthest from the tip of the endoscope, with the beam directed in a circular, paintbrush fashion to the malignant tissue as the scope is slowly withdrawn. When complete obstruction is encountered, the tissue is vaporized from the proximal edge for 2–3 cm of the length in one session (Figs 5.2.4 and 5.2.5). Further laser sessions are then performed at 2-day intervals, when the edema induced by the previous application has subsided, necrotic tissue has sloughed, and when the endoscopist is able to accurately assess the overall effect of the last session and predict the consequences of further applications. Laser application is at an output of 80–100 W and a distance from tip to tissue of 5–10 mm.

When a long, malignant stenosis is encountered, several treatment sessions should be performed rather than forcing recanalization in one session. Overly aggressive therapy may be associated with a higher incidence of perforation. In some cases, it may be helpful to predilate a stenosis with a bougie before starting laser therapy but this is not a requirement for successful treatment. Overtreatment must be avoided. The aim should be to safely establish luminal continuity but not to eradicate

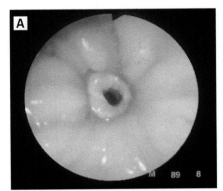

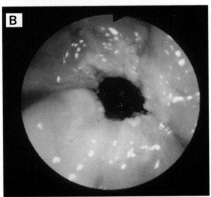

Fig. 5.2.4 Stenosis of a recurrent adenocarcinoma of the rectum. (A) Before laser vaporization. (B) Immediately after laser vaporization.

Fig. 5.2.5 Free passage through the stenosis for the 13 mm endoscope 5 days later.

the tumor. A good clinical result will be achieved when the lumen has been widened to allow the passage of a 13 mm endoscope. The energy applied in a single session varies between 2000 and 20 000 J.

Premedication with intravenous steroids and, if indicated, the placement of a decompression tube through the stenosis before removing the endoscope may be of value in reducing subsequent edema and to avoid complaints caused by bloating and accumulated gas.

The first series of treatments are performed in hospitalized patients until complete recanalization is achieved. The follow-up examinations are carried out at 4- to 6-week intervals on an outpatient basis whether retreatment is necessary or not.

Complete destruction in smaller malignancies may be accomplished by laser treatment in some cases when surgery cannot be performed.

Benign tumors

Between 30 and 50 W are used in the non-contact mode to coagulate adenomas. The energy applied may be as much as 3000 J per session depending on the size of the lesion. Irradiation is carried out under direct vision without preset pulse times using a paintbrush mode to cover the treatment area.

If, after previous polypectomy, adenomatous tissue remains in situ and complete removal with the high-frequency snare is not possible, complementary laser coagulation may eradicate the remaining tissue (Fig. 5.2.6A–D). In patients who are operable candidates in whom a tumor appears to be benign, it is important to obtain histopathologic evidence of the major part of the tumor by snare or biopsy prior to laser vaporization to avoid missing curative therapy in case of malignancy.

Non-neoplastic stenoses

In non-neoplastic stenoses, short-lasting laser pulses with no fixed time limit are applied under visual control in non-contact mode using an output of 80–100 W. The tissue of the cicatricial ring is cut stepwise with longitudinal stripes of vaporization of the tissue to a depth of 1–2 mm in two to four positions to open the stenosis. In case of a long stricture, additional bougienage with the endoscope may be necessary.

Actual and potential bleeding lesions

Hemostasis is achieved by applying the laser light at a distance of 5–10 mm from the metal tip to the bleeding lesion. With increasing temperatures, the denaturation, coagulation, and shrinkage of the tissue with the coincidental edema will lead to disruption, sealing and thrombotic closure of the nutrient artery.

The most important indication is the peptic ulcer with a visible vessel with or without active bleeding. Laser application is performed with a setting of 80–100 W in a paintbrush technique beginning around the bleeding vessel. After removal of debris or clot, the artery itself is coagulated directly, until bleeding ceases. If the hemorrhage persists, another attempt at hemostasis is performed after several minutes.

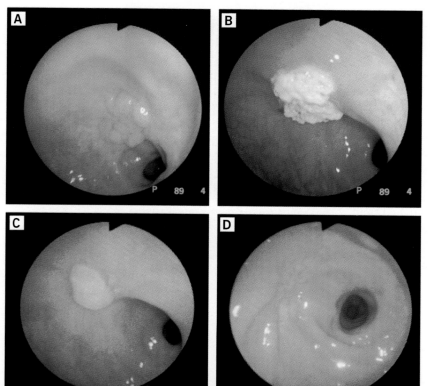

Fig. 5.2.6 Laser treatment of a recurrent villous adenoma in the rectum. (**A**) Before treatment. (**B**) Minutes after laser coagulation. (**C**) The healing ulcer 7 weeks later. (**D**) The scar 2 years later.

A previous injection of epinephrine solution 1:10 000 (1:20 000) into and around the lesion may help to improve the results regarding the incidence of rebleeding or emergency surgery.

Although the waterjet and the non-contact modes do not differ much with respect to technique, the energy applied per lesion is substantially higher when using the waterjet system (~3000 J) compared with the non-contact system (~1400 J) because of the limited surface damage associated with the water cooling effect.

When rebleeding occurs, a second laser treatment can be performed. Patients with a second rebleeding should probably undergo emergency surgery. Deep penetrating ulcers of the posterior wall of the duodenal bulb which show a visible vessel even without active spurting bleeding should be considered for an early elective surgical intervention without a previous endoscopic intervention.

Further indications such as bleeding Mallory–Weiss lesions, erosions, and angiomas are preferably handled with the non-contact technique (Fig. 5.2.7A and B). The waterjet system is useful for hemorrhage from tumors.

A special hemostatic laser technique is used in angiomas located in the proximal colon. Here a point coagulation of the lesions is required with short bursts of 30–50 W using the non-contact system with reduced gas flow. The treatment is continued until the color of the angioma has completely changed to white.

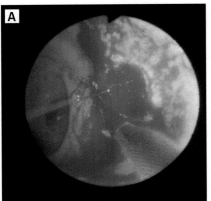

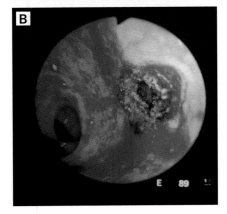

Fig. 5.2.7 (A) A spurting bleeding after polypectomy in the sigmoid colon, which stops after a single laser treatment (B).

COMPLICATIONS AND THEIR MANAGEMENT

Complications of laser application in the gastrointestinal tract are:

- perforation
- bleeding
- fistula
- stenosis.

Perforation

The risk of perforation is comparatively high in areas where there is a bend in the distal esophagus and sigmoid colon. When the endoscopist is unable to follow the lumen with the endoscope or pass a guidewire or probe through a stenosis, laser application may result in producing a false passage.

If a small perforation is produced in the upper gastrointestinal tract, conservative management is recommended primarily with parenteral nutrition and antibiotic therapy for approximately 1 week. In tumor patients, tumor overgrowth usually occludes the defect within a few days. In other cases, after withdrawal of the endoscope, a tiny hole in the wall of the organ spontaneously closes down when the gaseous distention of the organ is reduced and the lumen collapses.

In the event of a large perforation or any perforation in the colon, surgical intervention is often required to prevent the development of peritonitis, especially in patients with insufficient bowel preparation. Laser treatment of small or flat lesions such as angiomas or flat adenomas in either the esophagus or in the proximal colon have a comparatively high risk of perforation because the wall is relatively thin. Preceding intramural injection of saline solution makes coagulation safer by increasing the thickness of the wall.

To avoid the risk of explosion in the presence of inflammable gases (e.g. methane) in the insufficiently prepared colon, only sheathed fibers with coaxial gas or waterflow should be used.

Bleeding

Although the Nd:YAG laser is often used as a hemostatic tool, laser treatment sometimes induces hemorrhage as it destroys the superficial tissue overlying blood vessels, especially when using the non-contact modality.

Laser-induced bleeding usually stop spontaneously or upon continuing the laser application. When used for active hemorrhage from esophageal varices or for deep penetrating ulcers of the posterior wall of the duodenal bulb with a visible vessel, sometimes complementary measures such as banding, balloon-compression, or surgery may be required to achieve complete cessation of hemorrhage.

Fistula

A deep thermal injury may result in a fistula between two hollow organs such as between the esophagus (usually at a level of 25 cm from the incisor teeth) and the tracheo-bronchial system or between the rectum and the vagina or the urinary bladder. A small hole may be closed by injecting fibrin glue. In most cases, however, this measure does not work, especially when a fistula occurs during therapy of malignant tumors. In the esophagus, the implantation of a covered metal mesh stent or an endocoil may occlude the fistula so that swallowing saliva, or liquid and solid food can continue without aspiration.

Stenosis

Strictures may occur weeks to months following Nd:YAG laser treatment. These are caused by shrinkage of the tissue and the small feeding vessels of the submucosa and the muscularis along with fibroblastic proliferation induced by laser light. Dilation or implantation of a stent may be required to maintain lumenal patency.

RESULTS AND CONCLUSION

Results

From November 1978 to June 1999, 3105 patients were treated at the Municipal Hospital München–Harlaching in 6528 sessions. The indications were malignant tumors (708 patients, 3192 sessions), benign tumors (209 patients, 421 sessions), non-neoplastic stenoses (134 patients, 471 sessions), and bleeding (2057 patients, 2444 sessions).

Malignant tumors

Out of the 708 patients with malignancies, 433 were in the upper gastrointestinal tract and 275 in the lower tract. The reasons for palliation included tumor-related symptoms in non-resectable tumors, tumors with metastases, and patients who declined surgery. Major symptoms at the beginning of the laser treatment were dysphagia, obstruction, and abnormal rectal discharge. The results are shown in Table 5.2.1. Before treatment, 73% of the tumors could not be passed with the endoscope. About 98% of the malignant stenoses were completely re-opened within an average of 2.3 sessions per patient. The average length of the narrow segment was 6.0 cm (range 2–17 cm). In follow-up, each patient was treated with the laser an average of 6.4 times (range 1–39). The interval to the first restenosis was approximately 4 (upper gastrointestinal tract) to 6

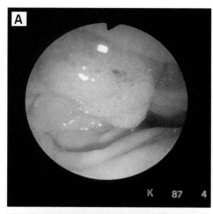

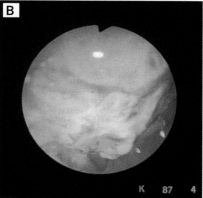

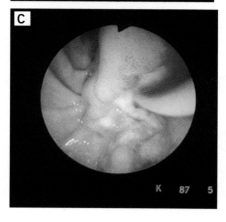

Fig. 5.2.8 (A) A protruding pancreatic carcinoma makes a primary cannulation of the duodenal papilla impossible. (B) Immediately after laser coagulation treatment of the tumor. (C) Placement of a stent is possible 10 days after the laser coagulation treatment.

(lower gastrointestinal tract) weeks. The malignancies were located in the esophagus (178), stomach (243), duodenum (12) (Fig. 5.2.8A–C), right colon (14), left colon (69), and rectum (192).

Twenty-nine major complications occurred in the upper gastrointestinal tract including fistulae (15), perforation (10), respiratory failure (3), and bleeding (1). Twenty-four of these patients received conservative management. Fistulae in the esophagus were treated with stents. In 5 out of 10 perforations after 1 week of parenteral nutrition, antibiotics, and monitoring, the patients received further laser treatment. Five patients underwent surgery, and one additional patient died from uncontrollable bleeding from a cervical esophageal carcinoma.

In the lower gastrointestinal tract, we observed 14 major complications, 10 were handled conservatively.

Laser-treated malignancies (n=578)		
	Upper GI (n=341)	Lower GI (n=237)
Treatment sucessful	305 (89.4%)	226 (95.4%)
Treatment not successful	36 (10.6%)	11 (4.6%)
— temporary success only	3	5
— non recanalization	4	5
— complication	29	1

Table 5.2.1 Laser-treated malignancies in the gastrointestinal tract (n=708); patients with complete follow-up (n=578)

38. MacLeod IA, Mills PR, MacKenzie JE, et al. Neodymium Yttrium Aluminium Garnet laser photocoagulation for major hemorrhage from peptic ulcers and single vessels: a single blind controlled study. BMJ 1983; 286:345–348.

39. Krejs GJ, Little KH, Westergaard H, et al. Laser photocoagulation for the treatment of acute peptic ulcer bleeding. N Engl J Med 1987; 316:1618–1621.

40. Escourrou J. In: Papp JP, ed. European clinical experience in laser photocoagulation in upper gastrointestinal tract. Endoscopic control of gastrointestinal hemorrhage. Boca Raton: FL CRC; 1981:103–110.

41. Swain CP, Bown SG, Salmon PR, et al. Controlled trial of neodymium YAG laser photocoagulation in bleeding peptic ulcers. Lancet 1986; i:1113–1114.

42. Cook D, Gyatt G, Salena B, et al. Endoscopic therapy for non-variceal upper gastrointestinal hemorrhage: a meta-analysis. Gastroenterology 1992; 102:139–148.

43. Sacks H, Chalmers T, Blum A, et al. Endoscopic hemostasis – an effective therapy for bleeding peptic ulcers. JAMA 1990; 264:494–499.

44. Rutgeerts P, Broeckaert L, Coremans G, et al. Randomized comparison of three hemostasis modalities for severe bleeding of peptic ulcers. Gastrointest Endosc 1987; 33:182.

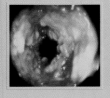

5.3

CLINICAL APPLICATION OF ARGON PLASMA COAGULATION IN FLEXIBLE ENDOSCOPY

KARL E. GRUND

GUNTER FARIN

INTRODUCTION

Argon Plasma Coagulation (APC) is a special electrosurgical modality in which high-frequency electric current (HF-current) is conducted 'contact-free' through ionized and thus electrically conductive argon (argon plasma) into the tissue to be treated. The aim of this technique is to create therapeutically effective temperatures in target tissues which are especially suitable and endoscopically applicable for thermal hemostasis and/or the ablation of pathologic tissue. Any biologic tissue can be treated whether in the gastrointestinal tract or in the tracheo-bronchial system. As a new therapeutic modality, APC's efficiency rivals other thermal methods like conventional electrosurgery and laser as well as other long-established and new interventional procedures as injection therapy and photodynamic therapy. A broad spectrum of indications has been found for APC since its introduction into flexible endoscopy in 1991.[1–10,13] This chapter describes the physical principle and the equipment required for APC as well as the indications, relevant techniques, and special points to be noted in its application. The advantages and disadvantages of APC in comparison to alternative interventional methods in flexible endoscopy are discussed for each indication on the basis of our own experience and that of other clinical centers.

PHYSICAL PRINCIPLES AND THERMAL EFFECTS

APC applies HF-current to tissue with defined thermal effects for hemostasis as well as for devitalization or destruction of pathologic tissue. In contrast to conventional electrosurgery, the HF-current is not conducted to the tissue through direct contact by active electrodes but via ionized and thus electrically conductive argon (argon plasma) (Fig. 5.3.1).

APC requires suitable APC applicators, an argon source, and an HF-current source (Fig. 5.3.1).

APC applicators consist in principle of a tube whose distal end contains an electrode (Fig. 5.3.2). When sufficient HF-voltage is applied between the electrode and the tissue, the argon gas flowing out of the tube becomes ionized in the electric field between this electrode and the tissue. In this way, electrically conductive argon plasma beams are created through which HF-current can flow into

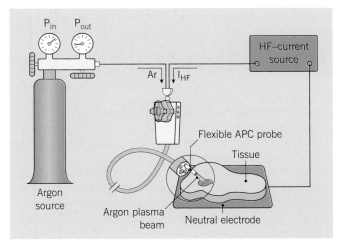

Fig. 5.3.1 Clinical application of argon plasma coagulation in flexible endoscopy, which consists of an argon source with controlled output pressure (P_{out}) for argon flow rate (Ar), an HF-current (I_{HF}) source and a flexible argon plasma coagulation probe.

87

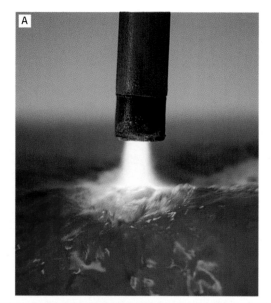

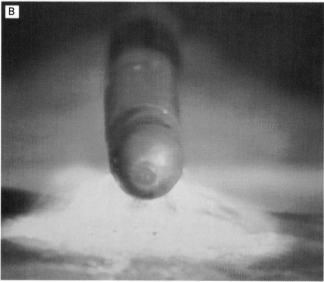

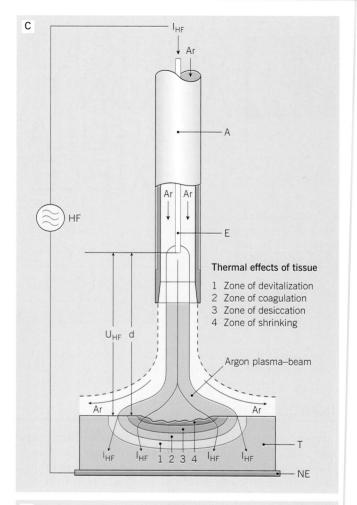

Thermal effects of tissue

1 Zone of devitalization
2 Zone of coagulation
3 Zone of desiccation
4 Zone of shrinking

Argon plasma–beam

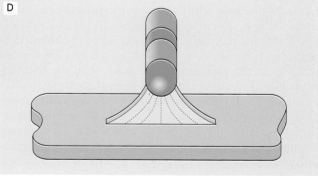

Fig. 5.3.2 Photographic (**A** and **B**) and schematic (**C** and **D**) depiction of argon plasma coagulation probes for frontal (**A**) and lateral (**B**) applications in flexible endoscopy. Ar=argon gas flow rate; E=electrode; d=distance between electrode and tissue; T=tissue; HF= high frequency source; I_{HF}=high frequency current; NE=neutral electrode; U_{HF}=high frequency voltage; A=applicator.

tissue and complete the electrical circuit back to the HF-current source via a neutral electrode. The HF-current generates heat in the tissue, causing devitalization, coagulation, desiccation, and hence tissue shrinking.

As soon as a point on the tissue surface loses electric conductivity because of desiccation, the plasma beam automatically moves to an adjacent surface which is still electrically conductive, and this process continues until the entire surface in the area close to the distal end of the APC applicator has been desiccated. As a result, APC creates zones of devitalization, coagulation, and desiccation of uniform depth. Even in large-area applications, the depth is automatically limited to 3 mm at most,[1,2,14–16] depending

mainly on application time (Fig. 5.3.3) when using the equipment described below.

An electric field strength of approximately 500 V/mm is needed to ionize argon. The field strength (FS) is defined mainly by the voltage (U_{HF}) and the distance (d) between the electrode (E) and the tissue (G):

$$FS = U_{HF}/d.$$

For example, a distance of 10 mm thus requires an HF-voltage with a peak value of approximately 5000 V. The HF-current needed for APC is comparable to that required for conventional contact coagulation. The direction of the HF-current in the argon plasma is mainly determined by

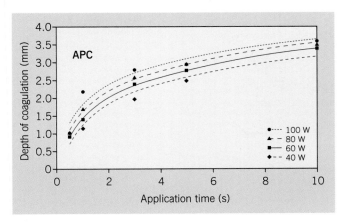

Fig. 5.3.3 Depth of the coagulation zone in relation to application time and power setting (flexible argon plasma coagulation probe: 2.3 mm, argon flow rate: 2 L/min, HF-current source: Erbe ICC 200).

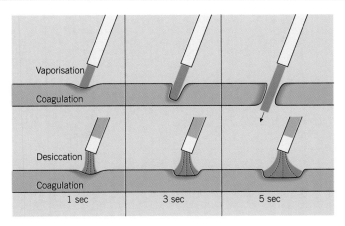

Fig. 5.3.4 Penetration of Nd:YAG laser (top row) and argon plasma coagulation (bottom row) during an application of 5 seconds. Note the differences: laser vaporizes and penetrates deeply while argon plasma coagulation covers a wider area with a limited penetration depth and does not vaporize tissue.

the direction and strength of the electric field and not by that of the argon flow. However, it is important that pure argon gas exists between the electrode and the target tissue. Hence special APC applicators, which direct the argon flow mainly at the target tissue, are advantageous in use. APC applicators can be used at nearly any angle to the tissue provided that the gas in the area of application is pure argon. The path of the HF-current beam is made visible by the luminescence of the argon plasma.

As argon is inert, APC causes neither carbonization nor vaporization and hence does not generate smoke, so that it is well suited for endoscopic applications. The absence of tissue vaporization and the automatically limited depth of thermal devitalization are advantageous, avoiding perforation of thin-walled organs during thermal therapy (Fig. 5.3.4). This same quality, however, also makes it difficult to remove large tumor masses with APC.[12,15,17–23]

EQUIPMENT

APC requires applicators suited to the intended task, an argon source, and an HF-current source (Fig. 5.3.1).

APC applicators for flexible endoscopy basically consist of a non-conductive flexible tube through which the argon is applied to the target tissue, and an electrode within the distal end of this tube. The electrode is connected by a wire through the lumen of this tube to the HF-generator (Fig. 5.3.2). The electrode is recessed from the end of the tube so that it cannot come into contact with tissue. Flexible APC applicators are available in different diameters and lengths as well as for axial or lateral application.

In its simplest version, an argon source consists of a gas cylinder with a valve that reduces the pressure from the gas cylinder to a level appropriate for the intended application. For safety reasons, in endoluminal applications the argon source must have automatically controlled flow rates and maximum gas pressure limitations. A relatively low argon flow rate or velocity is sufficient to produce plasma beams and should not be increased beyond the optimum flow to avoid overdistention of the intestine as well as to avoid argon embolism.

The HF-current source must provide both sufficiently high voltage for the ionization of argon gas and enough HF-current to generate adequate heat within the target tissue. This can be automatically controlled by the HF-generator.

PROCEDURE

Applications are performed according to the '10 rules of APC use' (see Checklist, p.98) and adapted to the individual circumstances. Application of the plasma beam can be frontal, lateral, and circumferential (Figs 5.3.5–5.3.7), anterograde, retrograde, or around the corner. In general, it should be used in a paintbrush-like manner under strict visual control without touching the tissue with the probe tip.

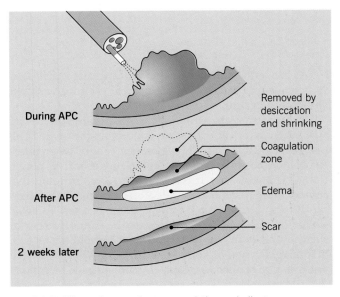

Fig. 5.3.5 Effects of argon plasma coagulation on bulky tumors: desiccation, shrinking, coagulation, secondary necrosis.

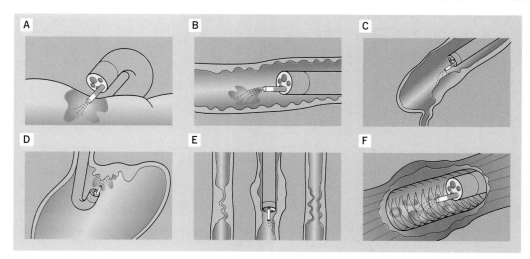

Fig. 5.3.6 Clinical application of argon plasma coagulation in technically difficult situations.

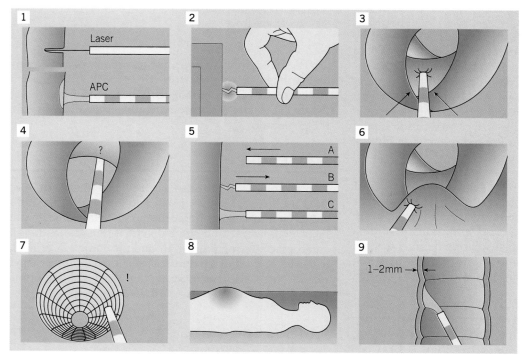

Fig. 5.3.7 Recommendations for use of argon plasma coagulation in flexible endoscopy.

As generally in high-frequency electric surgery, all safety precautions concerning the neutral electrode and the electrosurgical unit have to be followed.

If there is a combustible gas in the organ treated with APC, there is a danger of explosion within the organ. This plays an essential role when a patient cannot be prepared for colonoscopy, because the colon might harbor potentially flammable gas. It is essential to keep in mind that *behind* a tumor stenosis in the colon there may be a reservoir of methane in the prestenotic, dilated colon. To avoid explosion it is necessary to evacuate the flammable gas by suction and to inflate the colon with normal air or CO_2 before application of laser, HF-current or APC. A stenosis must first be opened *mechanically* (bougienage or balloon dilation) in order to evacuate the potentially explosive gas.

In bronchoscopy, there may also be a danger of explosion if the concentration of oxygen exceeds 25%. To per-form APC safely, one must disconnect supplemental O_2 and ventilate the patient with normal air for several seconds before starting APC.

Special problems, causes and remedies during the procedures are listed in Box 5.3.1.

Patient preparation

APC can usually be performed as an outpatient procedure. Only in special cases of extended use of APC (e.g. for tumor debulking) should the patient be kept in hospital under observation overnight after the treatment.

Patients must be informed before the APC session about the procedure, benefits, risks, and alternative treatments.

No special patient preparation in addition to the standard preparation for esophagogastroduodenoscopy (EGD), colonoscopy, and bronchoscopy is necessary.

BOX 5.3.1 Special problems, causes and remedies

Missing or weak ignition:
A. Test the electric arc outside the endoscope
B. Distance from the tissue is too great for ignition
C. Output setting is less than 40–50 W
D. Tip of the probe has coagulation debris

'Weak' plasma beam:
A. Insufficient argon gas flow
B. Low power setting
C. Debris on tip of the probe

Lumen distention:
A. Continuous suction using a double-channel endoscope
B. Intermittent suction via single-channel endoscope
C. Add a venting tube next to the endoscope

Wall contact with the tip of the probe:
A. Immediately interrupt application
B. Exclude perforation

INDICATIONS AND RESULTS

Database

Our own experience is based on the treatment of 1454 consecutive patients (799 men, 655 women, mean age 67 years (3 months to 97 years)) (Tables 5.3.1 and 5.3.3) who underwent treatment with APC (APC 300, Beamer two, ICC 200, ICC 350, different probes, all ERBE Elektomedizin, Germany) in the gastrointestinal tract or the tracheobronchial system in 2795 sessions from June 1991 to May 1999.

Primary indications for treatment (Table 5.3.2) are hemorrhages of various origin, malignant and benign tumors, tissue ingrowth and overgrowth of stents. Additional indications are: adenomata angiodysplastic lesions of all kinds, areas of dysplasia (e.g. Barrett's epithelium), premalignant lesions, and early cancer. Normally, these patients would all have been treated with the Nd:YAG laser, conventional electrosurgery, or an open surgical procedure.

The intention of the treatment is to achieve the following goals in each patient with a maximum of 2 to 3 sessions:

- *Hemorrhage*
  Reliable hemostasis according to endoscopic and/or clinical criteria, no recurrent bleeding.
- *Tumor stenosis*
  Restoration and preservation of the lumen for subsequent passage of the corresponding endoscope.
- *Tumors*
  Reduction of the intraluminal tumor mass by at least 50% and creating a sufficient lumen.
- *Adenoma*
  Total elimination of pathologic tissue.

Location of argon plasma coagulation applications

Location	No. of patients	No. of applications
Upper gastrointestinal tract	891	1693
Lower gastrointestinal tract	419	835
Tracheobronchial system	123	223
Other[1]	21	44
Total	1454	2795

[1] Anorectal area, oral cavity, pharynx, skin, vulva, cervix.

Table 5.3.1 Location of argon plasma coagulation applications (1991–1998) – personal series

Indications for argon plasma coagulation

Indication[1]	No. of patients	No. of applications
Tumor	772	1632
Acute hemorrhage	360	499
Stent (ingrowth, overgrowth)	160	436
Adenoma (or remnant)	215	279
Barrett's esophagus	55	103
Watermelon stomach	16	24
Granulation polyps	51	54
Kaposi's sarcoma	6	8
Other[1]	40	105

[1] Some items overlap (See Box 5.3.4 and Table 5.3.1)

Table 5.3.2 Indications for argon plasma coagulation

Parameters of application

No. of patients	1454
Male/Female	799/655
Age	67 years (3 months to 97 years)
No. of applications	2795
Applications per patient	2 (1–18)
Duration of application (seconds)	60 (0.5–600)
Insufflated argon (volume, liters)	1.3 (0.2–18)
Electric power (W)	79 (10–100)
Electric energy (kJ)	6.8 (0.08–30)

Table 5.3.3 Parameters of application (median range in parentheses)

- *Angiodysplastic lesions*
  Hemostasis and elimination of lesions with no recurrence of hemorrhage and elimination of chronic anemia.
- *Dysplasia and early cancer*
  Eradication of pathologic tissue according to endosonographic and histologic criteria.

Hemostasis and angiodysplastic lesions
Relationship between lesion and method

Hemostasis requires effective treatment with a minimum of damage to neighboring tissue, i.e. a controllable, uniformly shallow penetration depth, especially in the treatment of wide-area lesions.

A reliably reproducible restriction of penetration depth to less than 1 mm is necessary in the case of *angiodysplastic malformations*, especially in the right colon. In addition, contact-free application is desirable to prevent adhesion and sticking.

Hemostasis (see Table 5.3.4 and Box 5.3.2)

Hemostasis represents one of the most important problems in endoscopy. Many different endoscopic methods have been developed during the last 20 years, resulting in a revolution in the therapy of gastrointestinal bleeding. No single method, however, covers all kinds and sources of hemorrhage.

Bleeding sources in 360 patients and 499 episodes of treatment	
Tumors*	
Esophagus	71
Stomach	32
Duodenum/small bowel	11
Colon	17
Rectum	28
Other (pharyngeal, tracheobronchial)	14
Post-interventional	
Dilation/bougienage	22
Incision	4
Snare (polypectomy, mucosal resection)	26
Post-biopsy	12
Other	9
Other	
Angiodysplasia/watermelon stomach	65
Post-irradiation lesion	28
Mallory–Weiss lesion	13
Dieulafoy's ulcer	14
Other	17

* The majority of tumors were malignant ulcerating tumors with active bleeding. About one-third of the cases referred from other hospitals had previous unsuccessful attempts for hemostasis.

Table 5.3.4 Bleeding sources in 360 patients and 499 episodes of treatment

---

BOX 5.3.2 Hemostasis for acute and chronic bleeding: 360 patients/499 applications

- Tumor bleeding (80% malignant tumors) (Figs 5.3.8 and 5.3.9)
- Post-interventional (Fig. 5.3.10) (after polypectomy, mucosectomy, incision, bougienage, stenting, and stent removal)
- Angiodysplastic lesions
  - angiodysplasia sensu stricture
  - watermelon stomach (Fig. 5.3.11)
  - post-irradiation lesion
  - Dieulafoy's ulcer (Fig. 5.3.10)
  - others
- Coagulation disorders
- Others

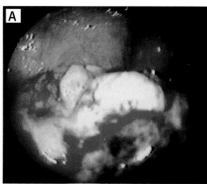
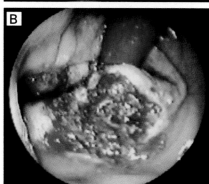
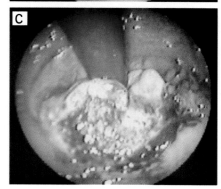

Fig. 5.3.8 Bleeding low rectal cancer, before (**A**), during (**B**) and after ~ 2 kJ argon plasma coagulation (**C**). Endoscope retroverted.

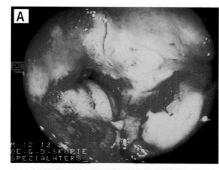
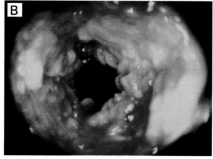

Fig. 5.3.9 Obstructing and bleeding esophageal cancer before (**A**) and 2 days after argon plasma coagulation (**B**). Hemostasis, lumen patent, secondary necrosis develops.

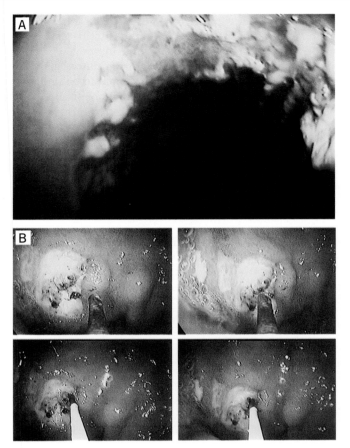

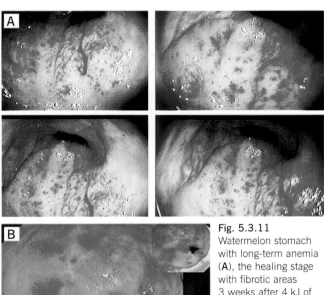

Fig. 5.3.11
Watermelon stomach with long-term anemia (**A**), the healing stage with fibrotic areas 3 weeks after 4 kJ of argon plasma coagulation (**B**) immediately after application of another 2.5 kJ argon plasma coagulation (**C**). Symptoms and bleeding signs completely abated.

Fig. 5.3.10 Hemostasis with argon plasma coagulation in a bleeding laceration after dilation (**A**) and in a Dieulafoy's ulcer (**B**).

APC is especially useful for diffuse bleeding arising from a large area, bleeding owing to coagulation disorders or tumor bleeding.[8]

In contrast to alternative methods, the plasma jet is easily kept in view during treatment and can be used in brush-like strokes over the tissue, so that wide-area, diffuse hemorrhages are easily treated. However, the underlying principles also permit the treatment of isolated, punctate hemorrhages (e.g. from ulcers). Our experience in this area is still limited, since we still regard the injection method (or clipping if possible) as the therapy of choice in treatment of spurting arterial bleeding. However, we were successful in permanently controlling eight spurting hemorrhages in Dieulafoy's ulcer with APC alone.

APC has proven to be extremely effective and safe in treating angiodysplastic lesions, especially in watermelon stomach and post-irradiation lesions, where wide areas are affected.

A special problem arises in endoscopic hemostasis in the tracheobronchial system because of the anatomical restrictions and the production of smoke and vapor. These treatments are technically very demanding, but APC seems to be an ideal therapeutic modality.[16]

Special points of application

Treatment of angiodysplastic lesions in the colon is difficult (especially in the right colon) because of weak ignition of the plasma beam owing to the need to have a relatively low power setting of the generator. Until improved generators and probes are available, we have found it helpful in these cases to perform submucosal injection with saline solution before APC treatment. By means of the submucosal saline-depot, it is possible to increase the power setting of the generator to improve the ignition, without an increased danger of perforation.

Results (see Table 5.3.5)

The data from all interventions were evaluated with regard to the previously defined goals of treatment, namely, to achieve successful therapy in 2 or 3 treatment sessions. In all but 1 patient, hemostasis was achieved (99.7%). In this case, as a result of forceful arterial bleeding from a gastric cancer, APC was tried after unsuccessful application of clips and injection. Bleeding was reduced but not stopped, so the patient underwent an emergency operation.

In 6 patients out of 360, recurrent bleeding was observed (1.7%); 2 of these patients required surgery, and in 4 others additional hemostatic endoscopic procedures (additional injection therapy, or more than three APC sessions) were successful. Intestinal emphysema occurred in

Results of 2795 procedures in 1454 patients	
Follow-up	25 (1–75) months
Failure rate	n=27 (1.9%)
Complications	
• Perforation	7/2795 (0.25%)
– immediately	1/2795
– delayed	6/2795
• Submucosal emphysema	10/2795 (0.35%)
• Mortality	1/1454 (0.07%)

Table 5.3.5 Results of 2795 procedures in 1454 patients

10 of 499 sessions (2%) during the treatment of bleeding caused by inadvertent activation of the APC probe during contact between the tip of the probe and the wall; this was asymptomatic in all instances and was no longer endoscopically visible during examinations 4 to 12 hours later. In these cases, no further complications or side effects were found during a mean follow-up period of 25 (1–75) months.

Besides the patients mentioned above, there were no severe side effects, complications, or mortality in the group of hemostatic procedures.

Approximately 30% of the patients noticed mild intermittent pain owing to heat sensation and/or over-distention. In no case was it necessary to interrupt the intervention.

The results in our series with primary hemostasis in 99.3%, recurrence of bleeding in 1.7%, a zero mortality and a complication rate <1% are promising (Table 5.3.5).

Results in the literature As with every new method, results may be dependent upon the physician's experience. First results from other clinical groups using APC, confirm our own findings (Table 5.3.6). All authors describe a successful hemostasis in all (or nearly all) patients with APC therapy. Complication rates for hemostatic indications are very low in all reports where APC is considered to be safe and cost-effective.[28,30] We found only one report about one case of bleeding caused by APC treatment.[55] In our own series we have never seen such a complication.

A number of studies have examined the treatment of telangiectasis (e.g. watermelon stomach and radiation proctitis) with APC with varying results. The majority of authors have confirmed our own results for this indication.[10,27,53] However, a few have described difficulties in

---

BOX 5.3.3 Devitalization of pathologic tissue: 1094 patients/2296 applications

Palliative
- Debulking and recanalization (Fig. 5.3.9 and 5.3.12)
- Tumor ingrowth and overgrowth in stents
- Giant adenoma

Curative
- Adenoma and remnants after snare resection
- Benign tumors
- Barrett's esophagus ± dysplasia (Fig. 5.3.13)
- Early cancer (Fig. 5.3.14) (pharynx, esophagus, stomach, colorectum, tracheobronchial system)
- Polyposis, familial adenomatous polyposis, papillomatosis (Fig. 5.3.15)
- Kaposi's sarcoma, carcinoid, granulation polyps

Results from other authors for hemostasis with argon plasma coagulation							
Authors	APC		Reports of bleeding		Bleeding lesion	Application parameters	Results	Complications
	Pat.	App.	Pat.	App.				
Johanns W, et al (1996)[33]	66	100	50	?	Angiodysplasia Polypectomy Erosions Ulcer, Tumor	40–155 W 2–7 L flow/min 1–10 seconds time of application	Successful hemostasis in 49/50 patients	Bowel wall emphysema (1 patient) Pneumomediastinum (2 patients)
Klump B, et al (1997)[60]	Case report				Angiodysplasia CREST Syndrome	?	1/1	None
Wahab PJ, et al (1997)[7]	125	400	20	60	Angiodysplasia Polypectomy	?	Successful hemostasis in all patients	1 perforation (colon)
Focke G, et al (1996)[61]	Case report		1		Angiodysplasia	?	Successful hemostasis	None
Cipolletta L, et al (1998)[13,28]	21	?	21	?	Peptic ulcer	60 ± 19 seconds time of activation to achieve hemostasis	Permanent hemostasis in 19/21 patients (90.5%)	1 perforation of treated ulcer

App. = no. of applications; Pat. = no. of patients.

Table 5.3.6 Results from other authors for hemostasis with argon plasma coagulation

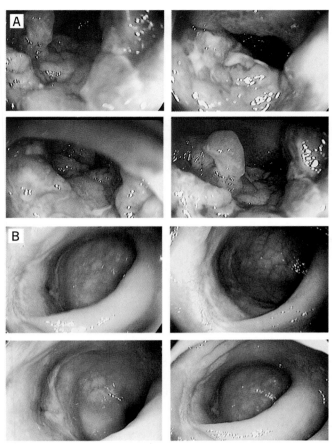

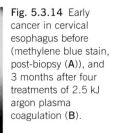

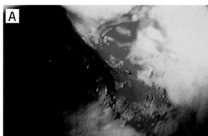

Fig. 5.3.14 Early cancer in cervical esophagus before (methylene blue stain, post-biopsy (**A**)), and 3 months after four treatments of 2.5 kJ argon plasma coagulation (**B**).

Fig. 5.3.12 Colonic cancer before (**A**) and after three sessions with argon plasma coagulation (in total 15 kJ) (**B**). Only small residual tumor remains at the site of India ink tattoo.

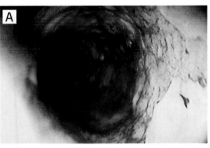

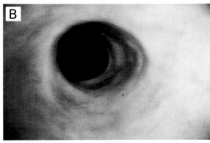

Fig. 5.3.13 Barrett's esophagus before (methylene blue stain (**A**)) and 6 weeks after argon plasma coagulation (**B**) (2 sessions of 2 kJ, side fire probe).

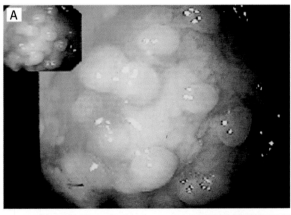

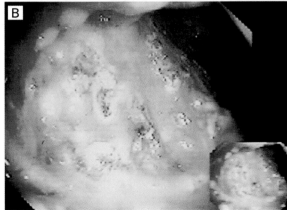

Fig. 5.3.15 FAP syndrome before (**A**) and immediately after (**B**) argon plasma coagulation (50 × 0.01 kJ in ultrashort single bursts).

handling the probe and in igniting the argon beam, especially under water, in comparison to the gold probe.[18] This problem may result from a low output setting below 50 W, which inhibits the ignition of the argon beam. In these cases, it can be helpful to perform submucosal injec-tion following which the power output of the HF-generator can be increased without danger of perforation. Especially in comparison to the treatment of teleangiec-tasis with the Nd:YAG laser,[29] APC seems to be more safe and effective.

Another reported problem is the development of strictures after APC treatment of radiation proctitis.[27] In our opinion, the formation of these strictures after radiation is more likely a result of the radiation itself, than of APC. No strictures were observed in our experience with more than 30 patients.

An ideal indication for APC seems to be the watermelon stomach which is treated safely, quickly, and effectively.[8,11,61]

Palliative tumor treatment
Relationship between lesion and method
Tumor treatment, especially in the case of bulky tumors, requires effective devitalization and a precisely defined depth of thermal effect for reducing tumor mass while simultaneously avoiding hemorrhages or perforations.

Various other problems must also be avoided: char formation and the development of smoke are very disadvantageous in endoscopy. The thermal effects should be independent of the color and form of the surface. Precise targeting requires that the coagulation process is visible through the endoscope.

The relatively high effectiveness of APC in palliative tumor treatment is *not* due to a vaporization effect – in contrast to the Nd:YAG laser – but rather to a highly effective desiccation and the ensuing, pronounced shrinkage of tumor volume (Fig. 5.3.5). Areas of thermal necrosis in the vicinity of the lumen peel away after 3 to 5 days like an onion skin, resulting in further predictable reduction of the tumor. Should it be necessary to eliminate a large tumor mass immediately, this can be performed in the first step via snare ablation or by means of vaporization with the Nd:YAG laser. Thereafter, APC is useful for further hemostasis and 'fine work' at the wall level, especially in the critical areas of the duodenum or colon. This method is suitable as a low-risk alternative to conventional laser vaporization of larger tumors.[46,47,50]

Results
Our clinical results, with a perforation rate of less than 0.5% (7 perforations in 1632 applications for tumor treatment) can be compared to the rate of complications, including perforation, with use of the Nd:YAG laser which range from 5 to 15%.[12,20,21,24,25]

Tumor treatment requires great care and an accurate eye during application as well as rigorous observation of the guidelines (see Checklist, p. 98).

Our data were evaluated according to the previously defined goals of therapy. These goals were attained with a mean of 2.0 sessions in nearly all patients (Table 5.3.3). In 11 patients (Table 5.3.5) the results were inadequate (inadequate tumor reduction).

In 7 of the 1632 sessions (0.5%) for palliative tumor treatment, visible wall damage or clinical signs of perforation were found either during intervention or later. Pneumoperitoneum developed during the procedure in 1 patient with peritoneal carcinomatosis with a lethal outcome. Delayed perforation (i.e. after 16, 24 and 48 hours) required subsequent laparotomy in 6 patients with no procedure-related mortality.

In comparison to other reports in the literature,[57,58] we consider the method as safe. However, the risk of perforation will never be totally excluded.

Curative tumor treatment
Suitability for the indication
Treatment of remnants after polypectomy,[48,49] debulking of large masses of adenoma or tumor, and precise superficial treatment of dysplastic epithelium or early cancer are possible using different techniques and parameters for the devitalization of pathologic tissues. APC is especially useful in the latter indication.[17,31] Preliminary results show that permanent ablation of pathologic epithelium is possible in a high percentage of cases, provided that application is performed carefully and precisely (Fig. 5.3.3) It must be stressed, however, that especially in Barrett's esophagus recurrences or residual Barrett's epithelium under the regenerated squamous epithelium have been observed.[19,20,32,35–40]

New applicator-tip technology and generator characteristics should lead to further improvements (Fig. 5.3.2) with better continuity and more precise devitalization. Nevertheless, such critical treatment should only be performed in highly experienced centers as experimental studies, following a strict study protocol with prospective controls and a meticulous endosonographic and histologic work-up.[16,19,20,22,23,31–43] Without retrospective studies, the observation of residual or newly developed islets of dysplastic epithelium below the re-established squamous epithelium[19,32,33,35–40] cannot be attributed to either the method itself or to an insufficient application technique.

At the present time, APC cannot be recommended as a standard procedure for these indications (nor can laser-treatment or photodynamic therapy). This is because the HF-generators and APC probes for flexible endoscopy have not yet been sufficiently optimized for this indication to ensure a homogeneous effect over the whole surface area of this very critical zone. Moreover, the application techniques (circumferential?, longitudinal?) and the application time, both of which are responsible for the local effects, may differ considerably. Either may influence the accuracy of devitalization. Since new HF-generators and optimized probes are in the initial stage of clinical trials, the use of APC for the treatment of Barrett's esophagus with or without dysplasia has to be further investigated.

Results
Many studies have recently been published dealing with the treatment of predysplastic and dysplastic changes in Barrett's esophagus and early carcinoma.[19,32,33,35–39,52] As in our own experience, these studies demonstrate that, in principle, ablation of such (pre)-malignant lesions is possible.[17,31] However, it must be stressed that the follow-up period in all these studies was too short to show whether the method as it is currently used is safe and effective.

6.
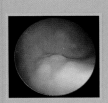
PHOTODYNAMIC THERAPY IN GASTROENTEROLOGY

L. GOSSNER

C. ELL

INTRODUCTION

Medical interest in the cytotoxic responses of photosensitizers has been recorded as early as 1900.[1-4] However, the synthesis of hematoporphyrin derivative (HPD), a complex porphyrin mixture with reported tumor-localizing properties, by Schwartz in the 1950s,[5] can be regarded as the beginning of modern photodynamic therapy (PDT). In the following years, experimental and clinical pilot studies evaluated hematoporphyrin and HPD for both diagnosis and therapy of malignant tumors.[6-11] Pioneering efforts in clinical HPD photosensitization were made by Dougherty,[12,13] whose reports of a series of cancer patients treated by this technique appeared from 1978 onwards. In 1980, Hayata et al[14] were the first to apply fiberoptic endoscopic laser irradiation to treat early endobronchial lung cancer with PDT. Reports concerning intraluminal photodynamic therapy in the gastrointestinal tract first began to appear as early as the late 1980s,[15,16] and were greeted with both enthusiasm and controversy. In that respect, little has changed even today. It is not that PDT has been outdated, nor that its technical potential has been fully exhausted, nor that it has been superseded by more modern procedures. On the contrary, PDT in the gastrointestinal tract is still going through a dynamic process of development, improvement, and standardization.

PHOTODYNAMIC PRINCIPLES: PHOTOCHEMISTRY AND PHOTOBIOLOGY

PDT represents a minimally invasive, organ-preserving therapeutic modality. PDT involves three separate components: light, oxygen, and a photosensitizing drug. PDT exploits the physical phenomenon that light is able to activate photosensitizing compounds that are incorporated by tissue. Light energy which is absorbed by the photosensitizer is transferred in several steps primarily to oxygen within the tissue and leads to tumor destruction through oxidation processes. Laser light with a specific wavelength lying within the absorption band of the applied photosensitizer is delivered endoscopically, through a flexible fiber, into the gastrointestinal tract. The laser light is not directly involved in tissue destruction but is employed as surface irradiation of the HPD-sensitized dysplastic or malignant tissue.

Type I and type II photochemistry

Upon absorption of a photon of light, a photosensitizer will be excited to a high energy singlet state. A singlet photosensitizer can decay back to its ground state, resulting in fluorescence emission (Fig. 6.1). Alternatively, it can form a triplet sensitizer, a slightly lower energy state, and longer lived excited species, by electron spin conversion in the process called intersystem crossover.[17] The fluorescent properties of photosensitizers have been useful for visualizing tumor localization and delineation of a malignant lesion. The most efficient photosensitizers for PDT have a high triplet quantum yield and long triplet half-life. A triplet photosensitizer can undergo either type I (electron or hydrogen atom transfer) or type II (energy transfer) photochemical reactions. Transfer of energy to

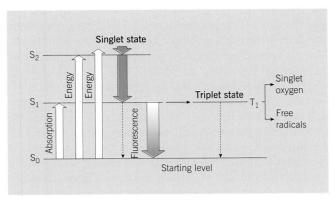

Fig. 6.1 The mechanism of photodynamic action.

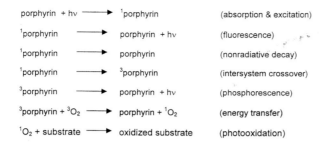

$$^1\text{porphyrin} \longrightarrow \text{porphyrin} + h\nu \qquad \text{(fluorescence)}$$

hv = light quantum
^{1}porphyrin = singlet excited state porphyrin
^{3}porphyrin = triplet excited state porphyrin
$^3O_2$ = ground state oxygen (triplet state)
$^1O_2$ = singlet oxygen

Fig. 6.2 Type II photochemical reactions involved in the cytotoxic action of PDT.

molecular oxygen is thought to be the primary photochemical reaction in porphyrin-mediated PDT which results in the in situ generation of singlet oxygen.[18,19] The scheme for type II photochemical reactions is shown in Figure 6.2.

Type I reactions which probably occur also as porphyrins are most likely to undergo electron transfer processes with production of superoxide anions.[17] Hydroxyl radicals and superoxide anions have been detected during PDT reactions.[20]

The highly reactive oxygen products of type I and II reactions produce damage initially at the *site of photosensitizer* localization, owing to their very short lifetimes in a biological environment. Unfortunately, it has been difficult to identify the initial target sites, because photochemical reactions can produce radical auto-oxidation and further oxidative reactions, leading to varying types of intracellular damage.[17]

Tissue distribution

Considerable information on porphyrin tissue distribution has been obtained from preclinical animal studies,[21–24] in addition to pharmacokinetic studies in humans.[25–27] Following intravenous injection, dihematoporphyrin ether/ester (DHE) has a biphasic plasma clearance in humans; an initial elimination half-life of 12 to 22 hours and a second half-life of 5 to 6 days have been reported.[26,27] The maximal therapeutic ratio for DHE between tumor and normal tissue is achieved between 24 and 96 hours. Many second-generation photosensitizers, such as monoaspartyl chlorin e6 (NPe6) and benzoporphyrin derivative (BPD), have a more rapid rate of clearance.[28,29] Consequently, photosensitizer injection and laser irradiation can be performed on the same day. DHE and NPe6 are primarily excreted unchanged through the feces.[22,28,29] Animal studies show that organ retention of these drugs is most persistent in reticuloendothelial tissues, such as liver, spleen, and kidney.[21,28] Levels in these tissues exceeded tumor levels at all time intervals after drug administration. Adrenal glands, pancreas, and bladder also retain high

amounts of DHE. Skin and muscle take up relatively low levels of porphyrin and normal brain tissue has minimal uptake.[22,23]

Transport in the blood of hydrophilic photosensitizers (hematoporphyrin monomers, tetrasulphonated porphyrins, and phthalocyanines) is mostly via albumin and globulins. These sensitizers localize in the stroma of tumor, vascular, and normal tissue. More hydrophobic photosensitizers (hematoporphyrin oligomers, mono and unsubstituted phthalocyanines) are preferentially incorporated in the lipid portion of plasma lipoproteins.[30] Dyes with affinity for low density lipoproteins (LDL) are taken up by cells, at least in part, by receptor-mediated endocytosis. Lipoprotein-carried dyes are mostly deposited in endocellular loci, including mitochondria, lysosomes, and plasma membrane.[30] Otherwise, tightly aggregated dyes partly circulate as unbound pseudomicellar structures, which can enter cells by pinocytosis and localize in macrophages.[30]

EQUIPMENT

Photosensitizers

Most clinical PDT experience comes from using the porphyrin variants, HPD and DHE. The active components of HPD were identified by Dougherty et al[30] to be DHE. The commercial preparation of DHE, known as porfimer sodium, or Photofrin, contains <20% of inactive monomers and >80% of the active porphyrin dimers and oligomers. However, Photofrin remains a complex mixture with inherent variability, and it has the further limitation of weak light absorption at wavelengths above 600 nm. In addition, Photofrin has the side effect of causing prolonged cutaneous photosensitivity. These properties provided incentives for developing new photosensitizers.

The next generation of clinical photosensitizers ideally will provide rapid plasma and tissue clearance, enhanced tumor to normal tissue selectivity, comparable photoactivation efficiency, and superior light absorption of visible red and near infrared light. Theoretically, these developments will lead to more selective treatment of malignant lesions than is currently possible with Photofrin-mediated PDT.

A growing number of second-generation photosensitizers are being synthesized which can be activated at wavelengths of light >650 nm. A non-exhaustive list of classes of compounds includes porphyrin and chlorin derivatives, purpurins, benzoporphyrins, phthalocyanines, and naphthalocyanines. Chlorins are derived either by modifying a porphyrin or from chlorophyll as the starting material for synthesis.[31,32] Second-generation photosensitizers undergoing clinical investigation include BPD, NPe6, meta-tetra(hydroxyphenyl)chlorin (mTHPC), tin etiopurpurin (SnET2), and 5-aminolevulinic acid (ALA). Light at 650 nm is used to activate mTHPC, 660–665 nm is used to activate the chlorin and purpurin derivatives NPe6 and SnET2, and 690 nm light to activate BPD.

More recently, photosensitizers with a specific chemical composition such as ALA have improved this situation.

ALA is a precursor of protoporphyrin IX (PPIX) in hemobiosynthesis, and endogenous PPIX produces effective photosensitization when activated by 630–635 nm light. PPIX, which is excessively formed through the exogenous supply of ALA in the framework of intracellular hemobiosynthesis via several enzymatic reaction steps, represents a potent photosensitizer exhibiting a high mucosa specificity and selectivity.[33] A longer-lasting phototoxicity of the skin is not expected in view of the rapid endogenous synthesis and decomposition of porphyrin.[33] This assumption is corroborated by initial clinical applications in gastrointestinal tumors carried out by our research group and by other authors as well.[34-36]

Foscan (mTHPC) was synthesized and evaluated in preclinical studies by Berenbaum.[37] In rodent models, mTHPC was found to have both improved tumor tissue selectivity and antitumor activity compared to DHE. It has an absorption peak at 652 nm. Initial clinical results with mTHPC were published by Ris et al[38] following treatment of patients with chest malignancies. Initially, two patients received an injection of mTHPC and 652 nm laser irradiation. Parameters were 0.3 mg/kg mTHPC, 48 hours prior to light exposure of 10 J/cm². Biopsy samples showed tumor infarction 10 mm deep owing to tumor vessel thrombosis, and the concentration of chlorin sensitizer was 14 times higher in mesothelioma tumor tissue than normal tissues. A further eight patients with diffuse malignant mesothelioma received intra-operative PDT to the thoracic cavity following unilateral pleurectomy and lobectomy.[38] The patients developed recurrences, although mostly in untreated areas. The conclusions drawn from the intra-operative treatments were that the procedure is feasible, but significant morbidity can occur when large areas are treated. Optimization of the therapeutic ratio is essential in order to prevent extensive damage to normal tissues during mTHPC-PDT.

Light sources

PDT instrumentation includes light sources, light delivery systems, and devices for light and drug dosimetry. For many clinical applications using current photosensitizers, the light 'dose' (energy fluence) required is substantial (e.g. typically 100 J/cm²). Thus, for reasonable treatment times, delivered powers of a few watts in a narrow wavelength are required. Until recently, the availability and clinical performance of light sources created significant impediments to the wider clinical use of PDT, but this situation is rapidly improving.

Initially, sources which could be found in the laboratory such as the argon-pumped dye laser or metal vapour laser (with or without a dye module to provide wavelength tunability) were used, despite their high costs and poor reliability. A few investigators also used filtered lamps (e.g. modified slide projectors) for superficial treatments. In the next phase, argon dye and metal vapour (-dye) lasers were 're-engineered' to be more suited to clinical use, but their main limitations remained.

In the last decade, the KTP laser superseded the argon laser as the means to pump the dye laser (Fig. 6.3). The

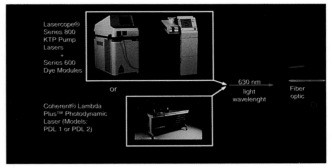

Fig. 6.3 The KTP/YAG XP 800 Laser (Laserscope Inc., San Jose, CA, USA). A solid state laser with an output power of 7.5 W and an Argonion-pumped dye laser with 3 W (Coherent Lamda Plus, Coherent Inc., Germany).

KTP (a solid-state, 1064 nm Nd:YAG laser, frequency doubled to give 532 nm light) is also clinically used as a surgical laser, so that many systems are in clinical use and simply require the addition of a dye module, retaining the flexibility of wavelength tunability. The KTP-dye laser is reliable and transportable, has a built-in calibration system, but is still expensive.

Alternatively, compact diode lasers now have adequate power (typically, a few Watts) and have many applications. Each operates at a single wavelength, which must be selected to match the photosensitizer. Recently, diodes around 630 nm for Photofrin and ALA have become available (Fig. 6.4). Diode lasers may also be pulsed with varying pulse width and shape, but very high peak powers are not attained. They can be 'stacked' to increase the total power and/or provide more than one wavelength. All laser sources can be coupled to small-diameter single optical fibers for endoscopic or interstitial treatments.

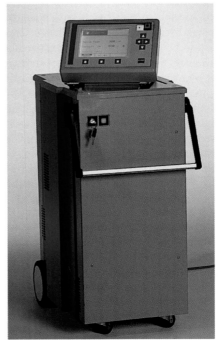

Fig. 6.4 The Visulas 630 (Carl Zeiss Jena GmbH, Germany). A new diode laser with a fixed wavelength of 630 nm and a power output of 1.8 W.

There are two main non-laser technologies: high-brightness lamps, filtered for specific wavelength bands, can be configured either for direct-beam illumination or for fiberoptic bundle/lightguide delivery. These sources have reasonable power and the wavelength can be changed easily. There is a trade-off between the wavelength spread and the delivered power. Novel lamp designs have also been introduced recently, e.g. high-pressure lithium-iodide or neon large-arc lamps provide very high continuous power levels in a relatively narrow wavelength band at low cost.

With the increasing variety of sources, an important issue is their 'photobiological equivalence'. A given delivered fluence from broadband sources may be significantly less effective than that from a laser with monochromatic light at the peak of the photosensitizer activation spectrum (measured in vivo) and it is important to determine the output characteristics in detail.

In the gastrointestinal tract, the need for fiberoptic light delivery devices which can be coupled to the source remains a critical issue so far and, therefore, the laser as a light source for PDT is unchallenged.

The ideal PDT light source should generate enough light of the correct wavelength(s) in a convenient and flexible way for delivery to the tissue, while being reliable, affordable, and 'clinic friendly'. At present, the KTP-pumped dye laser is the most powerful and reliable system, but if the diode laser can acquire more power, it will turn out to be a good, inexpensive alternative for clinical use.

Light application systems

Next to the development of suitable light sources and photosensitizers, the achievement of long-range homogeneous light application in hollow organs such as the esophagus presents a particularly difficult problem. Initially, flat-cut fibers were placed in the esophagus to carry out irradiation,[39,40] but cylindrical diffusers have now become established as standard light delivery systems for PDT in the esophagus.[41,42] However, cylindrical diffusers with a length of 2–3 cm that are placed freely in the esophagus fail to provide a defined, homogeneous field of irradiation, owing to inaccuracies in concentric positioning within the lumen. According to reports by other research workers and our own experience with this free light-delivery technique,[43,44] islands of cylindrical epithelium may partly persist when, e.g. Barrett's esophagus with severe dysplasia or early carcinoma is being treated, and incomplete destruction of the dysplastic or malignant mucosa may occur.

Inflatable clear balloons that accommodate a central linear diffuser seem to be the best option for PDT in the esophagus and cardia. They can be used to achieve homogeneous and circumferential irradiation in a single session, over a length of up to 7 cm (Figs 6.5 and 6.6).[36,42–44] Adequate centering and stable placement of the cylindrical light diffusers in the esophagus lumen is achieved by use of these balloons. Displacements of the applicator systems caused by both esophageal motility and cardial and respiratory movement disturb the irradiation procedure. To achieve better fixation and positioning, the group of van den Bergh[45] introduced an applicator system into the

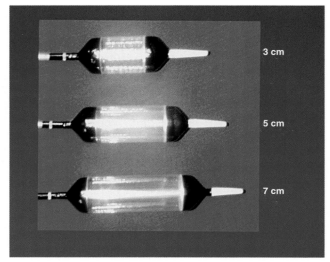

Fig. 6.5 A centering balloon system used over a guidewire with three different applicator lengths (Wilson–Cook, USA).

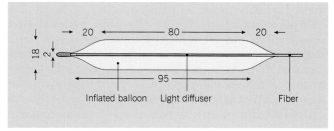

Fig. 6.6A Schematic diagram of a centering balloon system for PDT in the esophagus.

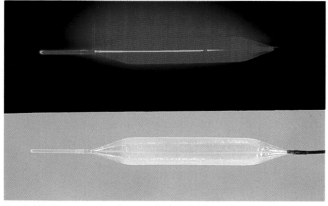

Fig. 6.6B The corresponding applicator which can be placed through the endoscope under direct vision (TTC PDT Balloon, Wilson–Cook, Germany) for surface illumination.

esophagus which is based on a Savary–Guilliard bougie with improved positioning and homogeneous irradiation characteristics. This applicator is placed, under general anesthesia, usually with rigid endoscopes. The distal esophagus and the cardia therefore cannot be directly visualized.

An inflatable balloon applicator has been developed by the research group of Overholt et al[46] which is able to minimize dislocation of the applicator by a slight distention of the esophagus wall. Unfortunately, this balloon cannot be delivered through the instrumentation channel of an endoscope, but has to be introduced into the esophagus via a guidewire under fluoroscopic control, or, under endoscopic control, through an additionally introduced pediatric endoscope (Fig. 6.6). Ablation of longer mucosal domains requires repeated segmental retraction of the balloon, which in turn automatically entails the risk of over- or underexposure to the incident laser light as a result of overlapping or insufficiently continuous illumination fields. In the event of an excessive accumulation of the photosensitizer in the tissue, an overdose of laser light could be a causative factor for the formation of strictures following PDT, as reported in over 50% of treated cases.[42]

Another centering balloon system with a diameter range of 18 to 20 mm can be directly implemented through the endoscope's instrumentation channel and also allows – apart from ensuring fixation in the esophagus – the flattening of the folds at the cardia or of folding in the tubular esophagus arising from peristalsis.[43]

Shadowing phenomena owing to a hill-and-valley effect caused by mucosal folds[24] and leading to inhomogeneous application of light can thus be reduced by the centering balloon with distention. Overdistention of the esophageal wall must be avoided during the flattening of mucosal folds, since excessive stretching can induce an alteration of microvascularization in the esophageal mucosa as tumor microvasculature plays a decisive role in photodynamic tissue destruction.[47,48] Balloon diameters of 18 and 20 mm preclude any such overdistention of the esophagus (Fig. 6.6).

In the stomach, laser irradiation is carried out in an antegrade fashion using a microlens with a 10 mm focus. If necessary, several fields can be irradiated[49] (Fig. 6.7). In order to reduce the inconsistencies in the distance to the target tissue, paintbrush hairs are useful as a gauge of distance.

The power output delivered by the applicators must be measured with a calibrated integrating sphere (e.g. Labsphere Inc. or Coherent Inc., USA) just before and after the PDT. A special integrated fiber detector can help to detect variations of the laser output power, defects of the fiber, or changes in the medium surrounding the fiber tip during laser treatment.[50] The appropriate wavelength relative to the photosensitizer must be cross-checked using a hand monochromator (e.g. PTR Optics Corp., Waldham, USA).

Dosimetry

One of the most critical and complex issues in PDT is dosimetry. Tumor characteristics such as size and the individual tumor geometry, vascularity, and photosensitizer uptake determine the depth of necrosis as much as the delivery of the optimal energy density (fluence) of light and the correct wavelength. Applying a given light intensity to the surface of an organ does not imply that we know precisely what happens to the light intensity as the photons penetrate the underlying tissue. The amount of light penetrating to a certain depth will depend on parameters related to both the tissue optics, i.e. its *absorption* and *scattering* coefficients, and the way we apply light to the surface: the light distributor itself, its position, and the wavelength. Thus, different models for light penetration into tissue have been developed and the optical properties of different tissues have been described.[51–53] When a homogeneous wide beam of light hits tissue, the radiation (space irradiance) is greater on the very surface of the tissue than that in the precalibrated beam itself owing to backscattering; the effect decreases exponentially with the depth of the tissue.

The space irradiance is defined as the fluence falling from all directions on an infinitesimally small sphere divided by the cross-sectional area of the sphere. Molecules are randomly oriented in biological tissues, and a 'mean molecule' does not mind from which direction the light comes, even though each individual molecule certainly minds. The penetration depth, defined as the depth at which the space irradiance is reduced from 1 to 1/e, is dependent on the scattering coefficient, as well as on the absorption coefficient of the tissue and the applied wavelength. The latter is notably large up to about 600 nm in tissues with increased vascularity. Tumors and tissues containing large amounts of melanin also have a large absorption coefficient. Penetration curves for different tissues in vivo have been measured.[54]

In clinical practice, the power density (irradiance) emitted by the selected diffuser must be measured before and after each treatment session. Power densities >400 mW/cm should be avoided so that thermal effects are not generated. The treatment time is determined by the desired energy density (fluence) divided by the intended power density (irradiance) and the diffuser length:

Treatment time (s) =

$$\frac{\text{desired energy density (fluence) in J/cm}^2}{\text{measured power density (irradiance) in W/cm}^2}$$

Using a centering balloon, the surface area of the lesion and respectively of the balloon has to be calculated:

$$\{A = r^2 \times \pi\}.$$

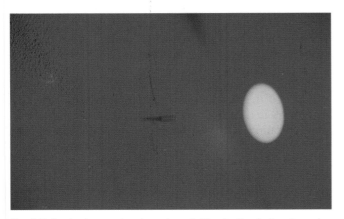

Fig. 6.7 A microlens system for antegrade illumination in the stomach (Laserscope Inc., San Jose, CA, USA).

An energy density of 150–300 J/cm^2 should be selected for ALA and Photofrin, while it can be reduced to 20 J/cm^2 for Foscan at 652 nm and power densities of 100 mW/cm^2.

INDICATIONS

Curative treatment

Early cancers of the upper gastrointestinal tract seem to be most suitable for this minimally invasive treatment modality with curative intention according to the unique effect of PDT on tumor tissue, although this application is based at present on only a limited clinical experience.

Reasoning in favor of local therapy of high-grade dysplasia (HGD) or early cancer (EC) of the upper gastrointestinal tract is borrowed from the experience with surgical therapy and local endoscopic treatment of early stomach cancer. Taking the generally accepted definition of low-risk early gastric cancer as a basis (mucosal type, 20 mm in diameter or less, type I–IIa, b, 10 mm in diameter or less for type IIc G1–G2), the 5-year survival rate after endoscopic local therapy is between 80% and 95%, hence in the same order as after surgical resection of the stomach.[55–58] Another argument for endoscopic local therapy can be derived from the low probability of lymph node metastases in low-risk early gastric cancer: the available surgical series indicate the prevalence of lymph node metastases in early gastric cancer to be between 0% and 4%, a risk that does not exceed the usual perioperative mortality of early stomach cancer.[58,59] Similar data are available for early esophageal cancer. The rate of lymph node metastasis in Barrett's EC of the mucosal type is approximately 0%, and in squamous cell carcinoma of the mucosal type about 1%.[60,61] In contrast to this low rate of lymph node metastases stands the unavoidably high rate of surgery-related mortality for esophagectomy (3–5% in HGD or EC) and high morbidity (18–48%).[60,61] Regarding the natural progression of HGD, it appears that, by careful surveillance, the transformation of HGD to carcinoma might be discovered in time, thus justifying continual interval surveillance.[62] On the other hand, there are often synchronous malignant foci in an established Barrett's HGD and the probability of progression to a carcinoma over the next few years appears to be more than 30%.[63] Because of the possibility of surveillance failure, endoscopic therapy would appear to be an acceptable therapeutic goal provided it is low risk and efficient.

The most frequent indication for PDT in the future may be Barrett's esophagus. Barrett's esophagus without dysplasia can be ablated by PDT, but it is of special value in treating low-grade and high-grade dysplasia and mucosal cancer. Similarly, PDT can be used for esophageal squamous cell HGD and EC. Another indication is early gastric cancer strictly confined to the mucosa. However, use of PDT in any situation must be evaluated in comparison with various methods of thermoablation and endoscopic mucosal resection (EMR). PDT is not likely to be useful for the treatment of villous rectal adenomas and flat (pap-illary) adenomas because of the alternative treatment procedures that are available.[64]

Palliative treatment

Stenotic tumors of the esophagus, stomach, colon and bile ducts are potential indications for palliative use of PDT. Owing to the limited penetration depth of the red light, large, bulky, malignant tumor stenoses may not respond to PDT therapy although an American multicenter study showed that fewer treatment sessions were required with PDT in comparison with Nd:YAG laser therapy, and that there was also a lower perforation rate.[65] In view of the high cost of PDT and the short life expectancy in this group of patients the treatment may not be economical.[65] The American health authorities (FDA) have just approved PDT exclusively for palliation, but in reality there are simpler thermodestruction modalities, and in the esophagus, self-expanding metal endoprostheses are available for simpler, less expensive, and more effective palliation.[66]

PDT can be used for stent overgrowth and ingrowth. The non-thermal nature of PDT obviates concerns about damage of the metal filaments or plastic covering of stents as observed with the Nd:YAG laser, monopolar electrocoagulation or APC.[67] Although APC damaged the plastic stent cover only at high energy levels >90 W, the thermal effect can be conducted along the metal filaments and lead to distant tissue vaporization.[67] As more and more covered stents are placed, tumor ingrowth will become a lesser problem in the future resulting in a decline in the use of PDT for this special indication.

With regard to the palliative treatment of malignant stenoses of the bile ducts using PDT, only one paper and one abstract have been published, with small numbers of cases. These reports require confirmation in larger studies – preferably multicenter prospective and comparative ones – before this therapeutic application can be recommended. There appear to be potential problems with the light application and dosimetry, which are carried out without direct endoscopic control. The high porphyrin concentration in the liver may be a factor in the therapeutic schema.[68,69] The different indications for curative and palliative treatment are summarized in Table 6.1.

CONTRAINDICATIONS

Patients with any of the following conditions are excluded from photodynamic treatment: patients with known porphyria or known hypersensitivity to porphyrins. Patients with white blood cell (WBC) count <2.5 × 10^9/L (minimum of 0.5 × 10^9/L granulocytes), platelet count <50 × 10^9/L or prothrombin time (PT) expressed as the international normalized ratio (INR) >1.5 times the upper limit of normal. Other contraindications are: known or suspected impaired renal and/or hepatic function with serum creatinine >1.5 the upper limit of normal, total serum bilirubin >1.5 times the upper limit of normal, aspartate-aminotransferase (AST), alanine-aminotransferase (ALT), or alkaline phosphatase of hepatic origin >2.5 times of the upper limit of normal. In addition, PDT should not be used in patients

Indications for the use of photodynamic therapy in the gastrointestinal tract
Curative treatment Barrett's esophagus with or without low grade dysplasia Barrett's esophagus with high-grade dysplasia/early cancer Squamous cell high-grade dysplasia/early cancer of the esophagus Early gastric cancer
Palliative treatment Advanced, obstructing cancer of the esophagus Advanced, obstructing cancer of the stomach Advanced, obstructing cancer of the colon/rectum Advanced, obstructing cancer of the bile duct Stent ingrowth/overgrowth

Table 6.1 Indications for the use of photodynamic therapy in the gastrointestinal tract

who are unable or unwilling to stay out of daylight for an interval according to the photosensitizer used or who cannot tolerate analgesia or endoscopy.

PATIENT PREPARATION

Intravenous sedation with midazolam and/or pethidine is often used since the patient may be required to remain motionless for a period of time in excess of 30 minutes. General anesthesia, however, is not necessary for the procedure. After ingestion or injection of the photosensitizer, the patient should remain in slightly darkened rooms. After oral application of aminolevulinic acid (ALA), vital signs should be monitored every 2 hours.

PRETHERAPEUTIC STAGING

The prerequisite for local endoscopic therapy of early malignancies of the upper gastrointestinal tract is precise clinical staging prior to treatment. Exact localization and measurement of the tumor size, its endoscopic classification according to the generally accepted classification of the Japanese Endoscopic Society, and the histopathological grading should be determined prior to local endoscopic treatment. The tumor should be of mucosal type without infiltration into the submucosa.

For initial staging, the following tests should be carried out: esophagogastroduodenoscopy, endosonography with the conventional radial-scanner as well as mini-endosonography with a 20 MHz-probe using a two-channel-video endoscope. Additionally, abdominal ultrasound and spiral computed tomography of thorax and abdomen should be completed.

Biopsies must be taken from all visible lesions and for Barrett's cases, four quadrant biopsies mapping the entire segment have to be taken. HGD should be evaluated by two pathologists aware of previous findings with regard to the grade of dysplasia, malignant degeneration, and grade of differentiation (G1–G3).

If lesions are very discrete or macroscopically not detectable, additional staging procedures that may be help-

ful are: chromo-endoscopy with methylene blue, indigo-carmine and Lugol's solution as well as fluorescence endoscopy with ALA-induced fluorescence (photodynamic diagnosis, PDD) to achieve a better and more accurate localization of the malignant process.[70,71] Discolorations, unstained or heterogeneously stained lesions, and fluorescent areas are then easily targeted for additional biopsies (Figs 6.8–6.14).

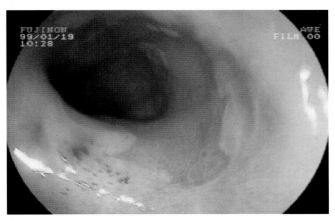

Fig. 6.8 Macroscopically invisible HGD in Barrett's esophagus.

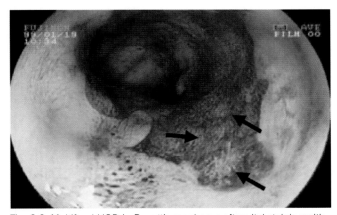

Fig. 6.9 Multifocal HGD in Barrett's esophagus after vital staining with methylene blue. Unstained areas or areas with stain heterogeneity had biopsy-proven HGD.

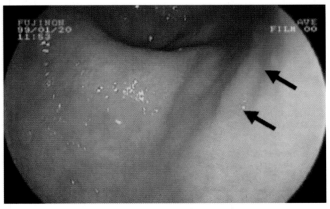

Fig. 6.10 Barrett's esophagus with early mucosal cancer type IIa.

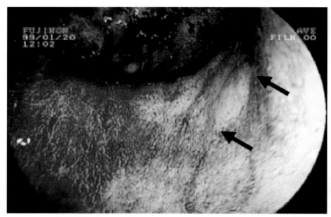

Fig. 6.11 Barrett's esophagus with early mucosal cancer type IIa after methylene blue staining.

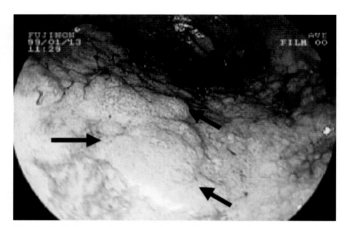

Fig. 6.12 Defining a type IIa early Barrett's cancer after indigocarmine application.

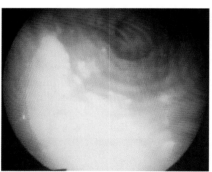

Fig. 6.13 Short Barrett with macroscopically invisible HGD.

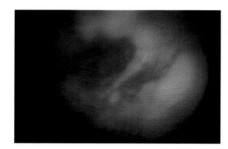

Fig. 6.14 Typical red porphyrin fluorescence after photodynamic diagnosis (PDD) with ALA.

The option of high-resolution ultrasound permits discrimination between mucosal (uT1m) and submucosal cancer (uT1sm) in up to 95% of the cases (Fig. 6.15).[72–74]

PROCEDURE

The exact procedure varies with each photosensitizer given: if the photosensitizer is applied intravenously, extravasation must be avoided. Photofrin is injected in a dosage of 2 mg/kg 48 hours prior to irradiation, whereas with 5-ALA, PDT is conducted 4 to 6 hours after oral ingestion of the sensitizer. For Foscan (mTHPC), the retention time is approximately 96 hours (Fig. 6.16). Endoscopy is performed with topical anesthesia and intravenous sedation. Before starting treatment, the patient's skin is covered to avoid inadvertent exposure. A dye laser delivers light of the specific wavelength according to the applied sensitizer (630–652 nm) through a quartz fiber (200–600 μm) inserted down the biopsy channel of a flexible endoscope. Special

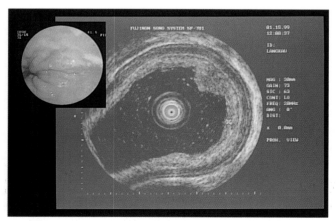

Fig. 6.15 Early Barrett's cancer type I strictly confined to mucosa determined by high-resolution endoscopic ultrasound (20 MHz).

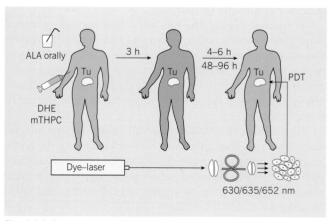

Fig. 6.16 The procedure of clinical photodynamic therapy: sensitizer application, retention times, and different wavelengths.

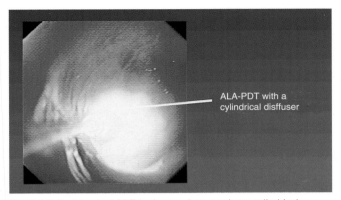

ALA-PDT with a
cylindrical disffuser

Fig. 6.17 Endoluminal PDT in the esophagus using a cylindrical diffuser: as a result of its high intensity the applied red light appears white using a videoendoscope.

applicators specific for the targeted lesion are connected to the fiber for endoluminal PDT. In the esophagus fiber, optical diffusers and centering balloons are used (Fig. 6.17). In the stomach, en face irradiation is done with a microlens system.

RESULTS

Barrett's esophagus

The number of patients having the diagnosis of Barrett's esophagus has rapidly increased in recent years.[75] The increasing rate of diagnosis is undoubtedly related to a broad awareness of the metaplasia–dysplasia–carcinoma sequence. It is useful to distinguish between Barrett's metaplasia with or without dysplasia on the one hand, and severe dysplasia or early Barrett's carcinoma on the other. The precondition for any local endoscopic therapy for Barrett's esophagus with or without mild dysplasia should be that the method used allows complete ablation of the undesirable epithelium and complete restitution of the

squamous epithelium. There have only been a few reports on PDT of Barrett's esophagus. The first publication in 1993 by Laukka et al[76] described 14 patients with Barrett's mucosa, and most of the other studies are case reports and lack a larger number of patients. The existing data do not yet allow firm conclusions to be made (Table 6.2). However, the data on the use of PDT in the treatment of Barrett's epithelium seem to be slightly better in comparison with those treated by thermoablation.[36,43,44,77–82] In addition, ablation using the spot effects of thermal procedures – whether laser coagulation or thermocoagulation – produces tissue injury of varying depths, and not infrequently causes tissue destruction that also affects the submucosa. By contrast, PDT with ALA is limited in its destructive effects to the mucosa, as has been adequately shown in animal experiments.[83] In this respect, ALA-PDT has a clear advantage over thermocoagulation procedures. In addition, suitable light applicators can be used to achieve homogeneous and circumferential irradiation in a single session, over a length of up to 7 cm.[36,43,44]

Summing up, it appears that ALA-PDT treatment of Barrett's mucosa with or without low-grade dysplasia has significant advantages over alternative procedures, although adequate clinical proof is still lacking. In addition, it has not been adequately shown whether ablation techniques in general do in fact provide the promised carcinoma prevention.

Although the case numbers concerned are smaller, the question of how to deal with Barrett's epithelium and severe dysplasia or early carcinoma is of much greater clinical relevance. The gold standard is undoubtedly still radical surgery, with partial gastric and esophageal resection. However, careful study of the published surgical data shows that there are good arguments for local therapy. When prior staging examinations are carried out, the histological and endoscopic ultrasound findings can be used to identify with a high degree of certainty those patients able to benefit from local curative treatment. The available

Results of local endoscopic therapy of Barrett's esophagus						
Author	Year	Method	Barrett without HGD/EC	Barrett with HGD/EC	Patients (n)	Complete remission (n)
Berenson[77]	1993	Argon laser	+	–	10	9
Sampliner[79]	1996	Electrocoagulation	+	–	10	9
Barham[80]	1997	KTP laser	+	–	11	6
Gossner[81]	1999	KTP laser	–(4)	+(6)	10	10
Laethem	1998	APC	31		31	25
Laukka[82]	1995	PDT	+	–	5	5
Overholt	1996	PDT	–	+	24	20
Gossner[35]	1995	PDT-ALA	–	+	5	4
Barr[34]	1996	PDT-ALA	–	+	5	5
Gossner[36]	1998	PDT-ALA	–	+	32	27
Overholt[40]	1999	PDT	65	35	100	87
Ell[88]	2000	EMR	–	+	64	53/54

ALA = 5-aminolevulinic acid; APC = argon plasma coagulation; EC = early cancer; EMR = endoscopic mucosal resection; HGD = high-grade dysplasia; KTP = potassium-titanyl-phosphate; PDT = photodynamic therapy.

Table 6.2 Results of local endoscopic therapy of Barrett's esophagus (published as full papers in western journals)

surgical and anatomical data indicate that the risk of lymph-node metastasis in HGD and in early mucosal carcinoma is almost zero. In any case, it is lower than the mortality rates with surgery. In choosing a local treatment procedure, endoscopic mucosal resection is undoubtedly the first option. However, EMR can only be used if the malignant lesions can be clearly localized. In addition, the resection cannot exceed a certain size, and when multifocal EMR is not a suitable form of primary therapy. Whenever a biopsy has demonstrated malignancy or severe dysplasia but precise macroscopic identification of the site is unclear, or in cases of long Barrett's segments with advanced histological changes, PDT should be considered as a primary form of local treatment.

With the original form of PDT, strictures occurred in up to half of the patients, but all of these were easy to treat endoscopically.[42] In Overholt's group, this somewhat more aggressive form of treatment was followed by complete remission in all patients, which was confirmed during a follow-up period of up to 5 years.[44] Using the 'milder' form of ALA-PDT, which is limited to selective destruction of the mucosa, Barr's group and our own group achieved long-term complete remission in all cases of HGD. However, long-term remission was seen in only around 75% of patients who already had early carcinoma[36] (Figs 6.18–6.20). When the mucosa is thicker than 2 mm, i.e. when mucosal changes are already visible macroscopically, ALA-PDT is very likely to be inadequate, and a more

intensive form of PDT should be used instead, e.g. with mTHPC as the photosensitizer.

Squamous Esophagus (HGD/early cancer)

With regard to the use of PDT in the treatment of squamous cell HGD and early carcinoma in the esophagus, only a few reports have appeared so far, at least from the Western hemisphere.[84–86] When ALA is used as photosensitizer, all patients with HGD experienced complete remission, but only about half of those with confirmed early carcinoma had remissions after ALA-PDT (Figs 6.21–6.23). No significant side effects of the treatment were observed.[84] By contrast, the results of the Lausanne group with mTHPC were better with regard to complete remission, although this was at the expense of increased morbidity.[41,85]

Summing up, PDT may become a significant factor in the treatment of high-risk patients with early squamous cell carcinoma, since in comparison with radical surgery or aggressive chemoradiotherapy, PDT represents a form of minimally invasive treatment.

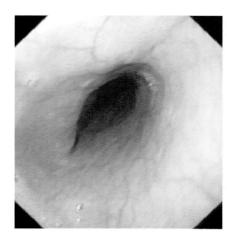

Fig. 6.20 Re-epithelialization with normal squamous mucosa after 1 year with proton pump inhibitors, biopsy-proven-free of dysplasia.

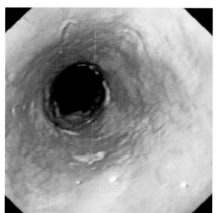

Fig. 6.18 HGD in a long segment of Barrett's esophagus prior to PDT.

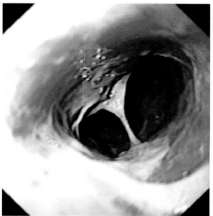

Fig. 6.19 Fibrinoid necrosis 24 hours after ALA-PDT.

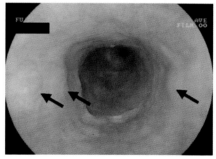

Fig. 6.21 Multifocal early squamous cell cancer in the upper third of the esophagus.

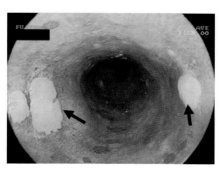

Fig. 6.22 Multifocal early squamous cell cancer after staining with Lugol's solution.

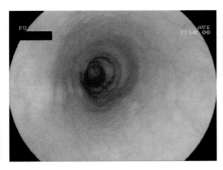

Fig. 6.23 Complete remission after PDT with ALA: macroscopically and microscopically tumor-free 18 months after PDT.

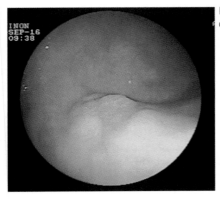

Fig. 6.24 Early gastric cancer type I.

Stomach

In Western countries, early gastric carcinoma is being diagnosed endoscopically with increasing frequency, and patients are receiving local curative treatment. When prior staging examinations are carried out, the histological and endoscopic ultrasound findings can be used to identify with a high degree of certainty those patients able to benefit from local curative treatment. When endoscopic mucosal resection is not possible or is not successful, PDT represents a good alternative.[49,87] In addition to the porphyrins, the photosensitizer mTHPC has proved its value (Figs 6.24 and 6.25). With no significant morbidity, and no cases of perforation, complete tumor destruction was achieved in about 80% of patients treated. In tumors that cannot be clearly located endoscopically ('biopsy carcinoma'), PDT of larger areas using mTHPC – or even with ALA, which is much less problematic in clinical practice – is a procedure that is fundamentally different from thermoablation

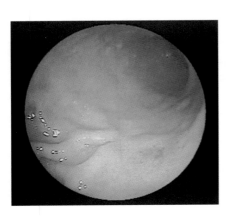

Fig. 6.25 Scar after PDT with mTHPC at the former tumor site, biopsy-proven-tumor-free 12 months after PDT.

methods and mucosectomy, and should therefore be considered as a potential treatment option.

COMPLICATIONS

The method-related mortality is almost zero and morbidity associated with severe complications appears to be very low. Of course, there is one predictable potential complication after PDT: all patients accumulate photosensitizer in their skin that, when exposed to light of sufficient energy, is activated inducing phototoxic side effects. The degree of skin reaction can vary from mild erythema to severe erythema and edema, to blistering and desquamation in the sense of third-degree burns. All skin reactions, however, can be prevented by appropriate precautions regarding clothing and adequate education of the patient.

Newer photosensitizers have shorter periods of cutaneous photosensitivity, especially ALA. A longer-lasting phototoxicity of the skin is not to be expected because of the rapid endogenous generation and decay of PPIX.[33–35] The fast decay kinetics of ALA, as proven by our fluorescence measurements in the blood plasma and the skin of patients with Barrett's esophagus,[36] has a clinically beneficial effect: it is not necessary to protect patients from sunlight for longer than 36 hours. Phototoxic side effects such as reddening of the skin or sunburn did not occur in the above mentioned study.

The most common symptomatic complications after PDT are transient retrosternal or epigastric pain in almost one-quarter of the patients. In addition, ductocircumferential, full thickness necrosis hematoporphyrin-derivative-mediated PDT is responsible for fibrotic stricturing that requires dilation. The relatively non-specific accumulation of this photosensitizer in all layers of the esophageal wall induces stenosis in the treated segments of the esophagus in up to 50% of cases.[42] In contrast, the high mucosal specificity and the preferential accumulation of ALA in dysplastic and malignant tissue[34,36,84] ensure selective, superficial destruction without damaging deeper layers of the wall, such as the muscularis propria. Thus, the formation of strictures by scarring and shrinkage of the esophageal wall can be avoided. It must be pointed out, however, that the superficiality of ALA therapy negatively affects the efficacy of destruction of malignant tissue.

Transient nausea and a mild increase of transaminases are documented after ALA-PDT in about 47% and 65% of patients, respectively.[36] The observed increase of transaminases falls to normal levels after 1 week and does not recur throughout long-term follow-up. Because of these minor and fully reversible side effects, PDT with ALA must be rated as the currently least invasive method for managing dysplasia and mucosal carcinoma in the upper gastrointestinal tract.

AFTERCARE

Patients should remain in slightly darkened rooms after PDT. Complete blood cell counts and blood chemistry studies (after ALA application) should be performed for 3 to 4 days after treatment. All patients who have received a photosensitizer will be photosensitive for various periods (ALA: 36 hours; Photofrin: 6 weeks to 3 months; Foscan: 4 to 8 weeks) and must observe precautions to avoid exposure of eyes and skin to direct sunlight or bright indoor light (from operating room or examination lamps). Ocular discomfort, commonly described as sensitivity to sun, is another side effect. When outdoors, patients should wear dark sunglasses. Exposure of the largest possible area of skin to ambient indoor light is, however, beneficial because the remaining drug will be inactivated gradually and safely through a photobleaching reaction. Because of the latter property, patients should not stay in a completely darkened room, but should be encouraged to expose their skin to ambient indoor light. Ultraviolet sunscreens are of no value in protecting against photosensitivity reactions because photoactivation is caused by visible light.

As a result of PDT treatment, patients may complain of nausea (especially after ALA) and substernal or epigastric pain because of inflammatory and necrotic responses within the area of treatment. Such pain may require the short-term prescription of opiate analgesics.

CONCLUSION

After decades of basic and clinical research, PDT is on the verge of becoming an established cancer treatment modality. Its role will be defined when current clinical trials are completed and access to therapy is generally available. The first product license approvals have been granted (outside the USA) for treatment of endobronchial, esophageal, and superficial bladder cancer. Certainly, some malignant diseases are more suitable than others to PDT treatment, e.g. Barrett's esophagus, with regard to whether complete eradication is possible. Very bulky lesions and tumors inaccessible to light irradiation remain untreatable by PDT. The efficacy and safety of PDT determined by clinical trials are not the only factors determining its future success, which will be measured in comparison with other therapies available. Development of resistance to PDT has not been noted in any patient, which is a distinct advantage over some other anticancer modalities. In addition, long-term morbidity is not a factor which would restrict the number of repeat treatments.

PDT is now being evaluated for wider applications, outside malignant solid tumor treatment, especially for precancerous conditions like Barrett's esophagus with or without dysplasia. Development of second-generation photosensitizers is continuing, and dyes have already been designed with improved photodynamic properties. The side effect of skin photosensitivity can be diminished by dyes that absorb only in the far-red spectrum. Non-systemic administration of drugs or targeting techniques may also eliminate photosensitivity side effects. Classes of sensitizers that have been evaluated photochemically and biologically include porphyrins, chlorins, purpurins, and phthalocyanines. The most promising examples are being developed commercially. The technical development of user-friendly light sources, whether laser or non-laser, is as important to the clinical applications of PDT as the choice of photosensitizer. Diode lasers generating sufficient power in the far-red visible region are only now becoming available for clinical use. In addition, specialized laser delivery systems continue to be developed, with respect to the specific site being treated. The methodology and technology used for photodynamic treatment of patients can be expected to change significantly for many years ahead as PDT continue to evolve.

In conclusion, PDT is a fascinating concept, which will continue to occupy many research groups around the world in the coming years. Although a widespread clinical application for the method has not yet emerged, there are good prospects that PDT will be able to establish itself at major gastroenterological centers as an endoscopic procedure with few or no side effects in the treatment of Barrett's esophagus (severe dysplasia and early carcinoma) and, in selected cases, for the treatment of early squamous cell carcinoma and early gastric carcinoma.

CHECKLIST OF PRACTICE POINTS

1. Gastrointestinal carcinomas can successfully be destroyed by PDT.
2. For selected precancerous conditions and early cancer, PDT can be applied with curative intent.
3. Precise pretherapeutic staging, including high-resolution ultrasound, in order to discriminate between mucosal and submucosal cancer is mandatory.
4. Advanced cancer of the gastrointestinal tract can be treated palliatively and local control of tumor growth seems to be possible. For debulking of large tumor masses, the Nd:YAG laser is the most reasonable option while stenting of malignant stenoses offers long-standing relief of dysphagia.
5. The photosensitizer should be chosen according to its photodynamic efficacy: ALA for dysplasia or tumors <2 mm; Photofrin or Foscan for thicker lesions requiring a more powerful sensitizer.
6. Power densities >400 mW should not be used in order to avoid thermal effects.
7. In the esophagus, centering balloon systems should be used for a homogeneous light application.
8. Patients must be warned to avoid exposure to direct sunlight or other strong light sources after photosensitization for a certain period of time according to the photosensitizer.

REFERENCES

1. Raab O. Über die Wirkung fluoreszierender Stoffe auf Infusorien. Z Biol 1900; 39:524–546.

2. Hausmaun W. The sensitising action of hematoporphyrin. Biochem Z 1911; 30:176.

3. Blum HF. Photodynamic action and diseases caused by light. New York: Rhinehholt; 1941 (reprinted, Haftier, 1964).

4. Figge FHJ, Weiland GS, Manganiello LOJ. Cancer detection and therapy. Affinity of neoplastic, embryonic and traumatized tissues for porphyrins and metalloporphyrins. Proc Soc Exp Biol Med 1948; 68:181–188.

5. Dougherty TJ, Henderson BW, Schwartz S, et al. Historical perspective. In: Henderson BW, Dougherty TJ, eds. Photodynamic therapy, basic principles and clinical applications. New York: Dekker; 1992: 1–18.

6. Lipson RL, Baldes EJ. The photodynamic properties of a particular hematoporphyrin derivative. Arch Dermatol 1960; 82:517–520.

7. Lipson RL, Baldes EJ, Olsen AM. Hematoporphyrin derivative: a new aid for endoscopic detection of malignant disease. J Thorac Cardiovasc Surg 1961; 42:623–629.

8. Gregorie HB, Horger EO, Ward JL. Hematoporphyrin derivative fluorescence in malignant neoplasms. Ann Surg 1968; 167:820–828.

9. Diamond L, Graneih SG, McDonah AF, et al. Photodynamic therapy of malignant tumors. Lancet 1972; ii:1175–1177.

10. Dougherty TJ, Grindey G, Fiel R. Photoradiation therapy II: cure of animal tumors with hematoporphyrin and light. J Natl Cancer Inst 1974; 55:115–121.

11. Kelly JF, Snell ME, Berenbaum MC. Photodynamic destruction of human bladder carcinoma. Br J Cancer 1975; 31:237–244.

12. Dougherty TJ, Kaufman JE, Goldfarb A, et al. Photoradiation therapy for the treatment of malignant tumors. Cancer Res 1978; 38:2628–2635.

13. Dougherty TJ. Photodynamic therapy (PDT) of malignant tumors. CRC Crit Rev Biochem 1984; 2:83–116.

14. Hayata Y, Kato H, Konaka C, et al. Hematoporphyrin derivative and laser photoradiation in the treatment of lung cancer. Chest 1982; 81:269–277.

15. McCaugham JS, Nims TA, Guy JT, et al. Photodynamic therapy for oesophageal tumours. Arch Surg 1989; 124:74–80.

16. Thomas RJ, Abbott K, Bhatal PS, et al. High-dose photoradiation of oesophageal cancers. Ann Surg 1987; 206:193–199.

17. Foote CS. Mechanisms of photooxidation. In: Doiron DR, Gomer CJ, eds. Porphyrin localization and treatment of tumors. New York: Liss; 1984: 3–18.

18. Weishaupt K, Gomer CJ, Dougherty T. Identification of singlet oxygen as the cytotoxic agent in photoinactivation of a murine tumor. Cancer Res 1976; 36:2326–2329.

19. Buettner GR, Need MJ. Hydrogen peroxide and hydroxyl free radical production by hematoporphyrin derivative, ascorbate and light. Cancer Lett 1985; 25:297–304.

20. Gomer CJ, Dougherty TJ. Determination of 3H and 14C hematoporphyrin derivative distribution in malignant and normal tissue. Cancer Res 1979; 39:146–151.

21. Bellnier DA, Ho YK, Pandey RK, et al. Distribution and elimination of Photofrin II in mice. Photochem Photobiol 1989; 50:221–228.

22. Pantelides ML, Moore JV, Blacklock NJ. A comparison of serum kinetics and tissue distribution of Photofrin II following intravenous and intraperitoneal injection in the mouse. Photochem Photobiol 1989; 49:67–70.

23. Quastel MR, Richter AM, Levy JG. Tumor scanning with indium-111 dihaematoporphyrin ether. Br J Cancer 1990; 62:885–890.

24. Gilson P, Ash P, Driver I, et al. Therapeutic ratio of photodynamic therapy in the treatment of superficial tumours of skin and subcutaneous tissues in man. Br J Cancer 1988; 58:665–667.

25. Brown SB, Vernon DL. The quantitative determination of porphyrins in tissues and body fluids: applications in studies of photodynaniic therapy. In: Kessel D, ed. Photodynamic therapy of neoplastic disease, vol 1. Boca Raton: CRC Press; 1990:109–208.

26. Kessel D, Nseyo U, Schulz V, et al. Pharmacokinetics of Photofrin II distribution in man. SPIE Optical Methods for Tumor Treatment and Early Diagnosis 1991; 1426:180–187.

27. Gomer CJ, Ferrario A. Tissue distribution and photosensitizing properties of mono-L-aspartyl chlorin e6 in a mouse tumor model. Cancer Res 1990; 50:3985–3990.

28. Richter AM, Jain AK, Canaan AJ, et al. Photosensitizing efficiency of two regioisomers of the benzoporphyrin derivative monoacid ring A. Biochem Pharmacol 1992; 43:2349–2358.

29. Jori G. In vivo transport and pharmacokinetic behavior of tumor photosensitizers. Ciba Foundation Symposium 1989; 146:78–86.

30. Dougherty TJ, Potter WR, Weishaupt KR. The structure of the active component of hematoporphyrin derivative. In: Doiron DR, Gomer CJ, eds. Porphyrin localization and treatment of tumors. New York: Liss; 1984:301–314.

31. Spikes JD. Chlorins as photosensitizers in bioiogy and medicine. J Photochem Photobiol B:Biol 1990; 6:259–274.

32. Pandey RK, Belinier DA, Smith KM, et al. Chlorin and porphyrin derivatives as potential photosensitizers in photodynamic therapy. Photochem Photobiol 1991; 53:65–72.

33. Loh CS, MacRobert AJ, Bedwell J, et al. Oral versus intravenous administration of 5-aminolaevulinic acid for photodynamic therapy. Br J Cancer 1993; 68:41–51.

34. Barr H, Shepherd NA, Dix A, et al. Eradication of high-grade dysplasia in columnar-lined (Barrett's) oesophagus by photodynamic therapy with endogenously generated protoporphyrin IX. Lancet 1996; 348:584–585.

35. Gossner L, Sroka R, Hahn EG, et al. Photodynamic therapy: successful destruction of gastrointestinal cancer after oral administration of aminolaevulinic acid. Gastrointest Endosc 1995; 41:55–58.

36. Gossner L, Stolte M, Sroka R, et al. Photodynamic ablation of high-grade dysplasia and early cancer in Barrett's esophagus by means of 5-aminolevulinic acid. Gastroenterology 1998; 114:448–455.

37. Berenbaum MC. Comparison of hematoporphyrin derivatives and new photosensitizers. In: Photosensitizing compounds: their chemistry, biology and clinical use. New York: Wiley. Ciba Foundation Symposium; 1989:33.

38. Ris HB, Altermatt HJ, Inderbitzl R. Photodynamic therapy with chlorins for diffuse malignant mesothelioma: initial clinical results. Br J Cancer 1991; 64:1116–1120.

39. McCaughan JS Jr, Nims TA, Guy JT, et al. Photodynamic therapy for esophageal tumors. Arch Surg 1989; 124:74–80.

40. Patrice T, Foultier MT, Yactayo S, et al. Endoscopic photodynamic therapy with hematoporphyrin derivative for primary treatment of gastrointestinal neoplasms in inoperable patients. Dig Dis Sci 1990; 35:545–552.

41. Sibille A, Lambert R, Souquet J, et al. Long-term survival after photodynamic therapy for esophageal cancer. Gastroenterology 1995; 108:337–344.

42. Overholt BF, Panjehpour M. Photodynamic therapy for Barrett's esophagus: clinical update. Am J Gastroenterol 1996; 91:1719–1723.

43. Gossner L, Sroka R, Ell C. A new long-range through-the-scope balloon applicator for photodynamic therapy in the esophagus and cardia. Endoscopy 1999; 31:370–376.

44. Overholt BF, Panjehpour M, Haydek JM. Photodynamic therapy for Barrett's esophagus: follow-up in 100 patients. Gastrointest Endosc 1999; 49:1–7.

45. Van den Bergh H. On the evolution of some light delivery systems for photodynamic therapy. Endoscopy 1998; 30:392–407.

46. Overholt BF, DeNovo RC, Panjehpour M, et al. A centering balloon for photodynamic therapy of esophageal cancer tested in a canine model. Gastrointest Endosc 1993; 39:782–787.

47. Ernst H, Sassy T, Sroka R, et al. Ultrastructural changes in normal rat colon induced by photodynamic therapy. Las Med Sci 1994; 9:17–25.

48. Wiemann TJ, Mang TS, Fingar H, et al. Effects of photodynamic therapy on blood flow in normal and tumor vessels. Surgery 1988; 104:512–517.

49. Ell C, Gossner L, May A, et al. Photodynamic ablation of early cancers of the stomach by means of mTHPC and laser irradiation. Gut 1998; 43:345–349.

50. Sroka R, Beyer W, Krug M, et al. Laser light application and light monitoring for photodynamic therapy in hollow organs. Laser Med Sci 1993; 8:63–68.

51. Svaasand LO. Optical dosimetry for direct and interstitial photoradiation therapy of malignant tumor. In: Doiron DR, Gomer CJ, eds. Porphyrin localization and treatment of tumors. New York: Liss; 1984:91–114.

52. Wilson BC, Jeeves WP, Lowe DM. In vivo and postmortem measurements of the attenuation spectra of light in mammalian tissues. Photochem Photobiol 1985; 42:153–162.

53. Cheong WF, Prahl SA, Welch AJ. A review of the optical properties of biological tissues. IEEE J Quantum Elect 1990; 26:2166–2185.

54. Iani V, Moan J, Ma LW. Measurements of light penetration into human tissues in vivo. SPIE 1996; 2625:378–383.

55. Inoue H, Endo M, Takeshita K, et al. Endoscopic resection of early esophageal cancer. Surg Endosc 1991; 5:59–62.

56. Torii A, Sakai M, Kajiyama T, et al. Endoscopic aspiration mucosectomy as curative endoscopic surgery: analysis of 24 cases of early gastric cancer. Gastrointest Endosc 1995; 42:475–479.

57. Takekoshi T, Baba Y, Ota H, et al. Endoscopic resection of early gastric carcinoma: results of a retrospective analysis of 308 cases. Endoscopy 1994; 26:352–358.

58. Winkler M, Jentschura D, Winter J, et al. Results of surgical therapy of early stomach cancer. Zentralbl-Chir 1995; 120:795–799.

59. Baba H, Maehara Y, Okuyama T, et al. Lymph node metastasis and macroscopic features in early gastric cancer. Gastroenterol Hepatol 1994; 41:380–383.

60. Hölscher AH, Bollschweiler E, Schröder W, et al. Prognostic differences between early squamous cell and adenocarcinoma of the esophagus. Dis Esophagus 1997; 10:179–184.

61. Heitmiller RF, Redmond M, Hamilton SR. Barrett's esophagus with high-grade dysplasia: an indication for prophylactic esophagectomy. Ann Surg 1996; 224:66–71.

62. Levine DS, Haggitt RC, Blount PL, et al. An endoscopic biopsy protocol can differentiate high grade dysplasia from early adenocarcinoma in Barrett's esophagus. Gastroenterology 1993; 105:40–50.

63. Sampliner RE. The Practice Parameters Committee of the American College of Gastroenterology. Practice guidelines on the diagnosis, surveillance and therapy of Barrett's esophagus. Am J Gastroenterol 1998; 93:1028–1032.

64. Bown SG. Photodynamic therapy of villous adenoma of the rectosigmoid. Endoscopy 1994; 26:234–242.

65. Lightdale CJ, Heier SK, Marcon NE, et al. Photodynamic therapy with porfimer sodium versus thermal ablation therapy with Nd:YAG laser for palliation of esophageal cancer: a multicenter randomized trial. Gastrointest Endosc 1995; 42:507–512.

66. Ell C, May A. Self-expanding metal stents for the palliation of stenosing tumors of the esophagus and cardia. Endoscopy 1997; 29:392–398.

67. May A, Gossner L, Hahn EG, et al. Treatment of tumor ingrowth/overgrowth in metal stents: a comparison of the argon-beamer, KTP- and Nd:YAG laser. Gastroenterology 1996; 110:A103.

68. Ortner A, Ernst H, Lochs H. Photodynamic therapy of malignant common bile duct stenoses. Gastroenterology 1998; 114:9–14.

69. Berr E, Mössner P. Photodynamische Therapie von cholangiocellulären Carcinomen (abstract). Z Gastroenterol 1997; 35:691.

70. Canto MI. Methylene blue staining and Barrett's esophagus. Gastrointest Endosc 1999; 49:S12–16.

71. Gossner L, Sroka R, Stepp H, et al. Photodynamic diagnosis versus random biopsies for dysplasia and invisible mucosal cancer in Barrett's esophagus – a prospective randomized trial. Gastroenterology 1999; 116:G0763.

72. Akahoshi K, Chijiwa Y, Hamada S, et al. Pretreatment staging of endoscopically early gastric cancer with a 15 MHz ultrasound catheter probe. Gastrointest Endosc 1998; 48:470–476.

73. Natsugoe S, Yoshinaka H, Morinage T, et al. Ultrasonographic detection of lymph-node metastases in superficial carcinoma of the esophagus. Endoscopy 1996; 28:674–679.

74. Yanai H, Masahiro T, Karita M, et al. Diagnostic utility of 20-megahertz linear endoscopic ultrasonography in early gastric cancer. Gastrointest Endosc 1996; 44:29–33.

75. Prach AT, MacDonald TA, Hopwood DA, et al. Increasing incidence of Barrett's oesophagus: education, enthusiasm, or epidemiology? Lancet 1997; 350:933.

76. Laukka MA, Wang KK, Cameron AJ, et al. The use of photodynamic therapy in the treatment of Barrett's esophagus. Gastrointest Endosc 1993; 39:A291.

77. Berenson MM, Johnson TD, Markowitz NR, et al. Restoration of squamous mucosa after ablation of Barrett's esophageal epithelium. Gastroenterology 1993; 104:1686–1691.

78. Sampliner RE, Hixon LJ, Fennerty MB, et al. Regression of Barrett's esophagus by laser ablation in an antacid environment. Dig Dis Sci 1993; 38: 365–368.

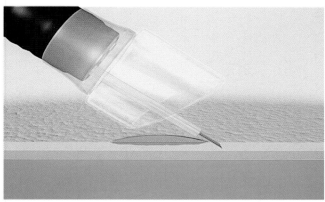

Fig. 7.4 Submucosal saline injection. Puncture the distal part of the lesion first.

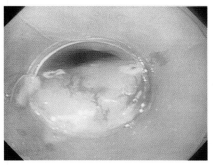

Fig. 7.5 Accurate submucosal injection causes mucosal surface lifting with a whitish color change.

4. A specially designed small-diameter snare SD-7P (1.8 mm outer diameter, Olympus Co.) is essential to the 'pre-looping' process. The snare wire is fixed along the rim of the EMRC cap. To prepare the area for looping, moderate suction is at first applied to the normal mucosa to seal the outlet of the cap (Fig. 7.6A), and then the snare wire that passes through the instrumental channel of the endoscope is opened (Fig. 7.6B). The opened snare wire is fixed along the rim of the cap, and the outer sheath of the snare placed onto the rim of the cap (Figs 7.6C and 7.7). This completes the pre-looping process of the snare wire.

5. When the endoscope approaches, the target mucosa, including the lesion, is fully sucked inside the cap (Fig. 7.8) and is strangulated by simple closing of the 'pre-looped' snare wire (Fig. 7.9). At this moment, the strangulated mucosa looks like a snared polypoid lesion.

6. The pseudopolyp of the strangulated mucosa is cut by the blend-current electrocautery (Fig. 7.10). The resected specimen can be easily taken out by keeping it inside the cap without using any grasping forceps (Fig. 7.11).

7. The smooth surface of proper muscle layer is observed at the bottom of the artificial ulcer (Fig. 7.12). In this case, a large vessel was observed at the center of the artificial ulcer, and a hemostatic clip was applied to it for prophylaxis of bleeding.[27] Bleeding is usually minor and it usually stops spontaneously by compression of the lateral wall of the transparent cap.

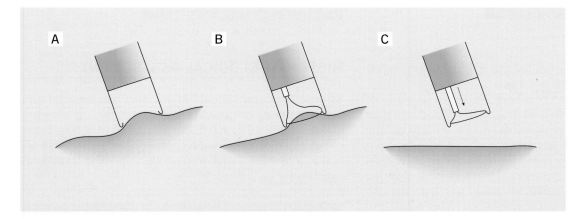

Fig. 7.6 Endoscopic mucosal resection using a cap-fitted endoscope – the 'pre-looping' procedure.
(**Left**) Suck the normal mucosa and seal the outlet of the cap.
(**Middle**) Open the snare wire and it goes along the rim of the cap.
(**Right**) 'Pre-looping' condition is created. Outer sheath of the snare is pushed up to the distal end of the cap.

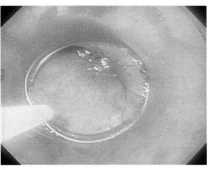

Fig. 7.7 Endoscopic view of the 'pre-looping' procedure. The snare wire is fixed along the rim of the EMRC cap. White snare sheath is pushed up to the tip of the cap.

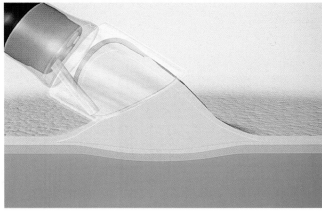

Fig. 7.8 After the 'pre-looping' procedure, the target mucosa is drawn inside the cap.

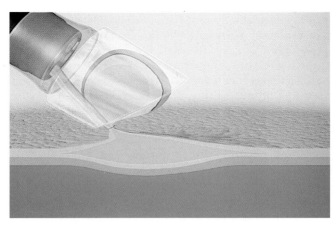

Fig. 7.9 In strangulated mucosa, injected saline acts as a cushion between mucosa and muscle layer. Large-volume injection makes the procedure safer.

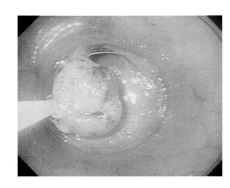

Fig. 7.10 Endoscopic view of the strangulated mucosa. Strangulated mucosa is observed as a large polyp.

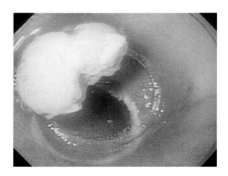

Fig. 7.11 Retrieval of the resected specimen by keeping it inside the cap.

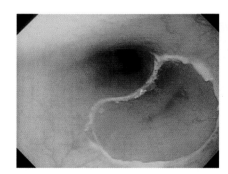

Fig. 7.12 Artificial ulcer induced by the EMRC procedure.

To confirm the complete resection of the lesion, iodine dye-spraying is useful (Fig. 7.13).

8. If additional resection is necessary to remove the residual lesion completely, all procedures including saline injection should be repeated step by step. Injected saline usually infiltrates and disappears within 5 minutes from the initial injection site and finishes up as a cushion between the mucosa and muscle layer. Repeated saline injection, therefore, becomes necessary to reduce the risk of muscle injury during the procedure. Our single experience of perforation in the esophagus happened at the second strangulation with no additional saline injection.

HISTOPATHOLOGICAL ASSESSMENT

Resected specimens should be stretched and fixed on rubber plates using fine needles, and then bathed in 10% formalin solution. The fixed specimen is divided into 2 mm columns. Histopathological analysis of semiserial sections makes it possible to reconstruct the superficial cancerous extension (Figs 7.14 and 7.15).

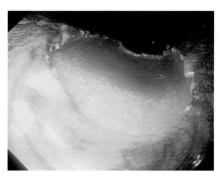

Fig. 7.13 Chromoendoscopy is effective to rule out the residual lesion.

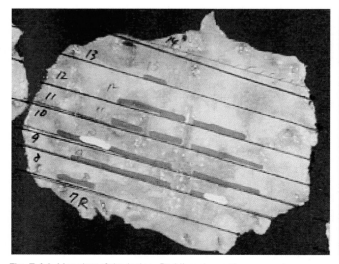

Fig. 7.14 Mapping of the lesion. Red line shows the mucosal cancer.

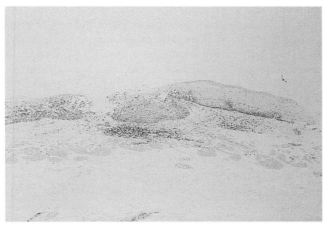

Fig. 7.15 Cancer invaded into lamina propria mucosae – m2 lesion.

HEALING PROCESS AFTER ENDOSCOPIC MUCOSAL RESECTION

Ulcer healing

Three days after EMR, the artificial ulcer is covered by a white coating (Fig. 7.16). Twelve days after EMR, the artificial ulcer is almost healed with thin but normal squamous epithelium (Fig. 7.17).

Symptoms after treatment

Almost all patients complain of mild retrosternal pain and mild throat pain which will disappear within a couple of days.

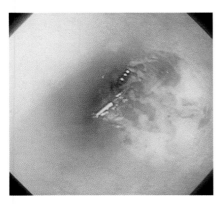

Fig. 7.16 Artificially induced ulceration 3 days after the EMRC procedure.

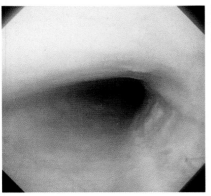

Fig. 7.17 Artificial ulcer 12 days after the EMRC procedure.

Medication

Just after EMR, a mucosal protective agent may be prescribed four times a day. Some experts administer antibiotics for a few days.

Food intake after resection

A few hours after treatment, the patient may start to drink liquids. On the following day, the patient receives soft meals. On the second day after treatment, the patient returns to a normal diet.

Quality of life after resection

In almost all cases of mucosal resection, the quality of life can be maintained adequately.[28]

RESULTS

In our institute more than 175 cases of early-stage esophageal cancer received mucosal resection.[29] Seventy-two percent of all cases were absolute indications for mucosal resection according to our criteria. The remainder were classified as poor risk for surgery or were patients who had refused surgery. In absolutely indicated cases, no local or no distant metastasis has occurred during the follow-up period. The 5-year survival rate was 95% including other causes of death. All patients who died during the 5-year follow-up period suffered from other lethal diseases such as myocardial infarction, liver cirrhosis, and stroke. As a major complication in the esophagus, one patient in our early series encountered perforation, which occurred during the second cauterization. That patient was treated conservatively with intravenous hyper-alimentation and antibiotics. Eight years later, she is well and has experienced no further side effects.

Another patient who received near total circumferential mucosal resection developed persistent stenosis that could not be controlled by repeated forceful balloon dilation and was finally treated by surgical esophagectomy. Five years after esophagectomy, the patient is fit and well. The other major complication is persistent stenosis after healing of the artificial ulcer. This disaster can happen when we perform near total circumferential resection in the esophagus and pre-pylorus, therefore, in principle, we should avoid near total or total circumferential mucosal resection.

We have carried out more than 100 EMR procedures involving the stomach and have encountered no major complications. In three cases where there were lesions on the lesser curvature of the gastric body, resected specimens included small particles of muscle component. All three cases were treated conservatively. In all cases but two, the lesions were completely resected. Two cases, however, had residual lesions after the initial EMR, that were successfully treated by laser ablation therapy. During more than a 5-year follow-up period, we encountered no local recurrence of tumor in cases of EMR in the stomach.[28]

In the duodenum, the wall is thinner than in the esophagus and stomach and therefore is considered to be more easily perforated. But the mucosal bleb induced by submucosal saline injection is prominently elevated, so that carrying out EMR in the duodenum is not technically difficult. Some results of EMR have been reported.[30,31] The author applied the EMRC procedure to three duodenal mucosal lesions, and the results were satisfactory. It is reported that the resection can also be carried out safely at the papilla of Vater.[32,33]

MECHANISM OF PERFORATION

In order to evaluate the mechanism of perforation during EMR objectively, the surgically resected specimens of human esophagus, stomach, and colon are included in this study. Those specimens were stretched on a rubber plate and then sunk into a basin filled with de-aerated water. The EMRC procedure was performed on the fixed specimens and the whole process was sonographically recorded on video tapes. In the EMR procedure without saline injection, the muscle layer beneath the surface

mucosa is also drawn into the cap together with the covering mucosa, which increases the potential risk of muscle involvement at the moment of closure of the snare loop (Fig. 7.18). Even if saline is injected, a small-volume injection is not sufficient to avoid muscle involvement. A small volume of saline only creates a small bleb (Fig. 7.19A). Full suction for a small bleb causes muscle movement into the cap, resulting in muscle strangulation with mucosa (Figs 7.19B and C, 7.20A). An extra-large-volume saline injection creates a large bleb (Fig. 7.19D). This large cushion mechanically prevents the muscle involvement during snare strangulation (Figs 7.19D and E; see also Fig. 7.9). In other words, snaring of the mucosa should not be done at the base of the lifted mucosa (Figs 7.19B and 7.20A) but should always be done at the middle part of the lifted mucosa (Fig. 7.19E; see also Fig. 7.8).

As mentioned above, the greatest risk factor that potentially causes perforation is the lack of submucosal saline injection (Fig. 7.20B). In order to prevent perforation,

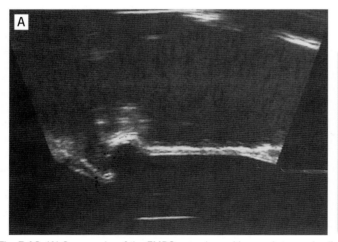
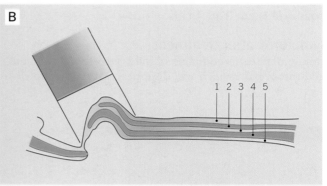

Fig. 7.18 (**A**) Sonography of the EMRC procedure with no submucosal saline injection. The fourth low echoic layer is also drawn into the cap, resulting in potential risk of muscle involvement. (**B**) 1–5: the first to fifth echoic layer.

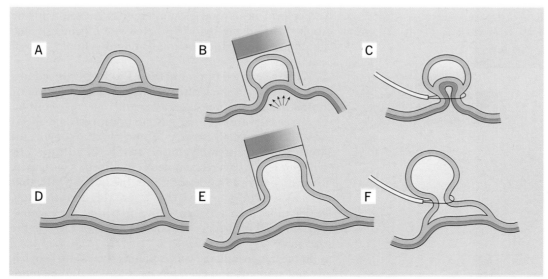

Fig. 7.19 (**A**) Small-volume injection of saline creates a small bleb. (**B**) During suction of the target mucosa, the muscle layer is also sucked into the cap. (**C**) Muscle layer involvement. (**D**) Large-volume saline injection creates a large bleb. (**E**) Even during full suction, only the top of the bleb is captured inside the cap. (**F**) Mucosa is strangulated at the middle part of the bleb, making the procedure safe.

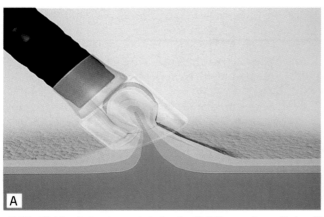
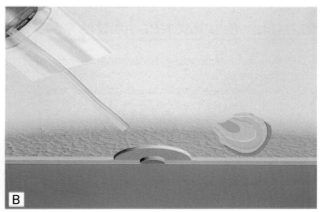

Fig. 7.20 (A) Muscle involvement during the EMRC procedure with insufficient-volume submucosal saline injection. (B) Full-thickness wall resection occurs at the center of the artificial ulcer.

large-volume saline injection is considered to be important. In the esophagus, around 20 mL saline causes more than half-circumferential mucosal dissection, keeping mucosal surface about 1 cm apart from the muscle layer (Fig. 7.21). In the stomach, EMR can be safely performed in general, because it has a relatively thick muscle layer. But at the lesser curvature in the upper and middle thirds of the stomach, special attention should be paid to avoid muscle involvement, because stretching of the mucosa is primarily limited. The use of either a small-capacity cap or reduction of the suction power makes the procedure safer. The risk of perforation is increased in the colon, because here a relatively large size cap is used for EMR and also the muscle layer in the colon is thinner than in the rest of the gastrointestinal tract.

When we perform this EMRC procedure, the most serious complication is perforation. As indicated in Figure 7.18, whole layers including muscle layer are totally sucked inside the cap when submucosal saline injection has not been used. We conclude that, a small volume of submucosal saline injection will increase the risk of perforation. In the esophagus, around 20 mL saline causes more than half-circumferential mucosal dissection from the muscle layer, which makes mucosal resection safer (Fig. 7.21). In the stomach, we have seen the same phenomenon. In conclusion, therefore, if saline is accurately injected into

the submucosa, lifting of mucosa or bulging of mucosa can always be observed in any part of gastrointestinal tract.

'With suction' techniques have potentially higher risk of muscle involvement than 'without suction' techniques (see Table 7.1), and therefore, larger volume of saline injection into the submucosa is highly recommended. The author usually injects at least 10 mL for each snaring, and, especially in the colon, larger volume injection and controlled suction power are recommended.

In our experience of removal of a creeping tumor in the rectum, about 100 mL of saline was injected in total, and the whole lesion was safely removed with inducing half-circumferential ulceration. In this case, the post-therapeutic course was uneventful, and therefore, we conclude that large-volume saline injection is a safe procedure.

CONTROL OF BLEEDING FROM ULCER BED

Low-concentration epinephrine–saline solution is effective to control bleeding during EMR. In the esophagus, submucosal injection of that solution results in almost complete hemostasis, but, in the stomach, bleeding from an artificial ulcer sometimes cannot be controlled. At present, the hemostatic clip is the most reliable and safe therapeutic modality to control spurting bleeding from the ulcer bed.[27] In the colon, bleeding is quite rare and here pure saline without epinephrine is enough to avoid bleeding. As a result, bleeding from the ulcer bed can be relatively easily controlled.

CONCLUSION

In general, mucosal cancer of the gastrointestinal tract has no risk of lymph node metastasis, and therefore it can be curatively managed by EMR.

Note
Figures 7.1, 7.3, 7.5, 7.7, 7.10, 7.11, 7.12, 7.13, 7.14, 7.15, 7.16 and 7.17 are consecutive photographs of the same case.

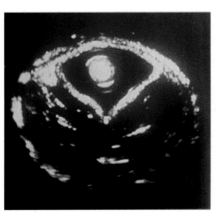

Fig. 7.21 Sonography. 20 mL saline is injected into the esophageal submucosa. More than half circumferential mucosa is lifted up to a maximum 1 cm from the muscle layer.

CHECKLIST OF PRACTICE POINTS

1. Did you fix the cap onto the tip of an endoscope by adhesive tape?
2. Did you prepare a special small-diameter snare? A small-diameter, crescent snare (Olympus) is essential to this procedure.
3. Can you observe mucosal-surface lifting during saline injection?
4. Did you create pre-looping condition of the snare wire? The outer sheath of the snare should be positioned to the tip of the cap.
5. Did you close the snare wire at the middle part of a created bleb? Never close at the base of the bleb.
6. Does strangulated mucosa by a closed snare move smoothly?
7. When you create a large artificial ulcer, antibiotics prescription is recommended.

REFERENCES

1. Lambert R. Endoscopic detection and treatment of early esophageal cancer: a critical analysis. Endoscopy 1995; 27:12–18.

2. Endo M, Takeshita K, Yoshida M. How can we diagnose the early stage of esophageal cancer? Endoscopic diagnosis. Endoscopy 1986; 18:11–18.

3. Endo M, Kawano T. Analysis of 1125 cases of early esophageal carcinoma in Japan. Dis Esoph 1991; 4:71–76.

4. Inoue H, Endo M. Endoscopic esophageal mucosal resection using a transparent tube. Surg Endosc 1990; 4:198–201.

5. Japanese Gastric Cancer Association. Japanese classification of gastric carcinoma. 2nd English edn. Gastric Cancer 1998; 1:10–24.

6. Takekoshi T, Baba Y, Ota H, et al. Endoscopic resection of early gastric carcinomas: results of a retrospective analysis of 308 cases. Endoscopy 1994; 26:352–358.

7. Takeshita K, Tani M, Inoue H, et al. A new method of endoscopic mucosal resection of metastatic lesions in the stomach: its technical features and results. Hepatogastroenterology 1997; 44:1602–1611.

8. Nakajima T. Tabular analysis of 10 000 cases of gastric cancer in CIH. Jpn J Cancer Chemother 1994; 21:1813–1897 (in Japanese).

9. Kudo S. Endoscopic mucosal resection of flat and depressed types of early colorectal cancer. Endoscopy 1993; 25:455–461.

10. Rosenberg N. Submucosal saline wheal as safety factor in fulguration of rectal and sigmoidal polypi. Arch Surg 1955; 70:120–122.

11. Tada M, Murakamai A, Karita M, et al. Endoscopic resection of early gastric cancer. Endoscopy 1993; 25:445–450.

12. Deyhle P, Largiader F, Jenny S, et al. A method for endoscopic electroresection of sessile colonic polyps. Endoscopy 1973; 5:38–40.

13. Martin TR, Onstad GR, Silvis SE, et al. Lift and cut biopsy technique for submucosal samplings. Gastrointest Endosc 1976; 23:29–30.

14. Hirao M, Masuda K, Asanuma T, et al. Endoscopic resection of early gastric cancer and other tumors with local injection of hypertonic saline-epinephrine. Gastrointest Endosc 1988; 34:264–269.

15. Monma K, Sakaki N, Yoshida M. Endoscopic mucosectomy for precise evaluation and treatment of esophageal intraepithelial cancer. Endoscopia Digestiva 1990; 2:501–506 (in Japanese).

16. Makuuchi H, Machimura T, Sugihara T, et al. Endoscopic diagnosis and treatment of mucosal cancer of the esophagus. Endoscopia Digestiva 1990; 2:447–452 (in Japanese).

17. Makuuchi H. Endoscopic mucosal resection for early esophageal cancer. Dig Endosc 1996; 8:175–179.

18. Kawano T, Miyake S, Yasuno M, et al. A new technique for endoscopic esophageal mucosectomy using a transparent overtube with intraluminal negative pressure (np-EEM). Dig Endosc 1991; 3:159–167.

19. Inoue H, Takeshita K, Hori H, et al. Endoscopic mucosal resection with a cap-fitted panendoscope for esophagus, stomach, and colon mucosal lesions. Gastrointest Endosc 1993; 39:58–62.

20. Inoue H, Noguchi O, Saito N, et al. Endoscopic mucosectomy for early cancer using a pre-looped plastic cap. Gastrointest Endosc 1994; 40:263–264.

21. Tada M, Inoue H, Endo M. Colonic mucosal resection using a transparent cap-fitted endoscope. Gastrointest Endosc 1996; 44:63–65.

22. Izumi Y, Teramoto K, Ohshima M, et al. Endoscopic resection of duodenal ampulla with a transparent plastic cap. Surgery 1998; 123:109–110.

23. Stiegmann GV. Endoscopic ligation: now and the future. Gastrointest Endosc 1993; 39:203–205.

24. Chaves DM, Sakai P, Mester M, et al. A new endoscopic technique for the resection of flat polypoid lesions. Gastrointest Endosc 1994; 40:224–226.

25. Freischer DE, Dawsey S, Tio TL, et al. Tissue band ligation followed by snare resection (band and snare): a new technique for tissue acquisition in the esophagus. Gastrointest Endosc 1996; 44:68–72.

26. Soehendra N, Binmoeller KF, Bohnacker S, et al. Endoscopic snare mucosectomy in the esophagus without any additional equipment: a simple technique for resection of flat early cancer. Endoscopy 1997; 29:380–383.

27. Hachisu T, Yamada H, Satoh S, et al. Endoscopic clipping with a new rotatable clip device and a long clip. Dig Endosc 1996; 8:172–173.

28. Takeshita K, Tani M, Inoue H, et al. Endoscopic treatment of early oesophageal or gastric cancer. Gut 1997; 40:123–127.

29. Inoue H. Endoscopic mucosal resection for esophageal and gastric mucosal cancers. Can J Gastroenterol 1998; 12:355–359.

30. Yoshikane H, Goto H, Niwa Y, et al. Endoscopic resection of small duodenal carcinoid tumors with strip biopsy technique. Gastrointest Endosc 1998; 47:466–470.

31. Hirasawa R, Ishi H, Tatsuta M, et al. Clinicopathologic features and endoscopic resection of duodenal adenocarcinomas and adenomas with the submucosal saline injection technique. Gastrointest Endosc 1997; 46:507–513.

32. Binmoeller KF, Boaventura S, Ramsperger K, et al. Endoscopic snare excision of benign adenomas of the papilla of Vater. Gastrointest Endosc 1993; 39:127–131.

33. Izumi Y, Teramoto K, Ohshima M, et al. Endoscopic resection of duodenal ampulla with a transparent plastic cap. Surgery 1998; 123:109–110.

8.

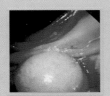

ENDOSCOPIC SPHINCTEROTOMY

MEINHARD CLASSEN

PETER BORN

Only a few years after the performance of the first endoscopic retrograde cholangiopancreatography (ERCP), Classen & Demling[1] and Kawai et al[2] virtually simultaneously introduced the technique of endoscopic sphincterotomy (EST) of the papilla of Vater and sphincter of Oddi.

Since its development in 1973, EST has gained widespread acceptance all over the world and has become an established therapeutic procedure for various pancreatobiliary disorders.

The number of applications has increased markedly, especially since the procedure which originally provided access to the biliary system has been extended to include the pancreatic duct, and more recently the minor papilla. Although the variety of new procedures would appear to compete with those performed surgically, there is no real competition between gastroenterologists and surgeons. Combined procedures as occurs with biliary stone treatment (endoscopic removal of bile duct stones followed by laparoscopic cholecystectomy) have proven beneficial for many patients.

INDICATIONS FOR EST (see also Table 8.1)

Since the introduction of EST, pancreatobiliary endoscopy, previously limited to diagnostic applications, began to cover an increasing spectrum of therapeutic applications. Whereas initially EST was performed predominantly for choledocholithiasis, a variety of endoscopic approaches to ductal obstruction are now available. In addition, access to the pancreatic duct system via the major and minor papilla is now an established procedure.

Choledocholithiasis is still one of the major indications for sphincterotomy to allow endoscopic stone extraction. Previous restrictions of EST to patients over the age of 50 and those deemed to be a high surgical risk are no longer valid; more recent data have not shown any relevant negative long-term effects.[3] Moreover, several studies have shown that EST can be carried out safely in young patients[4] and even in children.[5]

In choledocholithiasis, the presence or absence of the gallbladder has no bearing on the results since the aim of the intervention is decompression of the bile duct in order to treat and/or prevent serious complications. Whether there is a need for cholecystectomy following EST for choledocholithiasis is still a matter of debate and will be discussed below.

The indication for EST and stone extraction in patients with choledocholithiasis after cholecystectomy is unquestioned. The debate about the best approach to patients

Indications for endoscopic sphincterotomy
• Papilla
—tumors (benign or malignant)
—inflammatory stenosis
—sphincter of Oddi dyskinesia
• Bile duct
—biliary malignancies
—obstruction due to pancreatic cancer
—choledocholithiasis
—cholangitis
—biliary pancreatitis
—benign strictures unrelated to previous surgery (i.e. inflammatory, ischemic – primary sclerosing cholangitis)
—miscellaneous conditions (sump syndrome, choledochocele, parasites)
—complications after surgical interventions (i.e. leaks, strictures)
—choledochoscopy
• Pancreatic duct
—pancreatic cancer
—chronic (obstructive) pancreatitis
—pancreatic pseudocysts
—pancreatolithiasis
—pancreatoscopy
• Minor papilla
—chronic pancreatitis and pancreas divisum
—better access to main pancreatic duct in some cases

Table 8.1 Indications for endoscopic sphincterotomy

with choledocholithiasis and the gallbladder in situ was temporarily interrupted by the development and rapid spread of laparoscopic cholecystectomy that at least in the beginning needed endoscopy for the treatment of bile duct stones. The initial difficulty with laparoscopic access to the common bile duct (CBD) resulted in the so-called therapeutic splitting with endoscopic stone removal from the bile duct followed by laparoscopic cholecystectomy. With increasing experience, the minimal invasive surgeons are now able to perform laparoscopic cholangiography and even stone treatment.[6] Therefore, in the future, therapeutic splitting may be replaced by laparoscopic treatment of both gallbladder and bile duct stones in a one-step procedure.

Cholangitis, one of the most serious complications of choledocholithiasis, is an accepted indication for EST and subsequent re-establishment of the biliary flow.[7] Moreover meta-analysis of several important studies clearly shows the importance of an early intervention.[8] Therefore, cholangitis should be treated endoscopically within 8 hours of the patient's admission. Besides stones, the most common causes of obstructive cholangitis are tumors, post-surgical strictures, and occlusion of stents in previously endoscopically treated patients.

Less clear is the role of EST in the other most serious complication of choledocholithiasis, biliary pancreatitis. While there are convincing data in favor of early EST[9–11] in this disease, the study of Fölsch et al[12] in selected patients did not only yield no benefit but even showed a deterioration in some patients after EST.

Foreign material, such as food particles or parasites,[13] may occasionally be found in the bile ducts. EST and endoscopic clearance have been successfully performed in these circumstances, as well as for the rare but well-recognized sump syndrome, a complication of choledochoenterostomy with accumulation of debris in the distal part of the bile duct.[14] Further indications for EST and biliary drainage are complications such as strictures and leakages after surgical interventions (especially after laparoscopic cholecystectomy or liver transplantation).

Obstructing tumors of the papilla of Vater constitute another indication for EST. Besides its therapeutic effect, EST may also be of diagnostic value, as the diagnostic accuracy of endoscopic biopsy is increased after EST.[15] Histologic examination is important for confirming adenoma, which is considered a premalignant lesion. Selected cases of Vaterian adenomas being removed by endoscopic polypectomy combined with fulguration have been reported.[16] Infiltrative duodenal obstruction from cancer also has to be considered[15] when deciding upon appropriate drainage; in selected cases, percutaneous transhepatic access may be preferred.

In symptomatic patients with verified sphincter of Oddi dysfunction, Geenen et al[17] were able to show that endoscopic sphincterotomy is effective.

Papillotomy can be performed on not only the biliary but also the pancreatic sphincter via the major as well as the minor papilla (pancreas divisum). Indications are recurrent episodes of pancreatitis in patients with pancreas divi-

sum as well as strictures in obstructive chronic pancreatitis or intraductal concretions in symptomatic patients. In cases where pseudocysts are connected with the pancreatic duct, EST followed by the insertion of a stent or a nasocystic tube[18] is a successful therapeutic option.

EQUIPMENT

All duodenoscopes with side-viewing optics are suitable for EST. Improvements such as an increase in the viewing angle, a greater range of deflection angle at the instrument tip, as well as an increase in the diameter of the accessory channel, have further augmented therapeutic options. Instruments with working channels up to 4.2 mm diameter are suitable for implantation of endoprostheses with diameters up to 12 Fr.

A variation of the pull-type sphincterotome developed by Demling and Classen (Fig. 8.1A) is generally used for papillotomy. An outer Teflon catheter contains a thin steel wire which exits the catheter about 3 cm before the distal end and re-enters it about 3–5 mm from the tip (nose). Tension on the wire produces a bowing effect, with the wire forming the bowstring. When the instrument is correctly positioned in the papilla (Fig. 8.2), the exposed

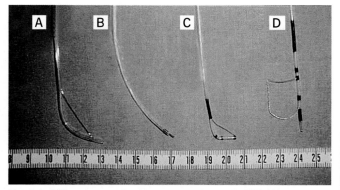

Fig. 8.1 Different types of sphincterotome for use in EST: (**A**) standard pull-type; (**B**) needle-knife; (**C**) precut; (**D**) push-type (shark-fin).

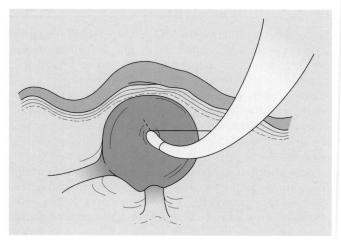

Fig. 8.2 Sphincterotome in situ immediately before cutting.

wire functions as a cautery-knife when high-frequency electrosurgical current is applied. The tip of the catheter without wire facilitates introduction into the duct system, with some investigators preferring papillotomes with a longer tip ('with a long nose') in situations with difficult cannulation.

Several modifications have been made to the basic sphincterotome design. One widespread modification is the so-called precut sphincterotome (Fig. 8.1C) which has a wire as short as 15–20 mm that re-enters the catheter at the tip (that means it has no nose) and is useful for performing short incisions. The technique of precut sphincterotomy is used when cannulation with the standard sphincterotome fails. Another alternative is the needle-knife sphincterotome (Fig. 8.1B). This instrument simply consists of a catheter and a protruding wire; the end of the wire can be extended 2–5 mm from the distal tip of the catheter. It can be especially useful for EST of the minor papilla. Push-type sphincterotomes (Fig. 8.1D), characterized by wires forming a bow when extruded from the catheter, are mainly used for EST after Billroth-II resections. Other developments for EST following a Billroth-II gastrectomy include a device[19] where the plastic catheter has a 'memory' that ensures that the sigmoid shape of the wire is retained after passage through the instrument channel. This enables a more precise incision compared to the shark-fin (push-type) papillotome. All sphincterotome catheters have a side or terminal hole to allow the instillation of contrast agent.

Using guidewires for insertion of the sphincterotome (Fig. 8.3) is helpful when previous intubation with the diagnostic catheter or the papillotome has proved difficult. A 0.035 inch (0.89 mm) guidewire is placed through the diagnostic catheter. The sphincterotome is then exchanged for the catheter over this guidewire. This technique reduces the risk of local tissue damage as well as the repeated filling of the pancreatic duct with contrast. The success of this method relies on close cooperation and interaction between the endoscopist and the assistant. Whether a so-called safety sphincterotome (wire-guided with a tapered tip including metal marker, a long nose, and an insulated cutting wire) will provide a further advantage has to be further evaluated.[20]

As the overall cost of medical care rises, the reuse of disposable sphincterotomes is becoming of special interest. In a prospective study, Kozarek[21] showed that reuse was safe, did not cause an increase of infections, and resulted in considerable financial savings. The legality of reusing equipment labeled as disposable has yet to be determined.

Most commercially available high-frequency electrosurgical generators with cutting and coagulation settings are suitable for EST. They should have a rapid-start function that helps initiate the incision so that delayed cutting and excessive local heating can be avoided.

In situations where EST is not possible or desirable, an alternative procedure is balloon dilation (Fig. 8.4) of the papilla. The balloon (usually 3–4 cm long with a caliber of 6–10 mm) is inserted over a guidewire under endoscopic and fluoroscopic control. After position is confirmed, it is inflated with diluted contrast for about 1 to 2 minutes until the waist of the balloon has disappeared.[22]

For stone extraction, Dormia baskets (Figs 8.5 and 8.6) and balloon catheters (Fig. 8.7) are used. Balloon

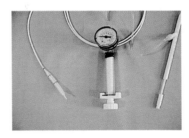

Fig. 8.4 Dilation balloon.

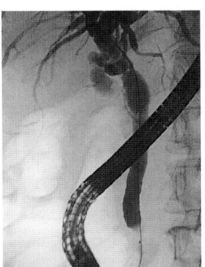

Fig. 8.3 Wire-guided sphincterotome in situ.

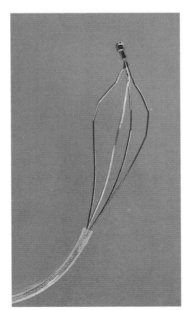

Fig. 8.5 Dormia basket.

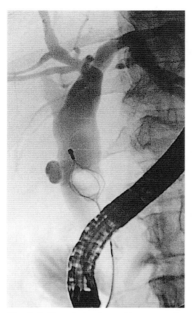

Fig. 8.6 Dormia basket with captured bile duct stone.

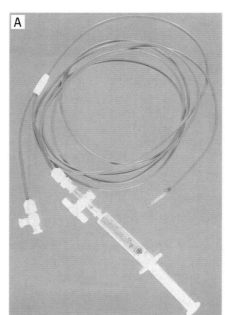

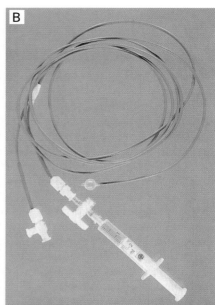

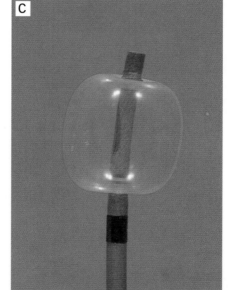

Fig. 8.7 Balloon catheter, used for stone extraction and to prevent contrast outflow from the bile duct during opacification after EST. (A) Balloon not filled. (B) Balloon filled. (C) Balloon filled (tip of the catheter).

catheters are also inserted to prevent contrast outflow from the bile duct if opacification is attempted after previous EST.

PATIENT PREPARATION

Informed consent is required for the procedure, as for all other invasive procedures. Indication, potential complications, and possible alternative methods should be discussed. A prothrombin time test and partial thromboplastin time should be done to check plasma coagulation; platelet count and bleeding time are required to rule out platelet dysfunction, especially after ingestion of aspirin or NSAIDs. Cardiopulmonary status should be assessed as before surgical interventions. Patients unfit for surgery can be treated endoscopically but both patient and endoscopist must be aware of the increased risk. Close monitoring of blood pressure, heart rate, and oxygen saturation are required, as it is for all patients in whom ERCP is performed.[23] The appropriate choice and dosage of sedation are prescribed individually for each patient, and the patient is fasting.

Antibiotic prophylaxis is not recommended generally for ERCP and EST. However, several international societies of gastrointestinal endoscopy recommend prophylaxis in patients with suspected biliary obstruction, previous cholangitis, and pancreatic pseudocyst. The European Society of Gastrointestinal Endoscopy (ESGE) is even recommending in its guidelines [24] prophylactic antibiotic application in all therapeutic ERCP interventions.

Because of the possibility of local complications, there should be a close cooperation with an experienced abdominal surgeon.

Although hemorrhage is a potential complication of EST, we do not recommend routine pre-sphincterotomy

crossmatching of blood. In order to minimize the risk of bleeding, endoscopic Doppler ultrasonography has been used to localize the retroduodenal artery;[25] but a study of our own group showed no significant benefit.[26]

PROCEDURE

Endoscopic sphincterotomy

Since its introduction, the technique of EST has not changed substantially. Following ERCP, the sphincterotome is introduced into the bile duct (Figs 8.2 and 8.3) and the position is checked fluoroscopically (Fig. 8.8), especially if it is not wire-guided.

If there is any doubt about the correct position, contrast medium should be instilled through the sphinctero-

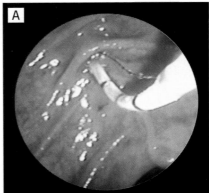

Fig. 8.9 (A) Sphincterotome in situ before cutting and (B) immediately after cutting.

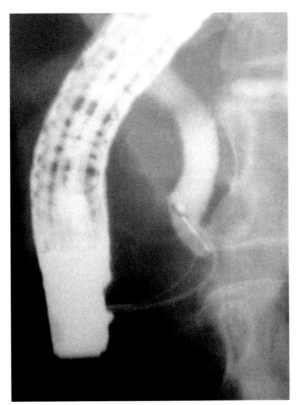

Fig. 8.8 X-ray of the sphincterotome in situ to check position before cutting.

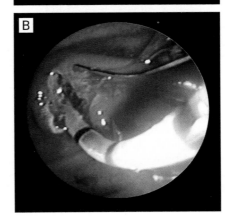

tome catheter. The roof of the papilla will be elevated when tension is exerted on the cutting wire. This allows the endoscopist to ascertain the correct direction of the cut (Fig. 8.9): at least one-third of the cutting wire should then be visible outside the papilla. This ensures that the cutting is carefully controlled. The cut should be directed toward 11 o'clock to avoid vascular injury. Common errors are to introduce the wire too deeply and to apply too much tension. This technique may produce an uncontrolled rapid and large incision with increased risk of bleeding and perforation. Usually blended current (cutting plus coagulation) is applied in short pulses, controlled by foot pedal activation. The correct length of the incision, which should be controlled endoscopically, varies, but should be about 10–15 mm and extends to the transverse fold for a normal papilla (Fig. 8.9). If the papilla is small and flat, the length of the cut is more difficult to determine.

There are a variety of methods to cope with more difficult situations after initial failure of duct cannulation. However, it should be pointed out that cancellation of the procedure and rescheduling ERCP at a later session should be considered in patients with no urgent indication. Repeat intervention by the same endoscopist has been reported to yield a considerable increase (87.5%) in the success rate.[27] In addition, a change of endoscopist should also be considered if that is a possibility.

Some centers[28] report that a small incision (precut) must first be performed in 10% of cases before the standard sphincterotome can be introduced. This special technique requires a precut sphincterotome distinguished by the absence of a 'nose' and a short cutting wire. The roof of the papilla is then incised as far as possible by the thermally activated wire. If the bile-stained mucosa of the bile duct can be seen, the procedure is completed by conventional EST with the standard instrument. An alternative precutting method is to make the incision with a needle-knife sphincterotome. Starting at the orifice, the papilla is incised along its roof by the activated needle-like wire. The cutting must be performed cautiously, proceeding stepwise in small increments. When the distal portion of the bile duct is opened, EST can be completed using a standard sphincterotome. Although considerable skill and practice are necessary, this method, at least in the hand of experts, bears no or only a slightly increased risk of complications while it significantly increases the success of diagnostic and therapeutic procedures at the papilla.[28,29] In patients with a previous Billroth-II gastrectomy, the safety of a needle-knife application can be augmented by insertion of a plastic stent prior to cutting, using the stent as a shelter against perforation.

Another method used to gain access to the CBD is endoscopic fistulotomy (choledochoduodenostomy), in cases where there is an obstructed orifice of the papilla of Vater. The distal obstruction results in a prominent impression of the duodenal wall owing to the dilated bile duct which can be visible endoscopically. The bulging intraduodenal segment of the choledochus is then punctured several millimeters proximal to the ostium of the papilla with a device such as a needle-knife. Depending on the anatomic position, the cut can be extended using a standard sphincterotome.[30] The success of this procedure requires considerable experience.

The technique of endoscopic papillectomy to gain access to the ducts is reserved for difficult situations and has its main indication in patients with papillary tumors.[31] In this procedure, a snare is placed around the papilla and tumor with cautery-transection of the lesion.

EST in patients with juxtapapillary diverticula is usually not more difficult nor does it carry a greater risk of perforation than when performed in a normal papilla. When the papilla is located within the diverticulum, cannulation might be impossible, and even if the sphincterotome is correctly positioned in the bile duct, control of the incision may be difficult.

After Billroth II operations, it is often difficult to reach the papilla, and introduction of the sphincterotome is also more difficult because of the reversed anatomic orientation. The use of forward-viewing endoscopes may sometimes be helpful. The application of pull-type and other modified papillotomes may be necessary.

In difficult situations of cannulation of the papilla, the application of a flexible guidewire can be a great help. The wire passed through the papillotome can be controlled by tightening or loosening the tension on the wire. This technique causes less local tissue damage and less unwanted contrast filling of the pancreatic duct, although there is a lack of controlled data.[32]

In cases where the papilla is accessible with the endoscope but cannulation is impossible for whatever reason, the so-called rendez-vous technique (Fig. 8.10) might be indicated. In these patients, percutaneous transhepatic puncture is performed, a thin tract established (usually only 7 Fr), and thereafter endoscopy repeated. A wire introduced from outside is captured and brought out through the endoscope accessory channel. The papillotome is then inserted over this wire. In patients with a Billroth II operation, it might even be preferable to perform papillotomy sheltered by a percutaneously inserted prosthesis.

Taken together, there are several different methods to gain access to the biliary duct after the failure of the standard procedure to perform EST. Most centers prefer one method and develop their own expertise; our hospitals rely heavily on needle-knife EST.

In contrast to biliary sphincterotomy, EST of the pancreatic sphincter is by far less commonly performed.[33] The technique is quite similar, and the recommended direction of the cut is toward 12–1 o'clock. Sphincterotomy of the minor papilla is more difficult as needle-knife papillotomy is more often necessary than with EST of the major papilla depending on its size and location.

Initially EST was only performed on an inpatient basis in institutions capable of coping with potential complications. Within the last few years, outpatient ERCP and EST are becoming more common. However, data are accumulating that in up to 25% of cases re-admission of patients because of complications or for observation is necessary.[34] In Ho et al's study,[34] pain during the investigation, a history of pancreatitis, and the performance of EST were risk factors indicating complications, while in the multicenter study of Freeman et al[35] sphincter of Oddi dysfunction, cirrhosis, difficult bile duct cannulation, precut sphincterotomy, and combined percutaneous–endoscopic procedures increased the need for patients' re-admission. In any case of outpatient EST as well as ERCP, the patient has to be informed about possible complications, which usually occur within several hours after the procedure[35,36] and what to do should complications arise. Howell's data on overnight hospitalization following EST,[36] showed a reduction of costs compared to the strategy of post-procedural discharge after 3 hours. The high quality outcome for patients treated this way reinforces our belief in the value of a one-night hospital admission following EST.

COMPLICATIONS AND THEIR MANAGEMENT AND PROPHYLAXIS

Apart from a myriad of complications published in case reports, hemorrhage, perforation, pancreatitis, and cholangitis are the main problems that arise following EST. The overall complication rate for EST as determined in large surveys ranges between 4% and 10%, while the mortality rate is between 0% and 2% (Table 8.2). In contrast to these older studies, Freeman et al[37] demonstrate in a large prospective multicenter study of EST in 2347 patients, a total rate of complication of 9.8% with a mortality (30 days) of 0.4%.

Usually complications become clinically manifest within several hours after the intervention.[35,36] Nevertheless, the late appearance of complications must also be considered.

In contrast to previous studies,[38] the study by Freeman et al[37] clearly showed that pancreatitis is the most common complication of EST (Table 8.2). However, the course is mild in most cases. Different statistics concerning bleeding might be explained by variations in its definition, as minimal self-terminating bleeding is seen in many patients after EST. Although a minimum increase of amylase and lipase is often seen after ERCP and EST, pancreatitis is defined as onset of pain after the procedure for at least 24 hours asso-

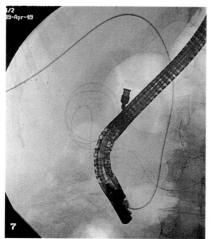

Fig. 8.10 Rendez-vous technique, a guidewire introduced percutaneously transhepatically and grasped via the endoscope.

Table 8.2 Details of complications

Details of complications				
	Lambert et al[38]	Freeman et al[37] All	Severe	Fatal
Bleeding	29 (4.8%)	48 (2.0%)	12 (0.5%)	2 (0.1%)
Acute pancreatitis	16 (2.6%)	127 (5.4%)	9 (0.4%)	1 (<0.1%)
Acute biliary sepsis	13 (2.1%)	24 (1.0%)	2 (0.1%)	1 (<0.1%)
Perforation	4 (<1%)	8 (0.3%)	5 (0.2%)	1 (<0.1%)
Miscellaneous	6 (1%)	25 (1.1%)	8 (0.3%)	5 (0.2%)
Total complications	68 (11.3%)	229 (9.8%)	38 (1.6%)	
Fatal complications	13 (1.2%)		10	(0.4%)

ciated with an increase of the serum pancreatic enzymes of three to five times above the normal value.[39]

Risk factors for pancreatitis after ERCP and EST are related to both the patient as well as the technique used. These factors include younger age, history of post-ERCP pancreatitis, sphincter dysfunction, and problems during cannulation, including the necessity for precutting and the number of pancreatic contrast injections.[37,40]

Pancreatitis is the most important complication of pancreatic sphincterotomy with rates exceeding 10% in several studies. Insertion of a drainage tube after EST has resulted in a dramatic reduction in this rate to levels below 1%.[33]

Several different efforts to prevent this complication have been reported. For patients with sphincter of Oddi dysfunction, pancreatic stenting may prevent pancreatitis after biliary sphincterotomy.[41] The application of pure cutting electrocautery current should cause less post-procedure pancreatitis than blended current.[42] But studies are needed to evaluate whether this may cause an increased risk of hemorrhage.

Several drugs, such as somatostatin (and the analogue octreotide), glucagon, gabexate,[43] or steroids[44] have been investigated in the prevention of post-ERCP and post-EST pancreatitis without conclusive results.[39] Markedly divergent results with somatostatin mandate further studies.[45] Rabenstein et al's[46] interesting observation of a possible protective effect of heparin deserves further evaluation. At this time, apart from controlled studies no recommendations can be given for routine use of any drug to prevent post-procedure pancreatitis.

The rates of bleeding reported in the literature are difficult to compare as the definition may vary. Self-limited oozing bleeding is not a rare event after EST but cannot be considered a clinically significant complication.[47] Hemorrhage is considered to be severe if there are clinical signs such as hematemesis and hematochezia, accompanied by a fall of hemoglobin of at least 2 mg/dL or if there is a need for blood transfusion. These criteria for severe bleeding are usually applied when patients present with delayed onset hemorrhage or in retrospective studies.[47] Severe hemorrhage may occur during the procedure with arterial spurting, but may often be controlled by the endoscopist at that time. The Freeman study[37] found significant hemorrhage in 2% of cases, with 0.6% defined to be mild (no

need of blood transfusion), 0.9% moderate (up to 4 units of blood being necessary) and 0.5% severe with the necessity of 5 or more units of blood.

In cases with immediate onset of bleeding, wire-guided papillotomes provide the advantage that the correct position of the instrument can be maintained in spite of loss of visual landmarks. This is of special importance in spurting bleeding, as in this situation the cut should be extended for some additional millimeters to complete the cutting of the artery and therefore facilitate the retraction of the two vessel stumps.[47]

In venous bleeding, the local application of coagulation current by the sphincterotome (with special care for the pancreas) may be successful. In most cases, injection therapy is preferred, most often using diluted epinephrine (1:10 000).

To reduce the risk of cholangitis after endoscopic treatment of post-EST bleeding, biliary drainage should be guaranteed by the insertion of a stent or a nasobiliary tube.

In most cases of post-EST bleeding, endoscopic therapy is successful but failure should lead to additional interventions such as radiologic embolization of the gastroduodenal artery or surgery.[48]

Late onset of bleeding can be seen up to 10 days after EST,[37] and patients, especially if treated as outpatients, should be informed about this possibility and how to react.

The best prophylaxis for hemorrhage is good technique and sufficient coagulation. The application of a Doppler before EST has not, as discussed above, gained general acceptance.

Retroperitoneal perforation is an infrequent but potentially dangerous complication[37,49,50] where symptoms are non-specific. The risk of perforation is influenced by the length of the EST incision, by the extraction of large stones, and by the diameter of the CBD. The occurrence of bile duct perforation does not necessarily require surgical intervention; many perforations heal spontaneously when effective biliary drainage is achieved either endoscopically or by a percutaneous transhepatic catheter.[51] Patients should be kept fasted and antibiotics should be administered. The diagnosis of perforation is made by plain abdominal X-ray and, if necessary, CT scan.[52] Although conservative treatment is often successful, close monitoring of the patient is mandatory to determine if surgical intervention is necessary.

When considering all complications, the Freeman study[37] clearly showed that the rates are strongly dependent upon the experience of the endoscopist. Those who are performing at least one EST per week have a significantly lower complication rate than endoscopists who rarely perform EST.

SHORT-TERM RESULTS

Success rates

Surveys from endoscopic centers all over the world reported cannulation success rates of more than 90% during the 1970s; currently, rates of up to 99% are reported.[53] These surveys reveal that choledocholithiasis was the indication for EST in most cases.

For patients with previous Billroth II gastrectomy, success rates 20 years ago were lower (falling to 50% if there was a Braun anastomosis) whereas technical difficulties and complications were higher[54] than in cases with normal anatomy. More recent studies[55] show success rates rising over 90% in patients with previous Billroth II resection, while Braun enteroenterostomy is no longer considered to be a negative factor. Even in patients with Roux-en-Y gastrojejunostomy, the papilla could be reached in 33% of attempts.[55] The experience of the endoscopist is of major importance in these difficult situations.

In abnormal situations such as post-surgical anatomy, a percutaneous radiologic approach to the biliary tree ought to be considered as a therapeutic alternative or at least as a facilitating factor (rendez-vous technique).

Sphincterotomy of the minor papilla is based on the assumption that there is an etiologic relation between pancreas divisum and recurrent episodes of pancreatitis.[56] Recently, the indication for EST has been extended to patients with incomplete pancreas divisum.[57] Although the technique is difficult, the procedure has been reported to have succeeded in all patients.[56,57]

Endoscopic treatment of choledocholithiasis

Since the introduction of EST, choledocholithiasis has remained the main indication. Although stones may pass spontaneously out of the bile duct after EST, clearing of the bile duct with a basket or balloon is strongly recommended. In cases where the stones cannot be removed immediately after EST (e.g. stone too big or local edema after EST), a stent or a nasobiliary tube should be inserted to maintain biliary flow and prevent the occurrence of cholangitis. Particularly in elderly and frail patients, especially if there are multiple or large stones or cholangitis, placement of a stent after EST may be the first treatment and elective stone removal might be performed after recovery of the patient. If stones cannot be removed, it is unwise to rely on a stent for long-term or definitive therapy, unless the patient is unfit for elective treatment later on after EST or the patient has a short life expectancy because of the occurrence of severe late complications, the most commonly reported of which has been cholangitis.[58] Insertion of a stent without EST as a temporary intervention has been described in pregnant women to reduce the risks of EST and to curtail the amount of radiation.[59]

Complete removal of bile duct stones is possible in at least 85% of cases with conventional means. Failure to clear the bile duct may be due to a variety of reasons, such as anatomic variations or abnormalities of the duodenum or the papilla in most cases following surgical interventions, e.g. Billroth II resection (Fig. 8.11) or biliary surgery. Large stones located above a stenosis or intrahepatically are further reasons for failure. The critical size of stones above which removal may be difficult is about 15 mm diameter, although removal of stones with a diameter of more than 25 mm has been reported.[60] Another limiting factor is the size of the sphincterotomy that can be performed safely. Large stones (Fig. 8.12) have to be disintegrated or pulverized before their extraction or their spontaneous passage through the papilla. For this purpose, mechanical lithotripsy is an easy and commonly used procedure. There are two systems available: one applicable via the endoscope, the other after its removal.

In mechanical lithotripsy (Figs 8.13 and 8.14), the stone is captured in a Dormia basket and then broken by application of considerable force. After the stone is trapped, the outer Teflon sheath of the Dormia basket catheter is removed because it cannot withstand the pressure required to break a stone. Only the wire remains in situ. A flexible metal rod is then passed over the wire and is advanced to

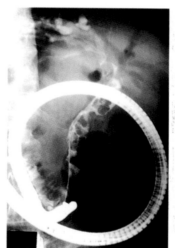

Fig. 8.11 Choledocholithiasis in a patient with Billroth II operation.

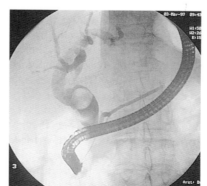

Fig. 8.12 Choledocholithiasis: a large stone in the common bile duct.

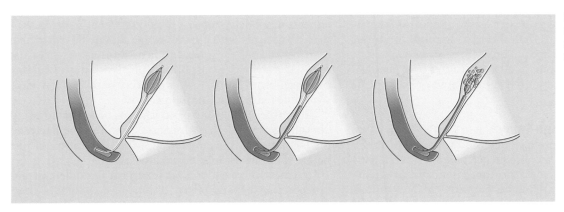

Fig. 8.13 Procedure of mechanical lithotripsy with the endoscope in situ.

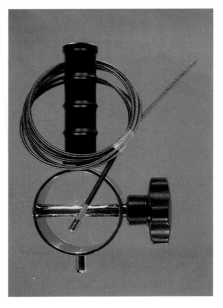

Fig. 8.14 Equipment for mechanical lithotripsy: Dormia basket and knurled wheel drive.

Stone disintegration can also be performed with electrohydraulic (EHL) or laser lithotripsy, which requires direct contact of the probe with the stone under strict visual control, which means that the application is performed under cholangioscopic guidance (Fig. 8.15) either transpapillary through a babyscope after EST or via a percutaneous transhepatic approach.

A more recent development is the pulsed rhodamine laser with a wavelength of 594 nm with an automatic stone detection system interrupting the pulses within nanoseconds when the back-scattered laser light detects tissue or material other than the stone ('intelligent laser'). This enables a broader and considerably safer application within the bile duct, although in most of these cases the application is performed through a cholangioscope as well.

Peroral cholangioscopy is currently performed with miniscopes (e.g. 3.4 mm) inserted through a standard therapeutic duodenoscope ('jumbo'). Although these newer 'mother–baby' systems are easier to handle than the older ones, the control of the baby cholangioscope within the biliary system is still a problem. The percutaneous transhepatic approach is technically much easier, but here the creation of the large tract causes significantly more complications.[65] Comparing ESWL and laser lithotripsy in an RCT, Neuhaus et al[66] showed a significant advantage of laser lithotripsy over ESWL. Practically the availability of both of these systems in specialized centers provides very high success rates in the non-surgical treatment of choledocholithiasis with rates up to 100%.

the basket under fluoroscopic control. Once the rod is in position, the Dormia wire is attached to a knurled wheel drive which is wound on to the cylinder of the lithotripsy device. The retraction of the basket holding the stone into the metal rod pulverizes the stone. The broken fragments can be removed easily.

Previously reported success rates are 79% for stones over 20 mm and 68% for stones over 25 mm diameter.[61] In a more recent study, the success rate was up to 93%, independent of the stone size.[62] One problem may be the impossibility of opening the basket sufficiently within the bile duct to grasp the stone.

Newer methods of stone fragmentation have resulted in a further increase of the success rates. Electroshockwave lithotripsy (ESWL) is an alternative to reduce the size of a stone that has been targeted by ultrasonography or X-ray, with the contrast applied through a nasobiliary tube. Stone-free bile ducts, especially if remaining fragments are removed by endoscopy, are reported in more than 90% of cases.[63,64] But this procedure is time-consuming – in many patients more than one session is necessary – and the concomitant pain may cause reluctance to continue treatment. However, it is a highly effective method without serious complications in most cases.

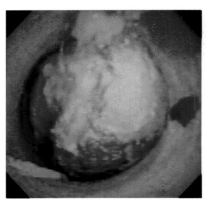

Fig. 8.15 Cholangioscopic (percutaneous transhepatical) view of a stone in the common bile duct (courtesy of PD Dr H.D. Allescher).

Therapeutic alternatives such as the application of solvents (e.g. methyl-terbutyl-ether) to dissolve or soften stones is restricted for special problem cases only.

In conclusion, in spite of all these endoscopic possibilities, the surgical alternative should always be kept in consideration.

Removal of a foreign body

A foreign body in the biliary tree is a rarity and is, in the majority of the cases, a consequence of surgery. EST with subsequent endoscopic duct clearance is an effective treatment. Using the same technique, parasites can be removed from the biliary or pancreatic duct, as reported in hydatid disease, a parasitic infection caused by *Echinococcus granulosus*. While diagnostic ERCP is sometimes performed to search for fistula between cysts and the biliary tree, EST with subsequent ductal clearance of daughter cysts and debris can be performed, particularly if pain or cholangitis occurs.[67]

Cholangitis is also the most dangerous clinical sign of the so-called sump syndrome. Spontaneously (as a consequence of e.g. a biliodigestive fistula) or as a result of a biliodigestive anastomosis, the distal segment of the CBD becomes a non-functional reservoir, where gastrointestinal contents and bile accumulate. Endoscopic ductal clearance after EST is successful[14,68] in treating this entity.

Acute obstructive cholangitis

Infection of the biliary system with the typical clinical symptoms of fever, right upper quadrant pain, and jaundice is an emergency that requires early intervention. The cause is an obstruction of the bile duct from a variety of causes including stones, stenoses after surgical interventions, e.g. biliobiliary or biliodigestive anastomoses, and occlusion caused by tumors of previously inserted stents. As the mortality of untreated patients is considerably high, early treatment is mandatory (Fig. 8.16).

Endoscopy with EST has replaced surgery as the first-line treatment. In an RCT in patients with cholangitis caused by stones the outcome of the endoscopically treated patients was significantly better than those who had surgical therapy. The mortality in the endoscopically treated patients was 10% compared to 32% in those in the surgical arm.[69] The aim of EST therapy is rapid decompression of the bile duct and maintenance of bile efflux by placing

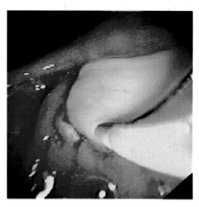

Fig. 8.16 Acute cholangitis with pus emptying after EST.

either a nasobiliary tube or a bilioduodenal stent. In seriously ill patients with difficult stones, it may be reasonable (in order to keep the intervention as short as possible) just to insert a stent or a nasobiliary tube (with the advantage of being able to flush).[70] After recovery of the patient, elective stone extraction can follow.

To further reduce the risks, it seems beneficial to avoid overfilling the system with contrast to limit the bacterial dissemination in the circulation. Initial aspiration of bile before the contrast injection is advisable.

In cases where endoscopic treatment has failed, percutaneous transhepatic biliary drainage is a valuable alternative to surgery.[70] As already pointed out,[8] the time factor plays an important role. Cholangitis has to be regarded as an emergency that needs early intervention – scheduled in our hospital within 8 hours of admission.

Simultaneous antibiotic therapy is mandatory as well, and must be started before endoscopy. Leung et al[71] studied 579 patients with documented bacteria in the bile duct along with choledocholithiasis. *E. coli*, species of *Klebsiella*, *Enterobacter*, *Enterococcus* and *Streptococcus* were the most relevant bacteria.

Biliary pancreatitis

Early in this century, Opie[72] claimed that a bile duct stone passing through the papilla with at least temporary blockage of the outflow of pancreatic juice was the main pathogenic mechanism leading to pancreatitis. Historical points in favor of a biliary origin of pancreatitis may include a history of gallstones,[73] the absence of alcohol abuse and, especially, signs of cholangitis. Elevated liver enzymes (especially alkaline phosphatase) and dilated bile ducts on ultrasonography offer further support for this diagnosis. The appearance of the papilla (edema, discharge of pus) may also be contributory (Fig. 8.17). ERCP is no longer considered to be contraindicated in biliary pancreatitis, and may substantially contribute to the diagnosis of a biliary cause.[74] Contrast injection into the pancreatic duct system should be avoided.

Although multiple reports described the beneficial effect of EST in biliary pancreatitis, it was Neoptolemos et al[9] who showed in a controlled study that patients with suspected gallstone pancreatitis and a severe course of the disease had fewer complications and reduced mortality when early EST was performed.

In another study from Hong Kong,[10] comparing early (within 24 hours) ERCP and EST with conventional therapy in patients with a predicted severe course of biliary pancreatitis, morbidity (from 54 to 13%) as well as mortality (from 18 to 3%) was reduced by the endoscopic intervention. This study, however, as well as the Neoptolemos study, did not show any benefit for patients with mild pancreatitis.

In a further study from Poland,[11] morbidity (17% vs 36%) and mortality (2% vs 13%) could be reduced by early endoscopic intervention in patients with biliary pancreatitis compared to conventional treatment. This study specially addressed the benefit of early (within 24 hours) intervention.

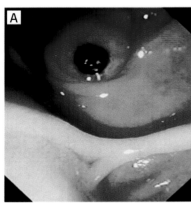

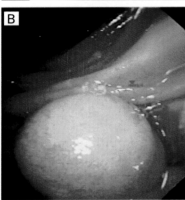

Fig. 8.17 (A) Stone impacted in the orifice of the papilla. (B) Ballooning of the papilla.

Contradictory to these results, a German study[12] reported an increase of mortality in endoscopically treated patients and concluded that ERCP and EST are not indicated in patients with biliary pancreatitis without biliary obstruction or sepsis, although there are some concerns about this report,[75] and further studies are required. At present, there is no debate that ERCP/EST is indicated in all patients with biliary pancreatitis and concomitant signs of cholangitis. Studies should aim to answer the questions whether much earlier intervention provides more benefit, what to do when no stones can be detected fluoroscopically or when the patient is seen early after onset of complaints and the bile duct is not (yet?) enlarged and so-called microliths might be overlooked without EST.

In all patients with biliary pancreatitis, antibiotic therapy should be started before endoscopy.[76]

Sphincter of Oddi dyskinesia

The etiology of sphincter of Oddi dyskinesia (SOD) is not clear with fibrosis or spasm of the papillary muscles being possible etiologic factors.[77] Diagnosis is performed with manometry. So-called biliary pain as well as idiopathic pancreatitis may be the indications for endoscopic intervention.

Following the Geenen–Hogan classification, the patients are divided into three groups: in Type 1 patients, there is at least a twofold increase of liver enzymes, a delayed biliary drainage (>45 minutes) and a widening of the CBD over 12 mm. Type 2 patients must have at least one of these findings while none of these diagnostic criteria is found in Type 3 patients.[78]

While there is an agreement about the efficacy of EST with a success rate between 80% and 95% in Type 1 patients,[77] success rates are lower and more divergent in the other groups, especially in Type 3 patients. A possible reason might be that the criteria for classification are partially inadequate.[78]

EST in SOD patients is accompanied by considerably more complications than EST for stone disease; subsequent pancreatic stenting might reduce these risks.[41] The combination of biliary and pancreatic sphincterotomy is reported to further increase the clinical success in Type 2 patients from 77 to 86%.[77]

Ampullary obstruction

Apart from SOD, a short ampullary stenosis is an indication for EST, although it may be more difficult and bears higher complication and mortality rates than EST for other indications.[50]

Benign papillary tumors are rare, and adenomas are found in less than 1% of cases in autopsy series. Adenoma is considered a premalignant lesion and is therefore treated by surgical resection. Endoscopic papillectomy combined with fulguration may be an alternative.[16] It should be pointed out that some tumors are more readily detectable by endoscopy and biopsy after EST.[15]

Ampullary carcinoma is the third most common tumor causing obstructive jaundice after carcinoma of the pancreatic head and of the CBD. As this tumor is often resectable, endoscopic diagnosis and therapy are steps in the preparation for surgery, the definitive treatment that should be the goal. Besides obtaining biopsies after EST, EST with subsequent biliary decompression may contribute to improvement in the preoperative condition of the patient. In patients for whom surgery is not appropriate, endoscopic implantation of biliary endoprostheses is a palliative therapy and often improves the quality of their remaining life. In cases where the papilla is not accessible for endoscopic treatment, percutaneous transhepatic biliary drainage is the palliation of choice to avoid or minimize surgery.

Biliary drainage

Following the introduction of EST to treat choledocholithiasis, Soehendra et al[79] extended the indication for the procedure to enable palliative stent placement (success rate over 90%) in patients with unresectable malignant biliary strictures. Cancer of the head of the pancreas and primary biliary malignancies as well as metastases are the most frequent indications for stent placement, and, in rare cases, also malignant ampullary tumors.

Usually the insertion of a 10–12 Fr plastic stent is intended, but stent occlusion and migration are the main problems of plastic stents. Self-expanding metal stents have been shown to have a longer patency than plastic stents (usually about three times longer) while dislocation is extremely rare. However, because of the high costs, palliative metal stent insertion (Fig. 8.18) is recommended to be used in patients with a longer life expectancy.[80]

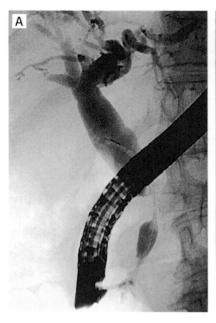

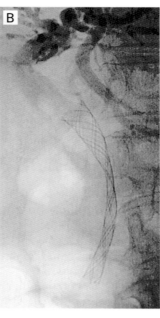

Fig. 8.18 (A) Malignant obstruction of the bile duct. (B) Palliative treatment with self-expanding metal stent.

Increasingly, endoscopic stent therapy has been extended to include patients with benign strictures. In some of these patients, the disease may be curable, with short-term relief of obstruction and a long-term possibility of cure.

Stenting produced a long-term beneficial effect (that means complete recovery of the patient) in up to 80% of the rising number of post-surgical (most important cholecystectomy and liver transplantation) strictures and leakages.[81] Inflammatory strictures in patients with primary sclerosing cholangitis also can be treated with stents, with the best success rates related to the more distal position of the dominant stricture.[81]

Long-term results of stenting in patients with biliary stenoses owing to chronic pancreatitis are not satisfactory with an incidence of about 30% of patients remaining free of the need for further stent insertion.[18,82] For these patients significantly more successful surgical approaches should always be considered in long-term treatment.[82]

Metal stents have been inserted in patients with benign strictures. As there is still a lack of controlled studies, no final recommendation can be given. But it should be kept in mind that these stents cannot be removed in most cases and therefore might provoke serious complications in patients with normal life expectancy.[83]

Pancreatic sphincterotomy

Interest in endoscopic incision of the pancreatic sphincter is developing after a long period of reluctance. Experience is not yet as extensive as with biliary sphincterotomy. Kozarek et al[84] showed that the method in the hand of an expert is safe. A concomitant biliary sphincterotomy is not necessary in the majority of patients and was performed in the above quoted study in only 35% of all patients.

Chronic obstructive pancreatitis

Pain is the most common cause for intervention; the assumed etiology is ductal hypertension, caused by a stric-

ture (Fig. 8.19). The indication for EST with subsequent dilation and/or stenting is derived from this assumption. Between 70% and 80% of the patients benefit from this procedure. However, long-term treatment with stents causes considerable side effects; therefore, in recurrent stenosis surgery always should be considered.[85]

Pancreatic duct strictures are often seen in combination with stones (Fig. 8.20). Endoscopy allows the capability of

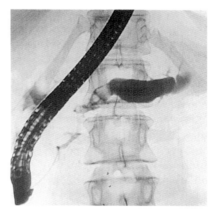

Fig. 8.19 Chronic pancreatitis with intraductal stones proximal to the stricture.

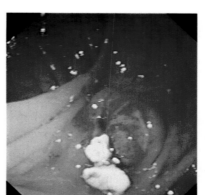

Fig. 8.20 Stones extracted from the pancreatic duct.

stone extraction after dilation of the stricture. In cases where extraction is not possible with a basket, ESWL is highly effective in the disintegration of the stone. Compared to biliary stones, in our experience, ESWL treatment is easier, particularly as the time required for the procedure is shorter. Stone visualization is mostly performed fluoroscopically, the contrast being injected through a nasopancreatic tube. In the same manner as in the biliary system, the remaining fragments after ESWL are removed endoscopically. Sufficient fragmentation is usually achieved in more than 80% and clinical improvement is seen in about 60% of the patients.[86]

Pancreas divisum

Since Cotton et al[87] claimed a relationship between pancreas divisum and pancreatitis in 1980, this association, and the question of endoscopic therapy (Fig. 8.21), has been argued in many subsequent papers.[18,85] Recent studies showed a success rate of about 75% for EST of the minor papilla in patients with pancreas divisum presenting with recurrent episodes of pancreatitis, while in patients with pancreatic-type pain, the success rate was only 25%. Taking all patients together, endoscopic treatment of the minor papilla in patients with pancreas divisum is reported to improve symptoms in 42 to 100%,[18] but this must be balanced against the risk of considerable complications (up to 15%[18]). Although again not undebated, pancreatic duct dilation seems to be a predictor for success of the therapy.[18,85]

Pancreatic pseudocysts

A recent indication for EST of the pancreatic sphincter is the endoscopic treatment of pancreatic pseudocysts. In cases with a proven connection between the ductal system and the pseudocyst, EST and subsequent insertion of a stent or nasopancreatic or nasocystic tube can be performed. Success rates between 60% and 90% are reported.[18,82,85]

A still more recent indication is the treatment in patients with pancreatic fluid collections that do not respond to conventional therapy. In these cases, a disruption or leakage in the main pancreatic duct is assumed (diagnosis by endoscopic retrograde pancreatography) and transpapillary drainage is proposed. Much more data are necessary to allow a final evaluation of this indication.

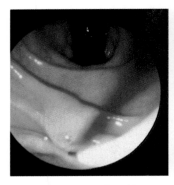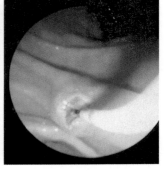

Fig. 8.21 Needle-knife sphincterotomy of the minor papilla.

LONG-TERM CONSEQUENCES OF EST

Functional alterations

After EST, the physiological barrier between the biliary system and the duodenum disappears. As a consequence, aerobilia can be found in more than 50% of all patients. But so far there have been no signs of any pathological effects.[88]

Biliary reflux after EST is common after oral contrast ingestion. However,[89] this reflux is abolished by 1 year after EST. It is unlikely that long-term problems such as malignancy might be provoked.

After biliary sphincterotomy, the duodenobiliary pressure gradient may be completely eliminated. There are, however, divergent long-term results with a partial re-establishment of the sphincter in some patients. The significance of these observations still remains unclear.[3]

After EST, the contractility of the gallbladder is enhanced, the nucleation time prolonged, and the cholesterol saturation index reduced. These data may explain the low occurrence rate of stones in the gallbladder after EST.[90]

In accordance with these results are data that patients after EST and subsequent cholecystectomy have no cholesterol crystals in spite of a high content of biliary lipids and cholesterol. A possible explanation is that the transit time is too short for cholesterol crystal formation.[91]

The composition of bile is influenced by changes in the anatomy of the extrahepatic biliary system. Cholecystectomy is followed by a rise in secondary bile acids in bile. After EST, the total bile acid pool is markedly reduced in patients with gallbladders in situ, whereas there is no significant change in pool size in patients after cholecystectomy.[92]

Bile acid composition was compared in women after EST and previous cholecystectomy with that of cholecystectomized women without EST. After EST, a significantly higher percentage of chenodeoxycholic acid was found in bile but no difference in the proportion of cholic acid. The concentration of secondary bile acids was lower in the EST group, but these differences were not statistically significant. The biliary lipid composition did not change. The authors[93] concluded that these findings are not deleterious to the biliary or gastrointestinal system.

Bacteria in the bile are found in up to 88% of patients after EST. However, the context with inflammatory alterations of the biliary system has to be further evaluated.[91]

There are no hints from follow-up studies that EST might promote occurrence of cancer of the biliary system or any other gastrointestinal organs. However, it has to be considered that the observation period still might be too short, as malignant degeneration may take a long period of time.[3] Long-term observation of patients after EST is necessary in the future.

COMPLICATIONS AND THEIR MANAGEMENT

The main complications related to EST are restenosis of the sphincter and recurrent CBD stones – in some cases accompanied by cholangitis.[3] In long-term follow-up studies, even if only patients without a gallbladder are considered, these complications are reported in 1 to 24%.[94]

In a study by Bergman et al[94] with a median follow-up of 15 years, 21/22 patients with complications suffered from symptoms of bile duct stones and the remaining one of pancreatitis. In 13 of these patients (13.8%) stones were found; moreover 9 of them also had a concomitant post-EST restenosis of the sphincter. Neither cholangitis nor malignancy was seen. Nearly all of the reported problems were managed endoscopically.

In another study by Tanaka et al[95] with a mean follow-up of 122 months, 410 patients were studied: 12.3% had stone recurrence within the bile duct, 1% had restenosis of the sphincter, about 5.5% had cholangitis, 1% had liver abscess, and 2% had cholangiocarcinoma. In patients with the gallbladder in situ, 7/32 who had gallbladder stones developed cholecystitis while this did not occur in any of the 88 patients with gallbladder in situ and no stones. In 6 patients, newly formed stones were detected. Overall 2% of these patients died, death being related to complications (1.5% cholangitis, 0.5% liver abscess).

Post-EST stenosis should be expected in 0.5 to 4% of patients. It may be associated with an inadequate primary incision, bleeding with subsequent injection of a sclerosant, but restenosis may occur in the absence of these factors.[3] A further factor of importance might be found in the primary indication for EST. Post-EST restenosis was seen about five times more frequently (16.8% vs 2.9%) in patients treated for papillary stenosis than in those treated for choledocholithiasis.[96]

Early recognition of these problems enables successful adequate endoscopic re-intervention and prevents more serious complications such as cholangitis.[3,97]

An unresolved question is what to do after EST when the gallbladder is still in situ. The necessity of cholecystectomy in a survey of several studies ranged from 2.3 to 33%.[3] In a large study, the incidence of post-EST cholecystectomy was 8.6%.[98] Risk factors for the development of gallbladder complications after EST include such events as a history of cholangitis, EST because of biliary pancreatitis, non-filling of the gallbladder during cholangiography, or the presence of stones, but the data from different studies are contradictory.[3] In accordance with Hammarström et al,[99] who reported some 31% of patients requiring cholecystectomy following acute pancreatitis, we recommend cholecystectomy for patients who have recovered from biliary pancreatitis and had been treated with EST.

In patients with the above-quoted risk factors, we tend to perform cholecystectomy after EST. In patients with none of these risk factors, age may be of importance. There are recommendations to leave the gallbladder in situ after EST in patients who are at an increased risk of surgery and in elderly patients. Hammarström[100] has suggested that the age over which cholecystectomy need not follow EST is 80 years.

ALTERNATIVES TO EST

Although it is obvious that EST causes changes in the physiology of the gastrointestinal tract, the clinical importance of these changes is unknown.

Alternative methods that produce more physiologic results are currently being investigated. Pharmacologic dilation of the sphincter for extraction of small stones has been attempted. Subsequent manometry confirmed intact sphincter function but the method did not gain widespread acceptance.[101] Balloon dilation of the papilla of Vater (Fig. 8.22) might be another alternative that could be combined with pharmacologic dilation with nitrates.

In a comparative randomized study, Bergman et al[22] showed that the success rate of balloon dilation is quite similar to EST. Also the risk of pancreatitis after dilation, as seen in an American study[102], was negligible. Therefore, and in consideration of several other studies with similar results, it can be concluded that this procedure is a valuable alternative to EST.

Combining balloon dilation with the application of isosorbide dinitrate, Minami et al[103] reported that this method can even be used in the treatment of larger stones where mechanical lithotripsy was performed before stone extraction. In this series, only 6% of patients developed mild pancreatitis.

In spite of a number of studies, all showing quite satisfactory results after balloon dilation of the papilla, Bergman & Huibregtse[104] state in a recent editorial that 'only the presence of risk factors for bleedings seems to be a clear-cut indication' for this method of stone extraction.

Besides impeded coagulation, there are some situations where dilation may be preferable to EST, such as the location of the papilla within a diverticulum or some other difficult anatomical situations, e.g. after Billroth II operation (Fig. 8.23). Moreover, it can be considered in patients with post-EST restenosis when repeated EST seems too dangerous.

At present, dilation without EST can be considered in patients with choledocholithiasis, but there is a lack of data for its use in other situations.

Finally, it should be pointed out that this seemingly easier and less dangerous appearing procedure should only be

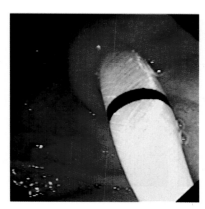

Fig. 8.22 Balloon dilation of the papilla: endoscopic view.

performed by endoscopists who are fully capable of performing EST in case a switch of the methods becomes necessary.

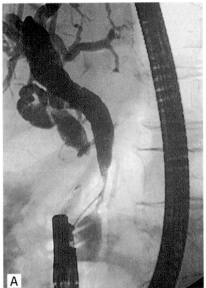

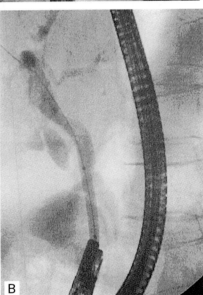

Fig. 8.23 Patient with Billroth II resection with distal common bile duct stenosis (**A**) treated with balloon dilation (**B**).

CHECKLIST OF PRACTICE POINTS

1. Before the investigation:
   - Check the patient's history, e.g. whether there has been previous surgical intervention
   - Check the patient's clinical status (general condition, clinical chemistry, coagulation parameters, risk factors for the planned intervention)
   - Check the necessity for the use of antibiotics
   - Check potential allergies (drugs, disinfectants, dressings)
   - Check that the patient has been fully informed and ask for written consent
   - Check the indication again
   - Check less risky, possible alternatives
   - Check instruments (especially the electrosurgical equipment)
   - Check available facilities for coping with an emergency, including endotracheal intubation and resuscitation.
2. Perform the ERCP. After sufficient filling of the ducts, re-evaluate the indication for EST.
3. Do not prolong the duration of investigation; it is preferable to schedule a second session if difficulties are encountered. A change of investigators should be considered early.
4. Avoid repeated cannulations of the pancreatic duct and overfilling with contrast agent.
5. Avoid papillary swelling by intramural injections of contrast agent – that means be patient with contrast application until the catheter or the papillotome is in a really good position.
6. Before EST, be sure that the correct duct is intubated (documentation).
7. Be sure that the direction of the cut is correct and that the sphincterotome is not introduced too deeply.
8. Make sure that after EST the efflux of contrast agent is sufficient, otherwise place a stent or a nasobiliary tube.
9. After endoscopy, ensure careful monitoring of the patient's condition.
10. If EST was performed on an ambulatory basis, inform the patient again after the procedure about the possible occurrence of symptoms, the most important of which are pancreatitis and delayed onset of bleeding. Explain to the patient what to do and where to go in these situations.

REFERENCES

1. Classen M, Demling L. Endoskopische Sphinkterotomie der Papilla Vateri und Steinextraktion aus dem Ductus choledochus. Dtsch Med Wochenschr 1974; 99:496–497.

2. Kawai K, Akaska Y, Murakami K, et al. Endoscopic sphincterotomy of the ampulla of Vater. Gastrointest Endosc 1974; 20:148–151.

3. Frimberger E. Long-term sequelae of endoscopic papillotomy. Endoscopy 1998; 30(Suppl 2):A221–A227.

4. Cotton PB, Geenen JE, Sherman S, et al. Endoscopic sphincterotomy for stones by experts is safe, even in younger patients with normal ducts. Ann Surg 1998; 227:201–204.

5. Tarnasky PR, Tagge EP, Hebra A, et al. Minimally invasive therapy for choledocholithiasis in children. Gastrointest Endosc 1998; 47:189–192.

6. Rhodes M, Sussman L, Cohen L, et al. Randomised trial of laparoscopic exploration of common bile duct versus postoperative endoscopic retrograde cholangiography for common bile duct stones. Lancet 1998; 351:159–161.

7. Gogel HK, Runyon BA, Volpicelli NA, et al. Acute suppurative obstructive cholangitis due to stones: treatment by urgent endoscopic sphincterotomy. Gastrointest Endosc 1987; 33:210–213.

8. Classen M, Sandschin W, Born P, et al. 20 years experience in the endoscopic therapy of acute biliary cholangitis: a meta-analysis. Endoscopy 1997; 29:E52.

9. Neoptolemos JP, Carr-Locke DL, London NJ, et al. Controlled trial of urgent endoscopic retrograde cholangiopancreatography and endoscopic sphincterotomy versus conservative treatment for acute pancreatitis due to gallstones. Lancet 1988; ii:979–983.

10. Fan ST, Lai ECS, Mok FP, et al. Early treatment of acute biliary pancreatitis by endoscopic papillotomy. N Engl J Med 1993; 328:228–232.

11. Nowak A, Nowakowska-Dulawa E, Marek TA, et al. Final results of the prospective randomized controlled study on endoscopic sphincterotomy versus conventional management in acute biliary pancreatitis. Gastroenterology 1998; 108:A380.

12. Fölsch UR, Nitsche R, Lüdtke R, et al, and the German Study Group on Acute Biliary Pancreatitis. Early ERCP and papillostomy compared with conservative treatment for acute biliary pancreatitis. N Engl J Med 1997; 336:237–242.

13. Al Karawi MA, El Sheikh Mohamed AR, Sultan Khurro M, et al. Bedeutung der Endoskopie in der Diagnostik und Therapie gastrointestinaler und biliärer Parasiten. Internist 1988; 29:807–814.

14. Baker AR, Neoptolemos JP, Carr-Locke DL, et al. Sump syndrome following choledochoduodenostomy and its endoscopic treatment. Br J Surg 1985; 72:433–435.

15. Huibregtse K, Tytgat GNJ. Carcinoma of the ampulla of Vater: the endoscopic approach. Endoscopy 1988; 20:223–226.

16. Bickerstaff KI, Berry AR, Chapman RW, et al. Endoscopic sphincterotomy for the palliation of ampullary carcinoma. Br J Surg 1990; 77:160–162.

17. Geenen JE, Hogan WJ, Dodds WJ, et al. The efficacy of endoscopic sphincterotomy after cholecystectomy in patients with sphincter-of-Oddi dysfunction. N Engl J Med 1989; 320:82–87.

18. Huibregtse K, Smits ME. Endoscopic management of diseases of the pancreas. Am J Gastroenterol 1994; 89:S66–S77.

19. Bethge N. EPT bei Patienten mit Billroth-II-Situation – Verwendung eines neuen modifizierten Erlanger Papillotoms mit B-II-Adaption. Endosk Heute 1993; 1:56.

20. Martin DF, England R, Martin O. The safety sphincterotome: the device, the technique and preliminary results. Endoscopy 1998; 30:375–378.

21. Kozarek RA, Raltz SL, Ball TJ, et al. Reuse of disposable sphincterotomes for diagnostic and therapeutic ERCP: a one-year prospective study. Gastrointest Endosc 1999; 49:39–42.

22. Bergman JJGHM, Rauws EAJ, Fockens P, et al. Randomised trial of endoscopic balloon dilatation versus endoscopic sphincterotomy for removal of bile duct stones. Lancet 1997; 349:1124–1129.

23. Lazzaroni M, Biancho-Porro G. Premedication, preparation and surveillance. Endoscopy 1999; 31:2–8.

24. Rey JR, Axon A, Budzynska A, et al. Guidelines of the European Society of Gastrointestinal Endoscopy (ESGE): Antibiotic prophylaxis for gastrointestinal endoscopy. Endoscopy 1998; 30:318–324.

25. Silverstein FE, Deltenre M, Tytgat G, et al. An endoscopic Doppler probe: preliminary clinical evaluation. Ultrasound Med Biol 1985; 11:347–353.

26. Neuhaus H, Hagenmüller F, Lauer R, et al. A prospective randomized trial of the influence of suprapapillary Doppler ultrasound on endoscopic sphincterotomy. Gastrointest Endosc 1991; 37:253A.

27. Ramirez FC, Dennert B, Sanowski RA. Success of repeat ERCP by the same endoscopist. Gastrointest Endosc 1999; 49:58–61.

28. Bruins Slot W, Schoeman MN, Disario JA, et al. Needle-knife sphincterotomy as a precut procedure: a retrospective evaluation of efficacy and complications. Endoscopy 1996; 28:334–339.

29. Rabenstein T, Ruppert T, Schneider TH, et al. Benefits and risks of needle-knife papillotomy. Gastrointest Endosc 1997; 46:207–211.

30. O'Connor HJ, Bhutta AS, Redmond PL, et al. Suprapapillary fistulosphincterotomy at ERCP: a prospective study. Endoscopy 1997; 29:266–270.

31. Farrell RJ, Khan MI, Noonan N, et al. Endoscopic papillectomy: a novel approach to difficult cannulation. Gut 1996; 39:36–38.

32. Sherman S, Uzer MF, Lehman GA. Wire-guided sphincterotomy. Am J Gastroenterol 1994; 89:2125–2129.

33. Elton E, Howell DA, Parsons WG, et al. Endoscopic pancreatic sphincterotomy: indications, outcome, and a safe stentless technique. Gastrointest Endosc 1998; 47:240–249.

34. Ho KY, Montes H, Sossenheimer MJ, et al. Features that may predict hospital admission following outpatient therapeutic ERCP. Gastrointest Endosc 1999; 49:587–592.

35. Freeman ML, Nelson DN, Sherman S, et al, the Multicenter Endoscopic Sphincterotomy (MESH) Study Group. Same-day discharge after endoscopic biliary sphincterotomy: observations from a prospective multicenter complication study. Gastrointest Endosc 1999; 49:580–586.

36. Howell DA, Oringer JA, Ku PM, et al. Overnight hospitalization following endoscopic sphincterotomy produces a higher quality outcome. Gastrointest Endosc 1999; 49:AB217.

37. Freeman ML, Nelson DB, Sherman S, et al. Complications of endoscopic biliary sphincterotomy. N Engl J Med 1996; 335:909–918.

38. Lambert ME, Betts CH, Hill JD, et al. Endoscopic sphincterotomy, the whole truth. Br J Surg 1991; 78:473–476.

39. Tittobello A. Diagnosis and prevention of post-ERCP pancreatitis. Endoscopy 1997; 29:285–287.

40. Mehta SN, Pavone E, Barkun JS, et al. Predictors of post-ERCP complications in patients with suspected choledocholithiasis. Endoscopy 1998; 30:457–463.

41. Tarnasky PR, Palesch YY, Cunningham JT, et al. Pancreatic stenting prevents pancreatitis after biliary sphincterotomy in patients with sphincter of Oddi dysfunction. Gastroenterology 1998; 115:1518–1524.

42. Elta GH, Barnett JL, Wille RT, et al. Pure cut electrocautery current for sphincterotomy causes less post-procedure pancreatitis than blended current. Gastrointest Endosc 1998; 47:149–153.

43. Cavallini G, Titobello A, Frulloni L, et al, and the Gabexate in Digestive Endoscopy Italian Group. Gabexate for the prevention of pancreatic damage related to endoscopic retrograde cholangiopancreatography. N Engl J Med 1996; 335:919–923.

44. Dumot JA, Conwell DL, O'Connor JB, et al. Pretreatment with methylprednisolone to prevent ERCP-induced pancreatitis: a randomized, multicenter, placebo-controlled clinical trial. Am J Gastroenterol 1998; 93:61–65.

45. Bordas JM, Toledo-Pimentel V, Llach J, et al. Effects of bolus somatostatin in preventing pancreatitis after endoscopic pancreatography: results of a randomized study. Gastrointest Endosc 1998; 47:230–234.

46. Rabenstein T, Ell C, Franke B, et al. Kann eine niedrig-dosierte Antikoagulation das Risiko einer akuten Pankreatitis nach endoskopischer Sphinkterotomie (EST) senken? Z Gastroenterol 1998; 36:721.

47. Costamagna G. What to do when the papilla bleeds after endoscopic sphincterotomy. Endoscopy 1998; 30:40–42.

48. Boujaoude J, Pelletier G, Fritsch J, et al. Management of clinically relevant bleeding following endoscopic sphincterotomy. Endoscopy 1994; 26:217–221.

49. Dunham F, Bourgeois N, Gelin M, et al. Retroperitoneal perforation following endoscopic sphincterotomy. Endoscopy 1982; 14:92–96.

50. Sherman S, Ruffolo TA, Hawes RH, et al. Complications of endoscopic sphincterotomy. Gastroenterology 1991; 101:1068–1075.

51. Lambiase RE, Cronan JJ, Ridlen M. Perforation of the common bile duct during endoscopic sphincterotomy: recognition on computed tomography and successful percutaneous treatment. Gastrointest Radiol 1989; 14:133–136.

52. Kuhlman JE, Fishman EK, Docidigan F, et al. Complications of endoscopic retrograde sphincterotomy: CT evaluation. Gastrointest Radiol 1989; 14:127–132.

53. Tanaka M, Konomi H, Matsunaga H, et al. Endoscopic sphincterotomy for common bile duct stones: impact of recent technical advances. J Hep Bil Pancr Surg 1997; 4:16–19.

54. Safrany L, Neuhaus B, Portocarreror G, et al. Endoscopic sphincterotomy in patients with Billroth II gastrectomy. Endoscopy 1980; 12:16–22.

55. Hintze RE, Adler A, Veltzke W, et al. Endoscopic access to the papilla of Vater for endoscopic retrograde cholangiopancreatography in patients with Billroth II or Roux-en-Y gastrojejunostomy. Endoscopy 1997; 29:69–73.

56. Lehman GA, Sherman S, Nisi R, et al. Pancreas divisum: results of minor papilla sphincterotomy. Gastrointest Endosc 1993; 39:1–8.

57. Jacob L, Geenen JE, Catalano MF, et al. Clinical presentation and short-term outcome of endoscopic therapy of patients with symptomatic incomplete pancreas divisum. Gastrointest Endosc 1999; 49:53–57.

58. Bergman JJGHM, Rauws EAJ, Tijssen JGP, et al. Biliary endoprostheses in elderly patients with endoscopically irretrievable common bile duct stones: report on 117 patients. Gastrointest Endosc 1995; 42:195–201.

59. Farca A, Aguilar ME, Rodriguez G, et al. Biliary stents as temporary treatment for choledocholithiasis in pregnant patients. Gastrointest Endosc 1997; 46:99–101.

60. Weizel A, Stiehl A, Raedsch R. Passage of a large bilirubin stone through a narrow papillotomy. Endoscopy 1980; 12:191–193.

61. Schneider MU, Metek W, Bauer R, et al. Mechanical lithotripsy of bile duct stones in 209 patients. Effect Tech Adv Endosc 1988; 20:248–253.

62. Nakajima M, Yasuda K, Cho E, et al. Endoscopic sphincterotomy and mechanical basket lithotripsy for management of difficult common bile duct stones. J Hep Pancr Surg 1997; 4:5–10.

63. Sauerbruch T, Holl J, Sackmann M, et al. Fragmentation of bile duct stones by extracorporeal shock-wave lithotripsy: a five year experience. Hepatology 1992; 15:208–214.

64. Harz C, Henkel TO, Köhrmann KU, et al. Extracorporeal shock-wave lithotripsy and endoscopy: combined therapy for problematic bile duct stones. Surg Endosc 1991; 5:196–199.

65. Born P, Neuhaus H, Classen M. Cholangioscopic laser lithotripsy of common bile duct stones – an overview. J Hep Pancr Surg 1997; 4:11–15.

66. Neuhaus H, Zillinger C, Born P, et al. Randomized study of intracorporeal laser lithotripsy versus extracorporeal shock-wave lithotripsy for difficult bile duct stones. Gastrointest Endosc 1998; 47:327–334.

67. Dumas R, Le Gall P, Hastier P, et al. The role of endoscopic retrograde cholangiopancreatography in the management of hepatic hydatid disease. Endoscopy 1999; 31:242–247.

68. Hallstone A, Triadafilopoulos G. 'Spontaneous sump syndrome': successful treatment by duodenoscopic sphincterotomy. Am J Gastroenterol 1990; 85:1518–1520.

69. Lai ECS, Mok FPT, Tan ESY, et al. Endoscopic biliary drainage for severe acute cholangitis. N Engl J Med 1992; 326:1528–1586.

70. Boender J, Nix GAJJ, de Ridder MAJ, et al. Endoscopic sphincterotomy and biliary drainage in patients with cholangitis due to common bile duct stones. Am J Gastroenterol 1995; 90:233–238.

71. Leung JW, Ling TK, Chan RC, et al. Antibiotics, biliary sepsis, and bile duct stones. Gastrointest Endosc 1994; 40:716–721.

72. Opie EL. The etiology of acute hemorrhagic pancreatitis. Johns Hopkins Hosp Bull 1901; 121:182.

73. Lux G, Riemann JF, Demling L. Biliäre Pankreatitis – Diagnostische und therapeutische Möglichkeiten durch ERCP und endoskopische Papillotomie. Z Gastroenterol 1984; 22:246–256.

74. Williamsen RCN. Endoscopic sphincterotomy in the early treatment of acute pancreatitis. N Engl J Med 1997; 328:279–280.

75. Tarnasky PR, Cotton PB. Early ERCP and papillotomy for acute biliary pancreatitis. N Engl J Med 1997; 336:1835.

76. Bassi C, Falconi M, Talamini G, et al. Controlled clinical trial of perfloxacin versus imipenem in severe acute pancreatitis. Gastroenterology 1998; 115:1513–1517.

77. Gottlieb K, Sherman S, Lehman GA. Therapeutic biliary endoscopy. Endoscopy 1996; 28:113–130.

78. Botoman VA, Kozarek RA, Novell LA, et al. Long-term outcome after endoscopic sphincterotomy in patients with biliary colic and suspected sphincter of Oddi dysfunction. Gastrointest Endosc 1994; 40:165–170.

79. Soehendra N, Reynders-Frederix V. Palliative bile duct drainage – a new endoscopic transpapillary drainage. Endoscopy 1980; 12:8–11.

80. Huibregtse J. Plastic or expandable biliary endoprostheses. Scand J Gastroenterol 1993; 28(Suppl 200):3–7.

81. Smith MT, Sherman S, Lehman GA. Endoscopic management of benign strictures of the biliary tree. Endoscopy 1995; 27:253–266.

82. Smits ME, Rauws EAJ, van Gulik TM, et al. Long-term results of endoscopic stenting and surgical drainage for biliary stricture due to chronic pancreatitis. Br J Surg 1996; 83:764–768.

83. Dumonceau JM, Deviere J, Delhaye M, et al. Plastic and metal stents for postoperative benign bile duct strictures: the best and the worst. Gastrointest Endosc 1998; 47:8–16.

84. Kozarek RA, Ball TJ, Patterson DJ, et al. Endoscopic pancreatic duct sphincterotomy: indications, technique, and analysis of results. Gastrointest Endosc 1994; 40:592–598.

85. Kaikaus RM, Geenen JE. Current role of ERCP in the management of benign pancreatic disease. Endoscopy 1996; 28:131–137.

86. Schneider HT, Andrea M, Benninger J, et al. Piezoelectric shock-wave lithotripsy of pancreatic duct stones. Am J Gastroenterol 1994; 89:2042–2048.

87. Cotton PB. Congenital anomaly of pancreas divisum as the cause of obstructive pain and pancreatitis. Gut 1980; 2:105.

88. Burmeister W, Wurbs D, Hagenmüller F, et al. Langzeituntersuchungen nach endoskopischer Papillotomie (EPT). Z Gastroenterol 1980; 18:527–531.

89. Sugiyama M, Atomi Y. Does endoscopic sphincterotomy cause prolonged pancreatobiliary reflux? Am J Gastroenterol 1999; 94:795–798.

90. Sharma BC, Agarwal DK, Baijal SS, et al. Effect of endoscopic sphincterotomy on gall bladder bile lithogenicity and motility. Gut 1998; 42:288–292.

91. Bergman JJGHM, van Berkel AM, Groen AK, et al. Biliary manometry, bacterial characteristics, bile composition and histological changes fifteen to seventeen years after endoscopic sphincterotomy. Gastrointest Endosc 1997; 45:400–405.

92. Sauerbruch T, Stellaard F, Baumgartner G. Effect of endoscopic sphincterotomy on bile acid pool; size and bile lipid composition in man. Digestion 1983; 27:87–92.

93. Stellaard F, Sauerbruch T, Brunholzl C, et al. Bile acid pattern and cholesterol saturation of bile after cholecystectomy and endoscopic sphincterotomy. Digestion 1983; 26:153–158.

94. Bergman JJGHM, van der Mey S, Rauws EAJ, et al. Long-term follow-up after endoscopic sphincterotomy for bile duct stones in patients younger than 60 years of age. Gastrointest Endosc 1996; 44:643–649.

95. Tanaka M, Takahata S, Konomi H, et al. Long-term consequence of endoscopic sphincterotomy for bile duct stones. Gastrointest Endosc 1998; 48:465–469.

96. Seifert E. Long-term follow-up after endoscopic sphincterotomy (EST). Endoscopy 1988; 20:232–235.

97. Sugiyama M, Atomi Y. Follow-up of more than 10 years after endoscopic sphincterotomy for choledocholithiasis in young patients. Br J Surg 1998; 85:917–921.

98. Siegel JH, Safrany L, Ben-Zvi JS, et al. Duodenoscopic sphincterotomy in patients with gallbladders in situ: report of a series of 1272 patients. Am J Gastroenterol 1988; 83:1255–1258.

99. Hammarström LE, Stridbeck H, Ihse I. Effect of endoscopic sphincterotomy and interval cholecystectomy on late outcome after gallstone pancreatitis. Br J Surg 1998; 85:333–336.

100. Hammarström LE, Holmin T, Stridbeck H. Endoscopic treatment of bile duct calculi in patients with gallbladder in situ. Scand J Gastroenterol 1996; 31:294–301.

101. Ibuki Y, Kudo M, Todo A. Endoscopic retrograde extraction of common bile duct stones with drip infusion of isosorbide dinitrate. Gastrointest Endosc 1992; 38:178–180.

102. Kozarek RA. Balloon dilatation of the sphincter of Oddi. Endoscopy 1988; 20(Suppl):207–210.

103. Minami A, Maeta T, Kohi F, et al. Endoscopic papillary dilatation and isosorbide dinitrate drip infusion for removing bile duct stone. Scand J Gastroenterol 1998; 33:765–768.

104. Bergman JJGHM, Huibregtse K. What is the current state of endoscopic balloon dilatation for stone removal. Endoscopy 1998; 30:43–45.

9.1

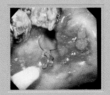

BILIARY TRACT STONE DISEASE: TRANSPAPILLARY ENDOSCOPIC MANAGEMENT

GREGORY B. HABER

ALESSANDRO REPICI

Among all therapeutic endoscopic procedures, perhaps the most gratifying is the sudden relief of symptoms following common bile duct (CBD) stone removal in the patient with acute cholangitis. A quarter of a century has passed since the first reports of this technique in the Western[1] and Japanese[2] literature in 1974 and many of the earlier challenges have now been resolved. Although 85 to 90% of the duct stones are removed in a 'routine' fashion, the *problematic* stones – intrahepatic, impacted, and giant – and *problematic* anatomy – Billroth II, diverticulum, and stones above strictures – are now the main challenge for current technology and endoscopic dexterity. This chapter will review the current state of the art in routine as well as advanced techniques of stone removal, with the exception of the management of intrahepatic stones which will be dealt with in Chapter 9.2.

INDICATIONS

In the post-cholecystectomy patient today, the presence of bile duct stones mandates an endoscopic approach because of the very high success rate,[3,4] efficiency and cost-containment when performed on an outpatient basis,[5] and acceptable complication rates for sphincterotomy for this indication.[6] There is rarely a role for laparoscopic or open surgery because of the widespread availability of advanced techniques and expertise in endoscopic stone removal. The failure of stone extraction owing to difficulties in cannulation, or because of the size and location of the stone at an initial attempt by routine endoscopy should no longer be considered as an indication for surgical intervention. Patients are best served in this situation by referral to an expert endoscopist with the necessary equipment to manage difficult stones, even when this requires substantial travel.

In the patient with a gallbladder in situ, in whom cholecystectomy is planned, the treatment algorithm may be quite different depending on the relative availability of endoscopic and laparoscopic skills and the relative probability of finding CBD stone(s). Other factors which impact on this decision include: the severity of symptoms such as septic shock, or severe biliary pancreatitis which may dictate immediate endoscopic decompression; the timing of surgery which may be due to patient factors such as pregnancy or comorbid illness as with a recent myocardial infarction or lack of available operating room time with surgery deferred for several weeks. In these situations, timely endoscopic removal may be in the best interests of the patient.

In an institution in which there are highly skilled endoscopists as well as laparoscopic surgeons experienced in CBD exploration, the treatment plan is predicated on the relative likelihood of finding a CBD stone, based on routine transabdominal ultrasound imaging and routine liver biochemistry. When the probability is low, operative cholangiography is performed followed by laparoscopic stone removal by those surgeons skilled in this technique or followed by postoperative endoscopic stone removal if laparoscopic removal is considered unusually difficult or would require laparotomy. When the probability is moderate or high, preoperative endoscopic removal is performed with laparoscopic common duct exploration reserved for those with failed extraction. The level of certainty in stone prediction clearly impacts on this approach and in the case of low or moderate probability, further imaging such as magnetic resonance cholangiopancreatography, tomographic intravenous infusion cholangiography or endoscopic ultrasound may be undertaken.

Many factors specific to the patient, physician, or institution may alter the strategies undertaken, not the least of which is the relative cost of the treatment chosen. This may vary by a factor of five- to tenfold in different countries, when the professional fees and costs of inpatient or outpatient management are considered.

Thus the treatment algorithm must be rationalized on the basis of factors specific to the individual situation.

CONTRAINDICATIONS

There are few contraindications to endoscopic transpapillary stone removal. The presence of a critical comorbid illness, especially cardiopulmonary, may limit the ability to safely administer sedation or to perform the procedure in the fluoroscopy suite. If the indication dictates urgent intervention, it can be performed in an intensive care unit setting, with C-arm portable fluoroscopy or without fluoroscopy. In the case of the latter, aspiration of bile may be sufficient to confirm biliary cannulation and to permit at least the insertion of a stent for relief of acute obstruction until the patient is stable enough for stone removal.

There may be anatomical factors which prevent endoscopic access to the papilla. The usual reason is a Roux-en-Y choledochojejunostomy with an intact stomach and duodenum. This requires passage of the endoscope past the ligament of Treitz into the jejunum.[7] The jejunojejunal anastomosis is approximately 20–40 cm beyond the ligament and the roux limb itself may be 30–60 cm in length. This distance can almost never be traversed by a duodenoscope and in only about 50% of the time when using a pediatric colonoscope or enteroscope.

Intubation may be impeded by a significant stenosis not amenable to dilation sufficient for scope passage. In a case of tracheoesophageal stenosis caused by radiation, we were only able to achieve endoscopic access through a percutaneous gastrostomy, following dilation of the tract and introduction of a 9 mm gastroscope which could be retroflexed in the duodenum to allow sphincterotomy and stone removal.[8] Common strictures in the esophagus or pyloric channel can usually be adequately dilated for passage of the diagnostic duodenoscope. The same is true for narrowing caused by a prior vertical-banded gastroplasty in morbid obesity.

Coagulopathy owing to underlying liver disease, or anticoagulant therapy is a contraindication for sphincterotomy. We do not cut with a prothrombin time of more than 15 seconds or with an international normalized ratio greater than 1.2 and platelets must be at least 50 000. In the presence of portal hypertension, more stringent guidelines should be applied. When these abnormalities are not correctable or there is not enough time for correction, endoscopic drainage is undertaken using stents or nasobiliary tubes. The option of balloon dilation of the sphincter can be considered and this is discussed elsewhere in this book.

EQUIPMENT

Endoscopes

The current generation of video duodenoscopes include two basic designs with a smaller caliber (11–11.5 mm) 'diagnostic' scope with an operating channel of 2.8–3.2 mm or a larger caliber (12–12.5 mm) scope with an operating channel of 3.7–4.2 mm. The therapeutic duodenoscope is used now as a multipurpose instrument and has a grooved elevator to enhance the control of the accessories, eliminating the need for smaller diagnostic scope for routine use. However, the smaller diameter scope may be needed for traversing strictured segments or to negotiate tightly angled loops as in the afferent limb of a Billroth II anastomosis. In addition, when fine movements are needed as with minor papilla cannulation, the smaller scope has an advantage with better elevator control of the accessory. Higher resolution video prototype systems should have an advantage for visualization and targeting the minor papillary orifice. Finally, in the pediatric population, the diagnostic scope is suitable for infants and children over 5 kg. For infants of less than 5 kg, a prototype specialized ultrathin pediatric duodenoscope is available as well.[9,10]

In 'mother–baby' endoscopy, babyscopes of 8 and 9 Fr diameter can be advanced through the therapeutic duodenoscope. The most widely used baby endoscope, the Olympus CHF-B20, is 4.5 mm in external diameter at its distal end with a 1.7 mm working channel and with two-way angulation of 160° up and 100° down. It requires a dedicated mother scope with a 5.5 mm channel (Fig. 9.1.1). The large operating channel in such a scope does not provide adequate control of the usual accessories which prevents using it for other purposes.[11]

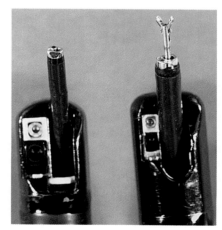

Fig. 9.1.1
(**Left**) Therapeutic duodenoscope with a 9 Fr babyscope. (**Right**) Motherscope with a 5.5 mm channel and a 4.2 mm babyscope.

To date, there has been limited experience with an Olympus video-chip baby cholangioscope (XCHF-B200, 4.5 mm outer diameter with a 1.2 mm working channel), that has remarkable image quality and a large field of view.[12]

Several prototype smaller caliber babyscopes have been developed with the purpose of incorporating the following features:

1. an external diameter small enough to permit passage through the accessory channel of a routine therapeutic duodenoscope (3.7–4.2 mm)
2. improved illumination and resolution
3. two-way angulation
4. incorporation of an operating channel with specialized ultrathin accessories. An example is a fine caliber flexible miniscope (2.09 mm external diameter with a 0.72 mm operating channel) recently developed for bile duct cannulation without papillotomy.[13] This miniscope is not steerable and is mainly for diagnostic purpose.

Accessories

Sphincterotomes or dilating balloons for sphincter ablation are dealt with in Chapter 8.

Baskets and balloons

Retrieval baskets are available in a variety of sizes and designs. There are four-wire square baskets with or without a Nitinol core, as well as spiral designs, used most often for entrapment of small stones. The baskets are available as a disposable single-use item or sterilizable and reusable. Standard retrieval baskets come in sizes of 2 by 4 or 3 by 6 cm in diameter but occasionally custom-made giant baskets 4 by 8 cm or larger can be ordered as needed. The baskets are constructed by design to break at the head or tip of the basket under excessive force. A rupture releases the stone from the basket when the breaking pressure, generated by the mechanical lithotriptor is reached.

Wire-guided baskets are available in two designs. A double-lumen catheter allows the basket and guidewire to be advanced down separate channels. When a single-lumen catheter is used, the tip of the basket must be small enough to allow complete withdrawal of the basket, then insertion of a guidewire to advance the catheter to the desired location followed by an exchange of the wire for the basket. Most of the wire-guided basket systems do not seem to function as well as the standard baskets. They are stiffer, deform easily, and do not have the durability of the regular baskets.

Wire-guided high-compliance retrieval balloons come in diameters of 5–18 mm. These are remarkably break-resistant considering the traction forces generated by pulling on them. Owing to the changing caliber of the duct at different levels, the balloon is often deformed as it is pulled into the more narrow distal duct and partial deflation of up to 25% of the volume is permissible without collapse of the balloon. In a double-lumen balloon, contrast may be injected through the wire channel when the wire is withdrawn or alongside the wire when a side-arm (Tuohy–Borst) valve is used. There are dedicated triple lumen balloons with a separate contrast injection port but the lumen size is very narrow and a small 5–10 mL syringe should be used to generate adequate pressure for injection. Hybrid devices such as the 'balloon-tome' have been developed incorporating a retrieval balloon onto the sphincterotome catheter. However, these are clumsy and expensive and have not been adopted for regular use.

Mechanical lithotriptors

The first effective mechanical lithotriptor was described by Demling et al in 1982.[14] It was composed of a hard wire basket, removable Teflon sheath, outer metal sheath, and a handle with a winding mechanism.

Nowadays, two principal designs of mechanical lithotriptor are available either for use outside the scope (OTS) or through the scope (TTS).

The OTS system was developed by Soehendra and is used as a rescue device when a stone is entrapped in a basket but cannot be pulled through the sphincter after sphincterotomy. This system requires removal of the handle usually by cutting it off with pliers or in other systems by unscrewing a detachable handle (Fig. 9.1.2). Once the handle is off, the scope is removed over the wire and under fluoroscopic guidance a semi-rigid tubular coil is advanced over the basket wire. A winch device is then used to tighten the wire attached to the basket. As the basket closes, it breaks the stone which is crushed against the metal coil (Fig. 9.1.3).

There are three types of TTS mechanical lithotripsy systems. The simplest of these is a dedicated single-use lithotriptor (Monolith, Microvasive, Natick, Mass.) with a basket inside a tubular steel coil attached to an ergonomically designed 'pistol-grip' handle. The basket is opened to capture the stone, and the stone is fractured by pumping the grip repetitively. The major flaw in this

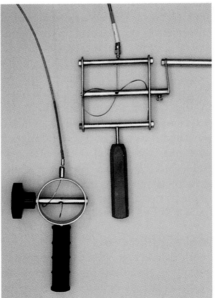

Fig. 9.1.2 Handles for outside-the-scope mechanical lithotripsy.

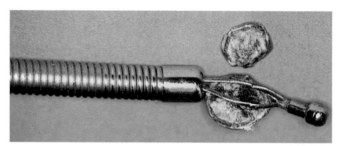

Fig. 9.1.3 Mechanical lithotripsy with a Soehendra outside-the-scope lithotriptor. The stone is fragmented by pulling the basket against the metal sheath.

design is the stiff straight nature of the metal sheath which poses difficulties in cannulation, much the same as during attempts at passing a biopsy forceps up the duct but with far less flexibility. Similarly, manipulation of the basket within the duct and around the stone is limited. However, when the anatomy is favorable, the simplicity of the design has merit.

The most commonly used device is the Olympus triple layer lithotriptor. This unit is comprised of a basket within a polyethylene sheath which is passed through the tubular steel coil. The basket and sheath can be employed in the usual manner as with standard baskets, allowing for greater manipulation and easier capture of the stone, prior to advancing the stiff outer steel coil. Contrast can be injected but with difficulty and smaller syringes should be used to generate greater force. The Olympus lithotriptor is supplied in two sizes, a smaller 7 Fr device which can be used with a 3.2 mm channel diagnostic scope and a larger size for a therapeutic scope (BML4Q and BML3Q respectively, Olympus, Tokyo). Initially, these were cumbersome to handle and to assemble but these problems have been minimized with the introduction of a pre-assembled single-use version.

There are also standard basket systems which can be supplemented by mechanical lithotripsy systems when the need arises during stone extraction. In order to permit any of the standard basket systems to be converted to use with the mechanical lithotripsy system, the essential elements are a detachable handle and a basket wire long enough (>400 cm) to permit removal of the plastic sheath outside the scope, allowing it to be replaced by a steel cable over the wire. One such system (Pauldrach, Germany) has a screw joint at the handle end of the basket wire to which a wire extension can be added. The other system (Erlangen, Germany) uses an extra-long wire basket over which the handle is advanced and secured by a pin-vise for routine use. When the lithotripsy coil is needed the vise can be loosened to remove the handle so that the coil can be advanced over the wire.

Intraductal shockwave lithotriptors

Specialized catheters with delivery of a shockwave to the surface of the stone permit intraductal fragmentation of large stones. Either electrical energy or laser wavelengths are used to fracture stones.

The most commonly utilized device is an electro-hydraulic generator (Northgate SD100, Northgate Technologies Inc., Arlington Heights, Illinois, USA; Lithotron EL-23, Walz Electronics, Germany) which delivers high voltage to the coaxial tip of a probe with a ring electrode around the circumference and a central wire electrode to form a spark-gap for delivery of the energy. The shockwave created is best transmitted and contained within a fluid medium. The shockwave energy rapidly disperses, requiring contact of the probe with the stone surface to be effective. Inadvertent contact with tissue can cause damage to the duct wall with possible perforation, limiting the use of this device to direct visualization under choledochoscopic control. The electro-hydraulic probes are 1.9, 3, or 4.5 Fr in diameter and can be passed through babyscopes with channels of 0.75, 1.2 and 1.7 mm, respectively. The 1.9 Fr probe delivers sufficient energy and is preferred as it may be used with channel sizes as small as 0.75 mm, and with larger channels permits easy coaxial irrigation of saline.

The earlier laser systems used either a thermal effect to rapidly vaporize fluid within the stone matrix or created a shockwave at the surface, by rapid expansion of gas or non-thermal shockwaves using very short laser pulse duration (Fig. 9.1.4). An example of the former is a traditional Nd:YAG laser which has been abandoned because of lack of efficacy, and more recently a Holmium

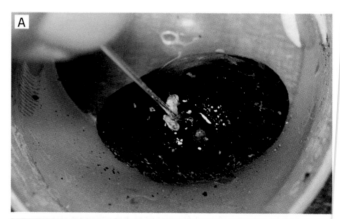

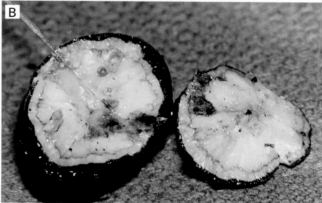

Fig. 9.1.4 (A) Quartz laser fiber applied to a pigment stone for delivery of Nd:YAG laser energy. **(B)** Fragmentation of a gallstone following laser lithotripsy.

laser, popular among urologists and more successful. An example of the latter is the pulsed flashlamp dye laser (504 nm wavelength) which is safer with much less risk of duct damage when there is inadvertent discharge during contact of the probe with the duct wall.

Two newer laser design systems have been developed which have eliminated the risk of soft tissue damage and thus do not require direct visualization with a babyscope but can be discharged under fluoroscopic control. One system is a pulsed flashlamp rhodamine dye laser which employs an automated stone-tissue recognition system based on the character of the laser light reflected from the target surface. The system shuts off within nanoseconds of hitting the duct wall or soft tissue thus eliminating the risk of damage. The latest device is a frequency-doubled Nd:YAG laser (532 nm wavelength) dubbed 'Freddy' which generates shockwaves of such short duration that no thermal damage occurs. Both systems are substantially more expensive than the electrohydraulic generators but have attractive design features which obviate the need for choledochoscopy.

Extracorporeal shockwave lithotriptors

There are three major types of extracorporeal shockwave systems: electrohydraulic or spark-gap, electromagnetic, and piezoelectric.

The *electrohydraulic* system has two electrodes placed underwater and as an electric current arcs between the electrodes, the water in the path of the current vaporizes. A shockwave generated is reflected off a hemi-ellipsoidal chamber and is propagated to a focal zone outside the ellipsoid, termed the second focus or F2 which is targeted on the stone. The principal manufacturer of this technology is Dornier.

The *electromagnetic* shockwave system employs an electromagnetic coil below a metallic membrane at the bottom of a long water-filled cylinder. When an electrical current is pulsed through the coil, the magnetic field deflects the metal plate creating a planar pressure front which passes up the cylinder to an acoustic lens which focuses the shockwave to a high intensity focal zone. Siemens has developed this technology.

The *piezo/electric* method for shockwave generation employs ultrasound piezo ceramic crystals mounted on a spherical dish in a mosaic array under water. Several hundred to several thousand crystals are simultaneously fired creating multiple small waves which converge at the focal point of the system. The principal manufacturer is Richard Wolf.

The mechanism of stone fragmentation is not completely understood. The variability of acoustic impedance at the surface and within a stone may cause the kinetic energy released by the shockwave to overcome the tensile strength of the stone matrix.

Stent

Endoscopic stenting has been used to treat retained CBD stones since its introduction in 1984. Both straight and double pigtail plastic stents have been reported to be effective and safe in relief of biliary drainage when endoscopic stone extraction has failed or is contraindicated.

The choice of the different stents mostly depends on the experience of the endoscopist since studies have shown no proven benefit of straight versus double pigtail stent placement. In this situation, even a small size stent (7 Fr) is enough to mantain drainage as bile can usually flow by the side of the stent.

PROCEDURE

Routine stone removal

The two most important factors which determine the ease of stone removal are the size of the stone relative to the duct diameter which affects the ability to capture a stone in a basket and the degree of tapering and compliance of the terminal end of the bile duct.

The ability to easily engage a stone in a basket depends upon adequate space around the stone to allow the wire arms of the basket to fully expand for stone entrapment. This usually requires a duct diameter approximately 25% larger than the stone. In a duct of uniform diameter, the basket can be deployed anywhere along the length of the duct for stone entrapment but usually the bile duct tapers at its distal end as it traverses the pancreas. Stone entrapment is best achieved at the level with the widest duct diameter, generally in the middle to upper third of the duct.

Pitfalls to avoid include careful contrast injection so as not to push the stone up into the liver or cystic duct; once the stone is clearly identified with the initial injection, completion cholangiography can be achieved after extraction of the most distal stone(s). Opening a basket underneath a stone may cause a similar problem if the basket tip pushes the stone up; it is preferable to advance the closed basket alongside or above a stone prior to opening the basket. Once opened, the basket should be shaken with a rhythmic back and forth motion to allow the arms of the basket to open fully and to engage the stone. During this maneuver the widest part of the basket should be aligned with the widest diameter of the stone. We do not routinely completely close the basket on the stone but leave it loosely entrapped so as to allow the stone to assume the best alignment for extraction as it is pulled down through the narrow distal duct. If the stone is not easily trapped, attempts should be made to advance the basket alongside the opposite side of the stone than at the initial attempt. Another maneuver is to push the basket wire deep into the duct to allow the basket to fold over on itself and then to push the folded basket above the stone and let it unfold over the stone as the basket is pulled down.

The second critical issue for ease of stone removal is the width, configuration, and compliance of the terminal bile duct. This should be carefully assessed on the initial cholangiogram because unexpected difficulty may be encountered in pulling a stone completely out of the duct. Anticipation of such a problem may lead to the use of alternate strategies such as the insertion of a TTS lithotripsy basket. A clue to a narrow distal duct is the absence of obvious stone impaction at the papilla in the jaundiced patient. If the papilla appears normal and cholangiography demonstrates a stone proximal to the papilla, the immediate consideration should be that the duct is too narrow to allow descent of the stone or that the intrapancreatic portion of the duct is non-compliant. A stenosis which is often overlooked may occur over a very short 2–3 mm segment at the very bottom end of the bile duct just above the sphincter secondary to inflammation possibly from prior episodes of transient stone impaction. Resistance to stone withdrawal at this level may be difficult to distinguish from an incomplete sphincterotomy. Regardless, the solution for this predicament is the same, which is the use of a TTS mechanical lithotriptor.

Balloon vs basket extraction

Different centers may employ either a balloon or basket as their routine extraction method. The inherent advantages of a balloon are the capability to advance the deflated balloon over a wire above the stone and the ability to abort the extraction by balloon deflation in the event of unexpected impaction. A basket, on the other hand, has a far greater tolerance for increased force of traction and can be reused more often than a balloon thus reducing the accessory costs of the procedure. For these reasons, we prefer basket extraction and reserve the balloon for special situations. These include the sweeping out of small fragments after lithotripsy of larger stones and removal of small stones which elude basket entrapment (Fig. 9.1.5). Moreover, in a duct which turns sharply at the bottom end (60°–120°) as it traverses the duodenal wall or skirts around a diverticulum, basket entrapment becomes more difficult and stones often slip out of the basket as it sweeps around this turn. On the other hand, a high compliance extraction balloon will 'hug' the curve in the duct and drag the stone through. Lastly, a balloon is often useful in pulling a stone out of an intrahepatic radicle down into the hepatic duct for basket extraction or for pulling the stone out completely. The balloon caliber used for intrahepatic

radicles is relatively small (<8 mm) and once the stone has been pulled down out of the liver, the balloon may not be large enough to prevent the stone from floating up again around the side of the balloon.

The elusive stone

There are a few situations in which stones may be missed or shadows misinterpreted. Pseudo-calculi may appear because of air artefact or anatomic deformity. The commonest of these is the inadvertent introduction of air through the cannula or papillotome or pneumobilia resulting from fistulae or prior bilio-enteric anastomoses. The spherical contour of an air bubble, the tendency to break up into smaller bubbles or conversely to coalesce into larger ones, and rapid migration of an air defect with tilting of the patient are helpful clues to distinguish air artefact from a stone. Aspiration with an appropriately positioned catheter may remove air bubbles and should help to resolve the dilemma.

Anatomic deformity is another reason for a mistaken diagnosis of a stone. Distortion of the sphincter segment may occur during cannulation with protrusion of the sphincter segment up into the duct creating a reverse meniscus sign, especially during forceful attempts at deep cannulation. The duct may also be compressed or distorted as the cystic duct spirals around or crosses the common duct and may mimic a stone defect. Awareness of these problems is often sufficient to avoid misinterpretation.

Polypoid tumors, benign or malignant, may initially be mistaken for stones but the presence of a pedicle, lack of movement up or down the duct, and inability to demonstrate contrast around the defect may help to distinguish such lesions. When unclear, the use of a balloon to dislodge or move the defect may avert the problem of basket wires becoming embedded in a polypoid mass if in fact the radiographically visualized defect is tumor and not stone. A biopsy sample is also helpful both to retrieve a bit of tissue or stone as well as to use the open jaw of the forceps as a sound to assess the firmness and mobility of the defect. The corollary of this problem is the true stone which has

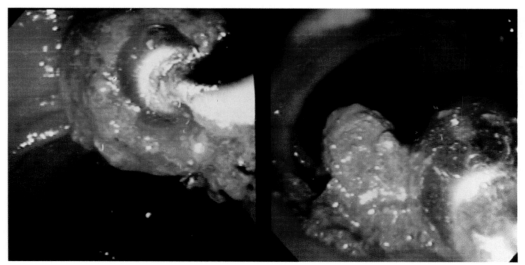

Fig. 9.1.5 Balloon extraction of a soft common bile duct stone.

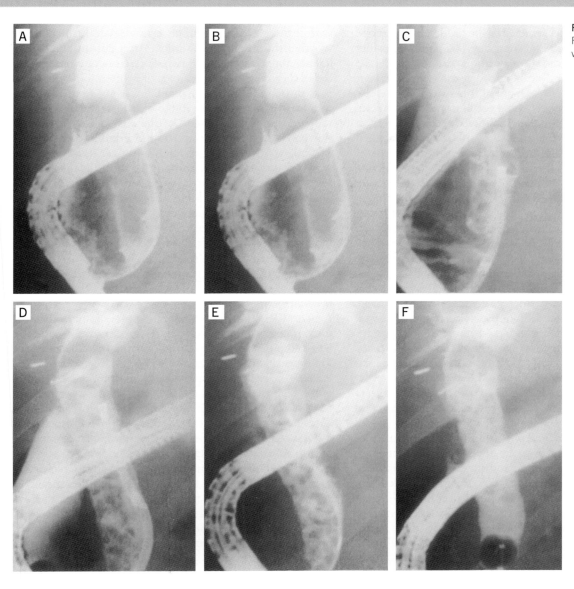

Fig. 9.1.6 (A to F) Fragmentation of a stone with a suture nidus.

formed over a suture nidus in the duct (Fig. 9.1.6) (generally at the level of the cystic duct) with a pseudo-stalk where the suture attaches to the duct wall mimicking the appearance of a polyp. The 'pseudo-polyp' may be detached from the duct wall when the suture is loosely attached because of partial erosion of the suture but otherwise choledochoscopy is required to clarify the diagnosis. Other defects which may mimic a stone include blood clots and parasites. An amorphous shape or a distinct shape is a helpful feature to identify these unusual problems.

The areas in which stones are often missed include the mouth of the cystic duct, the lower end of the cystic duct, or cystic duct stump, as well as within tertiary or higher order intrahepatic branch ducts. These problems mandate careful attention throughout the duration of the contrast injection, especially during the initial phases. During stone extraction, we recommend routine dredging of the lower end of the cystic duct so as not to leave a stone which may migrate back down into the common duct after the procedure. Care must be taken at the completion of common

duct stone extraction to carefully fill and inspect the right and left intrahepatic radicles. This often requires insinuation of the basket into branch ducts for further contrast injection, especially on the right side which may not fill well with the patient in the semi-prone position. Rotation of the patient onto the back may be required in rare instances to clarify apparent defects caused by overlapping ducts.

Finally, limitations of fluoroscopic resolution owing to the size of the patient, the quality of the equipment, or contrast which is too dense can cause small stones to be missed. This may mandate empiric sphincterotomy when the clinical presentation strongly favors the presence of a stone. Certain maneuvers are useful for identifying small stones. These include the use of dilute contrast or diluting the contrast even further with an additional injection of water. Torquing the endoscope in the short position will push the scope against the medial wall of the duodenum and cause extrinsic compression and flattening of the duct to highlight a small defect. Abdominal compression with an inflatable paddle may achieve a similar effect. Pushing the scope into the long position is important to uncover the

153

mid-section of the duct which may be hidden by the scope traversing the stomach and overlying this part of the duct when the scope is in the short position.

The appearance of a patulous orifice may suggest recent spontaneous passage of a stone. In this situation, it is relatively easy to use a wire-guided papillotome to cannulate and to place a wire up the duct followed by insertion of an extraction balloon which can be inflated and dragged down the duct to ensure stone clearance.

Difficult stone removal
Mechanical lithotripsy

Anticipation of a problem with routine extraction techniques is possible by careful assessment of the duct anatomy, the stone size and shape as well as the size of the orifice following sphincterotomy. The sphincterotomy should be assessed after cutting and this can be done by dragging an inflated retrieval balloon which approximates the size of the stone through the sphincter segment. An alternative, fast and simple technique we use is to pull the bowed sphincterotome down into the duodenum. We use a longer 30–35 mm sphincterotomy wire which when partially bowed has a radius of 10–15 mm for testing the opening. Moreover, there is a tactile sensation of the degree of resistance to withdrawal of the sphincterotome which reflects the differential compliance of the mucosa/submucosa and residual sphincter fibers.

The shape of the stone is a clue as to the ease of fracture during lithotripsy. Primary duct stones are often soft with an oval or round shape and these can be broken by simply tightening the ordinary basket or pulling the stone down into the sphincter segment and forcefully pulling the basket through the stone. Alternatively, the basket with the stone can be tightly withdrawn against the tip of the scope; advancing the scope with a clockwise rotation will drive the scope further down into the second part of the duodenum and drag the stone through the papilla or break it up. A stone with square edges usually reflects a greater cholesterol content, and a harder consistency. In such cases, a TTS lithotriptor should be used at the outset.

The OTS lithotriptor is often referred to as a 'rescue' device because it is employed when unexpected stone impaction occurs in the lower duct or at the sphincter segment. When the stone is impacted well above the sphincter, rather than pulling too hard and lodging the stone more tightly, the basket should be opened to dislodge the stone by advancing the catheter above the stone, then closing the basket to push the stone out of the wire arms. A TTS lithotriptor can then be used. The potential hazard of using the OTS lithotriptor for stones higher in the duct is that the steel coil tends to stiffen and straighten as the tension on the basket wire increases when being tightened with the winch. As the coil straightens, it may tear the mucosa at the angle where the duct enters the duodenal wall increasing the risk of bleeding or perforation.

When a stone impacts at the bottom of the duct, however, the OTS lithotriptor is suitable. As the use of this device requires cutting off the handle and destroying the basket, it is important to ensure that the stone is secure within the basket by pulling firmly several times to see whether the stone will dislodge. After cutting the basket handle, the scope is withdrawn. We do not attempt to keep the basket sheath on the wire as it is often too crimped to pass through the scope channel and is not needed to protect against wire damage to the alimentary mucosa. After scope withdrawal, the end of the basket wire is pushed through the lithotriptor coil and inserted into the winch. The coil is advanced into the mouth over the wire all the way down to the stone, and pushed until the distal tip of the coil curls up towards the stone under the sphincter. This aligns the tip of the coil under the stone to maximize the effect of the wire tension for stone fracture.

Following stone fracture, the fragments often impact at the distal end of the duct. It may be surprisingly difficult to re-enter the duct with the basket but repeated pushing at different angles should eventually dislodge the fragments upwards, and retrieval of individual pieces of stone is possible.

The TTS lithotriptor is used for stones impacted up the duct or above a narrowed segment or stricture (Fig. 9.1.7). The Olympus BML system allows initial passage of the Teflon catheter which can be manipulated to engage the stone. This basket has sufficient radial force for expansion and is reliable for stone capture, although it may be difficult to use for other stones in the same duct or for subsequent cases because it may lose its shape and the wires may not open widely. Large stones are often partially lodged in the mouth of the cystic duct. Expansion of the basket in the main duct may not be sufficient to trap a sufficient portion of the stone for fracture in which case the basket should be re-oriented to open into the cystic duct above the stone and then pulled down over the stone. Most of the time, entrapment of stones with the basket is best accomplished by opening the basket above the stone and then pulling it down over the stone.

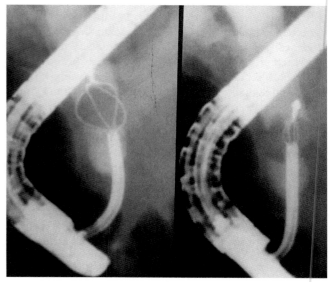

Fig. 9.1.7 Through-the-scope Olympus mechanical lithotriptor. (**Left**) Stone captured. (**Right**) Stone fragmentation.

Fracture of the basket cable can occur at a soldering point and may leave the trapped basket and part of the cable in the patient. There are several options for handling this complication. First is to try to retrieve the remaining cable and basket and remove these from the patient. The prominent nose on the tip of the Olympus lithotripsy basket and even the tip of the routine basket can be grabbed by passage of a second basket which is opened over the tip of the first basket, and closed to grip the tip which is then pulled off the stone. A second option is to ignore the trapped basket and repeat the procedure of trapping the stone with another basket and repeating the mechanical lithotripsy. Although the force of the first attempt was unsuccessful, and resulted in breaking the basket, the initial closure caused fracture lines or fissures which weaken the stone, usually sufficiently to allow a second attempt at fracture to succeed. The third option is to abandon mechanical lithotripsy and to arrange for shockwave treatment either intraductal with a babyscope or extracorporeal, placing a nasobiliary tube to permit a cholangiogram for radiographical targeting of the stone.

Intraductal shockwave lithotripsy

A uniquely challenging bile duct stone problem is that of the impacted stone which cannot be entrapped in a basket or dislodged with a balloon. We have employed direct contact shock devices with 'mother–daughter' peroral choledochoscopy employing the dedicated fiberoptic 'mother' duodenoscope with a 5.5 mm operating channel which allows passage of a 4.5 mm 'daughter' miniscope. The 'mother' duodenoscope elevator has limited mobility and is not useful for routine instrumentation. It is therefore advisable to perform cholangiography and sphincterotomy with a standard duodenoscope prior to insertion of the 'mother' endoscope. Given the limited maneuverability of the 'mother' endoscope, an ample sphincterotomy should be performed to facilitate passage of the 'daughter' endoscope through the papilla.

A 3.4 mm 'daughter' endoscope has been developed with a 1.2 mm operating channel and two-way angulation. This can be passed through a standard therapeutic duodenoscope, so that it is unnecessary to insert a variety of instruments during the procedure.

An important aspect of shockwave lithotripsy is the ability to irrigate the bile duct both to provide the appropriate fluid medium (half-normal saline) for the shockwave as well as to flush the sediment and debris which limit visibility. In addition, a fluid medium increases tenfold the fragmentation force of electrohydraulic lithotripsy. In our early experience, a previously inserted pigtailed nasobiliary catheter was used to provide drainage but it was an added step to the procedure, and the nasobiliary tube was easily dislodged during the subsequent insertion of the 'mother' endoscope. We have now adopted a much simpler approach using a Tuohy–Borst valve on the operating channel of the 'daughter' endoscope which allows passage of the laser waveguide or electrohydraulic probe and simultaneous instillation of half-normal saline or contrast through a side-arm. When the larger 3 Fr electrohydraulic

probes are used, there is considerable resistance to fluid instillation around the fiber in the operating channel and a tendency for fluid to back-up through the rubber cap on the valve.

The procedure demands the skills of two endoscopists, the more difficult role being that of the 'mother' endoscope operator. There is a limited range of motion of the tip of the 'daughter' endoscope and its correct positioning is accomplished by alterations in the angle of entry through the papilla. The choledochoscopic image is projected onto a monitor with a video-camera attachment to magnify the small field of vision (Fig. 9.1.8) and to permit the 'mother' endoscopist to orchestrate the movement of both endoscopes, as well as the shockwave probe, and to 'fire' when the stone is adequately targeted. All of the probes are particularly difficult to see endoscopically and it is critical to ascertain the position of the probe so as to avoid ductal injury. The probe may deflect outside the field of vision and it is best to retract and to re-advance it to bring it into view. Fluoroscopic tracking of the probe is also possible with the metallic tip on the electrohydraulic probe and with the metallic coating applied to the laser waveguide. With uncoated laser guides, preloading into a 3 Fr metal-tipped catheter, with the laser tip fixed 5 mm beyond the polyethylene catheter tip, facilitates localization of the laser tip both endoscopically and fluoroscopically. Another problem with the current electrohydraulic probes is their lack of stiffness making it difficult to push them through the operating channel. To

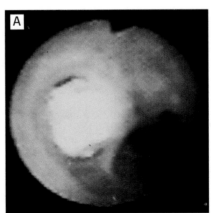

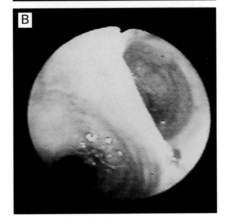

Fig. 9.1.8
(A) Cholangioscopic view of a white cholesterol stone impacted in the mouth of the cystic duct.
(B) Cholangioscopic view of the cystic duct take-off following electrohydraulic lithotripsy and clearance of a stone from the cystic duct (left).

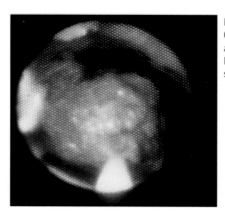

Fig. 9.1.9
Cholangioscopic view of an electrohydraulic lithotripsy probe on a stone in the bile duct.

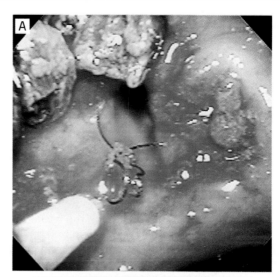

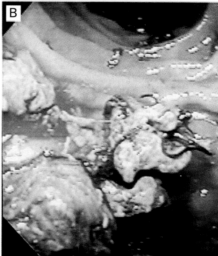

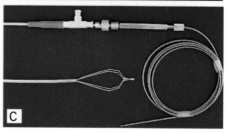

avoid kinking, it is necessary to pre-load the probe into the operating channel of the choledochoscope prior to insertion.

The probe should contact the stone lightly so as not to disperse the fluid interface (Fig. 9.1.9). On firing, there may be a very slight recoil which may displace the probe with the risk of inadvertent tissue injury. Provided the foot pedal is released promptly serious injury can be avoided. The objective of electrohydraulic lithotripsy is to break the stone into a few fragments which is sufficient for mechanical or standard basket extraction (Fig. 9.1.10). The holmium or candela dye lasers are not as powerful in that regard and tend either to drill into a stone or pulverize it more slowly rather than cracking the stone into large fragments.

Extracorporeal shockwave lithotripsy

Extracorporeal shockwave lithotripsy (ESWL) is a reasonable option for stone fragmentation but is often logistically more cumbersome. Targeting depends on X-ray imaging as accurate ultrasound localization is difficult. Moreover most ESWL units designed for urology have X-ray guidance only. This feature necessitates a preliminary endoscopic retrograde cholangiopancreatography (ERCP) for placement of a nasobiliary catheter, usually introduced at the same time as the ESWL treatment. In half of the cases with multiple or very large stones, two ESWL sessions are necessary with either hospitalization and maintenance of the nasobiliary catheter between sessions or removal of the nasobiliary catheter, placement of a stent, and repetition of this sequence prior to the next ESWL session. Following ESWL, ERCP is performed to remove fragments for duct clearance or to leave a prophylactic stent. Owing to the necessity of repeated procedures in two different units, ESWL is reserved for failures of intraductal lithotripsy because of failed targeting or fragmentation. This often occurs with stones above a stricture, an angulated duct, or with intrahepatic stones.

RESULTS

CBD stones represent the most common pathologic findings of the biliary system and the management of this

Fig. 9.1.10 (A and B) Electrohydraulic lithotripsy performed through a babyscope; and multiple small stone fragments removed with a Dormia basket (C) and with a balloon.

problem has undergone dramatic changes in both diagnosis and treatment in the last two decades.

Sphincterotomy and stone extraction performed by experienced endoscopists using conventional techniques are successful in 85 to 90% of cases.[15–18]

Although both the Dormia basket and the balloon catheter have been reported as equally effective in stone extraction, the majority of endoscopists prefer to use the more durable Dormia basket rather than the disposable balloon.

The maximal diameter of the CBD stone that can be extracted successfully using conventional methods depends principally on the diameter and the shape of the stone, the size of the duct, and the size of sphincterotomy. In general, stones greater than 15 mm are considered to be large, but equally important are other factors such as the consistency and the number of the stones and the presence of anatomical variants such as peri-ampullary diverticulum or Billroth II gastroenterostomy.

We retrospectively reviewed 400 consecutive patients seen for endoscopic removal of CBD stones over a 2-year period. These patients underwent 475 procedures performed by two experienced endoscopists at a tertiary referral center.

There were 164 males (mean age = 68 years, range 21–92) and 236 females (mean age = 68 years, range 24–97). Eighty-seven patients (21.8%) presented with jaundice and 24 (6.0%) presented with pancreatitis. The remainder were not symptomatic at the time of ERCP. Sixteen patients (4%) were referred with endoscopically or percutaneously placed biliary drains. Abnormal anatomy was a reason for referral in 21 patients. Sixteen patients had a Billroth II gastrectomy, 2 had a gastrostomy, 2 had choledochojejunostomy and 1 a Roux-en-Y anastomosis. Peri-ampullary diverticulae were present in 71 patients. The presence of an ampullary diverticulum was not associated with failure to cannulate, perform sphincterotomy, or clear the bile duct.

Successful cannulation and cholangiography were achieved in 397 (99.3%) and failure to cannulate occurred in 3 patients. One patient had a Billroth II gastrectomy. This patient subsequently had a cholecystectomy with CBD stone removal at surgery. The other two failed cannulations were due to an inability to cannulate a tight, narrow papillae. One of these patients had a cholecystectomy and stones removed at surgery. The other patient refused surgery, and had spontaneous clearing of jaundice and remained asymptomatic. The mean number of procedures per patient was 1.2 ±0.3 (range 1–5). In 319 patients only one procedure was required to clear the CBD duct. Two procedures were needed in 54 patients and three or more in the remaining 22 patients.

Of the 397 patients, in whom cholangiography was possible, 394 had a current or prior sphincterotomy. In 6 patients, pre-cut technique was utilized. In 48 patients, a papillotomy was already present, performed by the referring endoscopist. In 10 of the 48 patients, an extension of papillotomy was needed prior to stone extraction. Clearance was obtained after sphincterotomy using the Dormia basket in 435 procedures, compared with balloon catheter, which was used in 17 procedures. In 89 patients (22.3%), non-standard techniques were used including mechanical lithotripsy, electrohydraulic lithotripsy (EHL), and laser lithotripsy together with stent or nasobiliary tube placement. The mean stone diameter in this group of patients was 17 mm. The mean stone diameter for the total group was 10 mm.

When initial assessment or treatment attempts suggest a complex or difficult stone extraction, several techniques are available in order to fragment the stones and facilitate endoscopic removal.

Mechanical lithotripsy

The simplest endoscopic method for the management of stones that cannot be removed by conventional techniques is mechanical lithotripsy. Two types of mechanical lithotriptor are available: the OTS and the TTS. The emergency OTS also called Soehendra lithotriptor is more useful when a conventional basket with a grasped stone becomes impacted in the lower CBD. Binmoeller et al[19] reported 100% duct clearance using this lithotriptor in 33 patients with impacted Dormia baskets.

TTS lithotriptors, such as the Olympus BML series and the Microvasive Monolith, are preferable for elective lithotripsy. Using the first-generation mechanical TTS lithotriptor, Riemann et al[20] successfully fragmented 13 large stones (mean diameter 22.8 mm) in 8 patients. Unfortunately bile duct cannulation with this first-generation device was cumbersome owing to the large, stiff metal sheath that tended to point toward the pancreatic duct and impaired biliary cannulation. Improved design of the BML lithotriptor series by Olympus has since helped to overcome this problem.

Chung et al[21] using the BML-1Q lithotriptor basket successfully treated 55/68 patients (81.4%) with large CBD stones increasing their overall success rate for stone extraction from 84 to 97%. Failure resulted from the inability to either pass the stone or capture it in the basket.

Shaw et al[22] in 1993 reported their experience with the BML-3Q mechanical lithotriptor. They were able to successfully capture and break stones in 92% of their 116 patients and clear the bile duct in 85% of their cases. In a large series of 1722 patients, 162 (9.4%) failed to have their stones removed by standard techniques and had mechanical lithotripsy (mainly using the BML Olympus TTS lithotriptor).[23] Complete duct clearance was achieved in 136 patients (84%). Sorbi et al[26] reported their experience with the pre-assembled pistol-grip handle Monolith lithotriptor in 20 consecutive patients who underwent mechanical lithotripsy as part of a prospective multicenter study. The overall success rate to capture, fragment, and completely clear the bile duct was 80%. Clearance was incomplete in 10% of the cases and failure was reported in 2 patients.

In our previously described consecutive series (see above), mechanical lithotripsy was used in a total of 34 procedures with a success rate of 94%. In two procedures, failure resulted from an inability to capture the stone. For patients requiring non-standard techniques 9% had stones less than 10 mm in diameter and 61% had stones greater than 15 mm in diameter.

Similarly, multiple stones, especially with more than five stones present, were associated with a greater need for non-standard techniques and increased likelihood of multiple procedures. Thirty-eight percent of patients with more than five stones required more than one procedure.

The overall success rate of stone capture and fragmentation with mechanical lithotripsy has been reported in 92 to 96% of cases with complete clearance of the bile duct in 85 to 93% of patients.[21–26]

Electrohydraulic lithotripsy

Since its development for the mining industry in the Soviet Union 50 years ago as a method to fragment rocks, EHL has been adapted for medical use in the treatment of nephrolithiasis and choledocholithiasis.

Koch et al[27] in 1977 reported the first attempt of stone fragmentation with EHL in 17 patients. Since then, Leung & Chung[28] cleared nine large stones in 5 patients using EHL through the working channel of a cholangioscope. Bottari et al[29] also reported nine patients all successfully treated with EHL. Similar results were obtained by Ponchon et al[30] and Hixson et al.[31]

Siegel et al described complete stone clearance in 18/21 patients using EHL applied through a centering balloon catheter.[32] Binmoeller et al treated 65 patients with EHL obtaining a success rate of 99%.[19] One perforation of the bile duct occurred and was treated conservatively.

The largest series, consisting of 72 consecutive patients who underwent EHL using a peroral transpapillary mother–baby scope system, was published by our institution.[33] Two patients had incomplete records or failed follow-up, leaving 70 patients in this retrospective analysis.

Mean follow-up was 25.6 months (range 0–80). Prior to EHL, 69/70 patients (99%) had ERCP and failed standard stone-extraction techniques (mean 1.8 ERCPs/patient, range 0–5). Indications for EHL were large stones (63 patients) or a narrow caliber bile duct below a stone of average size (7 patients). Successful fragmentation (43 complete, 22 partial) was achieved in 65/69 patients (94%) (1 patient was excluded from analysis because of a broken endoscope). Fragmentation failures were due to targeting problems (2 patients) and hard stones (2 patients). Seventy-four percent of patients required one EHL session, 19% required two sessions, and 7% required three or more. All patients with successful stone fragmentation required post-EHL balloon or basket extraction of fragments, some requiring mechanical lithotripsy or ESWL. Complications included cholangitis and/or jaundice (10 patients), mild hemobilia (1 patient), mild post-ERCP pancreatitis (1 patient), and bradycardia (1 patient). There were no deaths related to EHL and no significant bile duct injuries. EHL via peroral endoscopic choledochoscopy is a highly successful and safe technique for use in the management of difficult choledocholithiasis and intrahepatic stones with a final stone fragmentation rate of 94% (65/69 patients).

The concerns regarding the potential complications of massive bleeding or duct perforation have not been borne out by the experience reported to date. The requirement for direct vision with the use of a scope and the presence of two experienced endoscopists have limited the dissemination of the technique.

Laser lithotripsy

Different types of laser have been described for bile duct stone lithotripsy. The Q-switched Nd:YAG laser is capable of pulverizing biliary stones into fragments smaller than 2 mm in diameter as shown in an in vitro study,[34] but the relatively large and stiff 600 μm quartz fiber makes it unsuitable for endoscopic applications.

Second-generation devices are based on high-energy flashlamp-pulsed dye technology with coumarin-green (wavelength 504 nm). These flashlamp-pulsed dye lasers use a thinner flexible fiber (200–320 μm) easily inserted into the bile duct under direct vision.

Cotton et al,[35] Ponchon et al,[36] Prat et al,[37] and Neuhaus et al[38] reported the results of laser lithotripsy using the flashlamp-pulsed dye laser either via endoscopic or percutaneous cholangioscopy. A successful clearance rate of 80 to 94% was reported and no serious complications were recorded. The percutaneous transhepatic approach was found to be more effective (96% vs 83% reported by Neuhaus et al and 100% vs 36% using a centering balloon or a laser basket reported by Ponchon et al) than the peroral route in these studies. The complication rate ranged from 0% in the studies of Cotton et al and Ponchon et al to 19% in the Prat et al study and 26% in the Neuhaus et al series. Most of the failures resulted from the inability to advance the quartz fiber because of the acute angulation of the bile duct and/or the catheter.

Recently a flashlamp-pulsed dye laser (rhodamine-6G, 595 nm) with an automatic stone-tissue discrimination system (STDS) has been developed.[39] The rhodamine-6G is comparable to the coumarin-green dye laser with respect to the emitted laser energy and the pulse length and repetition rate. The uniqueness of the rhodamine-6G laser is the STDS that allows safe stone fragmentation under fluoroscopic control alone, greatly increasing the speed and the ease of the procedure. When the tissue is contacted, the laser beam is automatically interrupted within nanoseconds, discharging only a negligible amount of laser energy. Neuhaus et al[39] reported with this system a 97% success rate in 38 patients, 18 treated perorally and 20 by the percutaneous approach. Ell et al[40] reported their experience treating 18 patients with the same laser. Eight patients were treated under fluoroscopic control and 8 using peroral retrograde cholangioscopy. CBD clearance was achieved in 13/18 patients. Of note is that patients treated under cholangioscopic control received significantly fewer laser pulses and had fewer misapplied pulses. One patient treated fluoroscopically developed hemobilia and cholangitis.

Jakobs et al[41] in 1996 reported on 30 patients with complicated intrahepatic and extrahepatic stones treated perorally with a rhodamine-6G STDS laser. Twenty-four (80%) patients were stone-free after laser therapy alone. Eighteen out of 19 patients with CBD stones were treated under fluoroscopic control whereas in 9/11 patients with intrahepatic stones choledochoscopy was necessary.

In the series of Hochberger et al,[42] 52/60 patients (83%) with impacted CBD stones refractory to conventional extraction or mechanical lithotripsy were successfully treated using the rhodamine-6G STDS laser. Complications included transient hemobilia, cholangitis, and pancreatitis in 5 patients all treated by conservative methods.

More recently, reports have been published regarding the use of the new frequency doubled Nd:YAG laser

(FREDDY) with an integrated piezoacoustic STDS.[43] A preliminary clinical study in 4 patients published by Hochberger et al,[44] showed promising results.

Finally, in a study published in 1999, Weickert et al,[45] using a Holmium laser under babyscopic monitoring, achieved stone fragmentation and bile duct clearance in 19/20 patients in whom conventional methods had failed to achieve stone fragmentation.

The only comparative study of laser and EHL was an in vitro study published by Birkett et al.[46] They compared the effect of a 504 nm coumarin-pulsed dye laser and EHL on in vitro porcine gallbladder and CBD stones. The authors' conclusion was that laser lithotripsy was likely to be safer than EHL.

Extracorporeal shock wave lithotripsy

Since 1986, ESWL has been successfully used for the treatment of CBD stones.

One of the first multicenter studies on the results of ESWL reported complete duct clearance in 86 patients with a 36% overall morbidity and 1.8% mortality.[47] Other study groups published success rates between 75% and 80%.[48–50] Yasuda & Tomita[51] evaluated ESWL without previous sphincterotomy in an attempt to preserve sphincter function. Complete fragmentation and clearance of the bile duct was achieved in 67.3% of patients without the need for repeat ERCP.

White et al[52] reported their experience with ESWL in a group of patients in whom bile duct stone removal failed because of stone size (38%), impaction (56%), or location proximal to a stricture (6%). Stone fragmentation was achieved in 94% of the patients while duct clearance was obtained in 81% either spontaneously or with techniques applied at ERCP. Adamek et al[53] compared the results of ESWL with those of EHL through peroral cholangioscopy in a group of 125 patients with difficult bile duct stones. This was a prospective study but the choice of therapy was decided by the availability of the facilities at the institutions involved. Although the success rate in stone fragmentation (97% vs 93%) and clearance of the bile duct (79% vs 74%) was similar for the two techniques, fewer sessions of lithotripsy were required in the group treated with EHL (1.1 sessions in EHL vs 2.0 in ESWL). In both treatment groups, additional endoscopic interventions were necessary to clear the bile duct.

In a prospective study by Neuhaus et al,[54] 60 patients with difficult stones were randomized to receive either ESWL under fluoroscopic targeting or intracorporeal lithotripsy using a pulsed dye laser with an automatic recognition system. Bile duct clearance was achieved in 22/30 (73%) in the ESWL group versus 29/30 (97%) in the intracorporeal laser lithotripsy (ILL) group ($P<0.05$). The number of treatment sessions (ESWL 3.0 ± 1.3; ILL 1.2 ± 0.4; $P<0.001$) and the duration of treatment (ESWL 3.9 ± 3.5 days; ILL 0.9 ± 2.3 days; $P<0.001$) were also significantly different in favor of ILL. Crossover to ILL led to stone removal in seven of eight cases in which ESWL failed, whereas ESWL fragmented the stone in the single patient in whom ILL failed. Two minor complica-

tions occurred in each group and there was no 30-day mortality.

The results of this prospective randomized trial are comparable with those previously reported by Jakobs et al[55] who compared ESWL with ILL performed under fluoroscopic control alone in a randomized prospective study involving 34 patients.

Therefore ESWL is not the preferred primary approach for difficult CBD stones. It represents an option before considering surgery when mechanical lithotripsy, EHL, or ILL have failed, particularly in patients with intrahepatic stones.

Utilization of stents for choledocholithiasis

Biliary stenting has been used to treat retained CBD stones since at least 1984 when the technique was first reported. Three major indications have been reported for stenting placement in presence of CBD stones. The first is for patients with severe comorbid illness and acute cholangitis which does not allow routine stone removal. The stent or nasobiliary catheter may help to stabilize the patient before further endoscopic treatment is performed.

The second indication is when initial ERCP fails to achieve complete bile duct clearance and a stent is inserted to prevent stone impaction until further endoscopic or alternative treatment is undertaken. In both cases, the stent serves as a temporary measure before a definite therapy.

In this clinical setting, short-term stenting affords excellent results. In the study of Cairns et al[56] endoscopic stenting increased the stone clearance rate from 80 to 88%. Maxton et al[57] placed endoscopic stents in 85/283 patients with failed stone extraction. Six patients died before a further endoscopic attempt but only one died of cholangitis. Subsequently, 50 patients (63%) had successful stone removal increasing the overall success rate to 91%. In the largest published study,[58] including 117 patients who received stents for difficult CBD stones, Huibregtse et al used stent insertion as a temporary measure before elective surgery (25 patients) or repeated endoscopic attempt to clear the bile duct (35 patients). In the latter group, 25/35 (71%) had complete clearance of the bile duct. Farca et al[59] used temporary stents in pregnant patients with duct stones. There were no complications to mother or fetuses. Stones were successfully removed within 4 months from stent placement.

Chan et al[60] observed that the stone size was significantly reduced in 21/30 patients (71%) who received a second ERCP after a mean time of 63 days (range 17–1002) from stent placement. Importantly, probably in part due to the stone size reduction, 25 patients had complete stone removal after ERCP was repeated. This result is comparable to those of previous studies published as abstracts by Vallera et al[61] and by Goldberg et al.[62] Although the exact mechanism is not known, the most likely explanation for the reduction of stone size is the constant mechanical friction of the stone against the stent. From this point of view, if mechanical action is important, Cotton supposed that two stents might be even more effective than one.[63]

There is a suggestion that the addition of oral ursodeoxycholic acid (UDCA) could help to speed up the process of stone size reduction. One retrospective un-blinded report showed good results in 9/10 patients who became stone-free with the use of stenting plus oral UDCA compared to none of the 40 patients who had stent alone.[64]

Another indication is the use of stents as a permanent treatment in elderly high-risk patients. The results in the long-term are sometimes controversial and not so favorable as those described for the short-term.

Cotton et al[65] reported long-term follow-up in 17 patients with retained CBD stones. Stone extraction was achieved in 2 patients in whom a second ERCP was repeated. Five of the remaining 15 patients died of non-biliary causes and only 2 patients required surgery for biliary symptoms.

van Steenbergen et al[66] followed 23 elderly patients with stent in place for up to 5 years. During this time, 3 patients (13%) developed biliary symptoms and 11 patients died of unrelated diseases. In the Amsterdam group study,[58] 58 patients were treated with permanent stents and were followed for a median period of 36 months (range 1–117). A total of 34 complications occurred in 23 patients (40%), cholangitis being the most frequent (22 patients). Forty-four patients died during the follow-up, 9 as a result of a biliary-related cause. The group's conclusion was that permanent stenting can be used with confidence only in patients with a very short life expectancy.

A randomized comparison of stent placement versus stone removal in patients with symptomatic CBD stones who were at high risk (older than 70 years or with severe comorbidities) was published by Chopra et al.[67] Forty patients were recruited in each treatment group. In the endoscopic stone extraction group, duct clearance was obtained in 81% of the patients. Early complications occurred in 7% of the stent group and in 16% in the bile duct clearance group ($P = 0.18$). However, the long-term complication rate was significantly higher in the stent group. Nine patients had 11 episodes of cholangitis in a median duration of 16 weeks after the stenting. At a median of 20 months' follow-up, 64% of patients who received stent placement and 86% of patients who had stone extraction remained free of symptoms ($P = 0.03$).

In our experience, 18 patients with expected short-term survival (mean age 86.4 years) had stents placed as a definitive measure for problematic stones. This series was compiled at a time when stents were occasionally used for large difficult stones as definitive therapy in the elderly (Fig. 9.1.11). Eight patients were without biliary-related symptoms despite no further intervention. Five patients had died in the follow-up period of unrelated causes. Four patients had a surgical procedure and 3/4 patients had stones found and removed. There was one peri-operative death. One patient in the stent group was lost to follow-up.

CONCLUSION

The current developments in endoscopic technology in concert with the thrust in developing instruments for minimally invasive procedures have provided the necessary tools for removal of almost all CBD stones. Limitations in expertise or equipment in smaller endoscopic centers may necessitate referral to a specialized unit.

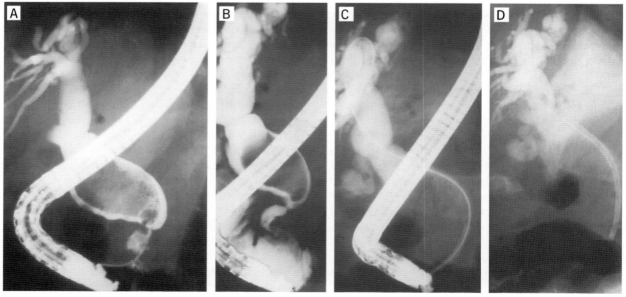

Fig. 9.1.11 (A) Giant stone in the common bile duct in an elderly high-risk patient presenting with cholangitis. (B, C, and D) Placement of a 10 Fr stent across the stone to ensure biliary drainage.

CHECKLIST OF PRACTICE POINTS

1. In the current endoscopic era, bile duct stones in the post-cholecystectomy patient should be managed endoscopically with referral to tertiary care centers for failed or difficult stones.

2. There is a role for emergency ERCP without fluoroscopy in the intensive care unit for biliary sepses employing a biliary stent or nasobiliary drainage.

3. Access to the biliary tract may be compromised by a Roux-en-Y choledochojejunal anastomosis or a severe upper gastrointestinal luminal stricture.

4. Basket extraction is preferred for routine stone removal. Ballon extraction is useful for removal of small fragments, or for larger stones when basket entrapment fails especially in patients with a sharply angulated termination of the duct.

5. A pseudocalculus radiographic image may result from air artefact, deformity at the cystic duct insertion, a polypoid tumor, or a hypertrophic sphincter prolapsing into the bottom of the bile duct.

6. Stones may be missed when situated in the mouth of the cystic duct, higher in the cystic duct stump, or when present in secondary or tertiary intrahepatic radicles.

7. The outside-the-scope (OTS) Soehendra mechanical lithotriptor is essential as a rescue device for a basket which becomes impacted at the bottom of the bile duct.

8. Through-the-scope (TTS) mechanical lithotripsy should be considered as an initial approach for very large stones or stones above a stricture or duct narrowing which may not be easily extracted with routine maneuvers.

9. Compared to various laser lithotripsy modalities, intraductal lithotripsy is best carried out with electrohydraulic lithotripsy (EHL), which is much less expensive, more efficient and proven to be safe after several clinical trials.

10. Biliary stents as a definitive measure should be reserved for those who truly have a short life expectancy with severe comorbid illness.

REFERENCES

1. Classen M, Demling L. Endoskopishe Sphinkerotomie der Papilla Vater und Steinextraktion aus dem Ductus choledocus. Dtsch Med Wochenschr 1974; 99: 469–477.

2. Kawai K, Akasaka Y, Marukani K, et al. Endoscopic sphincterotomy of the ampulla of Vater. Gastrointest Endosc 1974; 20:148–151.

3. Ponsky JL. Endoscopic management of common bile duct stones. World J Surg 1992; 16:1060–1065.

4. Seitz U, Bapaye A, Bohnacker S, et al. Adavances in therapeutic endoscopic treatment of common bile duct stones. World J Surg 1998; 22:1133–1144.

5. Elfant AB, Bourke MJ, Alhadel R, et al. A prospective study of safety of endoscopic therapy for choledocholithiasis in an outpatient population. Am J Gastroenterol 1996; 91:1499–1502.

6. Freeman ML, Nelson DB, Sherman S, et al. Complications of endoscopic biliary sphincterotomy. N Engl J Med 1996; 335:909–918.

7. Gostout CJ, Bender CE. Cholangiopancreatography, sphincterotomy and common duct stone removal via Roux-en-Y limb enteroscopy. Gastroenterology 1988; 95:156–157.

8. Gray R, Leong S, Marcon N, et al. Endoscopic retrograde cholangiography, sphincterotomy, and gallstone extraction via gastrostomy (letter). Gastrointest Endosc 1992; 38:731.

9. Guelrud M, Jaen D, Torres P, et al. Endoscopic cholangiopancreatography in the infant: a new prototype pediatric duodenoscope. Gastrointest Endosc 1987; 33:4–8.

10. Mauer K, Waye J. A new pediatric duodenoscope: successful cannulation without a cannula elevator. Gastrointest Endosc 1989; 35:437–439.

11. Bourke MJ, Haber GB. Transpapillary choledochoscopy. Gastrointest Endosc Clin North Am 1996; 6:235–252.

12. Meenan J, Schoeman M, Rauws E, et al. A video baby cholangioscope. Gastrointest Endosc 1996; 41:584–585.

13. Soda K, Shitou K, Yoshida Y, et al. Peroral cholangioscopy using a new fine-caliber flexible scope for detailed examination without papillotomy. Gastrointest Endosc 1996; 42:233–238.

14. Demling L, Seuberth K, Riemann JF. A mechanical lithotripter. Endoscopy 1982; 14:100–101.

15. Cotton PB. Endoscopic management of bile duct stones (apples and orange). Gut 1984; 25:587–597.

16. Ponsky JL. Endoscopic management of common bile duct stones. World J Surg 1992; 16:1060–1065.

17. Sauerbruch T, Feussner H, Frimberger E, et al. Treatment of common bile duct stones, a consensus report. Hepatogastroenterology 1994; 41:513–515.

18. Lee JG, Leung JW. Endoscopic management of common bile duct stones. Gastrointest Endosc Clin North Am 1996; 6:43–55.

19. Binmoeller KF, Bruckner M, Thonke F, et al. Treatment of difficult bile duct stones using mechanical, electrohydraulic and extracorporeal wave lithotripsy. Endoscopy 1993; 25:201–206.

20. Riemann JF, Seuberth K, Demling L. Clinical application of a new mechanical lithotriptor for smashing common bile duct stones. Endoscopy 1982; 14:226–230.

21. Chung SC, Leung JF, Leong HT, et al. Mechanical lithotripsy of large common bile duct stones using a basket. Br J Surg 1991; 78:1448–1450.

22. Shaw MJ, Mackie RD, Moore JP, et al. Results of a multicenter trial using a mechanical lithotriptor for the treatment of large common bile duct stones. Am J Gastroenterol 1993; 88:730–733.

23. Cippolletta L, Costamagna G, Bianco MA, et al. Endoscopic mechanical lithotripsy of difficult common bile duct stones. Br J Surg 1997; 84:1407–1409.

24. Shaw MJ, Dorsher PJ, Vennes JA. A new mechanical lithotriptor for the treatment of large common bile duct stones. Am J Gastroenterol 1990; 85:796–798.

25. Siegel JH, Ben-Zvi JS, Pullano WE. Mechanical lithotripsy of common bile duct stones. Gastrointest Endosc 1990; 36:351–356.

26. Sorbi D, Van Os E, Aberger FJ, et al. Clinical application of a new disposable lithotriptor: a prospective multicenter study. Gastrointest Endosc 1999; 49:210–213.

27. Koch H, Rosch W, Walz V. Endoscopic lithotripsy in the common bile duct. Endoscopy 1977; 9:95–98.

28. Leung JWC, Chung SSC. Electrohydraulic lithotripsy with peroral cholangioscopy. Br Med J 1989; 299:595–598.

29. Bottari M, Bertino A, D'Amore F, et al. Electrohydraulic lithotripsy of difficult biliary stones. G Ital Endosc Dig 1996; 19:127–130.

30. Ponchon T, Valette PJ, Bory R, et al. Evaluation of a combined percutaneous–endoscopic procedure for the treatment of choledocholithiasis and benign papillary stenosis. Endoscopy 1987; 19:164–166.

31. Hixson LJ, Fennerty MB, Jaffee PE, et al. Peroral cholangioscopy with intracorporeal electrohydraulic lithotripsy for choledocholithiasis. Am J Gastroenterol 1992; 87:296–299.

32. Siegel JH, Ben-Zvi JS, Pullano WE. Endoscopic electrohydraulic lithotripsy. Gastrointest Endosc 1990; 36:134–136.

33. Nelles SE, Haber GB, Kim YI, et al. Peroral endoscopic fragmentation of bile duct stones with electrohydraulic lithotripsy (EHL). Gastrointest Endosc 1998; A124.

34. Hochberger J, Gruber E, Wirtz P, et al. Lithotripsy of gallstones by means of quality switched giant-pulse neodymium:yttrium-aluminium-garnet laser. Basic in vitro studies using a highly flexible fiber system. Gastroenterology 1991; 101:1391–1398.

35. Cotton PB, Kozarek RA, Shapiro RH, et al. Endoscopic laser lithotripsy of large bile duct stones. Gastroenterology 1990; 99:1128–1133.

36. Ponchon T, Gagnon P, Valette PJ, et al. Pulsed dye laser lithotripsy of bile duct stones. Gastroenterology 1991; 100:1730–1736.

37. Prat F, Fritsch J, Choury AD, et al. Laser lithotripsy of difficult biliary stones. Gastrointest Endosc 1994; 40:290–295.

38. Neuhaus H, Hoffmann W, Zillinger G, et al. Laser lithotripsy of difficult bile duct stones under direct visual control. Gut 1993; 34:415–421.

39. Neuhaus H, Hoffmann W, Gottlieb K, et al. Endoscopic lithotripsy of bile cut stones using a new laser with automatic stone recognition. Gastrointest Endosc 1994; 40:708–715.

40. Ell C, Hochberger J, May A. Laser lithotripsy of difficult bile duct stones by means of a rhodamine-6G laser and an integrated automatic stone-tissue detection system. Gastrointest Endosc 1993; 39:755–762.

41. Jakobs R, Maier M, Kohler B, et al. Peroral laser lithotripsy of difficult intrahepatic and extrahepatic bile duct stones: laser effectiveness using an automatic stone-tissue discrimination system. Am J Gastroenterol 1996; 91:468–473.

42. Hochberger J, Bayer J, May A, et al. Laser lithotripsy of difficult bile duct stones: results in 60 patients using a rhodamine-6G dye laser with optical stone tissue detection. Gut 1998; 43:823–829.

43. Hochberger S, Bayer J, Tex S, et al. A frequency-doubled double-pulsed Nd:YAG laser (FREDDY) for the laser lithotripsy of gallstones: an interesting laser lithotriptor with an integrated piezo-acoustic stone-tissue-detection-system (paSTDS). Gastrointest Endosc 1997; 45:A133.

44. Hochberger J, Bayer J, Maiss J, et al. Klinische Ergebnisse mit einem neun frequenzverdoppelten doppelpuls Nd:YAG laser (FREDDY) fur die lithotripsie bei komplizierter choledocholithiasis. Biom Tech 1998; 43(Suppl):172.

45. Weickert U, Muhlen E, Janssen J, et al. The Holmium-YAG laser: a suitable instrument for stone fragmentation in choledocholithiasis. The assessment of the results of its use under babyscopic control. Dtsch Med Wochenschr 1999; 194:514–518.

46. Birkett DH, Lamont JS, O'Keane JC, et al. Comparison of pulsed dye laser and electrohydraulic lithotripsy on porcine gallbladder and common bile duct in vitro. Laser Surg Med 1992; 12:210–214.

47. Sauerbruch T, Stern M. Fragmentation of bile duct stones by extracorporeal shock wave lithotripsy: a new approach to biliary calculi after failure of routine endoscopic measures. Gastroenterology 1989; 96:146–152.

48. Adamek HE, Buttmann A, Jakobs R, et al. Extracorporeal piezoelectric lithotripsy of intrahepatic and extrahepatic biliary tract stones. Dtsch Med Wochenschr 1993; 118:1053–1059.

49. Martin LG, Ambrose SS, Elias DL, et al. Extracorporeal shock wave lithotripsy of intrahepatic stones. Case presentation and discussion of the literature. Am Surg 1988; 54:311–314.

50. Nicholson DA, Martin DF, Tweedle DEF, et al. Management of common bile duct stones using a second generation extracorporeal shockwave lithotriptor. Br J Surg 1992; 79:811–814.

51. Yasuda I, Tomita E. Extracorporeal shockwave lithotripsy of common bile duct stones without preliminary endoscopic sphincterotomy. Scand J Gastroenterol 1996; 31:934–939.

52. White DM, Correa RJ, Gibbons RP, et al. Extracorporeal shock-wave lithotripsy for bile duct calculi. Am J Surg 1998; 175:10–13.

53. Adamek HE, Maier M, Jakobs R, et al. Management of retained bile duct stones: a prospective open trial comparing extracorporeal and intracorporeal lithotripsy. Gastrointest Endosc 1996; 44:40–47.

54. Neuhaus H, Zillinger C, Born P, et al. Randomized study of intracorporeal laser lithotripsy versus extracorporeal shock-wave lithotripsy for bile duct stones. Gastrointest Endosc 1998; 47:327–334.

55. Jakobs R, Adamek HE, Maier M, et al. Fluoroscopically guided laser lithotripsy versus shock wave lithotripsy for retained bile duct stones: a prospective randomised study. Gut 1997; 40:678–682.

56. Cairns SR, Dias L, Cotton PB, et al. Additional endoscopic procedures instead of urgent surgery for retained common bile duct. Gut 1989; 30:535–540.

57. Maxton DG, Tweedle DE, Martin TF. Retained common bile duct after endoscopic sphincterotomy: temporary and long term treatment with biliary stenting. Gut 1995; 36:446–450.

58. Bergamn JJ, Rauws EAJ, Tijssen JGP, et al. Biliary endoprostheses in elderly patients with endoscopically irretrievable common bile duct stones: report on 117 patients. Gastrointest Endosc 1995; 42:195–201.

59. Farca A, Aguilar ME, Rodriguez G, et al. Biliary stents as temporary treatment for choledocholithiasis in pregnant patients. Gastrointest Endosc 1997; 46:99–101.

60. Chan ACW, Ng EKW, Chung SCS, et al. Common bile duct stones become smaller after endoscopic stenting. Endoscopy 1998; 30:356–359.

61. Vallera RA, McGee SG, Shearin M, et al. Biliary stents decrease the size of retained common bile duct stones. Gastrointest Endosc 1995; 41:A419.

62. Goldberg M, Huck HV, Ruchim M. Clearance of choledocholithiasis with indwelling biliary stents. Am J Gastroenterol 1993; 88:A1530.

63. Cotton PB. Stents for stones: short-term good, long-term uncertain. Gastrointest Endosc 1995; 42:272–274.

64. Johnson GK, Geenen JE, Venu RP, et al. Treatment of non-extractable common bile duct stones with combination ursodeoxycholic acid plus endoprostheses. Gastrointest Endosc 1993; 39:528–531.

65. Cotton PB, Forbes A, Leung J, et al. Endoscopic stenting for the long-term treatment of large bile duct stones: 2 to 5 year follow-up. Gastrointest Endosc 1987; 33:411–412.

66. van Steenbergen W, Pelemans W, Fevery J. Endoscopic biliary endoprosthesis in elderly patients with large bile duct stones. A long-term follow-up. J Am Geriatric Soc 1992; 40:57–60.

67. Chopra KB, Peters RA, O'Toole PA, et al. Randomised study of endoscopic biliary endoprosthesis versus duct clearance for bile duct stones in high risk patients. Lancet 1996; 348:791–793.

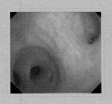

9.2

BILIARY TRACT STONE DISEASE: TRANSHEPATIC THERAPY

HORST NEUHAUS

Endoscopic sphincterotomy (EST) has become the method of choice for the majority of patients with bile duct stones and previous cholecystectomy. In addition, EST is widely accepted as a complementary procedure to laparoscopic cholecystectomy in patients with choledocholithiasis and gallbladder stones. Depending on selection criteria and the use of associated techniques, e.g. mechanical lithotripsy, the success rates vary from 85 to 95%. These results can be further improved by extracorporeal or intracorporeal lithotripsy of difficult bile duct stones. The few failures of transpapillary procedures are mainly caused by a difficult gastroduodenal or biliary anatomy, excessively large or impacted stones, or intrahepatic concrements.[1] Percutaneous transhepatic methods initially described by Nimura offer an alternative to surgery in these highly selected cases and allow mechanical removal of stones, electrohydraulic lithotripsy (EHL), or laser treatment under cholangioscopic control.[2] The percutaneous approach is more invasive and time-consuming than EST and should therefore be restricted to the small group of patients in whom advanced transpapillary procedures have failed. In view of the lack of controlled studies, the risks and benefits of transhepatic interventions should be compared with the surgical approach.

INDICATIONS

The indication for percutaneous transhepatic therapy of biliary tract stone disease should always be discussed by an experienced team of gastroenterologists, surgeons, and radiologists in view of various complementary or competitive therapeutic options.

Percutaneous treatment of bile duct stones is indicated in patients with previous cholecystectomy and extrahepatic or intrahepatic cholelithiasis in patients when transpapillary procedures have failed most often because of:

- inaccessibility of the papilla of Vater owing to:
  - previous gastroduodenal surgery, e.g. Billroth II resection or Roux-en-Y anastomosis with a long afferent loop
  - a stenosis in the upper gastrointestinal tract which cannot be sufficiently dilated for passage of a therapeutic duodenoscope
  - a difficult duodenal diverticulum
- inaccessibility of a biliodigestive anastomosis, e.g. hepaticojejunostomy
- bile duct strictures which cannot be passed or sufficiently dilated
- unsuccessful lithotripsy of giant, impacted, or inaccessible stones.

In some of these patients, the peroral access can be achieved by means of a combined endoscopic transhepatic technique ('rendez-vous maneuver').[3,4] A guidewire is inserted into the biliary tree through a thin sheath via the transhepatic route and grasped by the endoscopist with a basket catheter or a snare. The endoscope can then be advanced to the papilla or a biliodigestive anastomosis by traction on the percutaneous wire. When successful endoscopic bile duct clearance is achieved by this technique, this minimally invasive procedure is ideal because no further percutaneous interventions are required. However, problems can arise when the endoscope slips back during removal of stones requiring that the combined procedure has to be repeated. The approach is often difficult in patients with complicated stones because the endoscope is usually in an unstable position with limited maneuverability. Percutaneous treatment of bile duct stones may be more advantageous than the rendez-vous maneuver particularly in patients with a difficult gastroduodenal anatomy and multiple or impacted stones.

Percutaneous procedures can also be indicated in patients with gallbladder stones and endoscopic failure of removal of bile duct stones if:

- cholecystectomy is not planned because of a high surgical risk
- open cholecystectomy plus common bile duct exploration seems to be more difficult than a combination of percutaneous transhepatic bile duct clearance and laparoscopic cholecystectomy, e.g. in patients with intrahepatic stones. Alternatively, cholangioscopy can be performed via a T-tube tract after cholecystectomy and incomplete common bile duct exploration.[5]

CONTRAINDICATIONS

Percutaneous procedures are contraindicated in patients with a bleeding diathesis (prothrombin time <50%, platelet count <50 × 10[9]/L). The risk of bleeding is much higher in patients with liver cirrhosis. Ascites prevents establishment of a mature cutaneobiliary tract so that special precautions, e.g. the use of sheaths, are required. Transhepatic interventions should not be performed in uncooperative or restless patients because of an increased risk of failure and complications. A history of allergic reaction to contrast media requires prophylactic treatment with corticosteroids and antihistamines, and a consideration of the use of non-ionic contrast media.

EQUIPMENT

Accessories for establishment of a transhepatic tract

Needles
- Chiba needle with a diameter of 0.6 mm or 0.7 mm (various lengths from 90–400 mm)
- Uni-Dwell needle with a Teflon sheath and an outer diameter of 1.0 mm or 1.3 mm; accepts a 0.035 inch guidewire.

Guidewires
- Hydrophilic guidewires with a straight or J-shaped tip
- Flexible and stiff, kink-resistant torque-guidewires with a straight or J-shaped tip; outer diameter 0.035 inch, length 145 cm or 220 cm.

Catheters
- Vessel bougies with an outer diameter of 7, 8, 9, 10, 12 Fr
- Pigtail drainage catheters with a diameter of 7, 8.5, 10 Fr and 16 or 32 sideholes
- Nimura-type bougies with an outer diameter of 10, 12, 14, 16, 18 Fr (Fig. 9.2.1)
- Yamakawa-type transhepatic tubes with a stop-cock at the proximal end and a diameter of 10, 12, 14, 16, 18 Fr (Fig. 9.2.2).[6]

Cholangioscopes

A variety of cholangioscopes with different specifications are commercially available from several companies (Table 9.2.1). The insertion tube of a standard instrument (e.g.

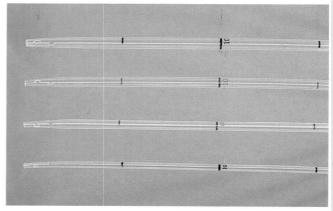

Fig. 9.2.1 Bougie catheters with an increasing diameter from 10 Fr to 16 Fr for sequential dilation of a percutaneous transhepatic tract.

Table 9.2.1 Cholangioscopes for the percutaneous transhepatic approach

Cholangioscopes for the percutaneous transhepatic approach				
	Diameter of the distal end(mm)	Diameter of the channel (mm)	Tip bending (deg.) (up/down/right/left)	Field of view (deg.)
Olympus[1]				
CHF P20	4.9	2.2	160/130	120
CHF XP20	3.5	1.2	160/130	120
CHF T20	6.0	2.6 and 1.2	130/100	120
CHF P20Q	5.0	2.0	160/130 (90/90)	120
Pentax[2]				
FCN-15X	4.8	2.2	180/130	125
ECN-1530 (Video)	5.1	2.0	180/130	120
Polydiagnost[3]				
PTC-Skop	3.0	1.2 and 0.6	90/-	70

[1]Olympus Optical Europe GmbH (Hamburg, Germany); [2]Pentax Europe GmbH (Hamburg, Germany); [3]Polydiagnost GmbH (Pfaffenhofen, Germany).

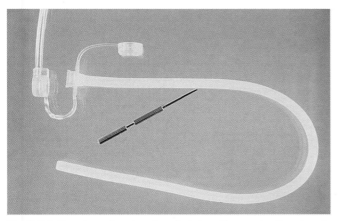

Fig. 9.2.2 Yamakawa-type transhepatic tube with an outer diameter of 16 Fr; the proximal end is provided with a stop-cock and a plate which is fixed on the skin; according to the biliary anatomy, sideholes are cut with a punch to allow bile drainage through the tube into the small bowel.

Olympus CHF P 20) has an outer diameter of 4.9 mm so that a transhepatic tract of at least 16 Fr is required for insertion. Ultraslim endoscopes with an outer diameter of 3.5 mm or less can be introduced through smaller fistulas and are more flexible which facilitates the approach to biliary side-branches[7] (Fig. 9.2.3). Most of the instruments have a two-way angulation system which allows easy maneuverability, enhanced by the short length of the insertion tube. The optical view is usually excellent and provides a clear image of the biliary tree which can be transmitted to a monitor by use of attached video cameras. The image size of ultraslim endoscopes is of course smaller and the working channel has a thinner diameter. In these latter instruments, irrigation of the biliary tree is less effective compared to large-bore choledochofiberscopes, especially after insertion of lithotripsy probes.

Instruments with two channels, a four-way angulation system or electronic cholangioscopes ('videoscopes') usually offer no clinically relevant advantage over standard devices for transhepatic treatment of bile duct stones. Large-bore fiberscopes or videoscopes require more sessions for establishment of the requisite wider cutaneobiliary fistula. Their better optical performance is rarely required for therapeutic purposes. However, instruments with a large channel may be needed for the use of stronger

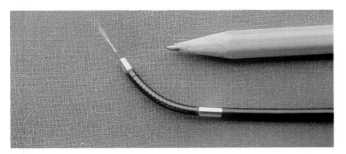

Fig. 9.2.3 Cholangioscope with an outer diameter of 2.8 mm and an inserted fiber with a diameter of 200 μm for pulsed dye-laser lithotripsy; a helium aiming beam produces red light for stone targeting.

basket catheters when there is no option for intracorporeal lithotripsy.

Lithotriptor systems

Extracorporeal shockwave lithotripsy

When extracorporeal shockwave lithotripsy (ESWL) was first carried out, first-generation lithotriptors required immersion of the patient in a waterbath.[8] Second-generation systems do not require a waterbath because the shockwave head is directly coupled to the skin by a hydrophilic gel. Three different types of shockwave generators (electrohydraulic, electromagnetic, and piezoelectric) are available and seem to be equally effective.[9] A biplanar fluoroscopy unit should be integrated for stone localization since ultrasonographic targeting can be difficult, especially in patients with distal concrements or in obese patients.

Electrohydraulic lithotripsy

This system includes a shockwave generator and probes with a minimal diameter of 0.8 mm for transmission of the energy to the stone surface. A spark discharge from a bipolar coaxial electrode at the tip of the probe induces shockwaves in a fluid medium. Absorption of the energy within the stone leads to build-up pressure gradients which subsequently cause stone fragmentation.[10] The frequency and the intensity of the shockwave generation can be adjusted depending on the size and composition of the stones. Although EHL probes with built-in balloon catheters for positioning in the central axis of the bile duct are available, cholangioscopic control of shockwave application is strongly recommended since perforation or bleeding may occur when the ductal wall comes in direct contact with the probe.[11–13]

Laser lithotripsy

Several systems for biliary laser lithotripsy have recently been reported in animal and clinical studies. A flashlamp, pulsed dye laser system has been used most frequently. The laser energy is transmitted via a 200 μm or 320 μm flexible quartz fiber (Fig. 9.2.3). Pulses with a duration of approximately 1 μs can be applied at a repetition rate of 1–10 Hz with an energy output up to 150 mJ. A fluid medium is required for initiation of a laser plasma leading to stone fragmentation. Although conventional laser lithotripsy is probably safer than EHL, direct visual control is recommended since bile duct perforation may occur when the energy is inadvertently applied to the ductal wall.

Intracorporeal cholangioscopic lithotripsy may be further improved by use of a new 'smart' laser with an automatic stone recognition system. This technique allows lithotripsy even under a limited direct visual control or under fluoroscopy.[14–16] This flash-lamp excited rhodamine 6G laser has a wavelength of 594 nm (Baasel Lasertech, Starnberg, Germany). The system provides an automatic cut-out upon tissue contact. The laser light which is backscattered by a surface in the first hundreds of nanoseconds of the pulse is conducted back through the fiber, decoupled by a beam splitter, and analysed.

Previous studies have demonstrated that tissue and ureter stones can be differentiated using this method. If, therefore, the intensity of the reflected laser beam is below a threshold value which indicates that the fiber is not in contact with a concrement, the pulse is immediately interrupted with the aid of a polarizer by rotating the plane of polarization by 90°. Up to the moment of interruption, less than 10% of the total power of the laser pulse has been emitted and tissue damage is thus safely excluded. The smart laser can therefore be used under fluoroscopic targeting without the need for cholangioscopic control. However, targeting of stones can be more difficult because the radiolucent fiber inserted through a catheter is not visible. In addition, steering of the catheter is limited compared with bidirectionally maneuverable miniscopes. However, the stone-tissue differentiation system is useful even if laser lithotripsy is performed under cholangioscopic guidance because the tip of the laser fiber may be difficult to visualize owing to clouds of stone fragments or ductal angulation.

PATIENT PREPARATION

A medical history and physical and laboratory investigation are required before any transhepatic procedure. Attention must be paid to the coagulation status. Transabdominal ultrasound should be performed for determination of intrahepatic bile duct dilation and measurement of the common bile duct size. In selected cases, e.g. suspicion of anatomical variations or undetermined lesions, magnetic resonance cholangiopancreatography (MRCP) can be helpful for guidance of the transhepatic access. Aims, risks, duration, and alternatives of the planned interventions should be explained to the patient at least 1 day before the procedure. The patient should ingest no solids and liquids for at least 6 hours prior to percutaneous interventions to minimize the risk of aspiration. An intravenous line is mandatory since repeated doses of sedation and analgesics may be needed whereas general anesthesia is rarely required. Monitoring of pulse oximetry, blood pressure, and level of consciousness is obligatory throughout and after the examination. Continuous ECG monitoring should be performed particularly in patients with heart disease and/or pulmonary problems. Equipment for resuscitation must be available. The cholangioscopes must have been sterilized by high level disinfection to reduce the risk of cholangitis. Peri-operative administration of antibiotics (mezlocillin, amoxicillin with clavulanic acid, cefotaxime, or cefuroxim) is strongly recommended for all percutaneous transhepatic interventions.

PROCEDURE

Transhepatic access
A high quality fluoroscopy unit with provisions for magnification and spot filming is essential for percutaneous treatment of bile duct stones. A transhepatic fistula (sinus tract) must be established in patients with no T-tube or a difficult T-tube tract which makes insertion of catheters or cholangioscopes impossible. The site of the transhepatic access depends on the findings of ultrasound or MRCP. An approach via the right lateral chest wall is usually preferred because the radiation exposure to the practitioner is lower compared to a ventral access. Percutaneous epigastric access through the left liver lobe is used in patients with strictures of the left biliary tract or intrahepatic stones in the right liver lobe which can only be approached by advancement of a cholangioscope from the left site via the hepatic bifurcation (Figs 9.2.4 and 9.2.5).

After determination of the puncture site, local anesthesia is performed and a Chiba needle is inserted towards the hepatic bifurcation under fluoroscopic guidance according

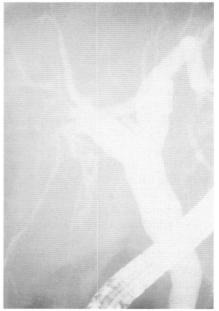

Fig. 9.2.4A Impacted intrahepatic stones in segment V in a patient with recurrent attacks of cholangitis.

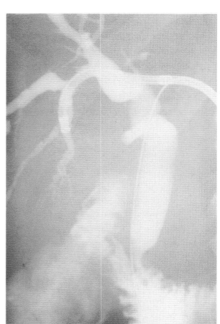

Fig. 9.2.4B Cholangioscopic approach via the left liver lobe to segment V with removal of the stone.

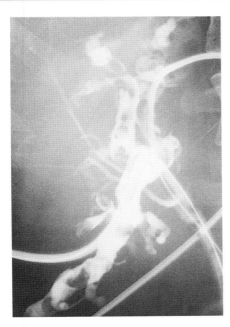

Fig. 9.2.5A Multiple intrahepatic stones in several liver segments in a patient with Caroli's syndrome; bilateral access with two external–internal drainage catheters.

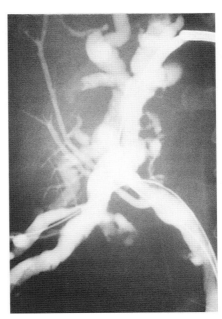

Fig. 9.2.5B Complete bile duct clearance after cholangioscopic flushing of the stones from the periphery to the bifurcation and then into the duodenum.

to the shape of the liver. The insertion site should avoid the pleural space. Guidance of the needle by transabdominal ultrasound can be helpful in difficult cases, especially when the the biliary tract is not dilated. Contrast medium is then carefully injected through the Chiba needle to avoid any extravasation. The needle is gradually withdrawn until a flow of contrast into the biliary system has been obtained. Further injection provides a complete cholangiogram. The procedure can be repeated in case of a failed puncture which is rare in patients with dilated ducts.

A Uni-Dwell needle is then inserted into a selected biliary segment which provides easy transhepatic access to the stones. A puncture into the central part of the biliary tree should be avoided because of the proximity of large vessels. After removal of the metal needle, a hydrophilic guidewire can be passed through the Teflon sheath into the biliary tree. These highly flexible guidewires can usually be inserted even via angulated or tight strictures into the distal part of the common bile duct or through the papilla or a biliodigestive anastomosis. The hydrophilic wire must be subsequently exchanged for a stiffer wire over which the transhepatic tract is sequentially enlarged with vessel bougies to a diameter of 8–10 Fr. Biliary strictures or papillary stenoses can be dilated with bougies or balloon catheters. The first session of percutaneous treatment is completed by placement of a pigtail catheter for temporary extrahepatic drainage. The number of sideholes depends on the anatomy and the distance of the intraductal portion of the catheter. The cutaneobiliary fistula can be dilated every second day in one to three sessions by replacing Nimura-type bougie catheters with inserted sideholes or pigtail catheters with progressively increasing diameters.[1,17,18] All of these procedures can be performed under conscious sedation and analgesia.

This gradual formation of a sinus tract is safer than dilation and cholangioscopy as a single-step procedure which requires the use of sheaths.[11] Stone extraction under

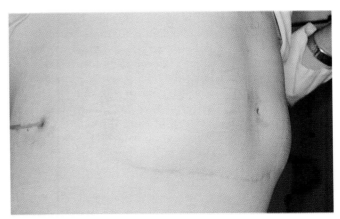

Fig. 9.2.6 Patient with percutaneous fistulas through both liver lobes via a right lateral and an epigastric access.

fluoroscopic or cholangioscopic control can be carried out as early as 7 to 8 days after the initial percutaneous procedure through the stabilized fibrous cutaneobiliary fistula[17,18] (Fig. 9.2.6). Covering plastic sheaths which require further dilation are only necessary when adequate sinus tracts have not been established or when sharp stone fragments must be removed percutaneously (Fig. 9.2.7). Yamakawa-type transhepatic tubes provide a flat stop-cock at skin level and can be left in situ for internal biliary drainage between treatment sessions (Fig. 9.2.8).

Percutaneous stone removal

Through a cutaneobiliary fistula or a large-bore T-tube tract, bile duct stones can be approached with baskets or balloon catheters under fluoroscopic control.[19,20] Because of the possibility of fistula disruption, stones should be extracted percutaneously only through sheaths unless the sinus tract was created at least 3 weeks prior to the procedure. A safe, rapid and effective alternative is the prograde

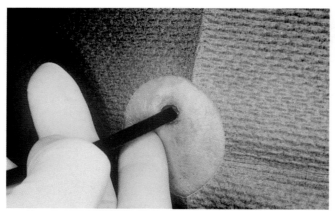

Fig. 9.2.7 Insertion of a cholangioscope through a mature percutaneous transhepatic fistula without use of a sheath.

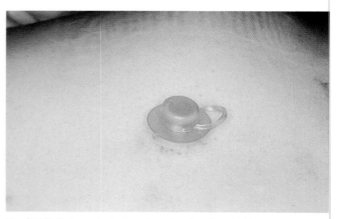

Fig. 9.2.8 Outer part of a transhepatic tube closed with a stop-cock at the skin level.

cholangioscopic removal of concrements through the papilla or through a pre-existent biliodigestive anastomosis preferably after intracorporeal lithotripsy.[11–13,15,18,21]

For stone extraction, the transhepatic catheter is removed over a guidewire which is left in situ. Contrast medium should be directly injected through the cutaneous stoma to confirm that the fistula is matured without any leakage into the abdominal cavity. A cholangioscope with an outer diameter smaller than the size of the established fistula can be inserted into the biliary system alongside the guidewire under direct visual control (Fig. 9.2.3). There is no need for sheaths or overtubes (Fig. 9.2.7). Effective irrigation is achieved by saline infusion through the instrumentation channel. Cholangioscopy facilitates mechanical removal of smaller stones by flushing or pushing them through the papilla or a biliodigestive anastomosis with the tip of the instrument (Fig. 9.2.9).

Transhepatic sphincterotomy is potentially hazardous and is not required after bougienage of the papilla.

Intrahepatic stones can often be approached only by positioning the endoscope above the stones where forceful flushing through the instrumentation channel can achieve migration of the concrements into the central parts of the biliary tree (Fig. 9.2.10). Alternatively, small stones can be grasped and carefully extracted via a mature cutaneobiliary fistula with baskets which are inserted through the instrumentation channel of the cholangioscope. Larger or impacted stones can be disintegrated by ESWL prior to the endoscopic procedure.

Intracorporeal lithotripsy is more promising and faster owing to the easy cholangioscopic approach and the option of complete bile duct clearance within a single session after establishment of the percutaneous tract.[21] For this purpose, the tip of the EHL probe or the laser fiber has to be positioned onto the surface of the stone. Continuous intraductal irrigation is required to establish a fluid medium. An advantage of laser therapy is that bile duct flushing can be easily performed even through tiny instrumentation channels of miniscopes because the laser fiber is much thinner than EHL probes. The use of miniscopes with an outer diameter of 3.5 mm or less requires fewer dilation procedures so that the treatment is more convenient for the patient and more cost-effective. The

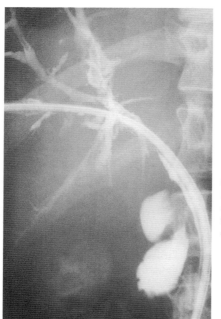

Fig. 9.2.9A Percutaneous transhepatic drainage in a patient with a benign stricture of the right hepatic duct and multiple filling defects in several segments with ductal irregularities; the left liver was previously resected because of infection with echinococcus; laboratory examinations and computed tomography showed no evidence of recurrence.

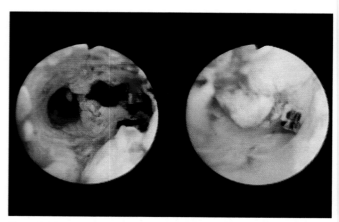

Fig. 9.2.9B (Left) Percutaneous transhepatic cholangioscopy reveals multiple black intrahepatic stones and echinococcus cysts. (Right) Close-up of a small intraheptic stone and a cyst.

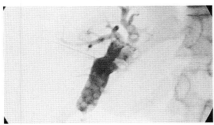

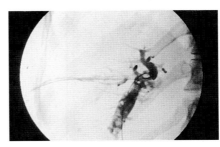

Fig. 9.2.10B Injection of contrast media through the cutaneobiliary fistula demonstrates a mature track 7 days after placement of a percutaneous transhepatic catheter.

Fig. 9.2.10A Percutaneous transhepatic cholangioscopy reveals multiple stones in segment VI in a 24-year-old patient with recurrent attacks of cholangitis after previous resection of a choledochocele and hepaticojejunostomy; there is no flow of contrast into the jejunum owing to a postoperative anastomotic stricture.

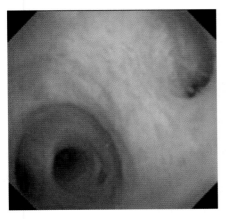

Fig. 9.2.10C Percutaneous transhepatic cholangioscopy with an electronic endoscope reveals stone-free radicles of segment VI after flushing intrahepatic stones into the right hepatic duct.

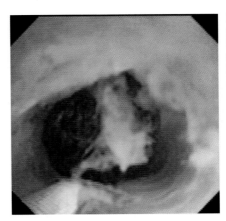

Fig. 9.2.10D Multiple pigment stones are flushed through the anastomosis after hepaticojejunostomy into the jejunum.

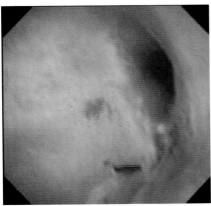

Fig. 9.2.10E Cholangioscopy finally demonstrates a fully opened biliodigestive anastomosis which allows excellent biliary drainage after complete ductal clearance of stones.

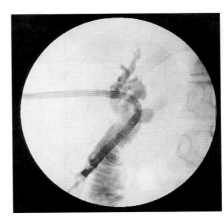

Fig. 9.2.10F The tip of the cholangioscope is in segment VI; cholangiography demonstrates complete bile duct clearance of stones and excellent drainage of contrast media into the jejunum.

resulting stone fragments from laser lithotripsy are smaller compared to EHL and can be more easily removed through a stricture, the papilla, or a biliodigestive anastomosis (Fig. 9.2.11).

The procedure is probably even safer when systems with an automatic stone recognition system are used since the cholangioscopic vision may be limited because of stone fragments or biliary sludge. In contrast to ESWL, there is no upper limit on the number of pulses during intracorporeal lithotripsy provided that ductal damage can be excluded by means of cholangioscopy or a 'smart' laser system. However, the procedure should not last more than approximately 2 hours as elderly patients in whom sedation must be carefully performed may not tolerate a longer treatment session. Large

amounts of irrigated saline solution must be considered as a risk for cardiovascular problems. Aspiration of fluid refluxed into the stomach can be avoided by placement of a nasogastric tube. Complete bile duct clearance can usually be achieved within a single treatment session. If clearance is not achieved, as in multiple intrahepatic stones, a transhepatic catheter must be inserted. Biliary sludge and smaller stone fragments usually pass spontaneously. Another procedure can be planned on the following day if cholangioscopy demonstrates residual stones.

Postprocedural care of the transhepatic tract

The transhepatic treatment of biliary stone disease is finished after cholangiographic documentation of complete

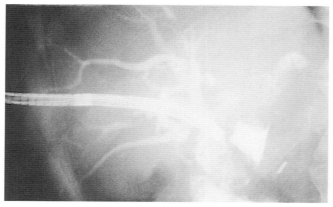

Fig. 9.2.11A Percutaneous transhepatic approach to the hepatic bifurcation with a cholangioscope in a patient with a benign anastomotic stricture after hepatojejunostomy and stones in the common hepatic duct and left hepatic duct.

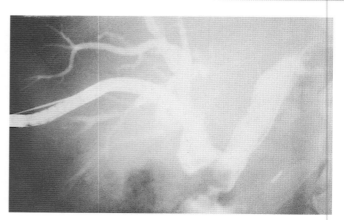

Fig. 9.2.11B Fluoroscopic control of cholangioscopic laser lithotripsy.

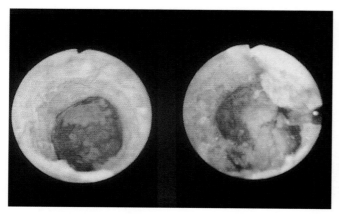

Fig. 9.2.11C (Left) Percutaneous transhepatic cholangioscopy shows a cholesterol stone at the hepatic bifurcation. (Right) The stone disintegrates by means of pulsed dye laser lithotripsy; the laser fiber can be seen at 3 o'clock; the tip is in direct contact with the surface of the stone.

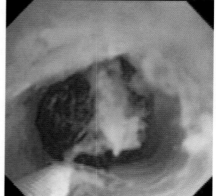

Fig. 9.2.11D Injection of contrast media through the cholangioscope demonstrates complete bile duct clearance after passage of all stone fragments through the anastomosis into the jejunum.

ductal clearance of stones and absence of bile duct stenoses. The transhepatic catheter can be removed and the cutaneobiliary fistula should spontaneously close within 1 or 2 days. Continuous bile leakage indicates biliary obstruction and requires cholangiographic examination by injection of contrast media through the unclosed fistula. In patients with benign bile duct strictures, Yamakawa-type transhepatic tubes which are occluded at the skin level can be left in situ for approximately 3 months to prevent early biliary restenosis after dilation[6,22–24] (Fig. 9.2.8). Cholangiography should be repeated after this period to decide if further treatment is required with these prostheses because of a persistent stricture. When problems are encountered, alternative methods, e.g. surgery or percutaneous implantation of metal stents in high surgical risk candidates or patients with incurable malignant stenoses, should be considered (Fig. 9.2.12). Indwelling transhepatic tubes should be regularly flushed with sterile saline solution once or twice a week to prevent blockage or stone formation by biliary sludge.

COMPLICATIONS AND MANAGEMENT

The main risks of the percutaneous transhepatic treatment of bile duct stones are related to the placement of the transhepatic catheter and the dilation of the cutaneobiliary fistula.[13,17,25,26] These procedures may cause hemobilia owing to biliovenous fistulas which close spontaneously when a transhepatic catheter of an appropriate size to compress the bleeding area is inserted far enough so that no sideholes are located within the fistulous tract. This tamponade technique is also used to stop rarely observed arterial bleeding into the biliary tract. However, in contrast to biliovenous fistulas, recurrent bleeding is frequently seen after removal of the catheter. Selective angiographic embolization is the treatment of choice for these cases of arterial fistulae. A subcapsular liver hematoma usually disappears spontaneously within a few days; forceful dilation procedures should be avoided during this time.

The incidence of cholangitis is increased in patients with incomplete biliary drainage in particular when multiple

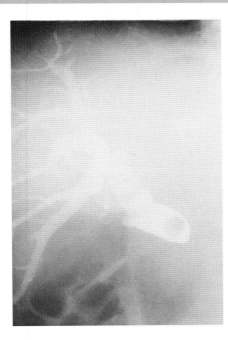

Fig. 9.2.12A Percutaneous transhepatic cholangioscopy reveals several biliary stones and complete obstruction of the distal common bile duct owing to pancreatic cancer; endoscopic retrograde cholangiopancreatography had failed because of a long afferent loop after previous Billroth II resection.

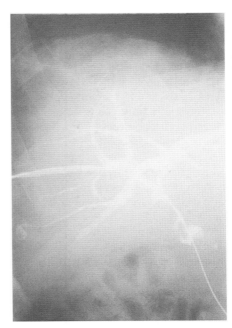

Fig. 9.2.12B Percutaneous placement of an external internal drainage catheter after successful cannulation of the stenosis with a hydrophilic guidewire.

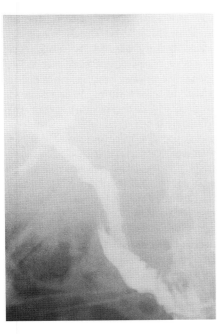

Fig. 9.2.12C Excellent internal biliary drainage after cholangioscopic removal of the ductal stones and implantation of a self-expandable metal stent as a palliative measurement.

drainage tract is required. These interventions can be difficult since the bile ducts are usually narrow owing to previous decompression or continuous leakage. Establishment of a large-bore transhepatic tract within a single treatment session is associated with a considerable risk of hemobilia because of arteriobiliary fistula formation and bile duct perforation. Although these complications can usually be managed by arterial embolization or bile duct drainage, gradual dilation is preferred.[11] Pancreatitis can be another complication of transhepatic drainage and is mainly observed when a large-bore catheter is positioned through the papilla without previous endoscopic sphincterotomy. Rapid improvement can usually be achieved by withdrawal of the tip of the catheter above the papilla with subsequent gradual dilation.

After maturation of a cutaneobiliary fistula, cholangioscopic procedures rarely cause serious complications. Minor hemobilia is seen in up to 20% of patients treated with EHL but can be managed conservatively.[11–13]

RESULTS

Fluoroscopically guided percutaneous transhepatic therapy of extrahepatic and intrahepatic bile duct stones with pre-shaped angulated catheters or baskets is time-consuming and has been reported only in a few series.[19,20] According to many Asian and some Western trials, percutaneous cholangioscopy is the non-surgical method of choice for hepatolithiasis and extrahepatic stones which are not amenable to transpapillary procedures. The endoscopic approach is frequently combined with intracorporeal lithotripsy. EHL and laser lithotripsy seem to show comparable effectiveness, with success rates of between 81% and 100%.[11–15,18,21]

The largest series have been reported from the Far East because of the high incidence of hepatolithiasis in these

stones or bile duct strictures cause obstruction of several liver segments. The risk can be reduced by preoperative application of antibiotics. Continuous cholangitis may require exchange of transhepatic catheters, drainage of obstructed segments, or rapid removal of stones.

If a sinus tract or a T-tube tract has not been stabilized, partial or complete migration of the catheter out of the transhepatic tract may cause bile leakage and biliary peritonitis. The risk of this serious complication is lower when the tip of a transhepatic catheter is inserted into the distal part of the common bile duct or through the papilla. Dislocation of a transhepatic catheter is more frequent when using the right lateral approach because of motion between the liver and the chest wall. Immediate replacement of the drainage catheter or establishment of a new

countries. The difficult application of treatment for this disease is a challenge for endoscopists, surgeons, and radiologists. The results are therefore less favorable compared to Western series which mainly include extrahepatic stones or more easily accessible intrahepatic stones above biliary strictures. Yeh et al[23] reported on 615 patients with hepatolithiasis of whom 450 initially underwent surgery with or without postoperative cholangioscopy in Taiwan. Percutaneous transhepatic cholangioscopy (PTCS) was the primary therapy for 165 patients because of a poor surgical risk, previous biliary surgery, or refusal of surgery. Cholangioscopy was performed 2 weeks after initial percutaneous transhepatic drainage and subsequent dilation of the tract. EHL was used for larger stones. No general anesthesia was required. A mean of 5.1 sessions of PTCS was needed for bile duct clearance which was completely achieved in 81% of the patients. One out of 5 patients had at least one episode of cholangitis and the mortality rate was 1.2%. In patients with difficult ductal strictures, large-bore transhepatic drainage catheters were left in situ for several months to avoid rapid restenoses. Follow-up after PTCS indicates a stone recurrence rate of 33% after a mean period of 58 months. All but one of the patients with recurrent stones could be managed non-surgically by PTCS or conservative treatment.

In a further study from Taiwan, Jan & Chen[24] reported on PTCS and EHL or laser lithotripsy in 48 patients with intrahepatic stones of whom 40 had previously undergone biliary tract surgery. A large-bore transhepatic fistula had been sequentially established often on an outpatient basis. Complete bile duct clearance was achieved in 83% of the patients with a mean of five PTCS sessions. Complications were seen in 15% of the patients and the short-term mortality rate was 2.1%. During a 4- to 10-year follow-up, 16/40 patients with initially successful PTCS developed symptomatic or asymptomatic recurrent stones. Only one of these patients underwent surgery. The recurrence rate was statistically higher in patients with associated bile duct strictures.

Jeng et al[27] reported on the important role of management of biliary strictures which are frequently associated with hepatolithiasis and also increase the risk of recurrence. They performed 208 sessions of balloon dilation in 57 consecutive patients with ductal strictures and intrahepatic stones. The success rate of complete clearance increased significantly from 0% predilation to 95% postdilation. The main complications consisted of septicemia and hemobilia. Subsequent temporary stenting was performed in 14% of the patients. The cumulative probability of restricture was surprisingly low with 8% at 3 years.

As a result of the more favorable selection of patients, the success rates of European series for biliary tract stone disease exceed 90%.[11,15,18] The main complication is temporary cholangitis which usually responds to antibiotic treatment.

There are only a few long-term results from Western trials in patients with associated biliary strictures. In a previous series from our group, 55 consecutive patients underwent percutaneous treatment of bile duct stones not amenable to transpapillary procedures.[22] After establishment of a cutaneobiliary tract, cholangioscopic laser lithotripsy was performed and fragments were flushed through the papilla or a biliodigestive anastomosis. Associated biliary or papillary stenoses in 30/55 patients were treated by dilation only, sphincterotomy, temporary prostheses, or metal stents in 8, 1, 15 and 6 cases, respectively. Fistula formation caused temporary bleeding or cholangitis in a total of 11 patients. Laser lithotripsy and bile duct clearance was safely achieved in 53/55 patients (97%). The 30-day mortality rate was 1.8%. During a median follow-up of 21 months, seven patients died of causes unrelated to biliary tract disease. Excellent (asymptomatic, normal liver enzymes) or fair (transient symptoms) responses were achieved in 42/46 patients (85%). Recurrence of stenoses required reinterventions in four.

We recently studied the efficacy and safety of percutaneous transhepatic interventions in a selected group of 29 patients with anastomotic stenoses after hepaticojejunostomy. Ten of these patients had ductal stones above the stenoses or in the intrahepatic biliary tree. Establishment of a transhepatic tract and internal biliary drainage was achieved in all cases. Removal of stones succeeded in all ten cases by PTCS and laser lithotripsy. The 30-day morbidity rate of 17% was mainly caused by temporary cholangitis. Yamakawa-type transhepatic tubes were left in situ until the disappearance of the strictures or decision for a surgical approach because of failure. During a mean follow-up period of 689 ± 444 days, 87 reinterventions were performed predominantly for exchange of catheters. The Yamakawa-type prosthesis could be removed in 14 patients after a mean of 167 ± 55 days without evidence of recurrent cholestasis during a follow-up period of 643 ± 306 days. The tubes are still in situ in eight cases. Metal stents were percutaneously implanted in four patients with a high risk for surgery. One of these patients and three further patients had to undergo surgery because of recurrent strictures. There was no mortality in this series.

CONCLUSIONS

Transhepatic treatment of bile duct stones offers an effective alternative to surgery when less invasive transpapillary maneuvers have failed or proved to be impossible because of an inaccessible papilla or large stones above a biliary stricture. The best approach is provided by a team of gastroenterologists, surgeons, and radiologists who have vast experience in the treatment of biliary tract diseases. Out of a variety of different percutaneous techniques, the most effective and safest approach seems to be the gradual establishment of a cutaneobiliary fistula which allows direct insertion of cholangioscopes. Extrahepatic stones can be easily approached even with less flexible large-bore instruments. The more difficult access to intrahepatic concrements can be improved by use of ultraslim cholangioscopes. Impacted or large stones can be disintegrated by EHL or laser lithotripsy under direct visual control. In general, transhepatic cholangioscopic lithotripsy is more effective than the peroral approach with a mother–babyscope system. The shorter instruments have a better optical system, can be more easily maneuvered to the stones, and allow fragments to be flushed progradely away from the tip of the endoscope. Bile duct clearance can usually be obtained within a single session by irrigation or pushing of stones and fragments through the papilla or a biliodigestive anastomosis. Failures are predominantly observed in difficult cases of Oriental hepatolithiasis. Severe complications are rare whereas mild courses of cholangitis can occur when there is incomplete drainage. The long-term results of transhepatic therapy of biliary tract stone disease are promising. Recurrences are mainly caused by associated strictures of the bile duct or a biliodigestive anastomosis. Temporary placement of large-bore transhepatic tubes capped at skin level promises to reduce the risk of recurrent strictures. Although transhepatic procedures seem to be technically easy, expertise is required for difficult cases and management of complications.

CHECKLIST OF PRACTICE POINTS

1. Before transhepatic procedures are performed:
   - review patient's history and all previous documents of gastroduodenal or biliary surgery, endoscopic or percutaneous transhepatic procedures, ultrasound, MRCP, and CT scan
   - evaluate the general condition of the patient with special attention to cardiopulmonary risk factors and clotting status
   - determine the indication or contraindication for percutaneous interventions and explain the procedure and alternatives to the patient
   - check the availability and function of all instruments and accessories required for percutaneous treatment of bile duct stones and monitoring of vital signs. Be prepared for cardiopulmonary complications including the need for resuscitation.
2. Select the site of the percutaneous access depending on the biliary anatomy and the location of stones or ductal strictures previously determined by transabdominal ultrasound or MRCP.
3. Consider ultrasonographic guidance of the transhepatic insertion of needles in patients with non-dilated bile ducts or a difficult biliary anatomy.
4. Avoid extravasation into the liver parenchyma by forceful injection of contrast media which impairs the quality of subsequent cholangiography.
5. Use hydrophilic guidewires for initial cannulation of the bile duct or passage through strictures and use stiffer wires for dilation procedures.
6. Avoid forceful dilation of the transhepatic tract, especially when bougie catheters cannot easily be advanced and fluoroscopy indicates bending of the guidewire towards the liver parenchyma; in this case, leave a smaller drainage catheter in situ and repeat the procedure after 2 days. Consider dilation of tight ductal strictures with balloon catheters.
7. Try to place transhepatic catheters in a stable position; the risk of dislocation is high when the tip is not advanced into the extrahepatic biliary tract.
8. Check by injection of contrast medium that the sideholes of the drainage catheter are in the biliary tree and that there is no leakage into the abdominal cavity and no flow via a biliovenous fistula.
9. Check maturation of the cutaneobiliary fistula by injection of contrast media before a cholangioscope is inserted without use of a sheath.
10. Select the type of cholangioscope according to the size of the transhepatic tract, the location of stones, and the diameter of accessories, e.g. basket catheters or probes for lithotripsy.
11. Limit the total amount of saline solution used for irrigation because of the risk of aspiration and overhydration.
12. Avoid extraction of stones through a cutaneobiliary fistula which was established less than 3 weeks previously. Avoid forceful pushing of stones through an intact papilla in lieu of lithotripsy for these cases.
13. Leave a guidewire in situ for all interventions in order to maintain rapid access in case of complications or failures.
14. Before definitive removal of catheters and guidewires, document complete bile duct clearance, absence of strictures, and maturity of the cutaneobiliary fistula by cholangiography. The fistula will rapidly close when there is no bile duct obstruction.
15. Consider temporary placement of large-bore Yamakawa-type transhepatic tubes to reduce the risk of early recurrence of biliary stenoses.

REFERENCES

1. Classen M, Hagenmueller F, Knyrim K, et al. Giant bile duct stones – non-surgical treatment. Endoscopy 1988; 20:21–26.

2. Nimura Y, Hayakawa N, Toyoda S. Percutaneous transhepatic cholangioscopy. Stomach Intestine 1981; 16:681–689.

3. Ponchon T, Valette PJ, Bory R, et al. Evaluation of a combined percutaneous-endoscopic procedure for the treatment of choledocholithiasis and benign papillary stenosis. Endoscopy 1987; 19:164–166.

4. Fujita R, Yamamura M, Fujita Y. Combined endoscopic sphincterotomy and percutaneous transhepatic cholangioscopic lithotripsy. Gastrointest Endosc 1988; 34:91–94.

5. Pitt HA, Venbrux AC, Coleman RN, et al. Intrahepatic stones. The transhepatic team approach. Ann Surg 1994; 219:527–537.

6. Yamakawa T. Percutaneous cholangioscopy for management of retained biliary tract stones and intrahepatic stones. Endoscopy 1989; 21:333–337.

7. Neuhaus H, Hoffmann W, Classen M. Laser lithotripsy of pancreatic and biliary stones via 3.4 and 3.7 mm miniscopes: first clinical results. Endoscopy 1992; 24:208–214.

8. Sauerbruch T, Holl J, Sackmann M, et al. Fragmentation of bile duct stones by extracorporeal shock-wave lithotripsy: a five-year experience. Hepatology 1992; 15:208–214.

9. Schneider HT, Fromm M, Ott R, et al. In vitro fragmentation of gallstones: comparison of electrohydraulic, electromagnetic, and piezoelectric shockwave lithotriptors. Hepatology 1991; 14:301–305.

10. Harrison J, Morris DL, Haynes J, et al. Electrohydraulic lithotripsy of gall stones – in vitro and animal studies. Gut 1987; 28:267–271.

11. Bonnel DH, Liguory CE, Cornud FE, et al. Common bile duct and intrahepatic stones: results of transhepatic electrohydraulic lithotripsy in 50 patients. Radiology 1991; 180:345–348.

12. Chen MF, Jan YY. Percutaneous transhepatic cholangioscopic lithotripsy. Br J Surg 1990; 77:530–532.

13. Jeng KS, Chiang HS, Shih SC. Limitations of percutaneous transhepatic cholangioscopy in the removal of complicated biliary calculi. World J Surg 1989; 13:603–610.

14. Ell C, Hochberger J, May A, et al. Laser lithotripsy of difficult bile duct stones by means of a rhodamine-6G laser and an integrated automatic stone-tissue detection system. Gastrointest Endosc 1993; 39:755–762.

15. Neuhaus H, Hoffmann W, Gottlieb K, et al. Endoscopic lithotripsy of bile duct stones using a new laser with automatic stone recognition. Gastrointest Endosc 1994; 40:708–715.

16. Schreiber F, Gurakuqi GC, Trauner M. Endoscopic intracorporeal laser lithotripsy of difficult common bile duct stones with a stone-recognition pulsed dye laser system. Gastrointest Endosc 1995; 42:416–419.

17. Neuhaus H, Hoffmann W, Classen M. Nutzen und Risiken der perkutanen transhepatischen Cholangioskopie. Dtsch Med Wochenschr 1993; 118:574–581.

18. Neuhaus H, Hoffmann W, Zillinger C, et al. Laser lithotripsy of difficult bile duct stones under direct visual control. Gut 1993; 34:415–421.

19. Mazzariello RM. A fourteen-year experience with nonoperative instrument extraction of retained bile duct stones. World J Surg 1978; 2:447–455.

20. Han JK, Choi BI, Park JH, et al. Percutaneous removal of retained intrahepatic stones with a pre-shaped angulated catheter: review of 96 patients. Br J Radiol 1992; 65:9–13.

21. Neuhaus H, Zillinger C, Born P, et al. Randomized study of intracorporeal laser lithotripsy versus extracorporeal shock-wave lithotripsy for difficult bile duct stones. Gastrointest Endosc 1998; 47:327–344.

22. Neuhaus H, Zillinger C, Illek B, et al. Percutaneous transhepatic cholangioscopy (PTCS) for laserlithotripsy of bile duct stones: medium-term follow-up in 55 patients. Gastroenterology 1994; 106:A352.

23. Yeh YH, Huang MH, Yang JC, et al. Percutaneous transhepatic cholangioscopy and lithotripsy in the treatment of intrahepatic stones: a study with 5 year follow up. Gastrointest Endosc 1995; 42:13–18.

24. Jan YY, Chen MF. Percutaneous trans-hepatic cholangioscopic lithotomy for hepatolithiasis: long-term results. Gastrointest Endosc 1995; 42:19–24.

25. Mueller PR, Van Sonnenberg E, Ferrucci JT Jr. Percutaneous biliary drainage: technical and catheter-related problems in 200 procedures. AJR Am J Roentgenol 1982; 138:17–23.

26. Stambuk EC, Pitt HA, Pais SO. Percutaneous transhepatic drainage: risks and benefits. Arch Surg 1983; 118:1388–1394.

27. Jeng KS, Yang FS, Ohta I, et al. Dilation of intrahepatic biliary strictures in patients with hepatolithiasis. World J Surg 1990; 14:587–593.

10.

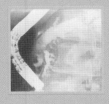

ENDOSCOPIC MANAGEMENT OF BENIGN PANCREATIC DISEASES

MICHAEL J. LEVY

JOSEPH E. GEENEN

Compared to therapeutic biliary endoscopy, the evolution of therapeutic endoscopy in the treatment of pancreatic diseases has been gradual, largely because of the concern for procedure-related complications. Once the safety of endoscopic sphincterotomy was observed in gallstone pancreatitis, interest flourished with regard to further applications of endoscopic treatment in pancreatic disorders. Today therapeutic endoscopic retrograde cholangiopancreatography (ERCP) is employed in various pancreatic diseases with the aim of improving upon the results of medical or surgical treatments, modalities which are often unsatisfactory in terms of efficacy, morbidity, and applicability (Table 10.1).

As with all new therapeutic endeavors, controlled trials are limited. Most of the available data apply to the success, efficacy, and safety of endoscopic treatments in various forms of acute and chronic pancreatitis. The generation of such data is anticipated, however, since therapeutic modalities, commonly utilized in the biliary tree, create new and specific technical problems when applied to pancreatic disease. Future studies are needed to better define the indications, efficacy, and complications of therapeutic pancreatic endoscopy.

INDICATIONS FOR ERCP IN BENIGN PANCREATIC DISEASE

ERCP has long been considered a useful diagnostic tool for evaluating benign pancreatic disease. Therapeutic application has been limited by concerns regarding safety and utility. The indications and acceptance of ERCP for benign pancreatic disease have expanded after establishing its utility and relative safety in acute gallstone pancreatitis. Endoscopic therapy is now commonly employed for the evaluation and therapy of acute and chronic pancreatitis, pancreatic strictures, pancreatic stones, and pseudocyst (Table 10.1). Further application will be fueled by carefully designed prospective, randomized, clinical outcome studies comparing endoscopic intervention to radiologic and surgical alternatives.

EQUIPMENT

Pancreatic therapeutic endoscopy requires accessory equipment such as minisphincterotomes, needle-tipped catheters, minibaskets for stone extraction, minisnares for extraction of migrated stents, nasopancreatic catheters, stents, and cytology brushes (Table 10.2). Most of these endoscopic accessories, up to and including 7 Fr stents, can be passed through a standard duodenoscope's accessory channel (2.8 mm diameter). Duodenoscopes with wider accessory channels (4.2 mm diameter) are required for insertion of stents larger than 7 Fr.

Accessory equipment is typically required for minor papilla cannulation. The needle-tip catheter, which is fitted with a blunt 23 gauge needle that projects 2–5 mm, is commonly used for minor papilla cannulation.[1] Others prefer the combined use of a 3 Fr, 200 cm angiographic catheter and a 0.018 inch (0.46 mm), 480 cm guidewire.[2] This latter technique requires gentle insertion of the angiocatheter into the minor papillary orifice. The guidewire is then passed through the catheter and into the dorsal duct. Once the guidewire is sufficiently in the pancreatic duct, the angiocatheter is slowly advanced over the guidewire

Table 10.1 Indications for ERCP in benign pancreatic disease

Indications for ERCP in benign pancreatic disease	
Pancreatic disease	**Endoscopic role**
• Acute gallstone pancreatitis (severe, cholangitis)	ES with bile duct clearance
• Acute recurrent pancreatitis	
— Choledocholithiasis	ES with bile duct clearance
— Microlithiasis	ES with bile duct clearance
— Sphincter of Oddi dysfunction	Sphincter of Oddi manometry
— Pancreas divisum	ES or stenting of minor papilla
— Choledochocele	ES to unroof cyst
• Acute pancreatitis and necrosis	
— Assessment of gland	Diagnostic ERCP
— Preoperative evaluation	Diagnostic ERCP
• Chronic pancreatitis (symptomatic)	
— Distinguish from acute	Diagnostic ERCP
— Abdominal pain	Diagnostic and therapeutic
— Cholestasis	Short-term bile duct stenting
— Stricture	Dilation/stenting (ES)
— Stones	ES with stone extraction (ESWL)
— Pseudocyst	Cystoenterostomy drainage
	Transpapillary drainage
— Neoplasm (ampulla, pancreas)	ES benign, non-surgical malignant
	Diagnosis
• Pancreatic duct disruption	Transpapillary stenting

ERCP = endoscopic retrograde cholangiopancreatography; ES = endoscopic sphincterotomy; ESWL = extracorporeal shockwave lithotripsy.

Accessories for pancreatic endoscopy	
• Sphincterotomes	• Stents
— Minisphincterotome (pre-cut)	— Plastic pancreatic duct stent
— Needle-knife sphincterotome	— Metal expandable Wallstent
— Conventional	
• Catheters (specialized)	• Extraction accessories
— Needle-tip catheters (pancreas divisum)	— Minibasket
	— Miniballoon
— 3 Fr angiocatheter with guidewire (pancreas divisum)	
— Cytology catheter/brush	
— Nasopancreatic catheter	

Table 10.2 Accessories for pancreatic endoscopy

and into the dorsal pancreatic duct. Over the past few years, the 5–4–3 contour catheter with an 0.018-inch road-runner guidewire has become the catheter of choice for minor papilla and dorsal duct cannulation.

The minisphincterotome or regular sphincterotome may be used for minor papilla sphincterotomy. This pre-cut papillotome is tailored with a tapered tip that assists cannulation efforts. On occasion, minor papilla insertion of the sphincterotome is difficult, a situation remedied by initial dilation of the minor papilla.[3]

The 'minibasket' is designed for extraction of pancreatic duct stones and proximally migrated pancreatic duct stents. This four-wire basket is much smaller than its biliary counterpart and is removable from its 5 Fr sheath. Wire-assisted sheath insertion beyond the stone (or stent) permits exact deployment of the basket. 'Minisnares', also

removable from 5 Fr sheaths, may be deployed in a similar fashion to capture and withdraw migrated stents.

The nasopancreatic catheter (5 Fr and 7 Fr) is similar to the nasobiliary catheter except for two important modifications: the distal end of the former is straight and furnished with multiple sideholes, including apertures outside the papilla. These design modifications minimize pancreatic duct injury and enhance pancreatic drainage. Pancreatic stents have similar structural features, including multiple sideholes. Single or double pairs of barbs (or flaps) are commonly added to anchor stents in place. Adequate stent therapy requires stent insertion beyond strictures and/or stones. As a result, stent length selection depends upon the location and length of ductal obstruction.

The cytology brush is uniquely adapted for sampling strictures. To permit easier passage through strictures, the brush is equipped with a 1–3 cm long flexible metal tip. Fluoroscopic visualization of the brush is enhanced by the addition of proximal and distal radiopaque markers at both ends of the brush. For brush deployment, a 6 Fr cytology catheter (also equipped with a radiopaque ring) is first inserted beyond the stricture over a guidewire. The guidewire is then exchanged for the cytology brush and sampling proceeds under fluoroscopic guidance.

PATIENT PREPARATION

Patient preparation begins with a careful search for potential complicating factors, including poor cardiopulmonary function, coagulopathies, and allergies to antibiotics or contrast dyes.

When the history suggests the possibility of a coagulopathy (family history, hemarthrosis, hematomas, excessive menses, and hemorrhagic tooth extractions), then further laboratory evaluation is indicated, especially if sphincterotomy is anticipated. Routine screening for coagulopathies is not advocated in otherwise healthy patients unless prolonged cholestasis is present.

Respiratory arrest may unfortunately occur with conscious sedation. Accordingly, narcotic and sedative/hypnotic drugs must be administered cautiously, especially in patients with diminished respiratory reserve. Cardiac and oxygenation status should be continuously monitored to ensure prompt recognition and treatment of any cardiopulmonary events. Naloxone and flumazenil should be readily available to reverse drug-induced respiratory depression.

The need for routine antibiotic prophylaxis during diagnostic and therapeutic ERCP remains controversial. While the benefit of routine antibiotic administration can be debated, there is general agreement that antibiotics are warranted when there is evidence of bile duct obstruction or a pancreatic pseudocyst.[4,5] In this setting, *Pseudomonas aeruginosa* and *Serratia marcescens* are of particular concern,[6,7] and commonly selected antibiotics include Augmentin, piperacillin or ciprofloxacillin. Endoscopic relief of obstruction is also necessary to help avoid sepsis.

Certain subgroups of patients have a more critical need for antibiotics. Such patients include those with diseased or artificial heart valves, systemic to pulmonary shunts, and synthetic vascular grafts less than 1 year old.

Non-ionic, water-soluble contrast agents have been developed in an attempt to reduce the incidence of post-ERCP pancreatitis. However, these agents are seldom used owing to cost and uncertain efficacy.[8] Many favor the use of non-ionic, water-soluble contrast agents in patients who are allergic to contrast and in those prone to post-ERCP pancreatitis.[9]

PROCEDURE

The technique of conventional ERCP is well established and yet technical success depends largely upon experience. In general, inexperienced endoscopists cannulate the pancreatic duct with relative ease, whereas common bile duct (CBD) cannulation is more difficult. With experience, however, selective cannulation of both ducts is successful in more than 90% of patients.[10] Endoscopic sphincterotomy also requires enhanced skill and should not be implemented purely for diagnostic purposes.

Pancreatoscopy

Initial use of peroral cholangioscopy and pancreatoscopy was described as early as 1975.[11] Miniscopes, passed through standard and larger channel duodenoscopes, were designed for direct intraductal inspection of the bile and pancreatic ducts and ultimately the application of endoscopic therapy or diagnostic sampling. Unfortunately, a number of factors contributed to a decline in interest and use, namely expense and fragility of the prototype miniendoscopes.

Enthusiasm for miniscope pancreatoscopy has returned, however, with the development of newer prototypes, including miniscopes with outer diameters of 0.8 mm (ultra-thin). Generally, larger miniscopes (3.1–3.7 mm diameter) offer greater diagnostic (tissue sampling) and therapeutic (laser lithotripsy) capabilities than ultra-thin versions, but scope insertion usually requires pancreatic duct sphincterotomy.[12,13] Ultra-thin miniscopes, on the other hand, have the advantage of smaller size, allowing insertion without prior sphincterotomy, and examination of more proximal segments of the pancreatic duct. From one report of initial applications of both miniscopes, pancreatoscopy enhanced the diagnostic accuracy of ERCP, especially in patients with indistinguishable benign or malignant strictures.[14] However, improvements in miniscope technology, namely directability, image quality, and photographic capability, are necessary before wider use is seen.

Diagnostic pancreatography (normal pancreatic duct)

The main pancreatic duct caliber decreases from the pancreatic head to the pancreatic tail. The normal mean duct diameter in the pancreatic head, body, and tail, is less than 5 mm, 4 mm, and 3 mm respectively.[15,16] However, the diameter of the main pancreatic duct is age-dependent. Beyond the age of 50, the width of the duct increases approximately 8% per decade.[17] Over time, the normal 'aged' pancreatic duct may resemble that of chronic pancreatitis. These changes are the result of several age-dependent histologic changes including ductal epithelial hyperplasia and intralobular and perilobular fibrosis.[18]

Normal pancreatic duct variants exist in which the duct caliber is altered in the absence of disease. Such anatomic variants include narrowing at the pancreatic genu and fusiform dilation of the distal pancreatic duct.[19] Ductal narrowing may also occur with inadequate contrast filling or as a result of compression by the superior mesenteric artery, vertebrae, or lymph nodes.[20] Narrowing is unlikely to be pathologic if adjacent side branches are normal in appearance and if proximal (upstream) ductal dilation is absent.[21]

Chronic pancreatitis

No consensus exists in regard to classifying pancreatographic changes of chronic pancreatitis. Many endoscopists use the classification system described by Kasugai,[22] which has been shown in one study to correlate with pancreatic exocrine function.[23] In an effort to unify terminology, an international workshop on chronic pancreatitis created a new classification system which emphasized the location and severity of pancreatic ductal changes.[24] The goal of the workshop was to develop a classification system that would be more widely accepted and in turn improve communication between centers and serve as a basis for future prospective and comparative trials (Table 10.3).

Table 10.3 International classification of pancreatograms (chronic pancreatitis)*

International classification of pancreatograms*			
Terminology	Main duct	Abnormal side branches	Additional features
Normal	Normal	None	
Equivocal	Normal	<3	
Mild	Normal	3 and >	
Moderate	Abnormal	>3	
Severe	Abnormal	>3	Any dilation, obstruction, or severe irregularity of the main pancreatic duct Filling defects, large cavity
Focal			Limited to $\frac{1}{3}$ of gland†
Diffuse			Affects > $\frac{1}{3}$ of gland

*Axon AT, Classen M, Cotton PB, et al. Pancreatography in chronic pancreatitis: international definitions. Gut 1984;25:1107–1112.
†Designated as in head, body, or tail.

Strictures

Distinguishing chronic pancreatitis from pancreatic cancer may be difficult when an isolated stricture is the only pancreatographic abnormality. Even a 'double duct sign', representing a distal stricture and obstruction of both the bile and pancreatic ducts, although highly suggestive, is not pathognomonic of malignancy. Similar morphologic changes are seen in patients with chronic pancreatitis.[25] Isolated strictures have also been reported in patients following acute pancreatitis, trauma, and surgery.[26] Ductal changes, including strictures, are also seen with pancreatic endocrine tumors.[27] Since endocrine tumors are parenchymal rather than ductal in origin, they remain virtually undetectable by pancreatography in the majority of cases.

PROCEDURAL ASPECTS OF THERAPEUTIC ERCP

Therapeutic techniques currently applied to benign pancreatic diseases include biliary and/or pancreatic duct sphincterotomy, minor papilla sphincterotomy, balloon or catheter dilation of pancreatic duct strictures, pancreatic drainage using a nasopancreatic catheter or endoprosthesis, bile duct and pancreatic stone extraction using balloons or baskets, and cystoenterostomy of pancreatic pseudocysts. Difficult cases may require combined techniques during a single endoscopic session.

Major papilla sphincterotomy (pancreatic duct)

Endoscopic sphincterotomy of the pancreatic duct sphincter is indicated in specific situations, including removal of pancreatic duct calculi, stent placement in chronic pancreatitis, and in selected patients with idiopathic acute recurrent pancreatitis who have not benefited from CBD sphincterotomy. Sphincterotomy of the pancreatic duct sphincter is performed after contrast enhancement of the pancreatic duct, using either a standard short-wire sphincterotome, precut sphincterotome, or needle-knife papillo-

tome.[28,29] The technique of pancreatic sphincterotomy differs from bile duct sphincterotomy in two important respects, namely the direction and length of the incision. After proper insertion and positioning of the sphincterotome, the pancreatic orifice is cut, usually over a non-current conducting catheter, in the 2 o'clock direction for a length of 5 mm or longer. The sphincterotomy is usually extended no further than the hood or covering fold (Fig. 10.1). Long incisions are generally avoided because sphincter fibers typically invest only a small portion of the distal pancreatic duct. In addition, since edema commonly accompanies the incision, access of the pancreatic duct should be established immediately after sphincterotomy, especially if further therapy is planned. Some endoscopists perform concurrent bile duct sphincterotomy with the hope of preventing procedure-related cholangitis.[29] A pancreatic stent is typically inserted before performing a needle-knife papillotomy. Prior pancreatic stenting insures both post-incisional ductal patency and easy access for cannulation. Even though needle-knife papillotomy is performed in a similar manner to sphincterotomy, the use of this acces-

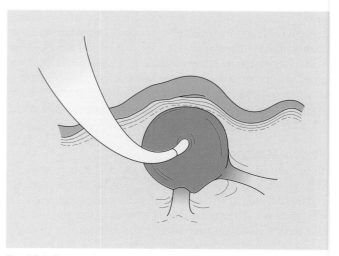

Fig. 10.1 Pancreatic sphincterotomy of the major papilla.

sory requires technical expertise and caution in order to limit potential risks.

Minor papilla sphincterotomy

Minor papilla sphincterotomy can be performed with or without prior minor papilla stenting, using a standard short-wire sphincterotome, precut sphincterotome, or needle-knife.[3] Catheter dilation of the minor papilla may be necessary to allow standard or precut sphincterotome insertion. A seldom used method to facilitate dorsal duct entry is pre-cannulation excision of the minor papilla. This technique results in complete removal of the minor papilla by use of a wire snare and applied diathermy. In one report, however, the rate of dorsal duct cannulation after minor papilla snare removal was disappointing.[30] Needle-knife minor papilla sphincterotomy is typically performed with the aid of a previously placed minor papilla stent (Fig. 10.2).[31] In order to avoid pancreatic duct tissue, the cut is made in a direction parallel to the stent (toward the 9 o'clock to 11 o'clock position) and should never exceed 6 mm. Because of the inherent risk of complications, such as pancreatitis and perforation, expertise in minor papilla sphincterotomy is mandatory. Short-term stenting of the minor papilla may also be helpful in preventing post-ERCP pancreatitis.

Pancreatic duct strictures

Dilating catheters, and less commonly hydrostatic balloons, are used to dilate pancreatic duct strictures.[28,32,33] Before dilation, a guidewire is passed through the cannulating catheter into and beyond the stricture. The cannulating catheter is subsequently exchanged for either a dilating accessory or a balloon with guidewire assistance. To optimize fluoroscopic localization within strictures, most dilating catheters and hydrostatic balloons are outfitted with radiopaque markers. The use of larger dilating accessories (>9 Fr) may require initial pancreatic sphincterotomy for duct access. As a result of the infrequent success of dilation alone, pancreatic duct stenting or nasopancreatic catheter insertion is often required.[33]

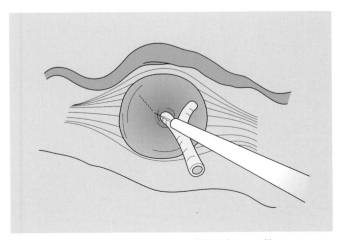

Fig. 10.2 Needle-knife sphincterotomy of the minor papilla.

Pancreatic duct stones

Pancreatic duct stones are usually located within 2–4 cm of the ampulla, a location accessible to endoscopic removal. Following pancreatic duct sphincterotomy, some stones pass spontaneously while others require balloon or minibasket retrieval. Occasionally, stone extraction is difficult owing to ampullary impaction, large stone size, or ductal adherence. In such cases, the stone can be mechanically disrupted by stent insertion or disintegrated by extracorporeal shockwave lithotripsy (ESWL).[28,34]

Stone removal by ESWL is usually preceded by sphincterotomy and nasopancreatic catheter insertion. The nasopancreatic catheter provides contrast localization of the stone or fragments before and after lithotripsy. Alternatively, ultrasound may be used to locate stones in some patients, thereby eliminating radiation exposure.[35] Although methodology varies, lithotriptors typically provide external shockwave energies equivalent to 18–19 EkV. Most patients are subjected to 100 shockwaves per minute for a total of 1000–4000 shockwaves per session.[28,34,36] Multiple lithotripsy sessions are needed if initial stone disintegration fails or is incomplete.

COMPLICATIONS AND THEIR MANAGEMENT

The frequency of ERCP-related pancreatic complications is difficult to determine when reviewing the literature. First, the majority of reports are small retrospective studies, which focus on therapeutic outcomes, rather than complications. Second, there is a lack of uniformity in defining complications.[37] Finally, many patients undergo many other treatment modalities in the same endoscopic session. In such patients, it is difficult to establish which procedure(s) contributed to the complication.

Early post-ERCP complications include perforation, hemorrhage, pancreatitis, sepsis, and stent-related problems.[38] Many of the post-ERCP complications are a result of performing sphincterotomy. The mechanism of pancreatic injury following pancreatic sphincterotomy, although not clearly established, is likely to be the same as after biliary sphincterotomy.[39] Implicated mechanisms include mechanical, thermal, hydrostatic, chemical, enzymatic, microbiologic, and allergic.[39] Over time, restenosis and pancreatic duct stricturing may develop.

Although studies differ in regard to the significance of various factors in the development of post-ERCP complications, there is general agreement that the skill and experience of the endoscopist are critically important.[38] Efforts to avoid or minimize complications should center around matching endoscopist skill and experience with the difficulty of the procedure, and careful patient selection.

Pancreatitis

Post-ERCP pancreatitis is a fairly common and potentially dangerous complication. Although data are conflicting regarding the risks, a number of factors have been implicated in the pathogenesis of ERCP-induced pancreatitis.

These factors include mechanical trauma to the papilla, acinarization, sphincter of Oddi manometry, pre-cut biliary sphincterotomy, thermal injury, sphincter of Oddi dysfunction, small bile duct caliber, current pancreatitis, a history of post-ERCP pancreatitis, a history of contrast media reaction, and the presence of a pseudocyst.[38,40]

Measures may be taken to reduce the risk of pancreatitis. These include limiting the number of cannulation attempts,[40] limiting the number of pancreatic duct injections, use of high resolution fluoroscopy to avoid overinjection, and limiting the current applied during sphincterotomy. Patients with contrast allergies may benefit from the use of non-ionic contrast and premedication with antihistamines and steroids. Pseudocyst-related complications may be avoided by refraining from overfilling, offering early drainage, and by administration of pre-procedure antibiotics. ERCP should be delayed, when possible, until pancreatitis resolves. Finally, placement of a pancreatic duct stent may be useful in the setting of sphincterotomy.

The risks of sphincter of Oddi manometry may be decreased by performing only biliary manometry, abbreviating the procedure time of pancreatic manometry, pancreatic duct drainage after manometry, and use of an aspirating catheter.[41] The aspirating catheter, a modified version of the conventional perfusion catheter, was developed in an effort to reduce the frequency of pancreatitis. With continuous aspiration of pancreatic fluid through its proximal tip, this catheter may be associated with a reduction in the incidence of post-ERCP pancreatitis. In one study, the use of an aspirating catheter reduced the incidence of pancreatitis to 3% of patients compared to 24% with a conventional catheter.[41]

Pancreatic duct stents may decrease the incidence and severity of post-sphincterotomy pancreatitis,[42–45] presumably by maintaining drainage. In an effort to avoid a second endoscopy to retrieve the stent, some advocate the use of a two-barb stent[43,44] or placement of a nasobiliary catheter.[42] Although opinions vary, our practice is to perform an abdominal plain-film approximately 1 week after stent placement. In the approximate 30% of patients in whom the stent does not spontaneously pass, the stent is at that time endoscopically retrieved. It is important to consider the risks of pancreatic duct stents when evaluating a patient for stent placement.

Stent-related complications
General
As with biliary stents, the use of pancreatic stents may result in complications, namely proximal stent migration and stent occlusion. Unlike biliary stents, stent-induced pancreatic ductal change is unique to pancreatic stents. The development of complications necessitates stent removal which may require the use of endoscopic accessories, such as a miniballoon or minibasket. Fortunately, serious complications develop in only about 3% of cases.[46]

Stent migration
Proximal stent migration (into the pancreatic duct) occurs infrequently. Migration appears to be directly related to the presence of barbs at the proximal end of the stent.[47] In one preliminary study of 318 patients, unmodified (four-barb) and modified (two-barb) pancreatic stent migrations were compared (Fig. 10.3). Although reports vary, removal of the proximal barbs is felt to lead to a greater likelihood of distal migration.[43,47] Approximately 5% of unmodified stents migrated into the pancreatic duct, whereas none of the modified stents migrated proximally.[47] Even though the mechanism for migration remains speculative, proximal barbs of an unmodified stent may serve to ratchet or pull the stent into the pancreatic duct. Since only few unmodified stents migrate proximally, however, additional factors may also be important, including the stent's physical characteristics and the anatomy of the pancreatic duct. Migration has also been reported more likely in the presence of sphincter of Oddi dysfunction, and with the use of longer stents.[48] In the event of proximal migration, the majority of stents are removable by endoscopic means. Rarely are pancreatic stents unretrievable endoscopically, but in such cases, surgical extirpation may be required.

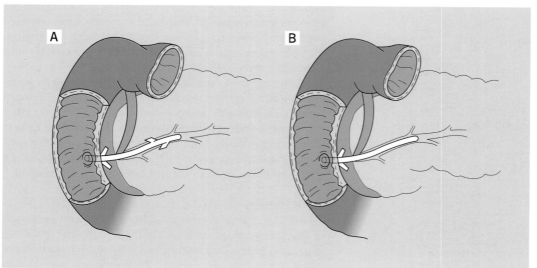

Fig. 10.3 (**A**) Unmodified four-barb pancreatic duct stent. (**B**) Modified two-barb pancreatic duct stent.

Stent occlusion

Pancreatic and biliary stents occlude at a similar rate, which is affected by time,[49] and stent caliber.[50] Stent occlusion (5 Fr, 6 Fr, and 7 Fr) occurs in 50% at 6 weeks and nearly 100% at 9 weeks after placement. The occluding substance is composed of a mixture of organic and inorganic material made up of cellular debris, calcium carbonate crystals, and calcium bilirubinate.[51] Duodenal reflux may also contribute to stent occlusion since intestinal contents have been identified within the occluding substance. Stent occlusion seldom leads to symptoms because the occluded stent acts like a wick, allowing sustained pancreatic secretory outflow alongside the occluded stent. Occluded stents may however lead to recurrent pancreatic pain, pancreatitis, or pseudocyst infection.

Pancreatic ductal alterations

The most problematic of all complications related to pancreatic stent therapy is the development of morphologic changes within the pancreas. The mechanism of injury likely relates to direct mechanical injury, side branch obstruction, stent occlusion, and reactions to the stent material.[52]

Reported pancreatic duct changes, following pancreatic duct placement, include focal scarring of the main pancreatic duct, and side branch abnormalities (including dilation, irregular stenosis, and ectasia).[53–56] Pancreatic parenchymal changes may also occur following pancreatic stenting, as has been demonstrated by endoscopic ultrasound.[57] Although most studies report these changes to be mild and temporary,[53] more severe and long-lasting morphologic alterations may develop.[54,55] These lesions have even been noted to progress after the stent has been removed.[54,56] It is unclear if the progression of morphologic changes reflects continued effects of the previous stent or the natural progression of the underlying disease. Nevertheless, these ductal changes have not proven to correlate with either symptoms or deterioration in pancreatic function.[55]

Nevertheless, based on the fact that chronic ductal changes may occur with stent therapy, and because of the lack of knowledge regarding long-term consequences of such changes, the widespread, chronic use of pancreatic duct stents cannot be advocated. Stent therapy should generally be limited to persons with a severe dominant pancreatic duct stricture or as part of a research protocol. A possible exception is in patients with chronic pancreatitis causing severe, disabling, chronic abdominal pain, in whom the risks of stenting may be warranted.

RESULTS OF ENDOSCOPIC THERAPY (ACUTE PANCREATITIS)

Endoscopic therapy can usually be successfully applied to patients with benign pancreatic disease. Technical success requires a high level of procedural competence and proper patient selection. Technically demanding procedures, especially those inherently risky, should be performed by endoscopists with sufficient experience. The requisite training and experience should include the ability not only to perform the diagnostic study but also to complete any necessary therapeutic intervention. There should also be clear familiarity with common and uncommon procedure-related complications, and the ability to adequately manage them. Through careful physician and patient selection, there will be enhanced ability to perform difficult interventions, with a high quality of care, and at a low complication rate.

Acute gallstone pancreatitis

Gallstones account for approximately half of all cases of acute pancreatitis,[58,59] and are believed to do so by transiently obstructing the ampulla of Vater.[60] This theory is supported by the fact that CBD stones or impacted stones are found in 62 to 75% of patients when surgery is performed within 48 hours of admission.[58] Interestingly, patients with gallstone pancreatitis may actually be predisposed to gallstone migration and ampullary obstruction. Smaller gallstones, wider cystic duct diameters, and longer common channels (>5 mm) are found more commonly in these patients than in asymptomatic patients with cholelithiasis.[61]

Acute gallstone pancreatitis is a common disease, affecting approximately 8% of patients with cholelithiasis.[62] Although most patients recover fully after an attack of pancreatitis, some develop significant morbidity with an estimated mortality rate of 10 to 20% at least twice that of alcoholic pancreatitis.[63] The mortality rate is even higher when patients develop concurrent cholangitis (13 to 50%).[64,65] Early assessment of disease severity is critical for determining which patients should undergo therapeutic intervention, and for estimating prognosis.[64] To aid in estimating disease severity recognized scoring systems are available for quick determination, namely the Ranson and modified Glasgow systems[66,67] (Table 10.4).

Establishing the diagnosis of gallstone pancreatitis during the early stages of disease may be challenging. While the presence of cholangitis strongly supports the diagnosis, it is usually necessary to rely on transabdominal ultrasound and biochemical tests to suggest gallstone pancreatitis. Transabdominal ultrasound is an excellent method for detecting gallstones and determining CBD caliber. Unfortunately, transabdominal ultrasound is of limited utility in detecting CBD stones owing to poor sensitivity, reported to range from 13 to 70%.[68] Biochemical indicators of CBD stones include serum bilirubin, transaminases, and alkaline phosphatase, and it is unclear which of these tests is most useful. A serum alanine aminotransferase level, at least threefold normal, is felt by some to be the best indicator.[69] Another study noted that the best indicator of CBD stones is serum total bilirubin >1.35 mg/dL or 23 mmol/L on the second hospital day.[70]

Endoscopic ultrasound is emerging as a valuable tool in identifying CBD stones. A number of studies have found endoscopic ultrasound to be of comparable or greater accuracy than ERCP for diagnosing choledocholithiasis.[71,72] While endoscopic ultrasound is of value

Severity scoring systems for acute pancreatitis		
Ranson criteria Non-gallstone pancreatitis	Gallstone pancreatitis	**Modified Glasgow criteria** Non-gallstone or gallstone pancreatitis
On admission Age >55 years WBC >16 000/mm³ Glucose >200 mg/dL 11.1 mmol/L AST >250 IU/L LDH >350 IU/L	*On admission* Age >70 years WBC >18 000/mm³ Glucose >220 mg/dL 12.2 mmol/L AST >250 IU/L LDH >400 IU/L	*Within 48 h* Age >55 years WBC >15 000/mm³ Glucose >180 mg/dL 10 mmol/L LDH >600 IU/L BUN >45 mg/dL 7.5 mmol/L Serum calcium ≤ 8 mg/dL 2 mmol/L PaO₂ <60 mmHg 8kPa Albumin <3.2 g/dL 32g/L
Within 48 h Hematocrit fall >10% BUN rise >5 mg/dL 0.83 mmol/L Serum calcium <8 mg/dL 2 mmol/L PaO₂ <60 mmHg Base deficit >4 meq/L Fluid deficit >6 L	*Within 48 h* Hematocrit fall >10% BUN rise >2 mg/dL 0.33 mmol/L Serum calcium <8 mg/dL 2 mmol/L PaO₂ <60 mmHg Base deficit >5 meq/L Fluid deficit >4 L	

Table 10.4 Severity scoring systems for acute pancreatitis

in establishing the diagnosis, it does not allow therapeutic intervention, and ERCP is still required in appropriately selected patients.

Surgery was once favored for severe gallstone pancreatitis because of concern over the safety of ERCP, and possible effects that ERCP may have on the course of pancreatitis. A prospective and randomized surgical study reported a mortality rate of 48% in patients in whom early operative treatment was performed for severe disease.[73] This unacceptable mortality rate shifted the focus of treatment to a safer, non-surgical technique for removing bile duct stones. The appropriate selection of patients to undergo therapeutic ERCP with endoscopic sphincterotomy and stone removal is critical.

Initial ERCP and endoscopic sphincterotomy trials in patients with gallstone pancreatitis reported dramatic clinical and biochemical improvements in the majority of cases.[74,75] These studies did little to change practices, partly because of flaws in methodology, and non-uniformity of disease severity, timing of sphincterotomy, and definition of complications. More recent studies, although having some significant design variations, have served to widely define the role of ERCP and sphincterotomy in this patient population.

Neoptolemos et al[76] in 1988 performed the first prospective randomized trial comparing urgent ERCP (within 72 hours of hospitalization) and sphincterotomy, with stone removal, to conservative therapy, in patients with gallstone pancreatitis. They not only established the safety of such therapy, but also noted improved morbidity (24% vs 61%) and shortened hospital stay (median 9.5 days vs 17 days), in the subset of patients with severe pancreatitis. They did not however find a statistically significant difference in mortality. Fan et al[77] conducted a similar prospective randomized study in 1993. They found that ERCP with sphincterotomy (within 24 hours of admission), was superior to conventional therapy in severely ill

persons with pancreatitis and cholangitis. They noted a reduction in morbidity (16% vs 32%) from biliary sepsis, irrespective of disease severity, but failed to detect a statistically significant difference in overall survival. Fölsch et al,[78] in a multicenter prospective trial in 1997, found no benefit to ERCP in acute biliary pancreatitis.[78] This study, however, excluded patients with biliary obstruction, jaundice, and cholangitis; those most likely to benefit from such therapy.

The Fölsch study[78] should not discourage the use of ERCP and stone removal in acute pancreatitis but instead serve to remind us of those patients most likely to benefit from such intervention. ERCP should be reserved for patients with severe acute biliary pancreatitis with an elevated or rising bilirubin or when cholangitis is suspected. If stone extraction fails, appropriate measures should be taken to maintain biliary drainage and to prevent recurrent stone impaction or worsening biliary sepsis. While ERCP is of benefit in this select group of patients, one should note that no study has demonstrated a positive influence on the course of biliary pancreatitis itself.

Finally, endoscopic therapy of gallstone pancreatitis appears to be safe. From endoscopic therapy in more than 600 patients with gallstone pancreatitis, the overall reported morbidity and mortality was 6% and 2% retrospectively, acceptable rates when compared to those of urgent surgical intervention.[59] Moreover, unintentional opacification of the pancreatic duct commonly occurred, but fortunately without consequence, in several large studies.[77,79] There was no evidence, in either report, that pancreatography exacerbated the underlying condition.

Acute recurrent pancreatitis

Alcohol and gallstones are the most common causes of acute pancreatitis in the Western world, accounting for nearly 70% of cases. Hypercalcemia, hyperlipidemia, and drugs are less often implicated. Approximately 30% of cases have no identifiable cause and are termed idiopathic acute recurrent pancreatitis.[80,81] ERCP is able to determine the etiology of pancreatitis 70% of the time when the rest of the evaluation is negative.[81–85] Evaluation most often leads to the diagnosis of microlithiasis, retained CBD stones, sphincter of Oddi dysfunction, pancreas divisum, choledochocele, ampullary or pancreatic tumors, or pancreatic duct strictures.[81–85]

At the time of ERCP one should perform, if appropriately trained, sphincter of Oddi manometry, bile aspiration for microcrystals when the gallbladder is intact, and minor papilla cannulation when pancreas divisum is suspected. The most appropriate timing for ERCP is unsettled. Most would agree that after one severe episode or two or more mild-to-moderate episodes, ERCP is indicated.

Endoscopic ultrasound has an emerging role in the evaluation of patients with idiopathic acute recurrent pancreatitis. Endoscopic ultrasound has been shown to have equal or superior sensitivity, to other commonly used tests, in the diagnosis of microlithiasis and macrolithiasis.[86,87] Sphincter of Oddi dysfunction may be detected by the secretin-stimulated endoscopic ultrasound test.[88] In persons with pancreas divisum, endoscopic ultrasound has been shown to have reasonable sensitivity and specificity.[88,89] Other less common causes of idiopathic acute recurrent pancreatitis, such as ampullary tumors, and pancreatic tumors, are also well evaluated by endoscopic ultrasound.[90–92] Finally, endoscopic ultrasound can help to detect those patients with chronic pancreatitis who may initially present with idiopathic acute recurrent pancreatitis.[93,94]

Microlithiasis

Microlithiasis is an important and frequent cause of idiopathic acute recurrent pancreatitis (Table 10.5).[81–83,85,95,96] Cholesterol or calcium bilirubinate crystals are felt to lead to pancreatitis by obstructing pancreatic outflow. Aspiration of bile, at the time of ERCP or via duodenal drainage tubes, detects crystals in about 70% of such persons.[82,83,95,96] The sensitivity of these studies is enhanced by the administration of cholecystokinin, which leads to gallbladder contraction. Cholecystectomy is the therapy of choice, but endoscopic sphincterotomy and urodeoxycholic acid are appropriate alternatives, in patients who are

Incidence of microlithiasis in idiopathic acute recurrent pancreatitis		
Authors	No. of patients enrolled	No. of patients with microlithiasis
Venu et al 1989[81]	116	8 (7%)
Ros et al 1991[96]	51	37 (73%)
Lee et al 1992[95]	29	21 (72%)
Sherman et al 1993[82]	13	7 (54%)
Kaw et al 1996[83]	25	15 (60%)
Geenen & Nash 1996[85]	88	5 (6%)
Total	322	93 (29%)

Table 10.5 Incidence of microlithiasis in idiopathic acute recurrent pancreatitis

poor operative candidates. Therapy has been shown to significantly reduce the risk of developing recurrent pancreatitis.[95,96]

Choledocholithiasis

Choledocholithiasis is an important and easily treatable cause of acute recurrent pancreatitis. Establishing the diagnosis is important since 20 to 50% of patients with prior pancreatitis and undiagnosed CBD stones develop recurrent attacks of pancreatitis.[97,98] Unfortunately, clinical, biochemical, and radiologic parameters are often unreliable in identifying patients with CBD stones. ERCP not only offers excellent sensitivity in establishing the diagnosis, but also allows duct clearance of stones.

Sphincter of Oddi dysfunction

Sphincter of Oddi dysfunction is another frequent and treatable cause of idiopathic acute recurrent pancreatitis, seen in about one-third of such persons (Table 10.6).[81–85,99,100] Pancreatitis is felt to result from either anatomic or functional obstruction of the distal pancreatic duct.[60,81] The diagnosis is established by finding an elevated sphincter of Oddi basal pressure (>40 mmHg) during manometry.

Endoscopic sphincterotomy is the therapy of choice, and may provide long-term clinical improvement in patients with this disorder.[3,11,81,101,102] There is some debate

Incidence of sphincter of Oddi dysfunction in idiopathic acute recurrent pancreatitis		
Authors	No. of patients enrolled	No. of patients with sphincter of Oddi dysfunction
Venu et al 1989[81]	116	17 (15%)
Sherman et al 1993[82]	55	18 (33%)
Pasricha et al 1994[99]	19	12 (63%)
Kaw et al 1996[83]	58	34 (59%)
Coyle et al 1996[84]	68	24 (35%)
Geenen & Nash 1996[85]	109	25 (23%)
Di Francisco et al 1997[100]	47	29 (61%)
Total	472	159 (34%)

Table 10.6 Incidence of sphincter of Oddi dysfunction in idiopathic acute recurrent pancreatitis

whether to cut one or both sphincters. CBD sphincterotomy does lead to a reduction in pancreatic duct segment pressure and is effective therapy in about 80% of patients with pancreatic duct sphincter hypertension.[103–107] Although sphincter dysfunction may be confined to the pancreatic duct alone, clinical improvement may occur with isolated biliary sphincterotomy.[108] Preservation of the pancreatic duct sphincter segment may account for the lack of clinical improvement after endoscopic biliary sphincterotomy.[105] In such cases, repeat manometry is appropriate to evaluate the pancreatic sphincter pressure and to help direct further therapy. We favor initially cutting the CBD sphincter and only if the course mandates, then later cutting the pancreatic duct sphincter. It should be remembered that the complication rate of endoscopic sphincterotomy, when performed for sphincter of Oddi dysfunction, is greater than when performed for other reasons.[38]

Surgical sphincteroplasty is an effective alternative,[109] but is more invasive and has been replaced by endoscopic sphincterotomy as the therapy of choice. Pancreatic duct stenting has been less well studied and results have usually been disappointing.[110,111] Balloon dilation and botulinum toxin injection of the pancreatic duct sphincter are no longer considered appropriate therapeutic options owing to the limited benefit, and because complications are common and often severe.[112,113]

Pancreas divisum

Whether minor papilla obstruction results in pancreatic disease (pancreatic pain, acute recurrent pancreatitis, or chronic pancreatitis) remains controversial. Although consensus has not been reached, the balance of opinion favors a relationship, with pancreas divisum reported in approximately 20% of such patients (Table 10.7).[81–84,99,100,114] Surgical specimens have noted histologic findings of isolated dorsal pancreatitis in patients with pancreas divisum.[115]

Pancreas divisum is the most common congenital malformation of the pancreas, and results from failure of the embryologic ventral and dorsal ducts to fuse (Fig. 10.4). As a result, the majority of the pancreas drains via the

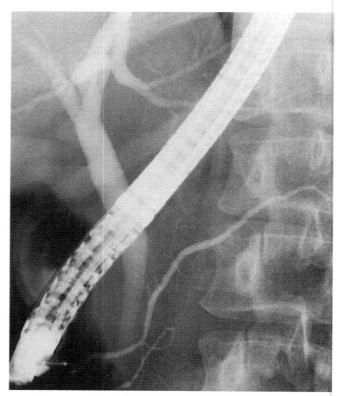

Fig. 10.4 Pancreas divisum.

minor papilla. The duct and papilla, which is often stenotic, may not accommodate the volume of secretions and may inhibit the flow of pancreatic juice. The diagnosis should be suspected if, at the time of ERCP and major papilla injection, a pancreatogram is not obtained or only a small ventral duct is visualized. The diagnosis can be confirmed by minor papilla cannulation which reveals the 'dorsal dominant' anatomy.

Endoscopic and surgical therapy favorably affects the long-term course of these patients.[116–120] Endoscopic treatment is directed toward relieving outflow obstruction at the level of the minor papilla. Therapeutic options include minor papilla sphincterotomy, catheter dilation of the minor papilla, stent placement across the minor papilla, and combination therapies. Importantly, the effectiveness of endoscopic or surgical therapy depends on the clinical presentation. In general, patients with acute recurrent pancreatitis respond more favorably to treatment than patients with chronic pancreatitis or pain alone.

Minor papilla sphincterotomy can be successfully performed in about 40 to 100% of cases, with an overall improvement noted in about 50% when followed over 1 to 40 months.[30,31,117,121] When patients are analysed from the perspective of clinical presentation, about 70% of patients with acute recurrent pancreatitis respond favorably, compared to roughly 20 to 40% with chronic pancreatitis or pain alone.[30,31,117,120,121]

Minor papilla stents can be successfully placed in up to 90% of patients.[110,116,122] In the setting of acute recurrent pancreatitis, stent therapy offers improvement in about 80 to 90% of patients during a follow-up period of 12 to 60

Incidence of pancreas divisum in idiopathic acute recurrent pancreatitis		
Authors	No. of patients enrolled	No. of patients with pancreas divisum
Venu et al 1989[81]	116	10 (9%)
Bernard et al 1990[114]	56	28 (50%)
Sherman et al 1993[82]	55	8 (15%)
Pasricha et al 1994[99]	43	10 (23%)
Kaw et al 1996[83]	58	6 (10%)
Coyle et al 1996[84]	68	11 (16%)
Geenen & Nash 1996[85]	196	41 (21%)
Total	592	114 (19%)

Table 10.7 Incidence of pancreas divisum in idiopathic acute recurrent pancreatitis

months.[116,123] The risk of developing pancreatitis is significantly reduced with the use of stents, 10%, compared to about 80% in untreated patients, over a follow-up period of nearly 3 years.[116] Stent therapy appears less effective for patients with pancreas divisum suffering from chronic pancreatitis or pain alone.

Choledochocele

A choledochocele is a rare congenital or acquired condition in which the intramural segment of the distal CBD herniates into the duodenal lumen (Fig. 10.5). Acute pancreatitis develops when the cyst or its contents (sludge or stones) obstruct pancreatic duct outflow. 'Unroofing' the choledochocele with endoscopic sphincterotomy has been shown to be effective treatment for this disorder.[124]

Ampullary and pancreatic tumors

Patients with ampullary or pancreatic tumors (Fig. 10.6) may also present with recurrent pancreatitis. Early diagnosis is important since in some patients surgical resection may be curative. ERCP is an excellent method for early detection since conventional testing (ultrasound, CT scan) often fails to detect small tumors. Papillary tumors may be treated endoscopically in high-risk surgical patients, using sphincterotomy, electrocautery, or laser ablation.[125,126] Another option for excision of symptomatic papillary adenomas is diathermy snare excision.[127] This therapy should be reserved for poor surgical candidates, with biopsy-proven benign tumors, owing to the high procedure-related complications (bleeding and pancreatitis) which develop in over 20% of patients.

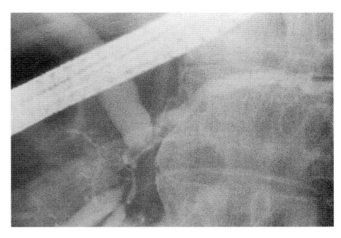

Fig. 10.6 Acute recurrent pancreatitis in a patient with cancer in the head of the pancreas.

Pancreatic duct strictures

Idiopathic or post-traumatic strictures may also lead to acute recurrent pancreatitis. Insertion of a pancreatic duct stent across the stricture may result in pain relief and a reduction in the frequency of pancreatitis.[28,33]

Acute pancreatitis and necrosis
Assessment of gland

Massive pancreatic necrosis may infrequently lead to exocrine insufficiency, endocrine insufficiency, or acute recurrent pancreatitis. Endoscopic retrograde pancreatography (ERP) typically reveals a normal pancreatic duct in patients with pancreatic necrosis, indicating that necrosis is peripancreatic, usually involving surrounding adipose tissue.[128] In the presence of complications, pancreatic function typically deteriorates comparable to the degree of ductal destruction. Infrequently, ductal damage leads to stricture formation and with resulting acute recurrent pancreatitis (Fig. 10.7). In such patients, post-inflammatory strictures are often amenable to endoscopic treatment.[129]

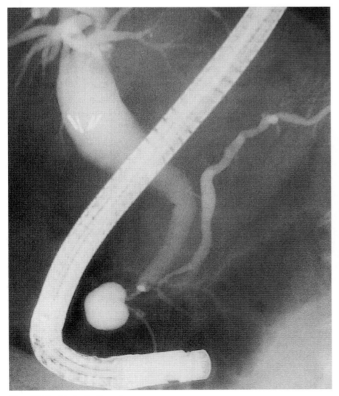

Fig. 10.5 Choledochocele.

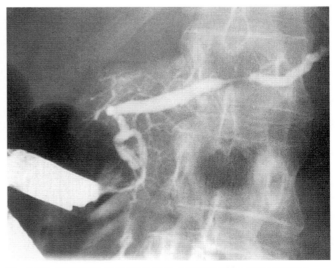

Fig. 10.7 Pancreatic duct stricture in a patient with acute recurrent pancreatitis.

Preoperative evaluation

Acute pancreatitis is complicated by pancreatic necrosis 4 to 5% of the time and caries a mortality rate as high as 20 to 50%.[130,131] Surgical intervention, either simple necrosectomy or regional pancreatic resection, remains the mainstay of therapy. Surgical resection of ductal or parenchymal fistulae is critical because of the association of residual fistulae with persistent or renewed inflammation.[132]

Preoperative ERP can provide valuable information. In one report of eight patients with necrotizing pancreatitis, the operative approach was selected based on the findings of ERP. Isolated necrosectomy of necrotic peripancreatic adipose tissue was performed in patients whose preoperative pancreatography was normal. However, pancreatic resection with removal of fistulae or necrotic pancreatic tissue was required when a pancreatic duct leak was demonstrated.[133] Experience with preoperative ERCP in pancreatic necrosis is limited, and further combined endoscopic and surgical trials are needed to determine the value and safety.

RESULTS OF ENDOSCOPIC THERAPY (CHRONIC PANCREATITIS)

Pancreatography and functional tests

The diagnosis of chronic pancreatitis can be established by pancreatography (Fig. 10.8) or pancreatic exocrine function tests (i.e. PABA test, secretin test). The pancreatic duct morphology may be normal with mild disease, therefore limiting the sensitivity of pancreatography. Pancreatic function testing may help to establish the diagnosis at an earlier stage. One study found an abnormal secretin test in 20% of patients with chronic pancreatitis who had normal pancreatograms.[134]

The intraductal secretin test was developed in the mid-1970s as an alternative method for measuring pancreatic function. Since intraductal secretin testing is conducted during ERCP, it is easier to perform than formal secretin testing.[135] Following secretin administration, aliquots of pure pancreatic juice are collected through an ERCP cannula positioned 5–20 mm in the pancreatic duct.[135–137] Intraductal secretin testing obviates several notable problems associated with formal secretin testing, including contamination of collected samples and patient discomfort.[137] Unfortunately, only limited data are available regarding its diagnostic value in patients with suspected chronic pancreatitis. Based upon the preliminary findings of one study, however, intraductal secretin testing was more sensitive than pancreatography in diagnosing mild chronic pancreatitis.[138]

Distinction between acute and chronic pancreatitis

Chronic pancreatitis may initially present as idiopathic acute recurrent pancreatitis. Given the increased morbidity and mortality of chronic pancreatitis, it is important to establish the correct diagnosis. The mortality rate for patients with chronic pancreatitis is at least three to four times greater than for controls, with mortality directly related to pancreatitis in 20% of both alcoholic and nonalcoholic patients.[139,140] By diagnosing chronic pancreatitis, ERCP can help to predict the long-term prognosis.

Abdominal pain

Pain is the most common symptom of chronic pancreatitis. Although the pathophysiology of pain remains undefined, surgical and endoscopic treatments have been directed toward removing ductal obstruction, with the goal of reducing pancreatic ductal pressure. Pancreatic duct stones, strictures, or papillary stenosis found in nearly half of these patients[141] may obstruct outflow and lead to intraductal hypertension. By removing these barriers to outflow, chronic pain and/or recurrent episodes of pancreatitis may be diminished or even completely alleviated.

ERP is useful to exclude pancreatic duct obstruction, and helps to select the most appropriate medical, endoscopic, or surgical therapy. Until recently, surgical duct decompression was the treatment of choice for pain. Nearly all surgical series reported immediate postoperative pain relief (≤1 year) in the majority of patients. However, the rates of long-term benefit (>5 years) were less impressive, as 30 to 50% of patients experienced recurrent postoperative pain.[142,143] In addition, the reported morbidity and mortality from various surgical series ranged from 9 to 40% and 0 to 5% respectively. Whether endoscopic treatment provides as effective pain relief as surgery is uncertain. The absence of any clinical trial directly comparing surgical and endoscopic therapy makes meaningful comparison impossible.

A variety of endoscopic techniques are available to treat chronic pancreatitis, including insertion of pancreatic duct stents, dilating strictures, removing stones with or without ESWL, sphincterotomy, and combination therapies. Alternative endoscopic methods have also been applied for treatment of painful pancreatic pseudocysts, including cystoenterostomy and transpapillary drainage. Most of these endoscopic techniques are designed to reduce intraductal pressures by alleviating pancreatic outflow obstruction.

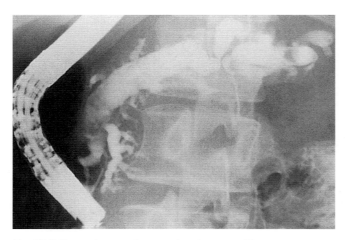

Fig. 10.8 Pancreatogram of severe chronic pancreatitis.

Cholestasis

Chronic pancreatitis is complicated by CBD strictures in approximately 10 to 27% of patients, with as many as 8% developing significant cholestasis.[144,145] In order to prevent cholangitis and/or secondary biliary cirrhosis, all symptomatic patients, or those with elevated liver function tests, should undergo biliary decompression. Endoscopic stent insertion provides effective decompression, albeit temporary, as stricture recurrence is common following stent removal.[146] However, endoscopic endobiliary stenting can provide immediate relief of symptoms and obviate the need for emergency surgery.

Pancreatic strictures

Although ductal strictures can be treated by catheter or balloon dilation alone,[28,32,33] subsequent pancreatic stent insertion is required in most cases since stricture recurrence is common (Fig. 10.9).[33] The technical success of stent placement for stricture dilation exceeds 95%, with or without prior pancreatic sphincterotomy (Table 10.8).[50,147–149] Typically 5–10 Fr stents are inserted for a period of 6 to 12 months. Abdominal pain is alleviated in the majority of patients 68 to 94% (average 83%) followed over a period of 1 to 69 months (average 22 months).[50,147–149] Although relatively uncommon, sustained pain relief following ther-

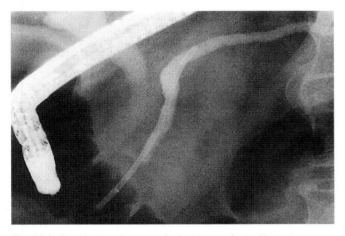

Fig. 10.9 Stent in dorsal pancreatic duct in a patient with acute recurrent pancreatitis.

apy has been observed.[33] An initial convincing response to therapy may be predictive of long-term response following surgical intervention.[33,147] Response to stricture therapy is also likely in patients demonstrating both obstruction and ductal dilation.[148] In a preliminary report, all stented patients (n = 13) with ductal obstruction (≤1 mm) and dilation (>6 mm) improved, as opposed to 58% of stented patients (n = 43) without ductal dilation or obstruction, obstruction alone, or isolated ductal dilation.[148]

Pancreatic stones

Debate continues as to whether pancreatic duct stones aggravate the clinical course of chronic pancreatitis or are the natural sequelae of on-going gland destruction. Pancreatic duct calculi may inhibit pancreatic outflow and lead to ductal hypertension, thereby inducing chronic pain or exacerbations of chronic pancreatitis. Clinical improvement following surgical removal of pancreatic stones supports this notion.[143,150] Endoscopic techniques for stone removal include pancreatic duct sphincterotomy followed by direct stone extraction, stent insertion or nasopancreatic catheter insertion, ESWL, and combination therapies.

Several important observations have been reported in the literature and are noteworthy. First, clearance of ductal calculi, although successfully performed in only 50% of cases, does correlate with immediate pain relief and reduction in ductal dilation.[151,152] Second, convincing symptomatic improvement is sustained longer in patients with exacerbations of chronic pancreatitis ('relapsing pancreatitis') than in patients with chronic pain.[151,153] Third, certain factors hinder stone clearance, including numerous stones, stones located proximally in the tail of the pancreas, the presence of distal ductal stricturing, impacted stones and stone diameter >1 cm.[151] Finally, as expected, multiple endoscopic sessions are typically required for difficult or incomplete stone removal.[36,152]

Successful endoscopic retrieval of pancreatic duct stones, in persons with chronic pancreatitis, has been reported in 27 to 100% of cases.[28,33,36,154,155] Success is directly related to the degree of difficulty of the cases enrolled. As expected, studies involving patients with distal ductal strictures or impacted stones show lower success rates. Approximately 85% of patients respond favorably to therapy when followed for approximately 1

Table 10.8 Endoscopic therapy for dominant strictures in chronic pancreatitis

		Endoscopic therapy for dominant strictures in chronic pancreatitis			
Authors	Patients (n)	Technical success rate (%)	Complication rate (%)	Improvement rate (%)	Mean follow-up (months)
Cremer et al 1991[147]	76	75 (99)	12 (16)	71 (94)	37
Burdick et al 1993[148]	56	56 (100)	ns	38 (68)	5
Ponchon et al 1995[50]	23	23 (100)	10 (43)	21 (91)	12
Smits et al 1995[149]	51	49 (96)	12 (22)	42 (82)	34
Total	206	203 (99)	34 (22)	172 (83)	22

ns=not stated.

to 2 years.[28,33,36,154,155] Complications occur infrequently, with an overall morbidity of roughly 10%. Patients typically develop transient pancreatic pain or hyperamylasemia. Sepsis developed in one-third of patients undergoing ESWL in one study, but antibiotics were not provided before or after the procedure.[152] The incidence of lithotripsy-induced bacteremia and infectious complications were reduced in another trial with prophylactic administration of antibiotics.[36] In reviewing the literature, pertaining to endoscopic therapy of pancreatic duct stones, no deaths were reported.

Pancreatic pseudocysts

Pancreatic pseudocysts have historically been treated by surgical means, cystoenterostomy (with or without resection) and/or lateral pancreaticojejunostomy, or more recently by percutaneous catheter drainage. Endoscopic techniques, such as endoscopic cystogastrostomy, cystoduodenostomy, and transpapillary drainage, have been available since the mid-1980s, and allow comparable efficacy and safety.[156–160] Endoscopic therapy, in properly selected patients, has approximately a 70 to 90% success rate, with complications developing in 20%, and cyst recurrence seen in 15% (Table 10.9).[156,158,161–163]

The preferred approach depends on cyst characteristics and anatomy, which is defined by ERCP and radiologic studies. Ideal candidates for endoscopic therapy include those with single cyst, mature cyst, size >4 cm, luminal compression by the cyst, absence of debris, necrosis and infection, and absence of portal hypertension. Endoscopic drainage is often unsuccessful in the presence of necrotic debris, tissue, or blood clots. Success has been reported with aggressive endoscopic therapy involving multiple large-bore stents and nasopancreatic lavage, given over an extended period of time.[160] This, however, is not a viable therapeutic option outside of highly specialized centers, with devoted teams offering close observation.

Patients with pancreatic duct obstruction or a communicating pseudocyst should undergo endoscopic or surgical intervention. In this situation, percutaneous treatment therapy is contraindicated because of the limited success and risk of cutaneous fistula formation.[68] Non-communicating pseudocysts are amenable to endoscopic, surgical, and percutaneous approaches.

Transpapillary drainage is indicated for pseudocysts that communicate with the main or dorsal pancreatic duct, especially in the presence of a stricture.[156] This technique involves placement of a stent or nasopancreatic catheter into the major or minor papilla, across the pseudocyst-ductal communication and sometimes into the pseudocyst itself (Fig. 10.10). The use of nasopancreatic catheters is generally reserved for initial drainage of large pseudocysts. Pancreatic stents are used to bypass structures which impede pseudocyst drainage, such as pancreatic strictures, stones, or duct disruption.[33,159] These stents are typically left in place for 4 to 6 weeks, or removed earlier if cyst infection is suspected, or if cyst resolution is suggested by CT.

Endoscopic cystoenterostomy (cystogastrostomy or cystoduodenostomy) is appropriately performed when the pseudocyst and pancreatic duct do not communicate. Before endoscopic cystoenterostomy is attempted, each patient should undergo abdominal CT, ultrasound, or endosonography to determine the size, location, and anatomic relationship of the pseudocyst to the intestinal wall. Demonstrating cystoenteric proximity (cyst to lumen distance <1 cm) helps to avoid blind puncture which may

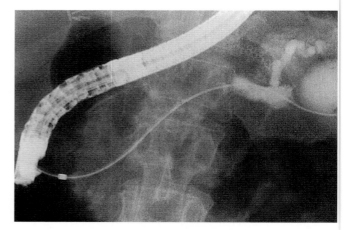

Fig. 10.10 Transpapillary drainage of pseudocyst with nasopancreatic catheter.

Table 10.9 Endoscopic therapy for pancreatic pseudocysts

	Cystoenterostomy*			Transpapillary drainage			Combined procedure		
Authors	No.	Respond	(%)	No.	Respond	(%)	No.	Respond	(%)
Barthet et al 1995[162]	0	0	(0)	20	16	(80)	10	7	(70)
Binmoeller et al 1995[163]	20	16	(80)	29	27	(93)	4	4	(100)
Catalano et al 1995[156]	0	0	(0)	21	17	(81)	0	0	(0)
Smits et al 1995[158]	17	10	(59)	12	7	(58)	8	7	(88)
Total	37	26	(70)	82	67	(82)	22	18	(82)

*Cystoenterostomy (either cystogastrostomy or cystoduodenostomy).

lead to inadvertent perforation or pancreatic parenchymal injury. In order to minimize the risk of complications and to help ensure technical success, puncture attempts should be restricted to endoscopically visible cysts that compress the gastric or duodenal lumen.[164,165]

At the site of maximal luminal compression, the enteric wall is punctured by a needle-knife, which is directed toward the cyst center. Following a puncture, the cyst is delineated with contrast. The pseudocyst is entered with a 19 gauge needle, and the location verified by fluid aspiration. The opening is enlarged by balloon dilation over a guidewire, using the Seldinger technique, or with a sphincterotome or cystoenterotome (Fig. 10.11). The use of a cystoenterotome is favored owing to its ability to sustain cyst access.[166] In order to maintain temporary patency of the cystoenterostomy, a nasocystic catheter or double pigtail stent(s) is inserted into the cystic cavity (Fig. 10.12).

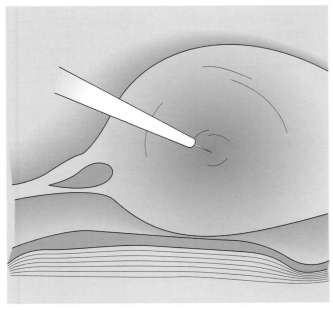

Fig. 10.11 Cystoenterostomy with needle-knife incision.

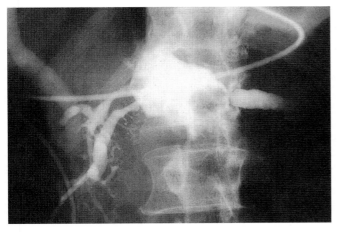

Fig. 10.12 Nasocystic catheter inserted in pseudocyst.

Endoscopic ultrasound has been advocated by some to be an effective and safe alternative for pseudocyst drainage.[167–169] Endoscopic ultrasound may allow more accurate characterization of the pseudocyst, and improved safety because of the greater ability to detect blood vessels. The inability to perform therapeutic intervention, such as dilation and stent placement, unfortunately, necessitates the exchange of endoscopes during the procedure. However, the ability to perform the entire procedure without the exchange of endoscopes, has been reported, with the use of a specialized ultrasound endoscope.[169]

Laser (argon or Nd:YAG) puncture is an alternative to puncture by diathermy needle or 19 gauge needle, particularly in patients with retrogastric pseudocysts.[170] Laser photocoagulation of the gastric mucosa overlying the cyst creates a necrotizing tract that eventually fistulizes and allows drainage of cystic contents. Because of the limited experience and uncertain risk, laser therapy has not been widely adopted.

Suspected pancreatic cancer

Patients with chronic pancreatitis are approximately two to thirteen times more likely to develop pancreatic cancer.[75,76] ERP may be useful in patients with suspected pancreatic cancer when conventional methods fail to establish the diagnosis. Unfortunately, the diagnostic yield of pancreatography is limited as ductal changes of chronic pancreatitis and carcinoma are frequently indistinguishable. Experts use stricture contour and neighboring side-branch morphology as references for differentiating benign from malignant disease. However, even close examination of these often inconspicuous features, is often insufficient to differentiate benign from malignant disease.[171] Pancreatic duct brush cytology may be a useful adjunct for establishing the diagnosis.

PANCREATIC DUCT DISRUPTION (POST-TRAUMATIC PANCREATITIS)

Pancreatic duct rupture may result from pancreatic trauma occurring at the time of blunt injury, gunshot wounds, and high-speed accidents.[172,173] Compulsory seat belt laws may have increased the incidence of this condition.[174] Ductal rupture is the most lethal of all pancreatic injuries, with a mortality rate as high as 17%.[175] The significant mortality results from delayed diagnosis commonly seen with retroperitoneal injuries, which often have vague or absent signs and symptoms until late in the course.

Preoperative ERP is the most accurate method for confirming the diagnosis of pancreatic duct rupture as shown in a prospective study of 14 trauma patients. ERP was compared to serum amylase, CT, and peritoneal lavage. ERP offered 100% sensitivity and specificity in establishing the diagnosis, which was superior to the combination of serum amylase, CT, and peritoneal lavage. Importantly, preoperative pancreatography was successful and safe in all patients.[176]

191

CHECKLIST OF PRACTICE POINTS

1. Certain indications for pancreatic therapeutic endoscopy are clearly beneficial, including severe gallstone pancreatitis, suspected gallstone pancreatitis with coexisting cholangitis, and idiopathic acute recurrent pancreatitis. Other indications, such as endoscopic treatment of pancreatic strictures, stones, and/or pseudocysts, may offer limited benefit and require considerable knowledge and skill to manage potential complications.

2. Endoscopic accessories are available to enhance the technical success of pancreatic endoscopy. Many of these accessories are smaller versions of counterparts used in therapeutic biliary ERCP, whereas some, including nasopancreatic catheters and pancreatic duct stents, have been developed specifically for this application.

3. Pancreatic duct sphincterotomy of the major or minor papilla demands endoscopic expertise and clear indications for application. Stent insertion before minor papilla sphincterotomy usually helps determine the direction of sphincterotomy.

4. Pancreatic stent therapy may be beneficial in patients with pancreas divisum who suffer from acute recurrent pancreatitis. Pancreatic stent may also benefit those patients with pancreatic ductal strictures, stones, or disruption. Knowledge of stent-related complications is mandatory since patients may develop acute pancreatitis and pseudocyst infection as a consequence of stent malfunction.

5. Technically challenging endoscopic approaches to pancreatic pseudocyst drainage exist, including cystoenterostomy and transpapillary drainage. These techniques must be applied to properly selected patients and circumstances in order to minimize complications.

6. The majority of reported experience in therapeutic pancreatic endoscopy is uncontrolled. To provide more meaningful data and a foundation for widespread acceptance, future studies must compare the results of endoscopic therapy to untreated subjects, regardless of the indications for treatment.

REFERENCES

1. O'Connor KW, Lehman GA. An improved technique for accessory papilla cannulation in pancreas divisum. Gastrointest Endosc 1985; 31:13–17.

2. McCarthy J, Fumo D, Geenen JE. Pancreas divisum: a new method for cannulating the accessory papilla. Gastrointest Endosc 1987; 33:440–442.

3. Soehendra N, Kempeneers I, Nam VC, et al. Endoscopic dilatation and papillotomy of the accessory papilla and internal drainage in pancreas divisum. Endoscopy 1986; 18:129–132.

4. Kullman E, Borch K, Lindstrom E, et al. Bacteremia following diagnostic and therapeutic ERCP. Gastrointest Endosc 1992; 38:444–449.

5. Niederau C, Pohlmann U, Lubke H, et al. Prophylactic antibiotic treatment in therapeutic or complicated diagnostic ERCP: results of a randomized controlled clinical study. Gastrointest Endosc 1994; 40:533–537.

6. Classen DC, Jacobson JA, Burke JP, et al. Serious *Pseudomonas* infections associated with endoscopic retrograde cholangiopancreatography. Am J Med 1988; 84:590–596.

7. Kullman E, Borch K, Lindstrom E, et al. Bacteremia following diagnostic and therapeutic ERCP. Gastrointest Endosc 1992; 38:444–449.

8. Johnson GK, Geenen JE, Bedford RA, et al. A comparison of nonionic versus ionic contrast media: results of a prospective, multicenter study. Midwest Pancreaticobiliary Study Group. Gastrointest Endosc 1995; 42:312–316.

9. Rambow A, Staritz M, Meyer zum Buschenfelde KH. Contrast media for ERCP. Endoscopy (letter) 1988; 20:126–127.

10. Cotton PB, Salmon PR. Endoscopic retrograde cholangiopancreatography (ERCP). In: Schiller KFR, Salmon PR, eds. Modern topics in gastrointestinal endoscopy. London: Heinemann Medical; 1976:213–227.

11. Takekoshi T, Maruyama M, Sugiyama N, et al. Retrograde cholangiopancreatoscopy. Gastrointest Endosc 1975; 17:678–683.

12. Kohler B, Kohler G, Riemann JF. Pancreoscopic diagnosis of intraductal cystadenoma of the pancreas. Dig Dis Sci 1990; 35:382–384.

13. Neuhaus H, Hoffmann W, Classen M. Laser lithotripsy of pancreatic and biliary stones via 3.4 mm and 3.7 mm miniscopes: first clinical results. Endoscopy 1992; 24:208–214.

14. Riemann JF, Kohler B. Endoscopy of the pancreatic duct: value of different endoscope types. Gastrointest Endosc 1993; 39:367–370.

15. Classen M, Hellwig H, Rosch W. Anatomy of the pancreatic duct. A duodenoscopic-radiological study. Endoscopy 1973; 5:14–17.

16. Cotton PB. The normal endoscopic pancreatogram. Endoscopy 1974; 6:65–70.

17. Kreel L, Sandin B. Changes in pancreatic morphology associated with aging. Gut 1973; 14:962–970.

18. Schmitz-Moormann P, Himmelmann GW, Brandes JW, et al. Comparative radiological and morphological study of human pancreas. Pancreatitis like changes in postmortem ductograms and their morphological pattern. Possible implications for ERCP. Gut 1985; 26:406–414.

19. Birnstingl M. A study of pancreatography. Br J Surg 1959; 47:128–139.

20. Sivak MV, Sullivan BH Jr. Endoscopic retrograde pancreatography: analysis of the normal pancreatogram. Dig Dis Sci 1980; 21:263–269.

21. Belber JP, Bill K. Fusion anomalies of the pancreatic ductal system: differentiation from pathologic states. Radiology 1977; 122:637–642.

22. Kasugai T, Kuno N, Kizu M, et al. Endoscopic pancreatocholangiography. II. The pathological endoscopic pancreatocholangiogram. Gastroenterology 1972; 63:227–234.

23. Tympner F, Rosch W, Lutz H, et al. Diagnostic methods in chronic pancreatitis. Value of the endoscopic retrograde pancreaticography, the volume-loss corrected secretin-pancreozymin test and ultrasonics. (German) Dtsch Med Wochenschr 1978; 103:805.

24. Axon AT, Classen M, Cotton PB, et al. Pancreatography in chronic pancreatitis: international definitions. Gut 1984; 25:1107–1112.

25. Ralls PW, Halls J, Renner I, et al. Endoscopic retrograde cholangiopancreatography (ERCP) in pancreatic disease: a reassessment of the specificity of ductal abnormalities in differentiating benign from malignant disease. Radiology 1980; 134:347–352.

26. Classen M, Phillip J. Endoscopic retrograde cholangiopancreatography (ERCP) and endoscopic therapy in pancreatic disease. Clin Gastroenterol 1984; 13:819–842.

27. Kaufman AR, Sivak MV Jr, Ferguson DR. Endoscopic retrograde cholangiopancreatography in pancreatic islet cell tumors. Gastrointest Endosc 1988; 34:47–52.

28. Grimm H, Meyer WH, Nam VC, et al. New modalities for treating chronic pancreatitis. Endoscopy 1989; 21:70–74.

29. Fuji T, Amano H, Harima K, et al. Pancreatic sphincterotomy and pancreatic endoprothesis. Endoscopy 1985; 17:69–72.

30. Russell RC, Wong NW, Cotton PB. Accessory sphincterotomy (endoscopic and surgical) in patients with pancreas divisum. Br J Surg 1984; 71:954–997.

31. Lehman G, O'Connor K, Troiano F, et al. Endoscopic papillotomy and stenting of the minor papilla in pancreas divisum. Gastrointest Endosc 1989; 35:167.

32. Siegel JH, Guelrud M. Endoscopic cholangiopancreatoplasty: hydrostatic balloon dilation in the bile duct and pancreas. Gastrointest Endosc 1983; 29:99–103.

33. Huibregtse K, Schneider B, Vrij AA, et al. Endoscopic pancreatic drainage in chronic pancreatitis. Gastrointest Endosc 1988; 34:9–15.

34. Sauerbruch T, Holl J, Sackmann M, et al. Disintegration of a pancreatic duct stone with extracorporeal shock waves in a patient with chronic pancreatitis. Endoscopy 1987; 19:207–208.

35. Kerzel W, Ell C, Schneider HT, et al. Extracorporeal piezoelectric shockwave lithotripsy of multiple pancreatic stones under ultrasonographic control. Endoscopy 1989; 21:229–231.

36. Sauerbruch T, Holl J, Sackmann M, et al. Extracorporeal lithotripsy of pancreatic stones in patients with chronic pancreatitis and pain: a prospective follow up study. Gut 1992; 33:969–972.

37. Cotton PB, Lehman GA, Vennes J, et al. Endoscopic sphincterotomy complications and their management: an attempt at consensus. Gastrointest Endosc 1991; 37:383–393.

38. Freeman ML, Nelson DB, Sherman S, et al. Complications of biliary sphincterotomy. N Engl J Med 1996; 335:909–918.

39. Sherman S, Lehman GA. Endoscopic pancreatic sphincterotomy: techniques and complications. Gastrointest Endosc Clin North Am 1998; 8:115–124.

40. Gottlieb K, Sherman S. ERCP and biliary endoscopic sphincterotomy-induced pancreatitis. Gastrointest Endosc Clin North Am 1998; 8:87–114.

41. Sherman S, Troiano FP, Hawes RH, et al. Sphincter of Oddi manometry: decreased risk of clinical pancreatitis with use of a modified aspirating catheter. Gastrointest Endosc 1990; 36:462–466.

42. Elton E, Howell DA, Qaseem T, et al. Nasopancreatic drainage following endoscopic pancreatic sphincterotomy (EPS): a safe alternative to stent placement. Gastrointest Endosc 1997; 45:157A.

43. Dahman B, Geenen JE, Hogan HJ, et al. Pancreatic stents: are two barbs better than four? Gastrointest Endosc 1996; 43:404A.

44. Barawi M, Olssen M, Sherman S, et al. Spontaneous dislodgement of unflanged pancreatic duct stents. Am J Gastroenterol 1996; 91:1928A.

45. Tarnasky PR, Palesch YY, Cunningham JT, et al. Pancreatic stenting prevents pancreatitis after biliary sphincterotomy in patients with sphincter of Oddi dysfunction. Gastroenterology 1998; 115:1518–1524.

46. Geenen JE, Rolny P. Endoscopic therapy of acute and chronic pancreatitis. Gastrointest Endosc 1991; 37:377–382.

47. Johanson JF, Schmalz M, Geenen JE. Simple modification of a pancreatic duct stent to prevent proximal migration. Gastrointest Endosc 1993; 31:62–64.

48. Johanson JF, Schmalz MJ, Geenen JE. Incidence and risk factors for biliary and pancreatic stent migration. Gastrointest Endosc 1992; 38:341–346.

49. Ikenberry SO, Sherman S, Hawes RH, et al. The occlusion rates of pancreatic stents. Gastrointest Endosc 1994; 40:611–613.

50. Ponchon T, Bory RM, Hedelius F, et al. Endoscopic stenting for pain relief in chronic pancreatitis. Results of a standardized protocol. Gastrointest Endosc 1995; 42:452–456.

51. Provansal-Cheylan M, Bernard JP, Mariani A, et al. Occluded pancreatic endoprosthesis – analysis of the clogging material. Endoscopy 1989; 21:63–69.

52. Binmoeller KF, Rathod VD, Soehendra N. Endoscopic therapy of pancreatic strictures. Gastrointest Endosc Clin North Am 1998; 8:125–142.

53. Kozarek RA. Pancreatic stents can induce ductal changes consistent with chronic pancreatitis. Gastrointest Endosc 1990; 36:93–95.

54. Eisen G, Coleman S, Cotton PB. Morphological changes in the pancreatic duct after stent placement for benign pancreatic disease. Gastrointest Endosc 1994; 40:107A.

55. Gulliver DJ, Edmunds S, Baker ME, et al. Stent placement for benign pancreatic diseases: correlation between ERCP findings and clinical response. Am J Roentgenol 1992; 159:751–755.

56. Smith MT, Sherman S, Ikenberry SO, et al. Alterations in pancreatic ductal morphology following polyethylene pancreatic stent therapy. Gastrointest Endosc 1996; 44:268–275.

57. Sherman S, Hawes RH, Savides TJ, et al. Stent-induced pancreatic ductal and parenchymal changes: correlation of endoscopic ultrasound with ERCP. Gastrointest Endosc 1996; 44:276–282.

58. Acosta JM, Pellegrini CA, Skinner DB. Etiology and pathogenesis of acute biliary pancreatitis. Surgery 1980; 88:118–125.

59. Houssin D, Castaing D, Lemoine J, et al. Microlithiasis of the gallbladder. Surg Gynecol Obstet 1983; 157:20–24.

60. Opie EL. The etiology of acute hemorrhagic pancreatitis. Bull Johns Hopkins Hosp 1901; 12:182.

61. Houssin D, Castaing D, Lemoine J, et al. Microlithiasis of the gallbladder. Surg Gynecol Obstet 1983; 157:20–24.

62. Armstrong CP, Taylor TV, Jeacock J, et al. The biliary tract in patients with acute gallstone pancreatitis. Br J Surg 1985; 72:551–555.

63. Trapnell JE, Duncan EH. Patterns in incidence in acute pancreatitis. BMJ 1975; 2:179–183.

64. Lawson DW, Daggett WM, Civetta JM, et al. Surgical treatment of acute necrotizing pancreatitis. Ann Surg 1970; 172:605–617.

65. Imrie CW, Whyte AS. A prospective study of acute pancreatitis. Br J Surg 1975; 62:490–494.

66. Ranson JHC. Etiologic and prognostic factors in human acute pancreatitis: a review. Am J Gastroenterol 1982; 77:633–638.

67. Ranson JH, Rifkind KM, Turner JW. Prognostic signs and nonoperative lavage in acute pancreatitis. Surg Gynecol Obstet 1976; 143:209–219.

68. Neoptolemos JP, Hall AW, Finlay DF, et al. The urgent diagnosis of gallstones in acute pancreatitis: a prospective study of three methods. Br J Surg 1984; 71:230–233.

69. Tenner S, Dubner H, Steinberg W. Predicting gallstone pancreatitis with laboratory parameters: a meta-analysis. Am J Gastroenterol 1994; 89:1863–1866.

70. Chang L, Lo SK, Stabile BE, et al. Gallstone pancreatitis: a prospective study on the incidence of cholangitis and clinical predictors of retained common bile duct stones. Am J Gastroenterol 1998; 93:527–531.

71. Chak A, Hawes RH, Cooper GS, et al. Prospective assessment of the utility of EUS in the evaluation of gallstone pancreatitis. Gastrointest Endosc 1999; 49:599–604.

72. Sahai AV, Mauldin PD, Marsi V, et al. Bile duct stones and laparoscopic cholecystectomy: a decision analysis to assess the roles of intraoperative cholangiography, EUS, and ERCP. Gastrointest Endosc 1999; 49:334–343.

73. Kelly TR, Wagner DS. Gallstone pancreatitis: a prospective randomized trial of the timing of surgery. Surgery 1988; 104:600–605.

74. Safrany L, Cotton PB. A preliminary report: urgent duodenoscope sphincterotomy for acute gallstone pancreatitis. Surgery 1981; 89:424–428.

75. Rosseland AR, Solhaug JH. Early or delayed endoscopic papillotomy (EPT) in gallstone pancreatitis. Ann Surg 1984; 199:165–167.

76. Neoptolemos JP, Carr-Locke DL, London NJ, et al. Controlled trial of urgent endoscopic retrograde cholangiopancreatography and endoscopic sphincterotomy versus conservative treatment for acute pancreatitis due to gallstones. Lancet 1988; ii:979–983.

77. Fan ST, Lai EC, Mok FP, et al. Early treatment of acute biliary pancreatitis by endoscopic papillotomy. N Engl J Med 1993; 328:228–232.

78. Fölsch UR, Nitsche R, Ludtke R, et al. German Study Group on Acute Biliary Pancreatitis. Early ERCP and papillotomy compared with conservative treatment for acute biliary pancreatitis. N Engl J Med 1997; 336:237–242.

79. Karjalainen J, Airo I, Nordback I. Routine early endoscopic cholangiography, sphincterotomy and removal of common duct stones in acute gallstone pancreatitis. Eur J Surg 1992; 158:549–553.

80. Soergel KH. Acute pancreatitis. In: Sleisenger MH, Fordtran JS, eds. Gastrointestinal disease; pathophysiology, diagnosis, and management. 4th ed. Philadelphia: WB Saunders; 1989: 1814–1842.

81. Venu RP, Geenen JE, Hogan WJ, et al. Idiopathic recurrent pancreatitis: an approach to diagnosis and treatment. Dig Dis Sci 1989; 34:56–60.

82. Sherman S, Jamidar P, Reber H. Idiopathic acute pancreatitis (IAP): endoscopic approach to diagnosis and treatment. Am J Gastroenterol 1993; 88:1541A.

83. Kaw M, Verma R, Brodmerkel GJ Jr. ERCP, biliary analysis, sphincter of Oddi manometry (SOM) in idiopathic pancreatitis (IP) in response to endoscopic sphincterotomy (ES). Am J Gastroenterol 1996; 91:1935A.

84. Coyle W, Tarnasky P, Knapple W, et al. Evaluation of unexplained acute pancreatitis using ERCP, sphincter of Oddi manometry (SOM) and endoscopic ultrasound. Gastrointest Endosc 1996; 43:378A.

85. Geenen JE, Nash JA. The role of sphincter of Oddi manometry and biliary microscopy in evaluating idiopathic recurrent pancreatitis. Endoscopy 1998; 30:237–241.

86. Amouyal G, Amouyal P, Levy P, et al. Value of endoscopic ultra sonography in the diagnosis of idiopathic acute pancreatitis. Gastroenterology 1994; 106:283A.

87. Amouyal P, Amouyal G, Levy P, et al. Diagnosis of choledocholithiasis by endoscopic ultrasonography. Gastroenterology 1994; 106:1062–1067.

88. Catalano MF, Lahoti S, Alcocer E, et al. Dynamic imaging of the pancreas using real-time endoscopic ultrasonography with secretin stimulation. Gastrointest Endosc 1998; 48:580–587.

89. Bhutani M, Hoffman B, van Velse A, et al. Diagnosis of pancreas divisum by endoscopic ultrasound (EUS). Gastrointest Endosc 1995; 41:298A.

90. Rosch T, Lorenz R, Braig C, et al. Endoscopic ultrasound in pancreatic tumor diagnosis. Gastrointest Endosc 1991; 37:347–352.

91. Rosch T, Lightdale CJ, Botet JF, et al. Localization of pancreatic endocrine tumors by endoscopic ultrasonography. N Engl J Med 1992; 326:721–726.

92. Chang KJ, Nguyen P, Erickson RA, et al. The clinical utility of endoscopic ultrasound-guided fine-needle aspiration in the diagnosis and staging of pancreatic carcinoma. Gastrointest Endosc 1997; 45:387–393.

93. Catalano MF, Lahoti S, Geenen JE, et al. Prospective evaluation of endoscopic ultrasonography, endoscopic retrograde pancreatography, and secretin test in the diagnosis of chronic pancreatitis. Gastrointest Endosc 1998; 48:11–17.

94. Sahai AV, Zimmerman M, Aabakken L, et al. Prospective assessment of the ability of endoscopic ultrasound to diagnose, exclude, or establish the severity of chronic pancreatitis found by endoscopic retrograde cholangiopancreatography. Gastrointest Endosc 1998; 48:18–25.

95. Lee SP, Nicholls JF, Park HZ. Biliary sludge as a cause of acute pancreatitis. N Engl J Med 1992; 326:589–593.

96. Ros E, Navarro S, Bru C, et al. Occult microlithiasis in 'idiopathic' acute pancreatitis: prevention of relapses by cholecystectomy or ursodeoxycholic acid therapy. Gastroenterology 1991; 101:1701–1709.

97. Welch JP, White CE. Acute pancreatitis of biliary origin: is urgent operation necessary? Am J Surg 1982; 143:120–126.

98. Satiani B, Stone HH. Predictability of present outcome and future recurrence in acute pancreatitis. Arch Surg 1979; 114:711–716.

99. Pasricha PJ, Lipsett PA, Kalloo AN. 'Idiopathic' pancreatitis: definition by endoscopic manometric and biliary analysis. Gastroenterology 1994; 106:313A.

100. DiFrancesco V, Tebaldi M, Angelini G, et al. Sphincter of Oddi manometry and microscopic bile examination in the aetiological definition of idiopathic recurrent acute pancreatitis. Gastroenterology 1997; 112:437A.

101. Lans JL, Parikh NP, Geenen JE. Applications of sphincter of Oddi manometry in routine clinical investigations. Endoscopy 1991; 23:139–143.

102. Williamson RC. Pancreatic sphincteroplasty: indications and outcome. Ann R Coll Surg Engl 1988; 70:398–399.

103. Raddawi HM, Geenen JE, Hogan WJ, et al. Pressure measurements from biliary and pancreatic segments of sphincter of Oddi: comparison between patients with functional abdominal pain, biliary, or pancreatic disease. Dig Dis Sci 1991; 36:71–74.

104. Silverman WB, Ruffolo TA, Sherman S, et al. Correlation of basal sphincter pressures measured from the bile duct and the pancreatic duct in patients with suspected sphincter of Oddi dysfunction. Gastrointest Endosc 1992; 38:440–443.

105. Funch-Jensen P, Kruse A. Manometric activity of the pancreatic duct sphincter in patients with total bile duct sphincterotomy for sphincter of Oddi dyskinesia. Scand J Gastroenterol 1987; 22:1067–1070.

106. Catalano MF, Sivak MV, Falk GH, et al. Idiopathic pancreatitis (IP): diagnostic role of sphincter of Oddi manometry (SOM) and response to endoscopic sphincterotomy (ES). Gastrointest Endosc 1993; 39:310A.

107. Sherman S. Idiopathic acute recurrent pancreatitis (IRP): endoscopic approach to diagnosis and therapy. Gastrointest Endosc 1992; 38:261A.

108. Lans JL, Parikh NP, Geenen JE. Application of sphincter of Oddi manometry in routine clinical investigations. Endoscopy 1991; 23:139–143.

109. Toouli J, Di Francesco V, Saccone G, et al. Division of the sphincter of Oddi for treatment of dysfunction associated with recurrent pancreatitis. Br J Surg 1996; 83:1205–1210.

110. McCarthy J, Geenen JE, Hogan WJ. Preliminary experience with endoscopic stent placement in benign pancreatic disease. Gastrointest Endosc 1988; 34:16–18.

111. Kozarek RA, Patterson DJ, Ball TS, et al. Endoscopic placement of pancreatic stents and drains in the management of pancreatitis. Ann Surg 1989; 209:261–266.

112. Kozarek RA. Balloon dilation of the sphincter of Oddi. Endoscopy 1988; 20:207–210.

113. Bader M, Geenen JE, Hogan WJ. Endoscopic balloon dilatation of the sphincter of Oddi in patients with suspected biliary dyskinesia: results of a prospective randomized trial. Gastrointest Endosc 1986; 32:158.

114. Bernard JP, Sahel J, Giovannini M, et al. Pancreas divisum is a probable cause of acute pancreatitis: a report of 137 cases. Pancreas 1990; 5:248–254.

115. Blair AJ, Russell CG, Cotton PB. Resection for pancreatitis in patients with pancreas divisum. Ann Surg 1984; 200:590–594.

116. Lans JI, Geenen JE, Johnson JF, et al. Endoscopic therapy in patients with pancreas divisum and acute pancreatitis: a prospective, randomized, controlled clinical trial. Gastrointest Endosc 1992; 38:430–434.

117. Lehman GA, Sherman S, Nisi R, et al. Pancreas divisum: results of minor papilla sphincterotomy. Gastrointest Endosc 1993; 39:1–8.

118. Russell RC, Wong NW, Cotton PB. Accessory sphincterotomy (endoscopic and surgical) in patients with pancreas divisum. Br J Surg 1984; 71:954–957.

119. Warshaw AL, Simeone JF, Schapiro RH, et al. Evaluation and treatment of the dominant dorsal duct syndrome (pancreas divisum redefined). Am J Surg 1990; 159:59–64.

120. Coleman SD, Eisen GM, Troughton AB, et al. Endoscopic treatment in pancreas divisum. Am J Gastroenterol 1994; 89:1152–1155.

121. Kozarek RA, Ball TJ, Patterson DJ, et al. Endoscopic approach to pancreas divisum. Dig Dis Sci 1995; 40:1974–1981.

122. Siegel JH, Ben-Zvi JS, Pullano W, et al. Effectiveness of endoscopic drainage for pancreas divisum: endoscopic and surgical results in 31 patients. Endoscopy 1990; 22:129–133.

123. Prabhu M, Geenen JE, Hogan WJ. Role of endoscopic stent placement in the treatment of acute recurrent pancreatitis associated with pancreas divisum. Gastrointest Endosc 1989; 2:165A.

124. Venu RP, Geenen JE, Hogan WJ, et al. Role of endoscopic retrograde cholangiopancreatography in the diagnosis and treatment of choledochocele. Gastroenterology 1984; 87:1144–1149.

125. Lambert R, Ponchon T, Chavaillon A, et al. Laser treatment of tumors of the papilla of Vater. Endoscopy 1988; 20:227–331.

126. Ponchon T, Berger F, Chavaillon A, et al. Contribution of endoscopy to diagnosis and treatment of tumors of the ampulla of Vater. Cancer 1989; 64:161–167.

127. Binmoeller KF, Boaventura S, Ramsperger K, et al. Endoscopic snare excision of benign adenomas of the papilla of Vater. Gastrointest Endosc 1993; 39:127–131.

128. Howard JM, Wagner SM. Pancreatography after recovery from massive pancreatic necrosis. Ann Surg 1989; 209:31–35.

129. Feller ER. Stenosis of the main pancreatic duct in acute pancreatitis of unknown etiology. Gastrointest Endosc 1988; 34:131–133.

130. Wilson C, McArdle CS, Carter DC, et al. Surgical treatment of acute necrotizing pancreatitis. Br J Surg 1988; 75:1119–1123.

131. D'Egidio A, Schein M. Surgical strategies in the treatment of pancreatic necrosis and infection. Br J Surg 1991; 78:133–137.

132. Tonak J, Lux G, Gebhardt C. A surgical approach to hemorrhagic necrotizing pancreatitis based on endoscopic retrograde pancreatography. Gastrointest Endosc 1986; 32:104–106.

133. Gebhardt C, Riemann JF, Lux G. The importance of ERCP for the surgical tactic in hemorrhagic necrotizing pancreatitis (preliminary report). Endoscopy 1983; 15:55–58.

134. Rolny P, Lukes PJ, Gamklou R, et al. A comparative evaluation of endoscopic retrograde pancreatography and secretin CCK test in

the diagnosis of pancreatic disease. Scand J Gastroenterology 1978; 13:777–781.

135. Clark DW, Geenen JE, Hogan WJ. Endoscopic secretin test: a rapid and accurate assessment of pancreatic exocrine function. Gastroenterology 1995; 106:5A.

136. Geenen JE, Meyerson SM. The intraductal secretin test. Clin Perspec Gastroenterol 1998; 1:1–3.

137. Burdick JS, Bedford R, Geenen JE, et al. Endoscopic secretin test: comparison with conventional duodenal secretin stimulation test. Gastroenterology 1993; 104:297A.

138. Gregg JA. Intraductal secretin test of pancreatic function in suspected pancreatitis. Gastroenterology 1981; 80:1163A.

139. Levy P, Milan C, Pignon JP, et al. Mortality factors associated with chronic pancreatitis. Gastroenterology 1989; 96:1165–1172.

140. Ammann RW, Akovbiantz A, Largiader F, et al. Course and outcome of chronic pancreatitis: longitudinal study of a mixed medical–surgical series of 245 patients. Gastroenterology 1984; 86:820–828.

141. Winstanley PA, Manning AP, Lintott DJ, et al. Endoscopic retrograde cholangio-pancreatography in pancreatitis with persistent or recurrent pain. Int J Pancreatol 1986; 1:407–412.

142. Morrow CE, Cohen JI, Sutherland DE, et al. Chronic pancreatitis: long-term surgical results of pancreatic duct drainage, pancreatic resection and near-total pancreatectomy and islet autotransplantation. Surgery 1984; 96:608–614.

143. Bradley EL III. Long-term results of pancreatojejunostomy in patients with chronic pancreatitis. Am J Surg 1987; 153:207–213.

144. Scott J, Summerfield JA, Elias E, et al. Chronic pancreatitis: a cause of cholestasis. Gut 1977; 18:196–201.

145. Littenberg G, Afroudakis A, Kaplowitz N. Common bile duct stenosis from pancreatitis: a clinical and pathologic spectrum. Medicine 1979; 58:385–412.

146. Deviere J, Devaere S, Baize M, et al. Endoscopic biliary drainage in chronic pancreatitis. Gastrointest Endosc 1990; 36:96–100.

147. Cremer M, Deviere J, Delhaye M, et al. Stenting in severe chronic pancreatitis: results of medium-term follow-up in seventy-six patients. Endoscopy 1991; 23:171–176.

148. Burdick JS, Geenen JE, Hogan W, et al. Pancreatic stent therapy in chronic pancreatitis; which patients benefit? Gastrointest Endosc 1993; 39:245A.

149. Smits ME, Badiga SM, Rauws EA, et al. Long-term results of pancreatic stents in chronic pancreatitis. Gastrointest Endosc 1995; 42:461–467.

150. Hansell DT, Gillespie G, Imrie CW. Operative transampullary extraction of pancreatic calculi. Surg Gynecol Obstet 1986; 163:17–20.

151. Sherman S, Lehman GA, Hawes RH, et al. Pancreatic ductal stones: frequency of successful endoscopic removal and improvement of symptoms. Gastrointest Endosc 1991; 37:511–517.

152. Delhaye M, Vandermeeren A, Baize M, et al. Extracorporeal shock-wave lithotripsy of pancreatic calculi. Gastroenterology 1992; 102:610–620.

153. Kozarek RA, Ball TJ, Patterson DJ. Endoscopic approach to pancreatic duct calculi and obstructive pancreatitis. Am J Gastroenterol 1992; 87:600–603.

154. Dumonceau JM, Deviere J, Le Moine O, et al. Endoscopic drainage in chronic pancreatitis associated with ductal stones: long-term results. Gastrointest Endosc 1996; 43:547–555.

155. Smits ME, Rauws EA, Tytgat GN, et al. Endoscopic treatment of pancreatic stones in patients with chronic pancreatitis. Gastrointest Endosc 1996; 43:556–560.

156. Catalano MF, Geenen JE, Schmalz MJ, et al. Treatment of pancreatic pseudocysts with ductal communication by transpapillary pancreatic duct endoprosthesis. Gastrointest Endosc 1995; 42:214–218.

157. Howell DA, Elton E, Parsons WG. Endoscopic management of pseudocysts of the pancreas. Gastrointest Endosc Clin North Am 1998; 8:143–162.

158. Smits ME, Rauws EA, Tytgat GN, et al. The efficacy of endoscopic treatment of pancreatic pseudocysts. Gastrointest Endosc 1995; 42:202–207.

159. Kozarek RA. Endoscopic therapy of complete and partial pancreatic duct disruptions. Gastrointest Endosc Clin North Am 1998; 8:39–53.

160. Baron TH, Thaggard WG, Morgan DE, et al. Endoscopic therapy for organized pancreatic necrosis. Gastroenterology 1996; 111:755–764.

161. Lehman GA. Pseudocysts. Gastrointest Endosc 1999; 49:S81–S84.

162. Barthet M, Sahel J, Bodiou-Bertei C, et al. Endoscopic transpapillary drainage of pancreatic pseudocyst. Gastrointest Endosc 1995; 42:208–213.

163. Binmoeller KF, Seifert H, Walter A, et al. Transpapillary and transmural drainage of pancreatic pseudocysts. Gastrointest Endosc 1995; 43:219–224.

164. Sahel J, Bastid C, Pellat B, et al. Endoscopic cystoduodenostomy of cysts of chronic calcifying pancreatitis: a report of 20 cases. Pancreas 1987; 2:447–453.

165. Cremer M, Deviere J, Engelholm L. Endoscopic management of cysts and pseudocysts in chronic pancreatitis: long-term follow-up after 7 years of experience. Gastrointest Endosc 1989; 35:1–9.

166. Cremer M, Deviere J, Baize M, et al. New device for endoscopic cystoenterostomy. Endoscopy 1990; 22:76–77.

167. Grimm H, Binmoeller KF, Soehendra N. Endosonography-guided drainage of a pancreatic pseudocyst. Gastrointest Endosc 1992; 38:170–171.

168. Savides TJ, Gress F, Sherman S, et al. Ultrasound catheter probe-assisted endoscopic cystgastrostomy. Gastrointest Endosc 1995; 41:145–148.

169. Wiersema MJ. Endosonography-guided cystduodenostomy with a therapeutic ultrasound endoscope. Gastrointest Endosc 1996; 44:614–617.

170. Buchi KN, Bowers JH, Dixon JA. Endoscopic pancreatic cystogastrostomy using the Nd-YAG laser. Gastrointest Endosc 1986; 32:112–114.

171. Ralls PW, Halls J, Renner I, et al. Endoscopic retrograde cholangiopancreatography (ERCP) in pancreatic disease: a reassessment of the specificity of ductal abnormalities in differentiating benign from malignant disease. Radiology 1980; 134:347–352.

172. Engrav LH, Benjamin CI, Strate RG, et al. Diagnostic peritoneal lavage in blunt abdominal trauma. J Trauma 1975; 15:854–859.

173. Gougeon FW, Legros G, Archambault A, et al. Pancreatic trauma: a new diagnostic approach. Am J Surg 1976; 132:400–402.

174. Balasegaram M. Surgical management of pancreatic trauma. Curr Prob Surg 1979; 16:1–59.

175. Balasegaram M, Joishy SK. Pancreatic resection. Key to the surgical approach to pancreatic lesions. Am J Surg 1981; 141:204–207.

176. Barkin JS, Ferstenberg RM, Panullo W, et al. Endoscopic retrograde cholangiopancreatography in pancreatic trauma. Gastrointest Endosc 1988; 34:102–105.

11.

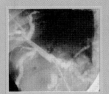

BILIARY STENTING

KEES HUIBREGTSE

VINOD DHIR

Obstructive jaundice caused by benign or malignant pathologies involving the bile duct deserves treatment to diminish the complaints of itching, nausea, and lack of appetite, and to prevent damage to the liver. Endoscopic biliary stenting, first described in 1979, has evolved into an important component of the multimodality management of these complex clinical problems.[1-7] It is important to emphasize that other techniques like surgical bypass and percutaneous stenting have also continued to evolve and the differences in results of these techniques reflect the available skills, expertise, and supportive care rather than the technique per se.

INDICATIONS

Malignant biliary tract obstruction caused by ampullary carcinoma, pancreatic carcinoma, bile duct carcinoma, and metastatic disease can be treated in a palliative way by the insertion of a biliary endoprosthesis. The prosthesis is often used as a measure to bring the patient into a better clinical condition before major surgery, although prospective data showing an advantage of preoperative stenting are not available. The prosthesis is mostly used as the definitive palliative treatment. Other indications of stenting are obstructive jaundice caused by chronic pancreatitis, operative trauma, or primary sclerosing cholangitis. A biliary prosthesis can also be used in patients with bile duct stones which cannot be removed after sphincterotomy, as a temporary measure to prevent cholangitis.

CONTRAINDICATIONS

There are no absolute contraindications. Coagulation disorders pose a relative contraindication in patients who need a sphincterotomy prior to stent placement. The use of stents in benign biliary strictures and in the pancreatic duct is still a subject of controversy. Metal stents cannot be removed and their use should be largely restricted to non-resectable malignant strictures.

EQUIPMENT

Endoscopes

Therapeutic biliary procedures are best performed with a side-viewing endoscope with a large (3.7, 4.2, or 4.5 mm) instrumentation channel (Olympus, Fujinon, Pentax).

Stents (Fig. 11.1)

The most commonly used biliary endoprosthesis is the Amsterdam-type, straight stent with side flaps to prevent dislodgement. These stents are made of polyethylene, polyurethane, or Teflon and are commercially available in 7, 8, 10, and 11.5 Fr diameter. The overall lengths vary from 5, 9 11, 14 to 19 cm (Wilson–Cook Med. Inc., Microvasive, PBN, Olympus). The double-pigtail prostheses are used for special indications like stone disease and drainage of pancreatic pseudocysts.

The Teflon 'Tannenbaum' stent without sideholes (Wilson–Cook Med. Inc.) (Fig. 11.2) and the three-layer Teflon stent (Olympus) (Fig. 11.3) have not shown a longer

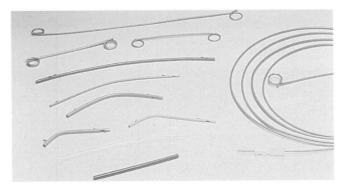

Fig. 11.1 Amsterdam-type endoprostheses, pigtail endoprostheses, and nasobiliary catheter.

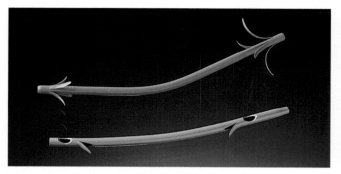

Fig. 11.2 'Tannenbaum' Teflon endoprosthesis (top) and Amsterdam-type endoprosthesis (bottom).

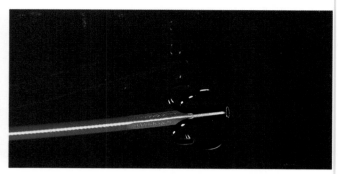

Fig. 11.3 Three-layer, Teflon 'Tannenbaum' stent. Note the metal wires.

patency in prospective randomized studies, when compared to the Amsterdam-type, polyethylene stents.[8,9]

Self-expanding metal stents

As the main drawback of plastic prostheses is the occlusion of these stents by biliary sludge, attempts have been made to develop stents with a larger diameter. Self-expanding metal stents (Wallstent, Microvasive: Spiral Z and Za-stent, Wilson–Cook Med. Inc., and Diamond, Microvasive) have the advantage of expanding after deployment to a diameter of up to 8–10 mm.

The Wallstent is made of cobalt alloy filaments, braided in a tubular fashion (Fig. 11.4).[10–14] It is pliable, self-expanding, and flexible in the longitudinal axis. The diameter of the prosthesis is substantially reduced by elongation. The delivery system comprises an 8 Fr coaxial catheter. The stent is loaded on the inner catheter while the outer catheter constrains the stent (Fig. 11.5). The space between the two catheters needs to be flushed with saline via a side-port. The prosthesis itself is radiopaque. Additional markers on the delivery catheter permit accu-

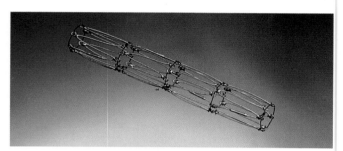

Fig. 11.6 Metal, self-expanding Z-stent.

rate placement of the stent. The stents have lengths of 6, 8, or 10 cm and a diameter of 8 Fr in the constrained form and of 30 Fr in the fully expanded form. The stent is inserted over a 4 m-long guidewire and is deployed by pulling the outer catheter over the inner catheter. Repositioning of the stent during deployment is possible by constraining the stent again, provided the stent is only deployed up to a mark shown on the catheter.

The Spiral Z and ZA-stents are cylindrical wire structures made of stainless steel or Nitinol that are constructed in a zigzag pattern. These stents are self-expanding and are released by withdrawal of the outer catheter of a double catheter system (Fig. 11.6).[15] The Ultraflex Diamond stents are made of Nitinol. A single wire is woven into a fine mesh and is constrained by an outer catheter. There are radiopaque markers at the proximal, middle, and distal ends as the stent itself is only faintly radiopaque.[16]

Catheters

The larger caliber plastic prostheses are inserted over a guiding catheter. In principle, two types of catheter are available (Fig. 11.7): the Huibregtse catheter (PBN,

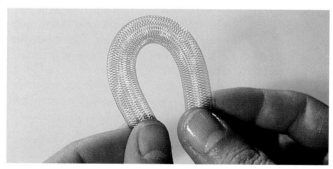

Fig. 11.4 Metal, self-expanding stent: Wallstent.

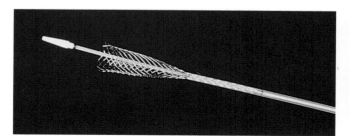

Fig. 11.5 Partially deployed Wallstent on delivery device.

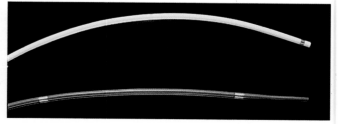

Fig. 11.7 (Top) Huibregtse catheter for stent insertion. (Bottom) Guiding catheter with two metal markers, 7 cm apart.

Wilson–Cook, Surgimed) with a blunt tip and a metal ring at the tip for visualization on the fluoroscopy screen; and one with a tapering tip with two metal rings, 7 cm apart to also allow the measurement of the distance from the stricture to the papilla and thereby the length of the desired endoprosthesis. The outer diameter of the guiding catheter is of significant importance. The catheter should fit snugly within the prosthesis. This facilitates prosthesis placement with the least amount of resistance at the site of the stricture.

Guidewires

The stainless steel, Teflon-coated guidewires, with or without an inner core, are of different lengths (260, 400, 480 cm) and of variable diameters (0.018, 0.025, 0.035, 0.38 inch). The tip of these guidewires is flexible and atraumatic. The length of the flexible tip can be adjusted by advancing or withdrawing an inner movable core. These guidewires are not torquable and kink easily. The torquable guidewire (Microvasive) has a flexible tip which can be readily seen fluoroscopically, but it is difficult to see the more rigid part. In spite of its name, the torque properties are limited.

The Terumo guidewire (Terumo Corporation, Japan) is coated over its full length with a hydropolymer, which makes the guidewire very slippery when in contact with water. This guidewire easily follows difficult bends and asymmetric strictures. It can also be used successfully in the pancreatic duct and for traversing the cystic duct for the positioning of nasocholecystic drains. The slippery distal end (when wet) is rather difficult to handle. The core is made of Nitinol and is therefore resistant to kinking.

A variety of coated wires have become available (Roadrunner, Tracer, and Hybrid tracer (Wilson–Cook), and Zebra, Jag, and Pathfinder (Microvasive)). They essentially consist of a Nitinol or stainless steel core having a Teflon or endoglide coating. In some wires, the hydrophilic coating is applied to a variable length at the tip (Tracer and Jag). The wires are available in diameters varying from 0.018 to 0.038 inch and the tip has a platinum core to make it radiopaque. These wires have graduated markings or stripes to facilitate detection of movement which facilitates exchange without fluoroscopy. The core of these wires is kink-resistant while the coating at the tip improves maneuverability through angulated strictures. The availability of these kink-resistant-coated wires allows passage through tortuous strictures and has enhanced success rates in difficult situations. Most guidewires are available with different shapes of the tip (J bend, U bend) (Fig. 11.8).

Most guidewires lack rigidity and are therefore not suitable to guide catheters used for dilation of proximal strictures. Pushing the dilating catheters often results in the formation of bends and curves in the distal bile duct preventing the force to be optimally conveyed to the more proximal stricture. Frimberger designed a guidewire (varioguidewire, B. Braum Melsungen Co., Germany) with a variable rigidity. The rigidity of this wire can be adjusted in situ by a factor of more than 50.

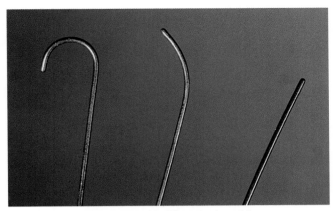

Fig. 11.8 Terumo guidewires with differently shaped tips.

Dilating devices

Dilating catheters are mostly used in the presence of firm strictures (Wilson–Cook, Microvasive) (Fig. 11.9). Such catheters of increasing diameter (from 5 to 10 Fr) have a long tapered tip and a metal radiopaque ring marking the location of the largest diameter. Some dilators (Microvasive) have a hydrophilic coating at the distal tip for 20 cm to improve passage through firm strictures. Use of dilating balloons after dilation of the stricture with catheters has been successful up to 7 Fr. Dilating balloons are available with diameters from 6 to 12 mm (Microvasive, Wilson–Cook, Surgimed) (Fig. 11.10).

Stent retriever

A commonly used stent retriever is a 200 cm-long, thin, metal spiral, the sheath of which resembles a biopsy forceps (Wilson–Cook) (Fig. 11.11). The tapered tip is threaded for 3–4 mm. This device can be passed over a guidewire. The other end has a small metal knob facilitating rotation of the whole device. The diameter of the threaded tip is selected to snugly fit into the lumen of the stent to be removed.[17] This device can also be used for dilation of very firm strictures (Fig. 11.12).[18–19] Specially designed snares are available to retrieve stents through the instrumentation channel of the endoscope.

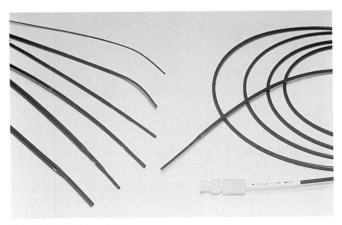

Fig. 11.9 Dilating catheters.

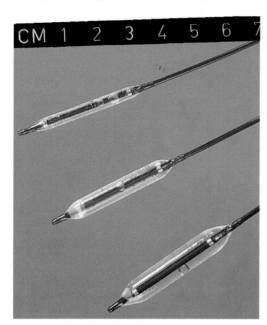

Fig. 11.10 Dilating balloons.

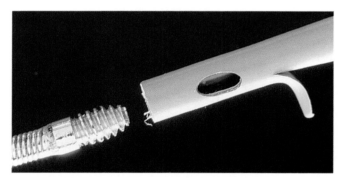

Fig. 11.11 Stent retriever in distal end of endoprosthesis.

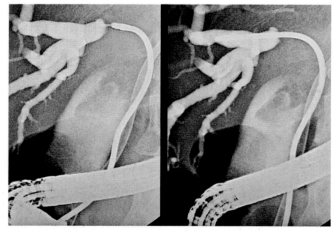

Fig. 11.12 Stent retriever is used to dilate a firm bifurcation stricture.

PATIENT PREPARATION

Patients are prepared as for diagnostic ERCP. Antibiotic coverage is mandatory, particularly in those patients in whom only incomplete drainage is anticipated.[20–23] Patients are routinely sedated with diazepam or midazolam, some-times combined with fentanyl or pethidine. The patients should be monitored by an assistant and by mechanical methods including pulse oximetry. Supervision by an anes-thetist may be required.[24–25]

TECHNIQUE

The procedure starts with a diagnostic ERCP. Preferably, both ducts should be filled in order to establish a firm diag-nosis and define the anatomy of both ductal systems. Knowledge of the exact location and nature of the bile duct stenosis is essential prior to endoprosthesis insertion. In case standard cannulation with a metal-ball-tip or metal-cone-tip catheter fails, cannulation can be attempted with a guidewire inserted in the metal-ball-tip catheter. Cannulation with a double-lumen sphincterotome with the guidewire (Cotton cannulotome, Wilson–Cook Med. Inc.) is the next step. Only in case of failure to cannulate by all these modalities should an attempt at pre-cutting with the needle-knife be made.[26–29]

Once a diagnostic catheter is inserted in the bile duct, contrast is injected and a guidewire can be introduced and maneuvered through the stricture. This guidewire should be left in place during subsequent manipulations in order to facilitate the introduction and exchange of subsequent accessories. In case a different guidewire is needed, the catheter should be advanced well above the stricture before guidewire exchange. Under all circumstances, either a guidewire or catheter should remain in place until the pro-cedure is successfully completed.

Some investigators routinely perform a limited sphinc-terotomy following the diagnostic ERCP to facilitate intro-duction of catheters, guidewires, and endoprostheses. Previously, it was believed that a sphincterotomy was nec-essary to avoid occlusion of the pancreatic duct by the prosthesis in order to prevent acute pancreatitis. However, the incidence of acute pancreatitis was not increased in a series of our patients in whom a 10 Fr prosthesis was inserted through an intact papilla. A sphincterotomy is no longer necessary to facilitate placement of drainage tubes, now that 'over-the-guidewire techniques' are used. Most endoscopists insert a 10 or 11.5 Fr prosthesis through an intact papilla without prior sphincterotomy. A sphinctero-tomy is still desirable or necessary when larger (>11.5 Fr) caliber prostheses or more than one prosthesis will be inserted.

Following successful cannulation and passage of a guidewire through the stricture, prosthesis placement is straightforward. Over the guidewire, the sphincterotome can be inserted when appropriate or a guiding catheter can be inserted over which the prosthesis can be pushed into correct position with help of the pusher tube (Figs 11.12 and 11.13). Successful deployment of an endoprosthesis requires that the catheter over which it is placed fits snugly in the prosthesis. For example, a 10 or 11.5 Fr prosthesis should not be advanced over a 5 Fr diameter catheter because there is too much space between the catheter and the inner wall of the prosthesis. The tip of the endopros-

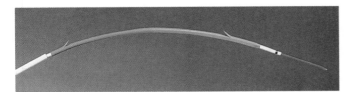

Fig. 11.13 The three-layer system for stent insertion: guidewire, guiding catheter, and stent plus pusher tube.

thesis tends to impact on the tissue instead of smoothly following the bends of the catheter. Substantial resistance may also be encountered during passage of the prosthesis through the intact papilla. When passage of a guidewire and diagnostic catheter through the stricture cannot be accomplished, a small sphincterotomy can be made to facilitate introduction of larger and stiffer catheters. Preferentially, the more rigid 6 Fr Teflon catheter with a radiopaque ring is used instead of the standard diagnostic catheter when difficult strictures are encountered. Guidewires are inserted through the catheter to intubate the stricture. The direction of the guidewire can be changed by manipulating the position of the guiding catheter with movements of the endoscope similar to those made for standard cannulation. The nurse/assistant can help to intubate the stricture by moving the guidewire in and out through the guidecatheter, but the endoscopist can also manipulate the guidewire by moving the guidecatheter when intubation is difficult. Different guidewires with various shapes of tip may be tried. Once the guidewire has been maneuvered through the stricture, the catheter can almost always be advanced through the stricture. It is imperative, especially in angulated strictures, that the more rigid part of the guidewire is passed through the stricture before the catheter is advanced. The guidewire should remain in position to stiffen the catheter during prosthesis insertion although it can be replaced by the Geenen cytology brush, which is withdrawn into the catheter after passing the brush through the stricture a few times (Fig. 11.14). The catheter with the brush still inside is removed after positioning the endoprosthesis.

Introduction of the prosthesis requires a carefully orchestrated series of manipulations. The prosthesis is first positioned over the guiding catheter and inserted into the instrumentation channel. It is then further advanced towards the tip of the endoscope with the help of a pusher tube. A combined system of catheter, endoprosthesis, and pusher tube is also available (Oasis system, Wilson–Cook), which can be used when no difficulties in positioning are anticipated. The elevator bridge is raised during advancement of the prosthesis through the endoscope to prevent deeper insertion of the Teflon guidecatheter into the intrahepatic bile ducts and to signal when the prosthesis has reached the end of the instrumentation channel. The length of the pusher tube is designed so that the catheter which traverses it can be held in place by the nurse while the endoscopist advances the pusher tube.

The elevator bridge, opened once the prosthesis reaches the tip of the instrumentation channel, allows the prosthesis to be gradually pushed out of the endoscope. The whole assembly (catheter, guidewire, and prosthesis) is moved forward by advancing the pusher tube. Under fluoroscopic control, the endoscopist can see the distance between the endoscope and the papilla widen by this initial movement (Fig. 11.15).

The endoprosthesis should be advanced not more than about 2 cm into the duodenal lumen. The stent is then raised by closing the elevator bridge, and the tip of the endoscope is moved closer to the papilla with the up–down knob. The nurse holds the pusher tube in a steady position but puts tension on the guidecatheter by withdrawing it a few centimeters. The endoprosthesis can be further pushed into the bile duct by an anticlockwise rotation of the endoscope and/or by slight withdrawal of the endoscope while both knobs are locked and the elevator bridge is fully raised. During these maneuvers, the endoprosthesis can be monitored visually as it moves into the papilla.

As the prosthesis enters the CBD the obtuse angle between the duodenoscope and the papilla is seen fluoroscopically to become more acute, and the distance between the scope and the papilla shortens.

Further insertion takes place by again opening the elevator bridge, advancing the prosthesis with the pusher tube

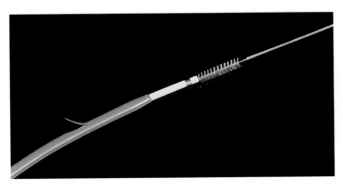

Fig. 11.14 The guidewire is replaced by the cytology brush.

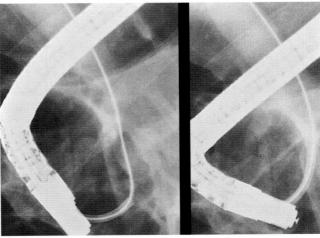

Fig. 11.15 (**Left**) The elevator bridge is open and the endoprosthesis is advanced a few centimeters in the duodenum. (**Right**) The elevator bridge is closed; the tip of the endoscope is angled up; the nurse pulls the guiding catheter and the prosthesis moves into the bile duct.

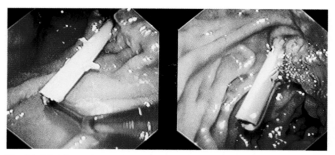

Fig. 11.16 The endoprosthesis hangs free in the duodenum.

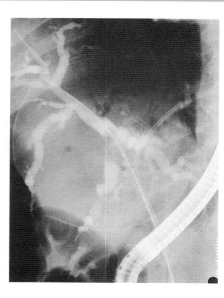

Fig. 11.17 Very firm bifurcation stricture. Stent of 7 Fr is inserted into the left hepatic duct. Dilating balloon is in the right hepatic duct.

and closing the bridge, while the nurse pulls on the catheter and the whole assembly is moved forward by bringing the tip of the endoscope as close as possible to the papilla. These steps are repeated until the distal barb of the prosthesis has reached the papilla (Fig. 11.16).

When the prosthesis has arrived at the desired position, the nurse can pull out the catheter and guidewire while the endoscopist keeps the prosthesis in position with the pusher tube. Care should be taken to avoid pushing the prosthesis too far into the CBD during the removal of the catheter. It is imperative that at least 1 cm of the prosthesis projects free into the duodenum. This allows easy retrieval in the event of clogging. Once adequate drainage can be seen endoscopically or fluoroscopically, the endoscope (containing the pusher tube, catheter, and guidewire) can be removed.

Malignant mid-CBD or distal CBD strictures can always be passed with a prosthesis after proper positioning of the catheter and guidewire without prior dilation. Benign strictures or malignant bifurcation tumors cannot always be passed by a prosthesis and may need prior dilation. Dilating catheters of increasing diameter are used for this purpose. These catheters can only be inserted through the stricture after positioning of a relatively rigid guidewire well above the stricture. Balloon catheters can be used for further dilation, once the stricture has been stretched up to a diameter of 2.1 mm. Occasionally, the insertion of a 10 Fr prosthesis may be difficult or impossible, even after balloon dilation. In these difficult, firm strictures, a small caliber prosthesis or nasobiliary drain should be left in place for a few days for gradual dilation. Generally, exchange for a 10 Fr prosthesis is easily possible a few days later (Fig. 11.17).

When an attempt to insert a 10 Fr stent through a firm stricture fails, it is impossible to retrieve the stent through the instrumentation channel. Stent retrieval can only be accomplished by removing the endoscope with the various devices inside. Frimberger designed a stent coupling device to be used when a difficult and possibly failed stent insertion is anticipated (Fig. 11.18).

Insertion of an expandable stent

The technique for insertion of a Wallstent is straightforward. A 4 m-long guidewire is positioned through the stricture by standard techniques. Following this, the insertion device with the constrained stent is inserted through the instrumentation channel over the guidewire. When the

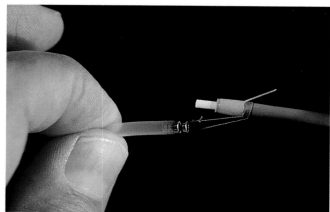

Fig. 11.18 Stent coupling device for retrieval of a stent when insertion fails.

insertion device is well positioned, the prosthesis can be released by removing the outer catheter while keeping the inner catheter steady. The stent shortens upon expanding. Correct positioning is easy in distal CBD strictures because the distal part of the stent can be seen endoscopically during placement. Positioning, however, is more difficult in high bile duct strictures because the positioning and deployment must be controlled fluoroscopically. Failure of stent expansion and inability to remove the inner catheter after stent release are rare technical problems.[30] Two Wallstents can be inserted in bifurcation strictures by first positioning two 4 m guidewires in the left and right hepatic duct. The first metal stent is inserted over one guidewire alongside the other guidewire and the second stent is inserted and deployed alongside the first inserted stent (Fig. 11.19). Combinations of a metal stent and a plastic stent are possible. A plastic stent can be inserted through the side mesh of the metal stent after prior opening of the mesh with a dilating balloon. The theoretical advantage of metal wire stents in bifurcation strictures is the capability for drainage of side branches via the open side meshes. This has not been studied in clinical studies.

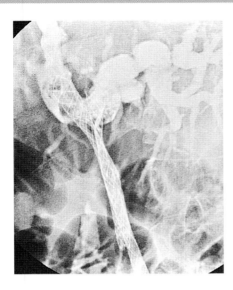

Fig. 11.19 Two Wallstents in a bifurcation tumor.

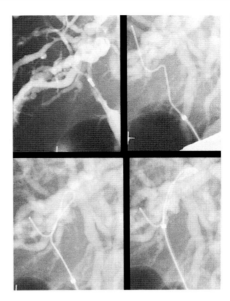

Fig. 11.20 Passage of a guidewire with a long floppy tip into the left hepatic duct.

Guidewire positioning: technical tips

Most bile duct strictures are in a direct line with the distal bile duct. These strictures can easily be passed with a guidewire and subsequently with the catheter and prosthesis. Some strictures, however, are asymmetrical and make an acute angle with the distal CBD. These strictures can usually be intubated by manipulation of the guide-catheter. The technique is that, under fluoroscopic control, while injecting contrast, the catheter is positioned in line with the stricture. The guidewire is then inserted in the guidecatheter which is jiggled to and fro to pass through the stricture. The catheter can then follow the guidewire, negotiate the stricture and finally be advanced beyond the stricture. Then the biliary prosthesis can be pushed into position over the catheter.

Insertion of a guidewire into the left hepatic duct in case of bifurcation tumor may be difficult. Following the placement of the floppy part of the guidewire in the left hepatic duct, further insertion of the stiff portion of the guidewire through the stricture may be impossible. The stiff portion of the guidewire tends to go to the right system. The guiding catheter can aid in directing the stiff portion of the guidewire into the left system. The sequence of movements requires a coordinated effort by the endoscopist and the endoscopy nurse to combine the advancement of the guiding catheter with a slow with-drawal of the guidewire which should ultimately result in placing the tip of the guidecatheter into the opening to the left hepatic system. An alternative technique is to use a guidewire with a long flexible tip. Continuous advance-ment may result in springing the guidewire into the left system (Fig. 11.20).

It may be difficult to pass the guidewire through asym-metric strictures, in particular those originating at the medi-al side of the bile duct. The stiff portion of the guidewire is normally pre-bent during advancement through the instru-mentation channel of the endoscope. This always results in pointing the tip of the guidewire toward the lateral side of the bile duct. When this occurs, a long flexible guidewire leader is used and as the wire advances into the common

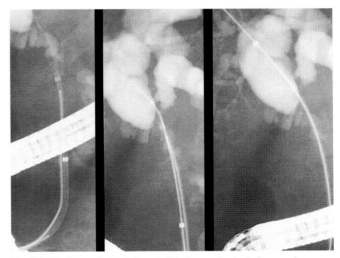

Fig. 11.21 One catheter is inserted in the cystic duct. A second catheter with a guidewire can now be passed through the bile duct stricture in the dilated common hepatic duct.

duct, a spring effect takes place to direct the catheter to the opposite side of the duct and through the obstruction.

Double strictures of the CBD and the cystic duct may create difficulties when the guidewire preferentially enters the cystic duct. A longer flexible portion of the guidewire may allow passage of the stiff portion of the guidewire through the CBD stricture. An alternative method is to temporarily occlude the cystic duct with a prosthesis or catheter to allow passage of the guidewire through the CBD stricture (Fig. 11.21).

Technique of removal of a clogged stent

For stent removal, the distal end of the clogged prosthesis is caught with a snare, a Dormia basket, or a foreign-body grasper and is then removed along with the endoscope. When using the Dormia basket, the prosthesis is pulled snugly close to the instrumentation channel, the control knobs of the endoscope are unlocked, and both endoscope and prosthesis are withdrawn (Fig. 11.22).

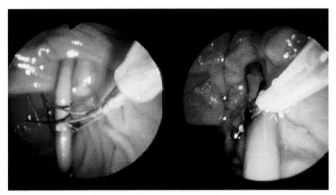

Fig. 11.22 Clogged endoprosthesis caught in a Dormia basket.

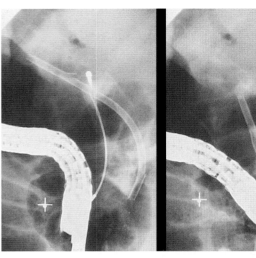

Fig. 11.24 An upward migrated stent is caught in a Dormia basket and retrieved.

Stent removal with a stent retriever starts with cannulation of the stent with a ball-tip catheter or a specially designed catheter with a hook. Once the prosthesis is cannulated, a 4 m-long guidewire is inserted through the catheter and the prosthesis, whereupon the catheter is removed. The retriever is then inserted over the guidewire up to the distal end of the stent. The thread of the retriever is then screwed into the stent by rotating the device (Fig. 11.23). The prosthesis can then be removed by slow withdrawal of the retriever while feeding the guidewire into the prosthesis. One of the advantages of the latter method is that the endoscope is not removed and that the guidewire remains in position, facilitating re-insertion of another prosthesis. Using the same technique, a small snare can be placed over the guidewire to grasp and remove the stent.

Removal of a dislodged or broken prosthesis

Retrieval of a prosthesis which has slipped into the CBD above the papilla may be exceptionally difficult.[31–32] One of the techniques available is to insert a balloon catheter into the prosthesis, to inflate the balloon, and to pull the

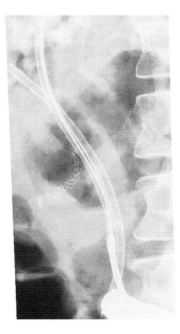

Fig. 11.23 Bifurcation tumor with two stents. The stent retriever is attached to one stent to be removed.

prosthesis back into the duodenum. Another technique is to insert a guidewire through the stent and then retrieve the stent with the special stent retriever. When a prosthesis has moved above a stricture and is high in the CBD, retrieval is only possible after snaring with a Dormia basket under fluoroscopic control (Fig. 11.24). When the duodenal part of the prosthesis is embedded in the opposite wall of the duodenum, a foreign body remover is useful for its retrieval.

Exchange of a prosthesis may be difficult or impossible because of massive tumor invasion and subsequent destruction of the duodenal wall. A blocked stent should not be removed when difficulties are anticipated in placing a new stent. It may be wiser to insert a new stent alongside the blocked stent. This procedure is possible in almost all patients. The blocked stent provides an indicator of the opening to the bile duct which can be cannulated alongside the original stent even when it cannot be clearly seen. The procedure is completed under fluoroscopic guidance.

Removal of metal stents

A metal stent can usually be removed within the first 2 to 3 days of deployment by grasping it with a forceps or a snare.[33] The stent should never be pulled within the endoscope channel. Attempts at stent removal after the first few days are not successful as the stent becomes embedded in the tumor tissue which may grow into each of the individual mesh openings.

RESULTS

Benign strictures

Biliary endoprostheses may play a role in the treatment of benign biliary disease. Postoperative leaks close more readily when drainage is improved through a prosthesis bypassing the intact papilla. Stricturing of the bile duct may be prevented by positioning of a prosthesis alongside the perforation site.[34,35]

Benign postoperative strictures can be dilated by leaving one or more biliary stents across the stricture for a period of 6 to 12 months. Several series have now been published with overall success of 60 to 85%.[36–38]

Bile duct strictures caused by chronic pancreatitis may be temporarily treated by a biliary prosthesis. Long-term results, however, show that only a small minority of the patients do well after removal of the stents.[39]

Biliary prostheses have also been used in the treatment of primary sclerosing cholangitis and in patients with bile duct stones, which cannot be endoscopically removed.[40–43]

Prostheses have been placed into the pancreatic duct to improve flow of pancreatic juice. Several series have been published showing clinical improvement in more than 60% of patients.[44,45] Stenting of the dorsal duct has been employed in the treatment of pancreas divisum.[46] Although the results of prosthesis placement are encouraging, potential risks, such as the induction of further ductal changes must be studied.[47] Further research is necessary before pancreatic duct stenting can be recommended as a standard routine treatment.

Malignant strictures

The goal of palliative treatment is to relieve pruritus, treat cholangitis if present, and lessen the physiologic impact of cholestasis. Successful drainage and complication rates vary according to the location of the stricture (Table 11.1).[4,48,49] Most studies have been performed in patients with pancreatic cancer. Table 11.2 shows the results and complications in two larger series. Three prospective RCTs have compared the results of endoscopic prosthesis and surgical

bypass (Table 11.3).[50–52] All show a lower immediate mortality rate and lower frequency of complications in the endoscopically treated patients. The early advantages of prosthesis placement are counterbalanced somewhat by the need for re-admission for the exchange of blocked stents and the surgical treatment of late duodenal obstruction. Mean survival remains approximately 6 months for those who have undergone either method of therapy.

Bifurcation tumors are extremely difficult to treat by any modality. Surgical access may be limited, as these tumors often spread proximally, deeply invading the parenchyma of the liver. Palliative surgical procedures are very difficult, and transhepatic access to the left hepatic

Results of endoscopic stents in patients with carcinoma of the pancreas in two large series		
	University of Amsterdam[48]	Middlesex Hospital[49]
No. of patients	632	403
Mean age	71 years	NA
Successful drainage	87%	85%
30-day mortality	10.8%	17%
Median survival	5 months	4–5 months
Duodenal stenosis	9%	5%
Stent blockage	29%	16%

NA = not available.

Table 11.2 Results of endoscopic stents in patients with carcinoma of the pancreas in two large series

Clinical results of endoscopic endoprosthesis placement in patients with cancer				
Type of tumor	Success rate (%)	Disappearance of jaundice (%)	Hospital mortality (%)	Median survival (months)
Ampullary	95–100	100	5	13
Pancreatic, distal CBD	90	95	7–12	6
Mid-CBD, bifurcation	70–75	70	20–25	5–6

CBD = common bile duct.

Table 11.1 Clinical results of endoscopic endoprosthesis placement in patients with cancer[4]

Results of three prospective RCTs comparing endoscopic stenting with surgical bypass for obstructive jaundice						
	Ref. 51		Ref. 50		Ref. 52	
	Stent	Surgery	Stent	Surgery	Stent	Surgery
No. of patients	23	25	25	19	101	103
Successful drainage (%)	91	92	96	84	94	91
Complications (%)	22	40	NA	NA	10	28
30-day mortality (%)	9	20	NA	NA	7	17
Duodenal bypass (%)	0	0	0	0	6	1
Recurrent jaundice (%)	17	2	28	16	18	3
Median survival	152 days	125 days	84 days	100 days	5 months+	5 months+
Range	39–411	52–354	3–498	10–642		

NA = not available; *statistically significant; +mean survival.

Table 11.3 Results of three prospective RCTs comparing endoscopic stenting with surgical bypass for obstructive jaundice

Results of three RCTs comparing metal stents with plastic stents					
	No. of patients	Drainage (%)	30-day mortality (%)	Occlusion (%)	Patency (days)
Davids et al[11]					
Metal	49	96	14	33	372
Plastic	56	95	4	54	126
Carr-Locke et al[12]					
Metal	86	98	5	13	111
Plastic	78	95	5	13	62
Knyrim et al[13]					
Metal	31	100	13	22	–
Plastic	31	100	9	43	–

Table 11.4 Results of three RCTs comparing metal stents with plastic stents

duct system may be virtually impossible. There has been much discussion lately concerning the proper endoscopic treatment of these lesions. The central question is whether adequate palliative relief of obstruction requires the placement of two endoprostheses, one to drain the left system and one to drain the right, or if one prosthesis placed in either system will suffice. It has been argued that adequate palliation of obstructive symptoms can be achieved if at least 25% of the liver parenchyma is drained.[53] Good results – successful drainage in approximately 80% of patients with Type II and III tumors – have been reported using a single prosthesis.[48,53,54] No difference in efficacy has been shown between single stent placement in the left or the right system. Some investigators advocate vigorous (including additional percutaneous stents, if necessary) means be taken to ensure drainage of both systems.[55] This recommendation pertains more to the prevention of post-procedure cholangitis than to the effective palliation of jaundice. In a recent study, it was found that patients with bilateral drainage had the longest survival, whereas patients with cholangiographic opacification of both lobes but drainage of only one had the shortest survival.[56]

Our approach is to attempt, under antibiotic cover, to stent both systems, understanding that we will be successful only about 30% of the time. We do not advocate that further measures, such as percutaneous drainage or the combined endoscopic–percutaneous approach, be applied to the non-drained system unless jaundice does not resolve or cholangitis supervenes. Patients with multiple intrahepatic strictures will probably not benefit from any type of drainage procedure, as several segments will always remain undrained. In the absence of intractable symptoms of cholestasis, we recommend that these patients should not be subjected to further therapeutic measures, as the risk of inducing cholangitis outweighs any benefit that could possibly be realized from the establishment of what could only be regarded as suboptimal drainage.

Results with metal stents

Many studies of endoscopically placed metal stents have been published. The overall conclusion is that the stent is easy to place with acceptable early complications and good initial drainage in 90 to 95% of patients. Late dysfunction owing to biliary sludge formation is significantly less than

with plastic stents, but late occlusion by tumor ingrowth or overgrowth occurs in up to 15% of patients. Three RCTs (Table 11.4)[11-13] have been published comparing metal stents with plastic stents. In all the studies, there was a higher obstruction rate, a higher cholangitis rate, and longer hospitalization time associated with plastic stents. A cost benefit in favor of the metal stents was also found. Theoretically, a metal stent should result in better drainage than a plastic stent in hilar strictures because the wire mesh does not block drainage from the side branches (Fig. 11.19). The few studies published show metal stents to be better than plastic stents in terms of patency rate and cost, and two metal stents appear to be better than one.[57,58]

COMPLICATIONS AND THEIR MANAGEMENT (TABLES 11.5 AND 11.6)

Early complications of prosthesis placement may be related to a small sphincterotomy or to the prosthesis insertion itself. In our experience, complications of persistent endoscopic sphincterotomy have been far less than the 6 to 8% generally quoted for endoscopic sphincterotomy for calculous disease, probably because the required size of the

Early complications of endoprosthesis placement	
Complication	Rate (%)
A. Papillotomy-related	
Bleeding	1–2
Pancreatitis	0–1
Perforation (duodenal, biliary)	0–1
B. Endoprosthesis-related	
Cholecystitis	0–1
Early clogging (blood clots)	1–2
Acute cholangitis	0–27
Papillary tumor	0
Pancreatic tumor	8
Mid-CBD tumor	14
Bifurcation tumor	27
Mortality	2

Table 11.5 Early complications of endoprosthesis placement (within 1 week)[4]

Late complications of endoprosthesis placement	
Complication	Rate (%)
Clogging (cholangitis, jaundice)	20–25 (mean 5 months)
Acute cholecystitis	0–1
Migration, duodenal or biliary	1–2
Perforation	1–2
Duodenal stenosis (tumor-related)	7–10 (mean 10 months)
Mortality	Unusual

Table 11.6 Late complications of endoprosthesis placement (over 1 week)[4]

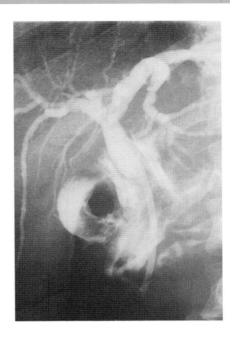

Fig. 11.26 Contrast around the common bile duct as a sign of perforation. A prosthesis was successfully inserted.

sphincterotomy is rather small (6–8 mm). Bleeding may be seen in 1 to 2% of patients, pancreatitis in 0 to 1%, while perforation of the duodenum or bile duct should be exceedingly rare events.

Acute cholangitis is the most important complication of the insertion procedure itself both in frequency and severity. Bacterial contamination of the biliary duct system during ERCP is unavoidable. Proper disinfection of the endoscope and any ancillary equipment is mandatory, but will not prevent the introduction of microorganisms from the mouth and the upper gut. The introduction of bacteria into the biliary tree only leads to the development of cholangitis when biliary drainage is incomplete. As a consequence, cholangitis is more frequently seen after drainage procedures of bifurcation tumors where complete biliary drainage is more difficult and nearly impossible to achieve than in adequately drained, more distally located bile duct strictures (Fig. 11.25).

Antibiotic treatment should be started or continued, when cholangitis develops. Furthermore stent function should be checked endoscopically. If the initial stent placement was not optimal, better and more complete drainage in case of bifurcation tumors should be re-attempted endo-

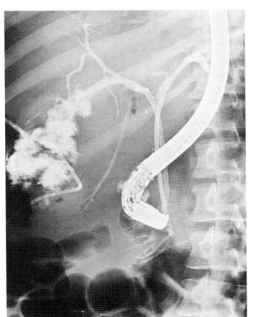

Fig. 11.25 Patient with liver abscess following partial drainage of a bifurcation tumor.

scopically. Percutaneous techniques are then used when endoscopic attempts are not successful.

Bile duct perforation may be caused by sphincterotomy, an attempt at precut needle-knife sphincterotomy, or by the guidewire. These perforations mostly heal spontaneously and usually do not result in clinical symptoms. If a perforation occurs during intubation attempts in a bile duct stricture, it is almost invariably distal to the stricture, and therefore in an area of low biliary pressure with little risk of bile leakage (Fig. 11.26). Many endoscopists prefer to continue the procedure and try to insert a stent even when a perforation and bile leakage are encountered because the stent may help in closing the perforation site. Antibiotic treatment should be continued for a few more days and the patients should not be allowed to drink or eat for 24 hours.

Acute cholecystitis may develop after stent insertion. This risk is high in patients with pancreatic cancer and involvement of the cystic duct in the tumor process. The stent further occludes the already partially occluded cystic duct. Cholecystectomy or percutaneous drainage of the gallbladder is then the treatment of choice.

The major late complication is clogging of the prosthesis, occurring in 21 to 36% of cases (Fig. 11.27). In our experience, clogging may occur from 8 days to over 15 months after placement with a mean of about 5 months. Clinically, patients with a clogged prosthesis present with a flu-like syndrome, malaise, low-grade fever, or deterioration of liver function tests. If the significance of this syndrome is not recognized early, frank cholangitis and jaundice will occur. Prompt recognition of these heralding symptoms should lead to immediate removal and replacement of the clogged prosthesis. In situ cleaning, brushing, and irrigation of a clogged prosthesis are technically possible, but re-obstruction of the prosthesis occurs quickly. Some endoscopists prefer to vent the biliary system after removal of a blocked stent by flushing and draining via a

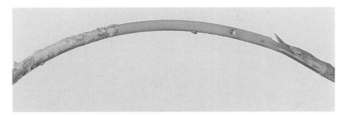

Fig. 11.27 Endoprosthesis clogged by biliary sludge.

nasobiliary drain for a few days prior to placement of a new stent. There are no studies to substantiate this policy or indications that the newly inserted stent remains patent for a longer period of time after a 'rest period'. Therefore we immediately exchange a blocked stent for a clean one, even in patients with suppurative cholangitis.

Other late complications are unusual and include acute cholecystitis, migration of a prosthesis into the more proximal bile ducts or bowel, and duodenal or bile duct perforation. Injuries of the CBD wall or the duodenal wall by the prosthesis or the side flap are possible. Also perforation of the duodenal wall may occur secondary to erosion by the stent. This complication is seen only when the inserted stent is too long. A shorter stent should be substituted. A very infrequent late complication is acute cholecystitis. This is probably the result of gradual cystic duct stenosis in the presence of infected bile in patients with a prosthesis in situ. The development of duodenal stenosis as a result of the ingrowing tumor is not a true complication of the procedure, but a consequence of the ingrowing tumor. The treatment of choice is then a gastroenterostomy and surgical biliary bypass procedure, or a duodenal stent in inoperable patients.[59]

Complications specific to metal stents

As mentioned earlier, about 10 to 15% of metal stents eventually get blocked because of tumor ingrowth through the wire mesh or tumor overgrowth above or below the stent.[11–14] The problem can be solved by inserting another prosthesis, either metal or plastic, through the blocked metal stent. A rare complication is trauma to the duodenal wall by the Wallstent.

Choice of stent: plastic or metal?

The advantages of the metal stent are its longer patency and its overall cost benefit. The disadvantages are its high initial cost and impossibility of removal. Only inoperable patients or patients with unresectable tumor are possible candidates for an expandable stent. Patency curves of expandable stents and plastic stents run parallel during the first 3 months. Thus patients with expected short survival should receive a plastic stent, while patients expected to live longer should receive a metal stent. Tumor size and general condition of the patient could guide the choice of stent.[60–62]

CONCLUSION

Endoscopic biliary stenting has evolved as a standard approach to treat obstructive jaundice caused by a variety of etiologies. The refinement in guidewire technology has made the procedure technically easier. Plastic stents remain an excellent option for relief of obstructive jaundice for short durations of up to 3 months. The problem of plastic stent occlusion has led to the development of self-expanding metal stents. The latter stents have shown improved patency rates, but problems remain in the area of tumor ingrowth and inability to remove them. Further improvements in technology are eagerly awaited to help improve the quality of life of patients with obstructive jaundice.

CHECKLIST OF PRACTICE POINTS

1. Review patient's history and results of prior laboratory data.
2. Review all documents of imaging techniques (ultrasound, Doppler, CT, MRCP).
3. Assess the general condition and operability of the patient.
4. Discuss with the surgeon, the radiologist, and the gastroenterologist or physician the various treatment options.
5. Check that all ancillary equipment that may possibly be needed is readily available.
6. Consider the use of antibiotics.
7. The patient should have an intravenous line for administration of sedatives, antibiotics, and hydration. Many patients undergo a series of investigations for which they have to be fasting and run the risk of being dehydrated.
8. Check prosthesis function fluoroscopically or radiologically. In case of malfunction, reposition the prosthesis.
9. Prevention of iatrogenic cholangitis is mandatory. When a prosthesis cannot be inserted for a drain and there is contrast proximal to the stricture, continue antibiotics and consider an alternative drainage procedure (radiologic or surgical) or schedule a second endoscopic attempt the next day.
10. In case of a bifurcation tumor and only partial drainage, continue antibiotics for 3 to 4 more days. The development of cholangitis should prompt further endoscopic or radiologic treatment.

REFERENCES

1. Soehendra N, Reynders-Frederix V. Palliative Gallengangdrainage. Dtsch Med Wochenschr 1979; 104:206–209.

2. Huibregtse K, Haverkamp HJ, Tytgat GNJ. Transpapillary positioning of a large 3.2 mm biliary endoprosthesis. Endoscopy 1981; 13:217–219.

3. Huibregtse K, Tytgat GNJ. Palliative treatment of obstructive jaundice by transpapillary introduction of a large bore bile duct endoprosthesis. Gut 1982; 23:371–375.

4. Huibregtse K. Endoscopic biliary and pancreatic drainage. Stuttgart: Thieme; 1988.

5. Cotton PB. Endoscopic methods for relief of malignant obstructive jaundice. World J Surg 1984; 8:854–861.

6. Cotton PB. Management of malignant bile duct obstruction. J Gastroenterol Hepatol 1990; 5(Suppl 1):63–77.

7. Sung JJY, Chung SCS. Endoscopic stenting for palliation of malignant biliary obstruction: a review of progress in the last 15 years. Dig Dis Sci 1995; 40:1167–1173.

8. Meyerson SM, Geenen JE, Catalano MF, et al. 'Tannenbaum' teflon stents versus traditional polyethylene stents for treatment of malignant biliary strictures: a multicenter, prospective randomized trial. Gastrointest Endosc 1998; 47:AB122.

9. Costamagna GG, Tringali AH, Perri VV, et al. Comparative trial of double layer stent versus polyethylene stent for malignant biliary strictures: interim results. Gastrointest Endosc 1999; 49:AB230.

10. Huibregtse K, Cheng J, Coene PPLO, et al. Endoscopic placement of expandable metal stents for biliary strictures. A preliminary report on experience with 33 patients. Endoscopy 1989; 2:280–282.

11. Davids PHP, Groen AK, Rauws EAJ, et al. Randomised trial of self-expanding metal stents versus polyethylene stents for distal malignant biliary obstruction. Lancet 1992; 340:1488–1492.

12. Carr-Locke DL, Ball TJ, Connors PJ, et al. Multicenter randomized trial of Wallstent biliary endoprosthesis versus plastic stents. Gastrointest Endosc 1993; 39:310.

13. Knyrim K, Wagner HJ, Pausche J, et al. A prospective randomized controlled trial of metal stents for malignant obstruction of the bile duct. Endoscopy 1993; 25:207–212.

14. Huibregtse K. The Wallstent for malignant biliary obstruction. Gastrointest Endosc Clin North Am 1999; 9:491–502.

15. Howell DA, Nezhad SG, Dy RM. Endoscopically placed Gianturco endoprosthesis in the treatment of malignant and benign biliary obstruction. Gastrointest Endosc Clin North Am 1999; 9:479–490.

16. Dumonceau JM, Devière J. The Ultraflex Diamond stent for malignant biliary obstruction. Gastrointest Endosc Clin North Am 1999; 9:513–520.

17. Soehendra N, Maydeo A, Eckmann B, et al. A new technique for replacing an obstructed endoprosthesis. Endoscopy 1990; 22:271–272.

18. Niall R, van Someren RNM, Benson MJ, et al. A novel technique for dilating difficult malignant biliary strictures during therapeutic ERCP. Gastrointest Endosc 1996; 43:495–498.

19. Brand B, Thonke SF, Obytz S, et al. Stent retriever for dilatation of pancreatic and bile duct strictures. Endoscopy 1999; 31:142–145.

20. Sauer G, Grabein B, Huber G, et al. Antibiotic prophylaxis of infectious complications with endoscopic retrograde cholangiopancreatography. A randomized controlled study. Endoscopy 1990; 22:164–167.

21. Motte S, Devière J, Dumonceau JP, et al. Risk factors for septicemia following endoscopic biliary stenting. Gastroenterology 1991; 101:1374–1381.

22. Alveyn CG, Robertson DAF, Wright R, et al. Prevention of sepsis following endoscopic retrograde cholangiopancreatography. J Hosp Infection 1991; 19(Suppl C):65–70.

23. van den Hazel SJ, Speelman P, Tytgat GNJ, et al. Acute and recurrent cholangitis: the role of antibiotics in the treatment and prevention. Clin Infect Dis 1994; 19:279–286.

24. Bell GD. Review article: Premedication and intravenous sedation for upper gastrointestinal endoscopy. Aliment Pharmacol Ther 1990; 14:103–122.

25. American Society for Gastrointestinal Endoscopy. Monitoring of patients undergoing gastrointestinal endoscopic procedures. Gastrointest Endosc 1991; 37:120–121.

26. Huibregtse K, Katon RM, Tytgat GNJ. Precut papillotomy via the needle knife papillotome: a safe and effective technique. Gastrointest Endosc 1986; 32:403–405.

27. Dowsett JF, Polydorou AA, Vaira D, et al. Needle knife papillotomy: how safe and how effective? Gut 1990; 31:905–908.

28. Shakoor T, Hogan WJ, Geenen JE. Needle knife papillotomy – efficacy and risks. Gastrointest Endosc 1992; 38:251.

29. Bruins Slot W, Schoeman MN, DiSario JA, et al. Needle knife sphincterotomy as a precut procedure: a retrospective evaluation of efficacy and complications. Endoscopy 1996; 28:334–339.

30. Jowell PS, Cotton PB, Huibregtse K, et al. Delivery catheter entrapment during deployment of expandable metal stents. Gastrointest Endosc 1993; 39:199–202.

31. Tarnasky PR, Cotton PB, Baillie J, et al. Proximal migration of biliary stents: attempted endoscopic retrieval in forty one patients. Gastrointest Endosc 1995; 42:513–520.

32. Lahoti S, Catalano MF, Geenen JE, et al. Endoscopic retrieval of proximally migrated biliary and pancreatic stents: experience of a large referral center. Gastrointest Endosc 1998; 47:486–491.

33. Chaurasia OMP, Rauws EAJ, Fockens P, et al. Endoscopic techniques for retrieval of proximally migrated biliary stent: the Amsterdam experience. Gastrointest Endosc 1999; 50:780–785.

34. Davids PHP, Rauws EAJ, Coene PPLO, et al. Postoperative bile leakage: the endoscopic management. Gut 1992; 33:1118–1122.

35. Ryan ME, Geenen JE, Lehman GH, et al. Endoscopic intervention for biliary leaks after laparoscopic cholecystectomy: a multicenter review. Gastrointest Endosc 1998; 47:261–266.

36. Davids PHP, Rauws EAJ, Coene PPLO, et al. Endoscopic stenting for postoperative biliary strictures. Gastrointest Endosc 1992; 38:12–18.

37. Meenan J, Rauws EA, Huibregtse K. Benign biliary strictures and sclerosing cholangitis. Gastrointest Endosc Clin North Am 1996; 6:127–138.

38. Dumonceau JM, Devière J, Delhaye M, et al. Plastic and metal stents for postoperative benign bile duct strictures: the best and the worst. Gastrointest Endosc 1998; 47:8–17.

39. Ng C, Huibregtse K. The role of endoscopic therapy in chronic pancreatitis-induced common bile duct strictures. Gastrointest Endosc Clin North Am 1998; 8:181–194.

40. Johnson GK, Geenen JE, Venu RP, et al. Endoscopic treatment of biliary tract strictures in sclerosing cholangitis: a larger series and recommendations for treatment. Gastrointest Endosc 1991; 37:38–43.

41. van Milligen de Wit AWM, van Bracht J, Rauws EAJ, et al. Endoscopic stent therapy for dominant extra hepatic bile duct strictures in primary sclerosing cholangitis. Gastrointest Endosc 1996; 44:293–299.

42. van Milligen de Wit AWM, van Bracht J, Rauws EAJ, et al. Lack of complications following short-term stent therapy for extra hepatic bile duct strictures in primary sclerosing cholangitis. Gastrointest Endosc 1997; 46:344–347.

43. Bergman JGHM, Rauws EAJ, Tijssen JGP, et al. Biliary endoprostheses in elderly patients with endoscopically irretrievable common bile duct stones: report on 177 patients. Gastrointest Endosc 1995; 42:195–201.

44. Smits ME, Badiga SM, Rauws EAJ, et al. Long-term results of pancreatic stent in chronic pancreatitis. Gastrointest Endosc 1995; 42:461–467.

45. Binmoeller KF, Rathod VD, Soehendra N. Endoscopic therapy of pancreatic strictures. Gastrointest Endosc Clin North Am 1998; 8:125–142.

46. Lehman GA, Sherman S. Diagnosis and therapy of pancreas divisum. Gastrointest Endosc Clin North Am 1998; 8:55–78.

47. Kozarek RA. Pancreatic stents can induce ductal changes consistent with chronic pancreatitis. Gastrointest Endosc 1990; 36:93–95.

48. Coene PPLO. Endoscopic biliary stenting – mechanisms and possible solutions of the clogging phenomenon (thesis). Meppel: Kripps Retro; 1990.

49. Dowsett JF, Polydorou A, Vaira D, et al. Endoscopic stenting for malignant biliary obstruction: how good really? A review of 641 consecutive patients. Gut 1988; 29:A1458.

50. Anderson JR, Sörensen SM, Kruse A, et al. Randomized trial of endoscopic versus operative bypass in malignant obstructive jaundice. Gut 1989; 30:1132–1135.

51. Shepard HA, Royle G, Ross APR, et al. Endoscopic biliary endoprostheses in the palliation of malignant obstruction of the distal common bile duct: a randomized trial. Br J Surg 1988; 75:1166–1168.

52. Smith AC, Dowsett JF, Russell RCG, et al. Randomised trial of endoscopic stenting versus surgical bypass in malignant low bile duct obstruction. Lancet 1994; 344:1655–1660.

53. Polydorou AA, Cairns SR, Dowsett JF, et al. Palliation of proximal malignant biliary obstruction by endoscopic endoprosthesis insertion. Gut 1991; 32:685–690.

54. Polydorou AA, Chisholm EM, Romanos AA, et al. A comparison of right versus left hepatic duct endoprosthesis insertion in malignant hilar biliary obstruction. Endoscopy 1989; 21:266–271.

55. Devieŕe J, Baize M, de Toeuf J, et al. Long-term follow-up of patients with hilar malignant stricture treated by endoscopic internal drainage. Gastrointest Endosc 1988; 34:95–101.

56. Change WH, Kortan P, Haber GB. Outcome in patients with bifurcation tumors who undergo unilateral versus bilateral hepatic duct drainage. Gastrointest Endosc 1998; 47:354–362.

57. Wagner HJ, Knyrim, Vakil N, et al. Plastic endoprosthesis versus metal stents in palliative treatment of malignant hilar obstruction. A prospective and randomized trial. Endoscopy 1993; 25:213–218.

58. Mehta S, Ozden S, Dhanireddy S, et al. Endoscopic single versus double Wallstents for palliation of malignant Bismuth type III/IV hilar strictures – comparison of clinical outcome and hospital costs. Gastrointest Endosc 1999; 49:A234.

59. Soetikno RM, Carr-Locke DL. Expandable metal stents for gastric outlet, duodenal and small intestinal obstruction. Gastrointest Endosc Clin North Am 1999; 9:447–459.

60. Prat F, Chapat O, Ducot B, et al. Predictive factors for survival of patients with malignant distal biliary strictures: a practical management guideline. Gut 1998; 42:76–80.

61. Prat F, Chapat O, Ducot B, et al. A randomized trial of endoscopic drainage methods for inoperable malignant strictures of the common bile duct. Gastrointest Endosc 1998; 47:1–7.

62. Schmassmann A, von Gunten E, Knuchel J, et al. Wallstent versus plastic stents in malignant biliary obstruction: effects of stent patency of the first and second stent on patient compliance and survival. Am J Gastroenterol 1996; 91:654–659.

12.

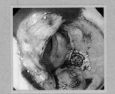

COLONOSCOPIC POLYPECTOMY

JEROME D. WAYE

Colonoscopy and the removal of colonic polyps are two of the major advances in gastroenterology in the 20th century. All of the accomplishments, innovations, and progress have been made in the past 30 years, since polypectomy was first introduced. Removal of colon polyps interrupts the adenoma–carcinoma sequence and has been reported by the National Polyp Study to markedly diminish the incidence of colon cancer.[1]

PATIENT PREPARATION

Visualization of the large bowel must be adequate to see the entire colon and to safely employ electrosurgical equipment during polypectomy. Almost any method of cleansing the colon, including castor oil and enemas, citrate of magnesia and enemas, phospho-soda or an electrolyte solution, is adequate to prepare the colon for electrosurgery.[2] A meta-analysis of the two major types of colonoscopic cleansing regimens revealed that sodium phosphate, when compared to the 4 L polyethylene glycol solution, is as effective, less costly, and a more easily completed preparation.[3] The phospho-soda preparation is taken in two 45 mL aliquots, with the second dose being mandatory and taken about 4 to 6 hours before the procedure. Fermentable sugars such as mannitol have been used to provoke an osmotic diarrhea which results in a clean colon but with the potential complication of an intracolonic explosion.[4] Carbon dioxide colonic insufflation, once thought necessary for avoidance of spark-induced explosion,[5] is now considered optional with most endoscopists not using CO_2, and the major reason for its use is to speed up gas absorption after the examination with a resultant decrease in post-colonoscopy cramps and distention.[6]

Routine testing for bleeding disorders prior to colonoscopic polypectomy is not necessary.[7,8] A history of a bleeding disorder should be obtained, including any tendency to bleed excessively following lacerations, a surgical procedure, or dental extraction. Patients do not need to be screened with a platelet count, prothrombin time, bleeding time, or clotting time. Aspirin, with its known antiplatelet properties, has not been shown to be detrimental to hemostasis during polypectomy, but many request that it be discontinued for 1 week prior to the endoscopic examination.[9] Diagnostic colonoscopy is relatively risk-free in the patient who requires continuous anticoagulation with Coumadin, but polypectomy should be avoided because of the possibility of bleeding. When polyps are to be removed in the anticoagulated patient at high risk for thrombotic episodes (such as prosthetic cardiac valves), a period of hospitalization is required with anticoagulation maintained substituting heparin with its short duration of action. When prothrombin levels return to the normal range, polypectomy may be performed within 4 hours after discontinuation of heparin therapy. If there is no bleeding during polypectomy, heparin may be given within 4 hours, and Coumadin may be resumed on the night of the polypectomy procedure. The patient should remain in the hospital on heparin until prothrombin times return to therapeutic levels. The introduction of low molecular weight heparin for prevention of deep vein thrombosis in orthopedic patients provides an out-of-hospital option for short-term warfarin substitution. It is tempting to consider its use for polypectomy patients, but it has not been studied for this purpose.[10]

EQUIPMENT

All of the available electrosurgical units (ESUs) are capable of producing continuous power output (cutting current), or an interrupted waveform (coagulation current). Most ESUs have the availability of combining the two waveforms with a setting called 'blended current'. Most experts use pure coagulation current during polypectomy, and eschew blended current, which tends to separate a polyp more rapidly than does coagulation alone. Once adjusted to the optimal setting, there is no need to change the power output during polyp removal, regardless of whether the base is large or small or when switching between the polypectomy snare and the hot biopsy forceps.

The injector needle is an important component of polypectomy equipment. It must be of sufficient length to traverse the colonoscope, the sheath should be strong enough to prevent buckling when pressure is applied to force it through several loops and convolutions of the scope when in the right colon, and the needle should lock in position when extended to prevent excess play of the needle when attempting to push it into the mucosa. In addition, the bevel of the needle is an important but often overlooked component, since a long bevel may pierce two or more layers and permit simultaneous injection into the submucosa while also spilling fluid into the peritoneal cavity. The distended bowel wall is relatively thin, with the total thickness about 1.5 mm;[11] each layer (mucosa, submucosa, and muscularis propria) is about 0.5 mm thick, so the bevel must be rather obtusely angulated to allow precise submucosal injection. Even without a sharply angulated bevel, a smaller diameter needle is of benefit when it is desired to deliver fluid into the submucosal layer without extravasation into the colon lumen.

A single-channel, 168 cm-long colonoscope with a 3.8 or 4.2 mm accessory channel is the instrument most preferred for colonoscopy by all experts and most colonoscopists. The double-channel scopes are somewhat less flexible, can be difficult to pass through the entire colon, and are associated with more patient discomfort than the one-channel type. There are only limited occasions when it is desired to pass two accessory devices simultaneously through a colonoscope, such as grasping a polyp and lifting it while placing a snare.[12–14] This maneuver would appear to be relatively easy, but in practice can be quite difficult, since the two accessories are obligated to move together rather than separately; it is desirable to lift up the portion grasped by the forceps while seating the snare downward over the polyp, but such manipulation is not possible. Attempts at use of instruments passed through both channels require that, before grasping the polyp, the forceps must be passed through the open snare, but even when this has been accomplished, moving the scope tip to lift up the forceps to elevate the polyp also causes the snare to rise up.

The hot biopsy forceps is an electrically insulated forceps through which electrical current flows to direct electrical energy around the tissue held within the jaws, enabling simultaneous cautery of a polyp base while obtaining a biopsy specimen.

Two contact thermal devices, the heater probe and BICAP electrode, can control post-polypectomy arterial spurting as well as lesser degrees of hemorrhage. When utilized for cessation of colonic hemorrhage, the current delivery should be decreased by approximately 50% from the power used for treatment of upper intestinal hemorrhage. Multiple applications at this power setting appear to be safe in the colon. It is not wise to push with a great deal of force as is recommended in the upper intestinal tract. The water jet from these probes is extremely useful for precise localization of the bleeding site to permit precise probe application.

The argon plasma coagulator is a device for the delivery of high-frequency current in a monopolar mode that does not require direct contact between the probe and tissue. When the distance from probe to tissue is optimal, the monopolar circuit is completed by the flow of electrons through the activated and ionized argon gas which transmits the electrical ions from the probe electrode to the tissue. The ionized argon gas is called the argon plasma. Utilizing a combination of voltage adjustment and motion of the probe tip, the thermal penetration of tissue can be varied between a range of fractions of 1–6 mm. In the colon, the power output setting should usually be at 40 W, with a relatively low gas flow (0.8 L per minute). Uses in the large bowel include treatment of post-polypectomy bleeding and ablation of residual adenomas following their piecemeal resection.[15–17] The delivery system for flexible endoscopy was developed in Germany (ERBE Inc., Tubingen, Germany).[18,19]

Two devices are available for polypectomy, but are underutilized. These are the detachable snare loop and clips. The loop, used for additional hemostasis during or after polypectomy, is a nylon ligature that can be placed over a lesion (such as a pedunculated polyp) like a wire snare, and tightened with a one-way, silicone-rubber stopper.[18] The stopper prevents opening of the loop once it has been closed. The fully assembled mechanism, with an accompanying over-sheath (to permit the soft nylon loop to pass through the instrument channel), is the same caliber as a snare. Once extruded from the end of the delivery system, the loop is maneuvered around the head of a polyp under direct vision. The tightened lasso is a self-retaining ligature; once deployed, the loop is separated from the insertion tube.[20] The loop is most often utilized for large polyps with a thick pedicle. When attempting to encircle large polyps, the floppy nylon loop – not having the same tensile strength of a wire snare – may become caught in the bumpy nodularity of the polyp head, resulting in the inability to pass the loop completely over the polyp. If the loop becomes inadvertently enmeshed in the interstices of the polyp head, closure of the loop will result in tangential placement interfering with snare positioning. If the head is encircled successfully, it is necessary that the loop be placed on the pedicle far enough toward the colon wall to allow transection of the stalk above the loop with sufficient margin to ensure safety if the polyp contains invasive cancer. After placement close to the bowel wall, polypectomy is performed above the loop-ligature (Fig. 12.1). Transection of the pedicle close to the loop may cause the loop to slip off with immediate bleeding as a

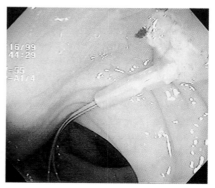

Fig. 12.1 This detachable snare was placed on a pedunculated polyp prior to transection. The plastic one-way stopper is in the foreground.

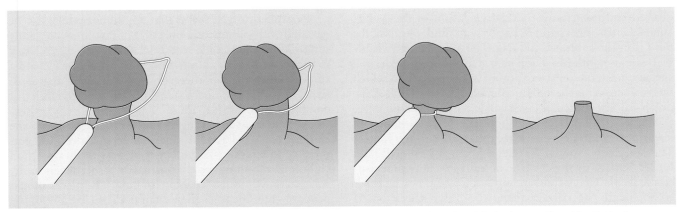

Fig. 12.7 Snare removal of pedunculated polyp. The tip of the sheath should be advanced to the point of desired transection. After tightening snare, retraction of the slide bar and heat application result in a clean polypectomy site.

The polyp with a wide attachment to the colon wall may be transected with one application of the wire snare, providing that it is located in the left colon and the base is less than 1.5 cm in diameter. In the right colon, where the wall is somewhat thinner, the endoscopist should consider piecemeal polypectomy or submucosal injection technique for any polyp whose base is over 1 cm. The heat produced by snare activation is localized to the area immediately around the wire loop, but also spreads toward the submucosa and serosa of the colon wall. The larger the polyp, the greater will be the volume of tissue captured within the wire loop, and a greater amount of thermal energy will be required to sever the polyp. This may result in a full thickness burn of colon wall, which can result in a perforation of the bowel. It is again noted that, once the polyp and mucosa have been captured in the loop, the submucosal layers and muscularis propria are in total about 1 mm thick.[11]

The submucosal injection technique can be used for removal of sessile adenomas, whether small or large.[45–47] Injection of fluid into the submucosa beneath the polyp will increase the distance between the base of the polyp and the serosa (Fig. 12.8). When current is then applied via a polypectomy snare, the lesion can be more safely removed because of a large submucosal 'cushion' of fluid which lessens the likelihood of thermal injury to the serosal surface. The fluid, injected through a long and stiff sclerotherapy needle, may be saline (normal or hypertonic),[48] with or without methylene blue to enhance visualization and with or without epinephrine.[49] Most endoscopists use normal saline only. Hypertonic solutions and epinephrine are used to retain the fluid at the site for a longer period, but saline blebs last for 10 to 15 minutes, which is sufficient time for removal of most polyps. There is a theoretical advantage to the injection of dilute epinephrine to prevent bleeding at the time of polypectomy or to prevent delayed bleeding. However, the incidence of immediate bleeding is low (1 out of 100 procedures),[21] and the long-term effect is nil because the action of epinephrine is measured in hours, not days.

The needle may be placed into the submucosa just at the edge of a polyp, or if the polyp is large and flat, multi-

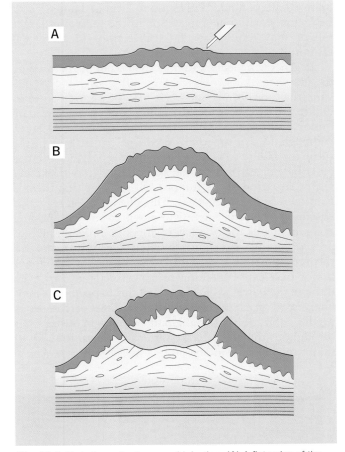

Fig. 12.8 Technique of submucosal injection. (**A**) A flat polyp of the colon. (**B**) Polyp lifted by injection of 2–10 mL of saline into the submucosa. (**C**) Polyp and portion of adjacent mucosa resected with snare.

ple injections may be given around the polyp or directly into the middle of the polyp. If a bleb does not form at the injection site when 1 mL of fluid has been given, the needle should be withdrawn since the tip may have penetrated the wall and pierced the serosal surface. When the needle is in the right plane, continuous injection of saline will result in a bleb. A large localized fluid collection is the desired endpoint, with marked elevation of the polyp. When the tissues expand in response to fluid injection, the fluid is in the submucosal layer. The absence of a visible bleb does not indicate that a bleb is forming on the serosal surface, since the only location of areolar tissue in which fluid can collect is the submucosa. Neither the mucosa, the polyp, nor the muscular layer will expand with fluid injection. If the needle placement is too superficial, the fluid will leak out from the beveled edge and spill into the lumen. This spilling is especially noticeable when a colored fluid is used, such as methylene blue or India ink. Several repeated needle placements and attempts at injector may be needed to locate the correct plane for polyp elevation. If possible, the approach by the needle injector should be tangential to the mucosal surface instead of perpendicular. The desired elevation of the polyp may take 3–4 mL of saline given in several places, although some authors use up to 30 mL of fluid.[50] Polyps up to 2 cm in diameter may be removed with one application of the snare, but larger polyps may require several transections in piecemeal fashion.[51]

In general, malignant tumors should not be removed by the submucosal injection technique. If a polyp fails to elevate (the 'non-lifting sign'),[52] it may be an indication of infiltration by cancer into the submucosa, with fixation by tumor limiting the expansion of the submucosal layer. Although deep or superficial needle placement may be the cause for failure to raise a bleb under a polyp, a submucosal bulging or bleb on one side of a polyp without any visible elevation of the tumor itself is a clue that there is fixation into the submucosa. This phenomenon may also be caused by a prior attempt at polypectomy with healing and scarring of the two layers, mucosa and submucosa, preventing their separation by fluid injection. There is a theoretic possibility that injection through a malignant tumor may cause tracking of cancer cells into or even through the bowel wall. The risk of this happening is minimal, based on experience gained from direct percutaneous needle aspiration of malignant tumors in other sites throughout the body. In the latter instances, the risk of tumor tracking is 1 in 10 000 to 1 in 20 000 cases.[53]

Parenthetically, it seems that any tumor which can be elevated with submucosal injection of fluid may be totally removed by endoscopic resection, even if invasive cancer is found on tissue examination. The ability to elevate a tumor indicates that there is only a limited degree of fixation to the submucosal layer, with the possibility of complete removal (Fig. 12.9).

Aspiration of air during attempted snare capture of the elevated polyp will result in an easier encirclement. It is permissible to remove a much larger piece with this injection technique than one would ordinarily resect when in the right colon without a 'cushion' of fluid. The pieces should probably not be larger than 2 cm in diameter.[50] With the fluid as protection against deep thermal tissue injury, it is even possible to fulgurate the base of the polyp resection site. The devices used for fulguration include a hot biopsy forceps, the tip of the snare, the argon plasma coagulator, or any other thermal device which delivers heat to the residual polyp site.

When attempting submucosal injection polypectomy, there is not a specific volume of fluid which is used, but rather, the desired endpoint is a large submucosal swelling beneath the polyp and adjacent portions of the mucosa. When part of the polyp is hidden from view behind a fold or wrapped around a fold in clamshell fashion, injection of the part nearest to the colonoscope may elevate that portion, but result in the inability to see the rest of the polyp because the mound of saline will block vision. This can be prevented. When the proximal edge of the polyp is hidden, an attempt should be made to pass the scope beyond the far edge of the polyp. While deflecting the tip toward the polyp, the injection should be made into the normal mucosa just at or near the edge of the polyp. Depending on the polyp size, several injections may be required to elevate the polyp so that snare placement is more readily accomplished. After the back portion of the polyp has been removed, then saline may be injected into the area closest to the scope to assist in completing the polypectomy.

During the technique of sessile piecemeal polypectomy with or without saline injection, an attempt should be made to place one edge of the wire snare at the edge of the

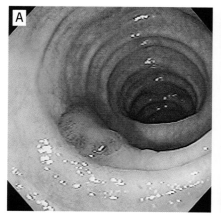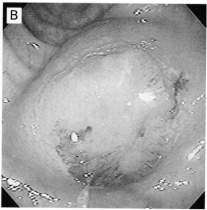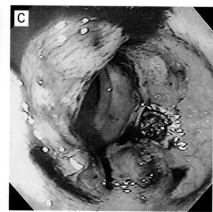

Fig. 12.9 (A) A flat polyp in the descending colon with a slight central umbilication which raises the suspicion of malignancy. (B) Following saline injection. (C) Following polypectomy and India ink injection for subsequent localization.

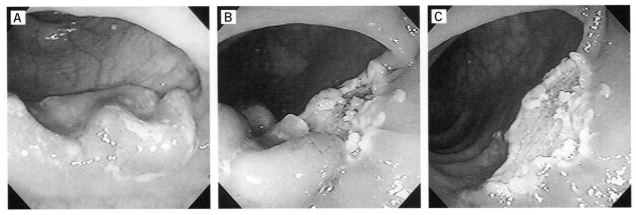

Fig. 12.10 (**A**) A flat irregular polyp. (**B**) Piecemeal resection of a portion of the polyp. The remaining polyp is to the left. (**C**) Total colonoscopic removal following submucosal saline injection.

adenoma or the junction between adenoma and normal mucosal wall.[7] The other wire of the loop can then be sited over a portion of the polyp to encircle a large piece of tissue (Fig. 12.10). Aspiration of air at this point will result in a decrease in the air-induced wall tension, resulting in a contracted segment of the wall. As the diameter decreases, the polyp becomes thicker and more pronounced, making it easier to ensnare. As the snare is closed slowly, the endoscopist's attention should be directed toward the tip of the loop as it slides over the mucosal surface behind the polyp. By so doing, it is often possible to see whether a portion of normal mucosa is caught and dragged up into the loop along with the polyp, or whether the tip slides over the mucosa and engages on the far margin of the polyp. This assessment is important, but in some instances of piecemeal polypectomy, the polyp itself may obscure direct vision.

When complete visualization is not possible as the loop is being closed, the assistant should close until resistance is met, or, if no closure sensation, then stop at the line. Once closed, the catheter sheath should be jiggled to and fro at the biopsy port while observing the colon walls around the polyp. If extraneous portions of the mucosa are not caught, the polyp will be seen to move independently of the surrounding colon walls as the sheath is jiggled. If the polyp and the surrounding wall move simultaneously, there is a strong probability that a portion of adjacent mucosa has been captured within the snare loop. Complete removal of the snare or partially opening the loop for repositioning is then advisable before application of electrocautery current. Transection of a large fragment of inadvertently captured normal mucosa is not a desirable outcome of polypectomy and may lead to perforation. If extra tissue is captured, there is no assurance that it will only consist of mucosa, for submucosa may also be entrapped, and when electrocautery current is applied, a deep burn may result.

After the wire is seated securely around the polyp, the sheath should be lifted slightly away from the wall, tenting it toward the lumen to separate the polyp from the submucosa.[54] This will limit the depth of thermal injury when current is applied because the local zone of heating has a lessened chance of damaging the muscularis propria and

serosa because the layers are pulled away from each other. Tenting of the polyp can be accomplished by a variety of movements with the success of any one being judged by its result; often a combination of efforts will be necessary: pushing the snare in or withdrawal, elevation with the thumb on the up/down dial, or torque.

When removing a sessile polyp, the characteristic whitening at the site of wire placement as electrocautery current is applied often cannot be observed because the wire is embedded in the polyp. After a few seconds of current, the wire snare should be slowly closed until separation occurs. During piecemeal polypectomy, the next placement of the snare may be immediately adjacent to the first, with the edge of the wire positioned into the denuded area just created by removal of the previous piece (Fig. 12.11). In this fashion, multiple portions can be sequentially resected in an orderly fashion, with removal of each succeeding piece being facilitated by its predecessor. Several applications may be required, removing fragments until satisfactory polypectomy is achieved.[55,56] After removing a sessile polyp in piecemeal fashion, the base may be somewhat irregular as a result of several individual passes of the snare. If only ragged fragments of tissue are seen at the base, a repeat examination after 4 to 12 weeks may reveal that the polyp has completely disappeared, since thermal energy delivered during polypectomy may slough the remnants. If visible adenoma is present, fulguration may be accomplished by using a variety of thermal devices, including the argon plasma coagulator, a BICAP, heater probe, current applied to the barely extended snare wire, or a hot biopsy forceps (Fig. 12.12).[57] In spite of all attempts to totally remove large sessile polyps (over 3 cm in diameter) when the polyp appears to have been completely removed with the snare, there is a 50% probability that there will be residual or recurrent adenoma at the site of original resection on the follow-up examination. If total polypectomy has not been achieved and there is visible residual adenoma left at the polypectomy site, there is no possibility of subsequent total involution and therefore residual polyp will be present on the follow-up examination. However, if visible residual adenoma is immediately

221

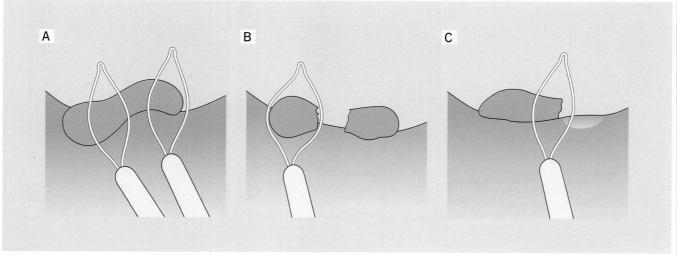

Fig. 12.11 Piecemeal resection. (A) Place the snare on any portion of the polyp and remove a piece, or position one wire at the edge of adenoma and capture polyp with other limb of wire loop. (B) Encircle isolated pieces, or (C) place one edge of loop in prior divot and proceed as in (A).

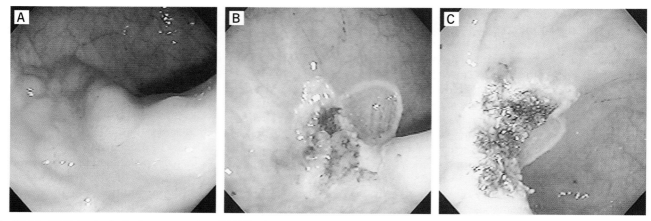

Fig. 12.12 (A) Flat polyp in the transverse colon. (B) Following partial piecemeal resection. Residual polyp is at the base, and represents the depressed portion of polyp initially seen. (C) The polyp following argon plasma coagulation to destroy residual polyp.

treated with the argon plasma coagulator, the risk of residual adenoma falls to the 50% mark.[58] Most of these recurrences can be subsequently endoscopically resected at the follow-up examination.

Problems during polypectomy

To capture a polyp, one of the most important factors is that it is in the proper position relative to the tip of the colonoscope. One of the most frustrating problems encountered during polypectomy is that the polyp is in a poor position. A polyp at the 5 o'clock position in the visual field is readily snared, since, in colonoscopes, the snare enters the field at this orientation. A polyp located between 9 and 12 o'clock in the visual field is much more difficult to lasso than a polyp in the right lower quadrant, and those in the 3 or 8 o'clock position are impossible. An attempt should be made to bring all polyps into the 5 o'clock position to facilitate snare placement.[7] This can usually be accomplished by rotation of the scope to reposition the face of the scope in relation to the adenoma.

Rotation of the scope may be difficult during intubation when the instrument shaft has loops and bends. Advantageous positioning may be best accomplished when the colonoscope shaft is straight, because a straight instrument transmits torque to the tip, whereas a loop in the shaft tends to absorb rotational motions applied to the scope. It is often difficult to capture a sigmoid polyp during intubation, when the obligatory sigmoid loop is present. It may not be possible to straighten the scope in the sigmoid because rotation and loop withdrawal result in losing the scope's position. With a loop in the scope, the dial controls may no longer work effectively to turn the instrument tip because the cables which transmit motion are maximally stretched by the loop. These two negative forces, the inability to torque effectively and the loss of cable-controlled tip deflection, combine to create an extremely difficult situation when attempting to maneuver the snare into position around a polyp. Maneuvering can be made considerably easier by passing the scope far beyond the polyp, even to the cecum (and thus visualize the rest of the colon) and attempting capture during the withdrawal phase of the examination. As the scope is withdrawn, the loops are removed and the polyp which proved difficult to position during intubation may be quite easily ensnared because both torque and tip deflection are responsive when the shaft is straight.

Small polyps (less than 5 mm) that are visualized during intubation should be removed at that time,[7] regardless of their position since it may be difficult to find them again upon withdrawal of the instrument. If a medium-sized pedunculated polyp (up to 2.0 cm) is encountered during intubation, is in excellent position, and looks like it will be easy and straightforward to lasso, it is wise to perform polypectomy at that time since it may not be in such good position on withdrawal. Small polyps that are transected during intubation should be collected in a polyp trap. The best trap is a multicompartmented trap available from Endodynamics. Polyps over 1 cm in diameter which are transected during intubation will be easily seen on endoscope withdrawal so there is no need to retrieve the polyp at the time of resection, since its retrieval will often necessitate removal of the instrument. There is no risk involved in passing the instrument beyond a fresh polypectomy site and performing total intubation of the colon.

In general, sessile polyps requiring piecemeal resection or pedunculated polyps larger than 1 cm in diameter that are not in good position should not be removed during the insertion phase since there may be a larger, more significant lesion proximally which would impact on the decision for polypectomy. It is possible to spend a considerable amount of time and effort to remove a large hepatic flexure polyp and then find an undetected carcinoma in the cecum which would require a surgical resection including the polypectomy site.

As noted previously, it is usually easier to properly position polyps for removal following total colonoscopy to the cecum. As the instrument straightens out by virtue of pulling the shaft out of the colon, clockwise or counterclockwise torque combined with dial control manipulation can result in unimpeded rotation of the colonoscope tip so that a polyp encountered at the 10 o'clock position (which

may be difficult to ensnare) can be moved to the 5 o'clock position even if it is located in the ascending colon. An additional consideration to shift a polyp into a more favorable position is to change the patient's position or apply abdominal pressure. Polyps partially hidden behind folds may come more prominently into view as the patient's position is altered. Polyps submerged in a pool of fluid can be rotated into a drier field by turning the patient so that fluid flows away from the base.

Rotatable snares are considered unnecessary by most endoscopists. With the wire loop extended, the combination of torque on the shaft and rotation of the dial controls affords much the same effect as snare wire rotation.

Some polyps may be extremely difficult to remove whether they are large or small. There is no substitute for skill and experience in colonoscopy when dealing with a difficult polyp since excellent control of the instrument will make polyps considered inaccessible readily removed by those with special training. All of the tricks of instrument handling will be helpful in trying to render a polyp more accessible when difficulty is encountered. Sometimes even a small polyp can be 'difficult', such as when located deep between two haustral folds or in an area distorted by diverticula, where the lumen is narrow and tip manipulation is almost non-existent.

The standard, regular-sized polypectomy snare may not be able to capture a small polyp in a difficult and 'tight' location where there is not a sufficient distance for the wire loop to open sufficiently wide to be placed over a polyp. A problem with the standard snare is that it must be completely extended to its full length of 6 cm in order for the loop to completely expand. During colonoscopy, it often occurs that the wire loop can only be extended a few centimeters beyond the scope because of a tight bend or because the tip of the loop impacts on an adjacent wall of the colon. When the snare loop cannot be fully extended, the two partially open parallel wires may not sufficiently spread apart to enable polyp capture. In this circumstance, a 'mini' snare 3 cm in length and 1.0 cm in width[7,59] is extremely valuable (Fig. 12.13). This snare will open fully when extended only 3 cm beyond the

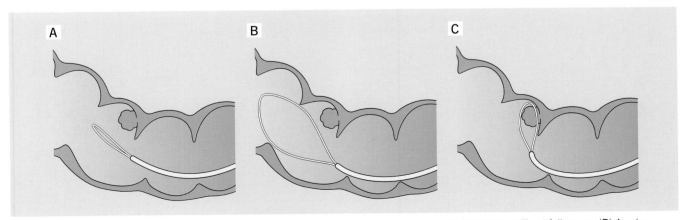

Fig. 12.13 Use of the minisnare. (A) When extended only a few centimeters beyond the sheath, the large snare will not fully open. (B) A polyp located in an area with multiple convolutions, or deeply placed between two haustral folds, may be difficult to capture with the large loop. (C) The minisnare is often useful for these situations because the loop opens fully when extended 3 cm beyond the sheath.

sheath making it useful in areas where multiple bends are present (such as in the sigmoid narrowed with diverticulosis), or when polyps are located in the depth between haustral folds. Since the vast majority of colon polyps are less than 1.0 cm in diameter, they are within the limits of this minisnare.

Even after total colonscopy has been performed and the colonoscope has been straightened, there may still be difficulty in the sigmoid colon when attempting to capture a polyp because of narrowing by diverticula and thickened hypertrophic folds. There are two maneuvers which may permit easier endoscopic polypectomy. The first is to use a minisnare, which will allow a full extension of the snare within a short segment of the bowel. The second maneuver is use of a narrow caliber scope to intubate the colon.[60,61] A pediatric colonoscope is useful, but not generally available. A standard upper intestinal gastroscope has been demonstrated to be of benefit.[62] The major attributes of the gastroscope is that it has a tighter bending radius of the tip than does a colonoscope and the tip beyond the bending portion is shorter in length. This will frequently allow easy snare positioning in the same location where the colonoscope was both cumbersome and difficult. There is a growing awareness among endoscopists that gastroscopes can easily and readily be used in the colon to intubate difficult and narrowed segments, to be passed through strictures, and to render a previously inaccessible polyp more readily manageable. The upper intestinal endoscope can be of use even in the rectum, where it may not be possible to snare a polyp on the proximal surface of one of the rectal valves. In this circumstance, the bending section of the colonoscope may be too long to permit a tight turn, whereas a gastroscope with its greater tip deflection capability and shorter 'nose' (or straight portion beyond the bending section) may permit easy visualization and removal of polyps.

Large sessile polyps wrapped around a fold in a 'clamshell' fashion usually permit the distal portion to be readily removed, but resection of the proximal portion on the far side of the fold may be considerably more difficult. This type of polyp is often located in the right colon and should be removed in piecemeal fashion. The piecemeal technique usually requires rotation of the colonoscope to place the polyp at the 5 to 6 o'clock position. Although it would be ideal to resect the total polyp at one session, it may only be possible to remove the portion nearest to the scope, leaving some of the polyp on the far side of the fold for an interval resection. Subsequent scarring may flatten the polypectomy site, bringing the residual polyp into a favorable location for subsequent polypectomy. If it is elected to attempt total polypectomy at the first session, the stiffness of the plastic snare catheter can be used as a probe. After endoscopic transection of the portion closest to the scope, and with the loop extended, the tip of the catheter can be positioned on the ridge of the fold in the polypectomy site where a portion of the polyp has just been removed. By a combination of torque and rotation of the large control knob, downward pressure on the ridge at the site of the polypectomy divot will often depress it sufficiently so that a portion of the residual adenoma will extend into the loop permitting capture under direct vision (Fig. 12.14). This maneuver is not dangerous. Several repeated snare applications and transections of this type will usually result in complete polypectomy. The tip of the instrument must be close to the polypectomy site for this technique to be effective, since the plastic polypectomy sheath becomes quite flexible when it is extended more than a few centimeters beyond the colonoscope. The sheath, with its tip barely protruded, is stiff and will depress a fold when torque or tip deflection is applied to the colonoscope shaft. Pushing on a fresh polypectomy site in this manner is not associated with any adverse results. The injection of fluid into the submucosa may assist in polypectomy attempts, and this has been previously described.

All polypectomy fragments must be retrieved and sent to the pathologist to determine whether the polyp is malignant. If the resected specimen is benign on histopathologic investigation, there is no rush to totally resect the polyp and several months may safely elapse before polypectomy completion. Even if some of the polyp is knowingly left behind, the interval between piecemeal polypectomies should range from 3 to 6 months to allow healing to take

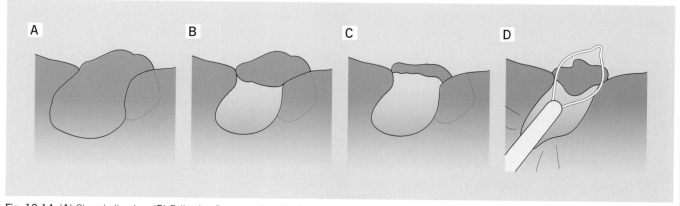

Fig. 12.14 (A) Clamshell polyp. (B) Following first resection. (C) Following second resection of top portion of polyp. (D) Position sheath within the divot, at the edge of existing polyp, and by pushing down on the sheath, the extended snare will encircle the residual polyp, rendering it easy to capture.

place. There is no medical necessity for a short interval (2 to 4 weeks) follow-up examination, and it is probably unwise to re-prep the patient and distend the colon with air shortly after the integrity of the wall has been compromised by a polypectomy.

An alternative technique for removal of a polyp located on the far side of a fold is to perform a U-turn maneuver. With standard instruments, this can only be accomplished in the cecum, ascending colon, and transverse colon. It is difficult but not impossible to resect a polyp in a U-turn mode because the tip deflection responses are opposite to those usually expected.

The size of the polyp is an obvious reason for difficulty with endoscopic resection. Most polyps are less than 1 cm in diameter, a size that should be well within the resection capability of any trained colonoscopist. Twenty percent of polyps are larger than 10 mm in diameter and only 1% greater than 35 mm in size. When polyps in the left colon grow to become larger than 1 cm in diameter, it is common for peristalsis to pull on the lesion, forming a tubular pedicle from the surrounding mucosa. A polyp of the same size in the right colon has a tendency to remain sessile, with a broad-based attachment.

If bleeding obscures vision during piecemeal polypectomy, the blood may be dispersed by squirting water through the biopsy channel. Mild bleeding may be controlled by continuation of piecemeal polypectomy where cautery of the next segment may heat seal the bleeding vessels at the previously cut edge. A BICAP, heater probe, or argon plasma coagulator may be useful to stop more severe bleeding, or a 1:10 000 solution of epinephrine can be injected into the site of bleeding to promote hemostasis. Injection therapy uses a standard, variceal sclerotherapy needle.

In spite of the knowledge and skill of modern endoscopists, not all colon polyps can be successfully removed with a colonoscope. Among these are carpet-like polyps which extend over several centimeters. An attempt can be made to fulgurate the surface of such polyps with the shank of the monopolar biopsy forceps, a BICAP probe, laser photocoagulation, or the argon plasma coagulator. A helpful maneuver to be considered when the lesion appears too flat to capture with the snare loop is to aspirate air from the colon with the snare device in place. This will collapse the distended colon, causing the colon wall and the polyp to fold up, rendering capture relatively easy so that piecemeal type resection is possible. Alternative possibilities include submucosal injection of fluid to elevate the polyp for safer transection and use of a two-channel colonoscope where a forceps can be passed through one channel to grasp the polyp over which the opened snare has been positioned. Once the forceps lifts up the polyp, the snare is tightened to capture the polyp.

If passage to the right colon has been arduous and prolonged, with the discovery of a large sessile polyp having a broad attachment that would require several attempts at piecemeal polypectomy, the wisest approach may be to suggest surgical resection to avoid the necessity for repeated difficult colonoscopies with repeated difficult polypectomies. The risk–benefit ratio will depend on the location of the polyp: the right colon is somewhat thinner than the left, increasing the risk of colonoscopic removal.

The advent of laparoscopic-assisted right hemicolectomy may markedly change the attitude of adventurous colonoscopists who attempt removal of large polyps. The ease of laparoscopic resection may make a significant difference in the willingness of the patient and endoscopist to embark on the repetitive number of colonoscopies required to ablate a right colon polyp. Both the risks and benefits of an aggressive endoscopic approach will need to be re-evaluated.

SITE LOCATION

In the era when laparoscopic-assisted surgical colonic resection is becoming as well accepted as primary colonoscopy, there is even greater urgency to have precise lesion location, since the laparoscopist does not have the capability of palpating the colon between the fingers at exploratory laparotomy.[63] For the laparoscopist, it is of great importance to have an easily visible marker which can be seen through the telescopic lens of the laparoscope. It is not acceptable for the endoscopist to state that 'a lesion is in the transverse colon', since a more specific localization is needed to avoid a subsequent open surgery to find the lesion.

Precise location of the tip position during colonoscopy is equally important when there is a need to relocate a lesion or an area of the colon at a later point in time. It may be desirable to know the precise site at which a polyp was removed in piecemeal fashion so that the area can be readily identified at the next follow-up colonoscopy, especially if the polyp were on the back-side of a fold or just around a difficult bend of the colon. Even under circumstances when open laparotomy is to be performed, site identification becomes necessary when a specific portion of the large bowel requires resection and the lesion may not be readily apparent by visual or palpatory exploration. Following endoscopic removal of a malignant adenoma, the site may heal completely in 8 weeks, and a locator mark may assist both the surgeon and the pathologist in identifying the place where the lesion had been.

Localization by measurement of centimeters of instrument introduced into the rectum is an extremely poor method for tip localization.[64] During introduction of the instrument, when loops are common, it is possible to advance the full length of a long colonoscope (180 cm) into the rectum, yet the tip may still be at the sigmoid/descending colon junction.[65] On the other hand, it is possible, by repositioning the instrument, removal of loops, and straightening, to reach the cecum in that same patient with a total length of only 60 cm of instrument. The actual number of centimeters inserted may bear no relationship with the actual tip location within the colon.[66]

Landmarks are notoriously imprecise for exact localization of areas between the rectum and cecum. Even the most experienced colonoscopists may err in their estimate of tip location.[63,65,67] Indeed, in a large tortuous sigmoid colon, it may be difficult to localize a lesion to even the mid- or upper sigmoid colon. Similarly, a lesion estimated by the endoscopist to be near the splenic flexure may be under the diaphragm, could be either proximal or distal to the flexure, or may even be actually located at the sigmoid descending colon junction. Precise location may be impossible because of tortuosity and multiple bends in that area of the colon. The only invariable localizing landmarks are when a lesion is located within 15 cm of the anus, there is no doubt that it is close to or in the rectum, and a lesion near the endoscopically identified ileocecal valve can be easily found by the surgeon. The problem in the last case revolves about the endoscopist's ability to recognize beyond a doubt that the cecum was indeed reached.

Clips may be placed through the colonoscope and onto the mucosa at any location. These will assist in radiographic or ultrasonographic location of the marked segment. However, clips tend to fall off at an average of approximately 10 days,[68] with some falling off earlier and some maintaining their attachment for longer intervals. Although it has been suggested that clips may be a helpful marker for surgical localization, it has been found that the clip devices are quite small to be palpated easily. In addition, the surgeon cannot be assured that a palpable clip had not been spontaneously detached just prior to surgery and is at some distance from the original placement during endoscopy. If, indeed, a surgeon palpates a clip in the sigmoid colon and resects that segment, it is possible that the clip actually had been placed at a location near the splenic flexure, had become detached, and migrated distally. A recent report of eight patients with pre-laparoscopic clip placement by colonoscopy stated that intra-operative ultrasound readily located the marked areas for surgical resection.[69]

The barium enema is still an acceptable method for determining the location of polyps or cancers,[66] but small lesions may not be readily identified on the barium enema X-ray examination. Certainly, if a malignant polyp were endoscopically resected, it may be extremely difficult to then try to locate the area where the polyp was removed, since only a small puckering may be present,[66,70] or the site may be almost completely healed within 3 weeks.

New methods of inductive sensing with a low-intensity magnetic field may aid in the moment-to-moment localization of the tip of the fiberoptic colonoscope as it progresses through the colon. The magnetic forces are attracted to sensors within the sheath of the colonoscope (or to sensors on a wand-like device inserted into the biopsy channel). Two different techniques have been developed in the UK, and will soon be ready for clinical trials.[71,72] These methods have replaced such devices as metal detectors for localization of the instrument tip.[73] Unlike a fluoroscopic image which demonstrates both the scope and air in the colon as a contrast media, the electromagnetic field method only shows the colonoscope itself, but is capable of a three-dimensional format. This technique may be of benefit in localizing the site of a colonic tumor or polyp, and is undergoing clinical trials for this purpose.

During colonoscopy in a suite where radiographic imaging is possible, either fluoroscopy or an X-ray of the abdomen during endoscopy may assist in locating the site of a lesion. Unfortunately, it may be difficult, with the instrument in a straightened configuration, to state that the tip of the colonoscope is in the distal descending colon or in the mid-portion of a long redundant sigmoid loop.

It is possible to localize the site of a tumor, or a resected polypectomy site, by performing intra-operative colonoscopy.[74–76] This technique has been avoided by most endoscopists because of the need to perform an endoscopic examination in the operating room with all the constraints of positioning the patient, handling the scope, and trying to use maneuvers such as torque and straightening techniques with the abdomen open. The amount of air insufflated for colonoscopy can create problems with surgical techniques once the endoscopist has completed the necessary localization. Because the site of a polypectomy may heal within a few weeks, there is a possibility that a polypectomy site may not be seen during an intra-operative endoscopy.

The ideal method for lesion localization is to have an easily identifiable marker which will immediately draw the attention of the surgeon or endoscopist.[67] This can be achieved with injection of dye solutions. An experimental study demonstrated that, of eight different dyes injected into the colon wall in experimental animals, only two persisted for more than 24 hours.[77] These were indocyanine green and India ink. The indocyanine green was visible up to 7 days after injection, and it is known that India ink is a permanent marker which lasts for the life of the patient by virtue of submucosal injection of carbon particles. Other dyes, such as methylene blue, indigocarmine, toluidine blue, lymphazurine, hematoxylin, and eosin, all were absorbed within 24 hours, leaving no residual stain at the injection site. Indocyanine green is approved by the FDA for human use, but India ink has not been so approved. Indocyanine green is not associated with any significant tissue reaction, and is relatively non-toxic.[77] It provides excellent staining of the serosal surface and draining lymphatics for up to 7 days following its injection.

Clinical experience with indocyanine green tattoo in 12 patients demonstrated that the dye was easily visualized on the serosal surface of the colon at surgery within 36 hours following injection.[78] The problem with a marker having such a relatively short time span is that the decision to operate after removal of a malignant polyp may require a few weeks, with slide reviews and multiple consultations. An injection at the time of polypectomy will have disappeared whereas the site will become more difficult to localize with the passage of time.

Most experience with dye injection technique has been accumulated with India ink as a permanent marker.[79,80] The stain lasts for at least 10 years with no diminution in intensity at that duration. A permanent marker may be worthwhile for several reasons. A lesion requiring surgery may be injected and, for clinical reasons, surgery may be postponed for several weeks at which time a vital dye such as indocyanine green will have been absorbed, leaving the operating surgeon with no visible evidence of its having been injected. Sometimes it is desirable to mark the site of a resected polyp for subsequent endoscopic localization when it is anticipated that the area will be difficult to find on a follow-up examination, especially when the lesion is located around a fold or behind a haustral septum. A stain with a permanent marker such as India ink will draw immediate attention to the site, enabling a more accurate and complete assessment. For the surgeon, a locator stain will aid immeasurably the efforts to seek and resect an area of the bowel containing the site of the lesion. When the lesion is relatively small, such as a flat cancer or a previously endoscopically resected malignant polyp which requires surgical resection, the site may not be evident from the serosal surface and may not even be palpable. If the area to be resected is in a redundant sigmoid colon or near the splenic flexure, it may be impossible to locate by either visual means or by palpation. Occasionally, even large lesions may not be palpable by the surgeon if they are soft and compressible.[75] As previously mentioned, visible marking can assist in precise surgical intervention for laparoscopic-assisted colon resections, or clips may be detected by an ultrasound probe.

There have been reported complications with India ink injection, but these are relatively rare.[81,82] The complications may in part be related to the wide variety of organic and inorganic compounds contained in the ink solution, such as carriers, stabilizers, binders, and fungicides.[83] It is possible that the toxic properties of India ink may be partially ameliorated by marked dilution of the ink. Ink diluted to 1:100 with saline produces as dark a spectrophotometric pattern as undiluted India ink, and in clinical tests, the tattoo made by 1:100 diluted India ink is readily visible by the endoscopist and by the operating surgeon. A small volume injection may increase the safety of the procedure.[84,85]

India ink is black drawing ink made with carbon particles. Permanent fountain pen ink is not an acceptable substitute. India ink is available from any stationery store, although it is supplied for medical use in non-sterile form as a stain to enhance the diagnosis of cryptococcosis in the cerebrospinal fluid. The India ink may be sterilized in an autoclave following dilution or can be rendered bacteriologically sterile by passing the diluted solution through a 0.22 μm Millipore filter which is interposed between the syringe containing the dilute solution of India ink and the injection needle.[86]

A standard sclerotherapy needle is utilized of sufficient length to traverse the accessory channel of a 168 cm colonoscope, and stiff enough so that the plastic sheath will not crinkle up as it is being forced through the biopsy port when the tip of the instrument is deep in the colon and the colonoscope shaft has several convolutions and loops. Ideally, the needle should enter the mucosa at an angle to permit injections into the submucosa, rather than to have the needle pierce the bowel wall. The edges of haustral folds should be targeted. If during an injection a submucosal bleb is not immediately seen, the needle should be pulled back slightly, since the needle tip may have penetrated the full thickness of the wall and the ink may be squirting into the peritoneal cavity. An intracavity injection is not a clinical problem,[70,78] but can scatter black carbon particles around the abdominal cavity, which may be somewhat disconcerting for the surgeon.

Since the colonoscopist cannot know which portion of the bowel is the superior aspect, multiple injections should be made circumferentially in the wall around a lesion to prevent a single injection site from being located in a 'sanctuary' site, hidden from the eyes of the surgeon as the abdomen is opened with the patient lying supine (Fig. 12.9C).[87] Each injection should be of sufficient volume to raise a bluish bleb within the mucosa at the injection site. The injection volume may vary from 0.1–0.5 mL. If injections are made a few centimeters from the lesion, the surgeon should be informed whether the injections are proximal or distal to the site. With the 1:100 dilution of India ink, endoscopic visualization is still possible should some of the ink spill into the lumen, whereas, with the more concentrated solutions, the endoscopic picture becomes totally black when ink covers the bowel walls.[70]

Most endoscopists who use India ink to mark colonic lesions do not prescribe antibiotics prior to its use, although it has been suggested that prophylactic antibiotics be given before injections of indocyanine green.[78]

The India ink is indeed a permanent marker, with endoscopic visualization of the tattoo site being possible in every case on follow-up examination without diminution in color up to an interval of 10 years following initial injection. Several reports have attested as to its safety as well as its efficacy.[81,88,89]

CAUSES OF BLEEDING AND THEIR MANAGEMENT

The major complications which occur with therapeutic endoscopy are perforation of the bowel, bleeding, and post-polypectomy syndrome. The combined incidence of significant hemorrhage and perforation in therapeutic colonoscopy is approximately 1.7%.[90,91] Perforation occurs in 0.04 to 2.1% of colonoscopic polypectomies, and is due to mechanically slicing across the wall with the wire snare, or causing thermal necrosis of the wall that perforates within hours post-polypectomy.[92]

Perforation

The presence of free air post-colonoscopy does not, in and of itself, mandate a surgical exploration if the clinical presentation is completely benign.[93,94] The literature states that the patient with neither signs nor symptoms of perforation post-endoscopy with only intraperitoneal or retroperitoneal air as the single sign of perforation should be treated with antibiotics, nothing by mouth, and watched carefully.[95] It is possible that a small leak may spontaneously seal and not require operative intervention.

'Benign pneumoperitoneum' post-colonoscopy has been described, where it is thought that air may 'leak' through a diverticulum. This was discovered on 1/100 consecutive post-colonoscopy flat abdominal and X-ray films. The patient was completely asymptomatic, treated conservatively, and the pneumoperitoneum resolved. The amount of free air on X-ray or CT scan may bear little relationship to the clinical picture.

On the other hand, if the endoscopist is sure that a perforation has occurred by virtue of seeing the peritoneal cavity or the serosal side of other organs, then immediate exploration is necessary. There is no justification in waiting until symptoms develop, since they surely will with a large through-and-through perforation. Whenever there is visible evidence of fat protruding through a hole in the colon, this also is evidence of a free perforation and mandates surgical exploration.

In between the two extremes of the asymptomatic person and the obvious large hole in the wall, there is a subset of patients who have a high probability of perforation, who may or may not have free air, but have localized peritonitis, without any signs of generalized peritonitis. These patients may have localized and rebound tenderness, leukocytosis and a low-grade fever. Often treatment with intravenous fluids, nothing by mouth, and antibiotics will permit the symptoms of acute inflammation to resolve.[96,97] If watchful waiting is the choice, then the patient must be closely monitored in the hospital setting by the gastroenterologist and a surgeon. If the situation deteriorates, and it is deemed that the signs or symptoms of inflammation are spreading, then surgery should be performed. Under these circumstances, a water-soluble contrast enema may be worthwhile in an attempt to localize the site of perforation. Such an enema may be especially valuable in patients who have had multiple polyps removed, and there is some doubt as to the site of perforation.

Laparoscopic treatment of iatrogenic colon perforations has been successfully accomplished,[98] and may be a useful first-line surgical approach to this problem. A small perforation at polypectomy, if recognized immediately, may respond to transcolonoscopic clip application with closure of the hole.[99]

Post-polypectomy coagulation syndrome – serositis/transmural burn/post-polypectomy syndrome

This syndrome is known by several names, and is the result of a transmural burn causing irritation of the serosa with localized inflammatory response. This reaction to electrocautery current causes symptoms similar to any other intra-abdominal localized inflammatory response,[100] such as appendicitis or diverticulitis. The difference is that an illness like appendicitis is a response to an infectious process causing inflammation, whereas a transmural burn is a result of thermal injury to the colon wall. The post-polypectomy inflammatory response may result in localized pain, tenderness, guarding, and rigidity. There may or may not be fever, tachycardia, and leukocytosis. This syndrome occurs in 1% of colonoscopic polypectomies[21] and symptoms begin 6 hours to 5 days post-polypectomy (average 2.3 days). As with all other syndromes in medicine, there are several gradations of severity, with some patients having spontaneous discomfort with deep tenderness on palpation, while others may have a full-blown inflammatory response with fever. Most patients with this syndrome have a mild ache or tenderness in the area overlying the polypectomy site. About 20% of patients will have more severe symptoms such as guarding, rigidity, and fever, and should be treated with intravenous fluids and close observation in the hospital. All symptoms usually resolve in 2 to 5 days. The major differential diagnosis of the post-polypectomy coagulation syndrome involves perforation of the bowel.[94] Surgeons frequently consider this symptom complex as a 'mini-perforation', although the major distinguishing characteristic between a free perforation and the post-polypectomy coagulation syndrome is that the latter does not reveal radiographic evidence of free air in the peritoneal cavity. Whenever the endoscopist is concerned about the integrity of the colon wall, an X-ray should be taken. Should free air be seen under the diaphragm, the diagnosis is a perforation, and treatment decisions should be made in conjunction with a surgical consultation.

The worst outcome in this syndrome is a through-and-through burn of the wall with rapidly developing necrosis and free perforation. The patient may have early evidence of localized peritonitis which becomes increasingly severe, and, when the necrotic wall perforates, air and bowel contents enter the abdominal cavity. There is no question that surgery is necessary at that time and should be performed urgently. In a recent prospective series of 777 polypectomies, this occurred in two patients (0.3%) from 1 to 9 days post-polypectomy.[21]

Post-polypectomy hemorrhage

This is the most common post-polypectomy complication.[101] In a series of colonoscopic resection of large sessile polyps, 2.3% required blood transfusions.[102] Severity of bleeding ranges from arterial pumping post-polypectomy to a slight ooze. Whatever is the severity of bleeding, an attempt should be made at that time to ensure hemostasis. Approximately 1.5% of patients will have bleeding immediately after the polyp is resected and should be controlled at that time.

Immediate bleeding

Most bleeding which occurs immediately upon resection can be controlled by the endoscopist.[21] This may require several modalities performed in sequential fashion. If a pedunculated polyp bleeds following transection, bleeding can be stopped by regrasping the pedicle with a snare and holding pressure on the pedicle to stop blood flow, initiating the hemostatic clotting cascade. Retransection of the pedicle can be performed, but is not the preferred approach since there may be too little of the pedicle remaining to regrasp if rebleeding ensues. Most often, holding a snare around a bleeding pedicle tightly for 5 minutes will result in hemostasis. If bleeding occurs upon loosening the snare after 5 minutes, a second 5 minute pressure application will always result in cessation of bleeding. A detachable loop may be useful, since it can often be applied after transection.

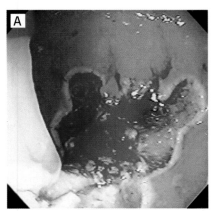

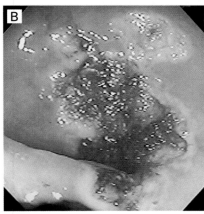

Fig. 12.15 (A) Bleeding from a sessile polypectomy site. (B) Following argon plasma coagulation with complete cessation of bleeding.

Bleeding following a sessile polypectomy may require several modalities for control, but a flexible injector needle is the single most useful tool. Bleeding can often be controlled by injection of a 1:10 000 solution of epinephrine. Several milliliters may be required to stop bleeding. The desired effect is a large bleb at the bleeding site. Multiple injections may be made around the bleeding site. The heater probe, BICAP electrode or argon plasma coagulator are helpful adjuncts to the hemostatic armamentarium (Fig. 12.15). The hot biopsy forceps may be used as a cautery probe by direct application of monopolar current. Repeated light touching with the activated hot biopsy forceps to the tissue results in better fulguration than continuous pressure, since the latter may cause heating of tissue without hemostasis, whereas creating a spark-gap results in a better coagulum.

Delayed bleeding

Delayed bleeding occurs in approximately 2% of patients who have polyps removed.[21] If the patient comes into the hospital and is actively bleeding as assessed by frequent bloody bowel movements, colonoscopy should be performed immediately.[101] Blood is a good cathartic, and usually cleans residual stool out of the colon. Even if the lesion is on the right side, patients can usually be endoscoped with adequate visualization of the site enabling treatment to be delivered. If, however, the frequency of bowel motions seems to be decreasing, this is the best clinical sign that bleeding has slowed or stopped, and emergency colonoscopy need not be carried out. If, during observation, the patient begins to bleed again, urgent endoscopic examination should be performed. An electrolyte preparation may provide an easier colonoscopy,[103] but is not an absolute necessity for ongoing bleeding. A report of intra-operative colonoscopy for localization of acute severe lower gastrointestinal tract bleeding has demonstrated the effectiveness of intra-operative on-table irrigation via a catheter placed in the cecum.[104] Angiography may be of benefit in the presence of severe bleeding, with infusion of pitressin causing hemostasis.[105]

A band ligation device can be attached to the tip of a colonoscope to create hemostasis.[106,107] The ligator is a modification of the standard apparatus used to band esophageal varices.

Delayed post-polypectomy hemorrhage occurs on an average of 1 week after the procedure, but can be seen from a few hours to 12 days later.[21]

The hot biopsy forceps

This modality must be used in a specific fashion to decrease the incidence of complications.[108] Under no circumstances should the hot biopsy forceps be pushed toward the colon wall when current is applied, since this will tend to push away the areolar tissue in the submucosa, and decrease the distance between the mucosal surface where the burn is occurring and the serosal surface. The coaption of the two layers may lead to a full thickness burn effect, and even a subsequent perforation of the wall. Hemorrhage after use of the hot biopsy forceps technique has been reported to occur on a retrospective survey in 0.41% of cases and perforation in 0.05%.[41] A recent prospective series failed to detect any excess risk for either complication with the hot biopsy forceps.[109] An alternative technique is to guillotine small polyps using a snare without electric current.[42]

OVERVIEW

Colon cancer is preceded by a benign precursor phase, which is the adenomatous polyp. There is no primary prevention for colon cancer, and colonoscopy with polypectomy is the only means for secondary prevention of colon cancer. Specifically, prevention of colon cancer is achieved through the removal of polyps before they have malignant degeneration. The vast majority of polyps throughout the colon can be removed with endoscopic techniques. Modern colonoscopes can inspect every portion of the colon, and, with training and experience, the use of multiple polypectomy techniques will result in clean and bloodless polyp removal with a minimum of complications.

The best results occur when the operator and assistant work together as a team dedicated to removal of colon polyps. It makes little difference whether the colonoscopic suite is large and modern or small and cramped. The type of colonoscope does not play a great role in safe polypectomy, nor does the type of ESU or the shape or brand of the snare wires. The critical factors are the capability of the endoscopist and the interaction between endoscopist and gastrointestinal endoscopy assistant. A good team ensures quality performance in endoscopic polypectomy endeavors.

Not all polyps can be removed by all endoscopists. It is necessary to continually assess one's operative skills and, if the proposed polypectomy has a high risk of complication, or the endoscopist is concerned that the lesion is too large or cannot be approached in a safe manner, it should not be performed. As in all medical therapeutic endeavors, the safety of the patient must be foremost at all times.

CHECKLIST OF PRACTICE POINTS

1. Most polyps can be removed by various techniques of colonoscopic polypectomy.
2. A clean colon is mandatory. Fermentable sugars are not the ideal pre-polypectomy preparation.
3. A bleeding tendency should be assessed by taking a history of any abnormal bleeding.
4. Assess the entire colon before beginning to remove a large polyp, although small polyps should be removed whenever they are encountered.
5. Prior to snaring a polyp, torque the colonoscope to place the polyp at 5 o'clock in the visual field.
6. Mark the snare handle prior to beginning polypectomy.
7. A minisnare (3×1 cm) is suitable for the vast majority of polypectomies.
8. Place the tip of the plastic sheath at the desired point of separation prior to closing the slide bar.
9. As the wire loop is being closed, observe the tip of the wire loop as it slides across the mucosa. This will ensure that excess mucosa is not captured within the closed wire loop.
10. Obtain a full view of the polyp and surrounding areas. This may require torquing the instrument, further air insufflation, abdominal pressure, or moving the patient's position.
11. Polyps with a base larger than 1.5 cm in the right colon should have a submucosal injection of fluid prior to polypectomy. This makes the polypectomy safer and easier.
12. During transection, closure of the handle should be slow and steady while the operator gives continuous power application by standing on the foot switch.
13. Post-polypectomy bleeding is rare and can be controlled with epinephrine injection, heater probe, BICAP, hot biopsy forceps, argon plasma coagulator, application of a detachable snare, or the use of clips.
14. Lesions suspicious for malignancy, flat lesions, or those in a position where re-localization may be difficult should be marked with a permanent surgical marker (India ink) to facilitate future localization either by the surgeon or at repeat interval follow-up colonoscopy.
15. Teamwork is essential during colonoscopic polypectomy.

REFERENCES

1. Winawer SJ, Zauber AG, Ho MN, et al and the National Polyp Study Workgroup. Prevention of colorectal cancer by colonoscopic polypectomy. N Engl J Med 1993; 329:1977–1981.

2. Bond JH, Levitt MD. Colonic gas explosion – Is a fire extinguisher necessary? Gastroenterology 1979; 77:1349.

3. Hsu CW, Imperiale TF. Meta-analysis and cost comparison of polyethylene glycol lavage versus sodium phosphate for colonoscopy preparation. Gastrointest Endosc 1998; 48:276–282.

4. Monahan DW, Peluso FE, Goldner F. Combustible colonic gas levels during flexible sigmoidoscopy and colonoscopy. Gastrointest Endosc 1992; 38:40–43.

5. Bigard MA, Gaucher P, Lassalle C. Fatal explosion during colonoscopic polypectomy. Gastroenterology 1979; 77:1307.

6. Stevenson GW, Wilson JA, Wilkinson J, et al. Pain following colonoscopy: elimination with carbon dioxide. Gastrointest Endosc 1992; 38:564–567.

7. Waye JD. Endoscopic treatment of adenomas. World J Surg 1991; 15:14–19.

8. American Society for Gastrointestinal Endoscopy Guidelines. Guideline on the management of anticoagulation and antiplatelet therapy for endoscopic procedures. Gastrointest Endosc 1998; 48:672–675.

9. Kadakia SC, Angueira CE, Ward JA, et al. Gastrointestinal endoscopy in patients taking antiplatelet agents and anticoagulants: survey of ASGE members. American Society for Gastrointestinal Endoscopy. Gastrointest Endosc 1996; 44:309–316.

10. Rutgeerts P, Wang TH, Llorens PS, et al. Gastrointestinal endoscopy and the patient with a risk of bleeding disorder. Gastrointest Endosc 1999; 49:134–136.

11. Tsuga K, Haruma K, Fujimura J, et al. Evaluation of the colorectal wall in normal subjects and patients with ulcerative colitis using an ultrasonic catheter probe. Gastrointest Endosc 1998; 48:477–484.

12. Valentine JF. Double-channel endoscopic polypectomy technique for the removal of large pedunculated polyps. Gastrointest Endosc 1998; 48:314–316.

13. Akahoshi K, Kojima H, Fujimarua T, et al. Grasping forceps assisted endoscopic resection of large pedunculated GI polypoid lesions. Gastrointest Endosc 1999; 50:95–98.

14. Kawamoto K, Yamada Y, Furukawa N, et al. Endoscopic submucosal tumorectomy for gastrointestinal submucosal tumors restricted to the submucosa: a new form of endoscopic minimal surgery. Gastrointest Endosc 1997; 46:311–317.

15. Waye JD. New methods of polypectomy. Gastrointest Endosc Clin North Am 1997; 7:413–422.

16. Johanns W, Luis W, Janssen J, et al. Argon plasma coagulation (APC) in gastroenterology: experimental and clinical experiences. Eur J Gastroenterol Hepatol 1997; 9:581–587.

17. Farin G, Grund KE. Technology of argon plasma coagulation with particular regard to endoscopic applications. Endosc Surg Allied Technol 1994; 2:71–77.

18. Grund KE, Storek D, Farin G. Endoscopic argon plasma coagulation (APC) first clinical experiences in flexible endoscopy. Endosc Surg Allied Technol 1994; 2:42–46.

19. Storek D, Grund KE, Gronbach G, et al. Endoscopic argon gas coagulation – initial clinical experiences. Z Gastroenterol 1993; 31:675–679.

20. Rey JF, Marek TA. Endo-loop in the prevention of the post-polypectomy bleeding: preliminary results. Gastrointest Endosc 1997; 46:387–389.

21. Waye JD, Lewis BS, Yessayan S. Colonoscopy: a prospective report of complications. J Clin Gastroenterol 1992; 15:347–351.

22. Matsushita M, Hajiro K, Takakuwa H, et al. Ineffective use of a detachable snare for colonoscopic polypectomy of large polyps. Gastrointest Endosc 1998; 47:496–499.

23. Ellis KK, Fennerty MB. Marking and identifying colon lesions. Tattoos, clips, and radiology in imaging the colon. Gastrointest Endosc Clin North Am 1997; 7:401–411.

24. Nagasu N, DiPalma JA. Bleeding ulcer: inject or clip? Am J Gastroenterol 1998; 93:1998.

25. Hachisu T, Yamada H, Satoh S, et al. Endoscopic clipping with a new rotatable clip-device and a long clip. Dig Endosc 1996; 8:127–133.

26. Uno Y, Satoh K, Tuji K, et al. Endoscopic ligation by means of clip and detachable snare for management of colonoscopic postpolypectomy hemorrhage. Gastrointest Endosc 1999; 49:113–115.

27. Iida Y, Miura S, Munemoto Y, et al. Endoscopic resection of large colorectal polyps using a clipping method. Dis Colon Rectum 1994; 37:179–180.

28. Cohen LB, Waye JD. Treatment of colonic polyps – practical considerations. Clin Gastroenterol 1986; 15:359.

29. McNally DO, DeAngelis SA, Rison DR, et al. Bipolar polypectomy device for removal of colon polyps. Gastrointest Endosc 1994; 40:489–491.

30. Geenen JE, Fleischer D, Waye JD. Techniques in therapeutic endoscopy. 2nd ed. New York: WB Saunders and Gower Medical Publishing; 1992.

31. Van Gossum A, Cozzoli A, Adler M, et al. Colonoscopic snare polypectomy: analysis of 1485 resections comparing two types of current. Gastrointest Endosc 1992; 38:472–475.

32. Waye JD, Lewis BS, Frankel A, et al. Small colon polyps. Amer J Gastroenterol 1988; 83:120–122.

33. Mitooka H, Fujimori T, Ohno S, et al. New methods – new materials: chromoscopy of the colon using indigo carmine dye with electrolyte lavage solution. Gastrointest Endosc 1992; 38:373–374.

34. Mitooka H, Fujimori T, Maeda S, et al. Minute flat depressed neoplastic lesions of the colon detected by contrast chromoscopy using an indigo carmine capsule. Gastrointest Endosc 1995; 41:453–459.

35. Fleischer DE. Chromoendoscopy and magnification endoscopy in the colon. Gastrointest Endosc 1999; 49:S45–49.

36. Fennerty MB. Should chromoscopy be part of the 'proficient' endoscopist's armamentarium? Gastrointest Endosc 1998; 47:313–315.

37. Jaramillo E, Watanabe M, Slezak P, et al. Flat neoplastic lesions of the colon and rectum detected by high-resolution video endoscopy and chromoscopy. Gastrointest Endosc 1995; 42:114–122.

38. Peluso F, Goldner F. Follow-up of hot biopsy forceps treatment of diminutive colonic polyps. Gastrointest Endosc 1991; 37:604–606.

39. Woods A, Sanowski RA, Wadas DD, et al. Eradication of diminutive polyps: a prospective evaluation of bipolar coagulation versus conventional biopsy removal. Gastrointest Endosc 1989; 35:536.

40. Vanagunas A, Jacob P, Vakil N. Adequacy of 'hot biopsy' for the treatment of diminutive polyps: a prospective randomized trial. Am J Gastroenterol 1989; 84:383.

41. Wadas DD, Sanowski RA. Complications of the hot biopsy forceps technique. Gastrointest Endosc 1988; 34:32–37.

42. Tappero G, Gaia E, DeFiuli P, et al. Cold snare excision of small colorectal polyps. Gastrointest Endosc 1992; 38:310–313.

43. Uno Y, Obara K, Zheng P, et al. Cold snare excision is a safe method for diminutive colorectal polyps. Tohoku J Exp Med 1997; 183:243–249.

44. Waye JD. Techniques of polypectomy: hot biopsy forceps and snare polypectomy. Am J Gastroenterol 1987; 82:615–618.

45. Karita M, Tada M, Okita K, et al. Endoscopic therapy for early colon cancer: the strip biopsy resection technique. Gastrointest Endosc 1991; 37:128–132.

46. Karita M, Tada M, Okita K. The successive strip biopsy partial resection technique for large early gastric and colon cancers. Gastrointest Endosc 1992; 38:174–178.

47. Karita M, Cantero D, Okita K. Endoscopic diagnosis and resection treatment for flat adenoma with severe dysplasia. Am J Gastroenterol 1993; 88:1421–1423.

48. Uchikawa H, Hirao M, Yamagutio M, et al. Endoscopic mucosal resection combined with local injection of hypertonic saline epinephrine solution for early colorectal cancers and other tumors. Gastroenterol Endosc 1992; 34:1871–1878.

49. Shirai M, Nakamura T, Matsuura A, et al. Safer colonoscopic polypectomy with local submucosal injection of hypertonic saline-epinephrine solution. Am J Gastroenterol 1994; 89:334–338.

50. Kanamori T, Itoh M, Yokoyama Y, et al. Injection-incision-assisted snare resection of large sessile colorectal polyps. Gastrointest Endosc 1996; 43:189–193.

51. Waye JD. Saline injection colonoscopic polypectomy (editorial). Am J Gastroenterol 1994; 89:305–306.

52. Uno Y, Munakata A. The non-lifting sign of invasive colon cancer. Gastrointest Endosc 1994; 40:485–489.

53. Schiano TD, Pfister D, Harrison L, et al. Neoplastic seeding as a complication of percutaneous endoscopic gastrostomy. Am J Gastroenterol 1994; 89:131–133.

54. Waye JD. Polyps large and small (editorial). Gastrointest Endosc 1992; 38:391–392.

55. Nivatvongs S, Snover DC, Fang DT. Piecemeal snare excision of large sessile colon and rectal polyps: Is it adequate? Gastrointest Endosc 1984; 30:18.

56. Christie JP. Colonoscopic removal of sessile colonic lesions. Dis Colon Rectum 1978; 21:11.

57. Walsh RM, Ackroyd FW, Shelito PC. Endoscopic resection of large sessile colorectal polyps. Gastrointest Endosc 1992; 38:303–309.

58. Zlatanic J, Waye JD, Kim PS, et al. Large sessile colonic adenomas: use of argon plasma coagulator to supplement piecemeal snare polypectomy. Gastrointest Endosc 1999; 49:731–735.

59. McAfee JH, Katon RM. Tiny snares prove safe and effective for removal of diminutive colorectal polyps. Gastrointest Endosc 1994; 40:301–303.

60. Bat L, Williams CB. Usefulness of pediatric colonoscopes in adult colonoscopy. Gastrointest Endosc 1989; 35:329–332.

61. Rogers BHG. The use of small caliber endoscopes in selected cases increases the success rate of colonoscopy. Gastrointest Endosc 1989; 35:352.

62. Kozarek RA, Botoman VA, Patterson DJ. Prospective evaluation of a small caliber upper endoscope for colonoscopy after unsuccessful standard examination. Gastrointest Endosc 1989; 35:333–335.

63. Hancock JH, Talbot RW. Accuracy of colonoscopy in localization of colorectal cancer. Int J Colorectal Dis 1995; 10:140–141.

64. Dunaway MT, Webb WR, Rodning CB. Intraluminal measurement of distance in the colorectal region employing rigid and flexible endoscopes. Surg Endosc 1988; 2:81–83.

65. Waye JD. Colonoscopy without fluoroscopy (editorial). Gastrointest Endosc 1990; 36:72–73.

66. Frager DH, Frager JD, Wolf EL, et al. Problems in the colonoscopic localization of tumors: continue value of the barium enema. Gastrointest Radiol 1987; 12:343–346.

67. Hilliard G, Ramming K, Thompson J Jr, et al. The elusive colonic malignancy. A need for definitive preoperative localization. Am Surg 1990; 56:742–744.

68. Tabibian N, Michaletz PA, Schwartz JT, et al. Use of endoscopically placed clip can avoid diagnostic errors in colonoscopy. Gastrointest Endosc 1988; 34:262–264.

69. Montorsi M, Opocher E, Santambrogio R, et al. Original technique for small colorectal tumor localization during laparoscopic surgery. Dis Colon Rectum 1999; 42:819–822.

70. Shatz BA, Thavorides V. Colonic tattoo for follow-up of endoscopic sessile polypectomy. Gastrointest Endosc 1991; 37:59–60.

71. Bladen JS, Anderson AP, Bell GD, et al. Non-radiological technique for three-dimensional imaging of endoscopes. Lancet 1993; 341:719–722.

72. Williams C, Guy C, Gilles D, et al. Electronic three-dimensional imaging of intestinal endoscopy. Lancet 1993; 341:724–725.

73. Leicester RJ, Williams CB. Use of metal detector for localisation during fibresigmoidoscopy or limited colonoscopy. Lancet 1981; ii:232–233.

74. Forde KA, Cohen JL. Intraoperative colonoscopy. Ann Surg 1988; 207:231–233.

75. Richter RM, Littman L, Levowitz BS. Intraoperative fiberoptic colonoscopy. Localization of nonpalpable colonic lesions. Arch Surg 1973; 106:228.

76. Sakanoue Y, Nakao K, Shoji Y, et al. Intraoperative colonoscopy. Surg Endosc 1993; 7:84–87.

77. Hammond DC, Lane FR, Welk RA, et al. Endoscopic tattooing of the colon: an experimental study. Am Surg 1989; 55:457–461.

78. Hammond DC, Lane FR, Mackeigan JM, et al. Endoscopic tattooing of the colon: clinical experience. Am Surg 1993; 59:205–210.

79. Ponsky JL, King JF. Endoscopic marking of colon lesions. Gastrointest Endosc 1975; 22:42–43.

80. Cohen LB, Waye JD. Colonoscopic polypectomy of polyps with adenocarcinoma: when is it curative? In: Barkin JS, ed. Difficult decisions in digestive diseases. Chicago: Year Book Medical Publishers; 1989:528–535.

81. Nizam R, Siddiqi N, Landas SK, et al. Colonic tattooing with India ink: benefits, risks, and alternatives. Am J Gastroenterol 1996; 91:1804–1808.

82. Gopal DV, Morava-Protzner I, Miller HAB, et al. Idiopathic inflammatory bowel disease associated with colonic tattooing with India ink preparation. Gastrointest Endosc 1999; 49:636–639.

83. Lightdale CJ. India ink colonic tattoo – blots on the record (editorial). Gastrointest Endosc 1991; 37:68–71.

84. Poulard JB, Shatz B, Kodner I. Preoperative tattooing of polypectomy site. Endoscopy 1985; 17:84–85.

85. Shatz BA. Small volume india ink injections (letter to editor). Gastrointest Endosc 1991; 37:649–650.

86. Salomon P, Berner JS, Waye JD. Endoscopic India ink injection: a method for preparation, sterilization, and administration. Gastrointest Endosc 1993; 39:803–805.

87. Hyman N, Waye JD. Endoscopic four quadrant tattoo for the identification of colonic lesions at surgery. Gastrointest Endosc 1991; 37:56–58.

88. Shatz BA, Weinstock LB, Swanson PE, et al. Long-term safety of India ink tattoos in the colon. Gastrointest Endosc 1997; 45:153–156.

89. McArthur CS, Roayaie S, Waye JD. Safety of preoperation endoscopic tattoo with India ink for identification of colonic lesions. Surg Endosc 1999; 13:397–400.

90. Habr-Gama A, Waye JD. Complications and hazards of gastrointestinal endoscopy. World J Surg 1989; 13:193–201.

91. Rankin GB. Indications, contraindications and complications of colonoscopy. In: Sivak MV, ed. Gastroenterologic endoscopy. Philadelphia: WB Saunders; 1987.

92. Shinya H. Complications: prevention and management. In: Shinya H, ed. Colonoscopy: diagnostic and treatment of colonic diseases. New York: Igaku-Shoin; 1982:199–208.

93. Kavin H, Sinicrope F, Esker AH. Management of perforation of the colon at colonoscopy. Am J Gastroenterol 1992; 87:161–167.

94. Waye JD, Kahn O, Auerbach ME. Complications of colonoscopy and flexible sigmoidoscopy. Gastrointest Endosc Clin North Am 1996; 6:343–377.

95. Carpio G, Albu E, Gumbs MA, et al. Management of colonic perforation after colonoscopy. Report of three cases. Dis Colon Rectum 1989; 32:624–626.

96. Christie JP, Marrazzo J. 'Mini-perforation' of the colon – not all postpolypectomy perforations require laparotomy. Dis Colon Rectum 1991; 34:132–135.

97. Hall C, Dorricott NJ, Donovan IA, et al. Colon perforation during colonoscopy: surgical versus conservative management. Br J Surg 1991; 78:542–544.

98. Wullstein C, Koppen M, Gross E. Laparoscopic treatment of colonic perforations related to colonoscopy. Surg Endosc 1999; 13:484–487.

99. Yoshikane H, Hidano H, Sakakibara A, et al. Endoscopic repair by clipping of iatrogenic colonic perforation. Gastrointest Endosc 1997; 46:464–466.

100. Waye JD. The postpolypectomy coagulation syndrome. Gastrointest Endosc 1981; 27:184.

101. Rex DK, Lewis BS, Waye JD. Colonoscopy and endoscopic therapy for delayed postpolypectomy hemorrhage. Gastrointest Endosc 1992; 38:127–129.

102. Nivatvongs S. Complications in colonoscopic polypectomy: lessons to learn from an experience with 1576 polyps. Am Surg 1988; 54:61–63.

103. Jensen DM, Machicado GA. Diagnosis and treatment of severe hematochezia. Gastroenterology 1988; 95:1569–1574.

104. Cussons PD, Berry AR. Comparison of the use of emergency mesenteric angiography and intraoperative colonoscopy with antegrade colonic irrigation in massive rectal hemorrhage. J R Coll Surg Edinb 1989; 34:91–93.

105. Carlyle DR, Goldstein HM. Angiographic management of bleeding following transcolonoscopic polypectomy. Am J Dig Dis 1975; 20:1196–1199.

106. Slivka A, Parsons WG, Carr-Locke DL. Endoscopic band ligation for treatment of post-polypectomy hemorrhage: case report. Gastrointest Endosc 1994; 40:230–232.

107. Smith RE, Doull J. Treatment of colonic post-polypectomy bleeding site by endoscopic band ligation. Gastrointest Endosc 1994; 40:499–503.

108. Williams CB. Diathermy-biopsy: a technique for the endoscopic management of small polyps. Endoscopy 1973; 5:215.

109. Mann NS, Mann SK, Alam I. The safety of hot biopsy forceps in the removal of small colonic polyps. Digestion 1999; 60:74–76.

13.
ENDOSCOPIC TREATMENT OF LOWER INTESTINAL BLEEDING

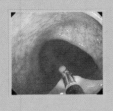

CHRISTOPHER B. WILLIAMS

INTRODUCTION

'Bleeding per rectum' is one of the classic ways in which a patient may present, and is a matter of some concern. In over 90% of cases of minor or recurrent bleeding, the cause will be due to the results of trauma to the region of the squamocolumnar junction at the anal opening, and especially the underlying hemorrhoidal plexus. There is nonetheless always concern that there could be other serious pathology proximally. 'Bleeding' therefore early became a prime indication for colonoscopy. Almost always this meant a *history* of one or more episodes of minor bleeding, with little or no bleeding visible at the time of the procedure.

For acute or severe bleeding, the relative technical difficulty of colonoscopy, especially in the tortuous sigmoid and particularly in the presence of active bleeding and clots, meant that early publications extolling the feasibility of 'emergency' colonoscopy for active bleeding[1,2] were received with incredulity. However, in the last few years, trail-blazing publications of Jensen et al,[3–5] supported by other large series,[6–10] literature reviews,[11–14] and the American Society for Gastrointestinal Endoscopy policy statement[15] have all emphasized the primary role of colonoscopy in management of major colonic bleeding (in preference to angiography or isotope scanning and avoiding early surgery).

Current recognition of the prime role of colonoscopy in management of bleeding patients is partly due to improvements in the mechanical and visual excellence of endoscopes. It also reflects the range of therapeutic modalities introduced over three decades, the 'tricks of the trade' in applying them successfully, and published proof of the cost-effectiveness and safety of the direct endoscopic approach over other means. It must be said that the literature series are decidedly heterogeneous, reflecting case selection bias and variable criteria in different institutions plus the impossibility of collecting sufficient numbers of matched cases for RCTs. This chapter is primarily concerned with the methodologies available for treating bleeding patients and practical endoscopic aspects of their management.

CLINICAL ASSESSMENT AND THE TIMING OF ENDOSCOPY

Lower gastrointestinal bleeding is in at least 95% of adults typically both minor and self-limiting, rather than either severe or likely to continue.[3] Some patients will present only with suspected blood loss, inferred because of positive occult blood tests or iron deficiency anemia, but mandating examination of the upper gastrointestinal tract by gastroscopy (even enteroscopy in appropriate cases) as well as requiring careful visualization of the whole colon. Confident exclusion of pathology is important even in those in whom endoscopic therapy proves unnecessary. Even cases of acute or 'massive' bleeding can be expected to stop spontaneously in between 70%[8] and 85–90%.[12] It therefore frequently makes sense, rather than reflexly rushing into emergency endoscopy, to temporize, assess (and, if necessary, transfuse) the patient with a view to a more controlled, fully-prepared, and high-quality examination later on. However, if transfusion requirements rise to 4 units or more and the patient remains hemodynamically unstable, the indication for urgent colonoscopy is indisputable – but a relatively rare event.

It makes good sense to anticipate relevant factors which can be divined from the preliminary *clinical history* and *examination*, both to facilitate management and ensure that the best available person is undertaking it. So-called 'telephone triage' will often decide who can be reassured and endoscopy planned as an elective event, whereas two or more large bloody stools within an hour indicates hospitalization. 'Acute bleeding' is defined as abrupt onset with multiple passages of bloody stool over 1 to 3 days, classified as 'moderate' if manageable without transfusion but 'severe' when resuscitation is required. A history of profuse, bright red, painless bleeding suggests a possible anorectal origin and 14% of one series of acute bleeds (over 4 units tranfused) proved to be hemorrhoidal in origin.[8] There is therefore a need for skilled proctological assessment or particular care in examining the anorectal area by *proctoscopy* (or possibly flexible sigmoidoscopy, to allow retroversion in the rectum) before venturing upstream for what may be an extremely tedious, but eventually fruitless and potentially inconclusive, examination. Abdominal pain and sudden onset of bleeding suggest a possible ischemic origin, almost always self-limiting and an indication not to take any risks during colonoscopy if the mucosal surface is found to be severely ulcerated or gangrenous. Placement of an aortic graft in the preceding year can be the cause of erosion and major bleeding. Any medication taken by the patient may have relevance. Non-steroidal anti-inflammatory agents (NSAIDs) may either cause or aggravate bleeding lesions. Anti-coagulants generally require reversal before undertaking a therapeutic procedure and a history of alcohol abuse warns that underlying liver disease may complicate management.

The patient's account of the colour and volume of bleeding is an obvious indicator of probable site and severity of the problem. It can also be grossly misleading. Blood in the lavatory pan is frightening and, once diluted, tends to be over-estimated. Color is a subjective assessment, but few clinicians bother to confront the patient with a standard color chart. Even so, 'bright' red blood can, if in sufficient volume, present at the anus from an upper gastrointestinal source – 10 to 15% arising above the ligament of Treitz.[11] Different series report small intestinal sources, usually angiodysplasia, in 3 to 5%,[11] 9%[20,33] or 18%.[16] Conversely, hemorrhoidal bleeding can reflux to the proximal colon and emerge altered and dark. The *clinical status* of the patient must be established, both in assessing the individual and when comparing different published series describing colonoscopic management of bleeding. It is common sense that, before undertaking bowel preparation and a demanding procedure, the patient should be in a stable condition and 'resuscitation' or replacement of fluid volume is a prerequisite, when indicated. Hemodynamically unstable patients are likely to have lost over 15% of blood volume, so tranfusion of 2 or more units will be the minimum requirement, and sometimes much more. However, emergency colonoscopy may occasionally be needed (and be potentially life-saving) in a destabilized, hypovolemic, and massively-bleeding patient, providing that the fullest possible resuscitatory measures are simultaneously applied, with intensive care and surgical teams involved or alerted. In intermediate cases, the volume of blood lost and the success of its replacement by transfusion will determine the urgency with which colonoscopy must be undertaken, especially if an experienced endoscopist is not available. It is reasonable to delay up to 24 hours for 'elective' colonoscopy if 2–3 units of blood or fluid infusion have stabilized the patient. However, if 4 or more units are required or the patient remains hemodynamically unstable, the hemorrhage is considered 'severe' or 'massive' and immediate emergency colonoscopy is indicated (within 4 to 6 hours at most, and if necessary in the intensive care facility or even peroperatively).[3,5]

PATIENT PREPARATION

Preparation of the colon in a bleeding patient depends on circumstance and clinical assessment. Ideally, full oral preparation is given, according to the regimen usually employed in the particular endoscopy facility. In a few severely bleeding cases there is no time for this and colonoscopy is attempted *without* preparation, relying on the purgative tendency of blood to clear the bowel distal to the bleeding point. Unprepared colonoscopy (or flexible sigmoidoscopy) is particularly likely to be successful for post-polypectomy bleeding when the removed polyp(s) were situated in the distal colon, but some series have reported entirely on unprepared colons.[8] In actively bleeding patients, the PEG-electrolyte purge regimen[17] is ideal, providing maximal washout clearance, avoiding the tendency of enemas to reflux blood proximally, and the possibility of stimulant laxatives worsening bleeding, also safeguarding the patient's volumetric status. Patients with minor or moderate active bleeding can drink the solution, but for more severe bleeding it is quicker and more effective to administer it through a nasogastric tube (warm solution, 2 L per hour, up to 6–8 L or more required).[5] In extreme circumstances, some authors have described good results from cecostomy-tube lavage to clear the view for intra-operative colonoscopy.[18,19]

Investigation options

Gastroscopy ('top and tail' endoscopy at the same examination) is required in any patient with significant blood loss, whether demonstrated as anemia or clinically as hypovolemia and transfusion requirement.[11] Gastroscopy, to exclude the presence of blood or a visible source for bleeding, need take no longer than 2 to 3 minutes and is significantly quicker and more accurate than the previous routine of aspirating a nasogastric tube and looking or testing for blood.

Barium studies are now no longer indicated, since they have a much lower diagnostic yield than endoscopy, no therapeutic potential, and the disadvantage of leaving a barium residue which impedes other investigations.

Isotope scanning or *angiography* may have a role in some large institutions and selected problematic patients with moderately severe bleeding, but now usually only *after* colonoscopy has been attempted.[5,13] Colonoscopy is more accurate than either modality and allows immediate therapy, significantly more safely than most angiographic methods. Angiographic selective intra-arterial infusion of *vasopressin* is usually only a temporary measure, with rebleeding in 50%,[20,21] although significantly more effective than the crisis measure of vasopressin administered intravenously.[22]

Enteroscopy is an adjunctive investigation in the 5 to 15% of patients with continuing blood loss in whom no diagnosis is made by first-line investigations.[6,16,23] It is preferably performed with a 'push enteroscope', long, floppy, and with a supporting overtube available if needed.[24] A pediatric or standard colonoscope (disinfected and used orally) makes a reasonable substitute. Few centers have experience of the 'sonde' or balloon enteroscope.[23] Successful enteroscopy ensures that the maximum possible extent of jejunum (orally) and ileum (peranally) are examined. Forty-five percent of one series had angiodysplasias, treatable by electrocoagulation and resulting either in cure or significant reduction in transfusion requirements long-term.[24] Adding enteroscopy to the investigation of the 5% of patients with recurrent bleeding who are undiagnosed after first-line investigation is said to be diagnostic in 70 to 100%.[23]

Surgery as a life-saving crisis measure was the norm for patients with massive and uncontrollable hemorrhage. In 10 to 16% of recent series, surgery was employed in management, but with 4 to 5% mortality.[6-8] In one surgical series, 4/12 patients with massive bleeding died.[25] In spite of the much greater safety of colonoscopy, emergency surgery should still be considered (and the surgical team given early warning)[5] in patients in whom:

1. resuscitation measures fail to control hypovolemia
2. 6 or more units have been transfused but *no* diagnosis made by all available means
3. bleeding site has been identified but is uncontrollable by colonoscopic therapy.

Blind resection is not advised without an attempt at per-operative endoscopic diagnosis,[9,12] using on-table lavage if necessary.

COLONOSCOPY TECHNIQUE

Colonoscopic technique in actively bleeding patients is little different from that usually employed, except that maximum dexterity will be needed to pass residual blood or clots. Selecting a *large-channel colonoscope* (3.2 or larger instrumentation channel) maximizes suction, especially of residual clots. Removing the suction button and covering the hole with a finger increases suction pressure or the suc-

tion tube can be connected directly to the channel at the biopsy port. Ideally, an *irrigation pump* facility (dental Water-pik or similar) should be available to clear the mucosal surface of adherent residues or clot. If not available, a 50 mL syringe is a reasonable substitute, hand-activated down the suction channel or used with a spray-catheter for greatest local effect. Other accessories and therapeutic modalities used are described later.

Position change is a fundamentally valuable trick in bleeding patients, particularly effective in obtaining at least a partially air-filled view of the sigmoid and descending colon by the simple means of turning the patient from the usual left lateral position to the back or to the right lateral position (Fig. 13.1). The gravitational re-distribution of air, fluid, and clots resulting should create just enough airspace to insert proximally. Once in the more capacious proximal colon, often clot-free, there is less problem in seeing but a change back to the left lateral position should optimize the view. Appropriate re-positioning during the examination phase similarly increases the percentage of mucosal surface inspected if full aspiration or evacuation of bowel contents has not been possible. Position change can be similarly important in successfully targeting and managing an active bleeding point, ensuring that it will remain visible (above the rising tide of blood) during the therapeutic process.

Retroversion of the endoscope is often possible in the cecum and ascending colon, so minimizing the 'blind spots' to examination which otherwise occur behind haustral folds, although retroversion is technically impossible in many patients and has the potential to traumatize any local lesions, such as angiodysplasia.

Rotation of the endoscope if necessary, so as to ensure that therapeutic instruments emerge 'on target' (at 5 o'clock in the endoscopic view) (Fig. 13.2), is another small but important maneuver, likely to increase the speed and success of therapeutic attempts.

EQUIPMENT

The endoscopist undertaking colonoscopy in a patient with bleeding should, as well as being experienced, have the fullest reasonable array of accessories for treatment and be

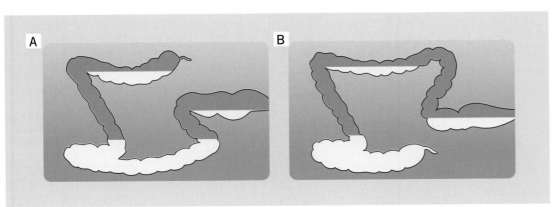

Fig. 13.1 Position change during colonoscopy. **(A)** In left lateral position, blood obscures the distal colon. **(B)** Changing to right lateral position improves the view.

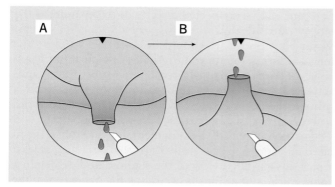

Fig. 13.2 Rotation of the endoscope to target correctly. (**A**) Instrument channel inconveniently placed. (**B**) Rotation to 5 o'clock position facilitates therapy.

familiar with their use. In practice, most of the items required are those regularly used for polypectomy (see Chapter 12). However, in treating colonic bleeding the view is generally worse than in 'routine' colonoscopy and the need for precise targeting greater. For this reason, the availability of a choice of alternative techniques, or the application of several modalities to the abnormal or suspect area, can be particularly desirable.

Sclerotherapy injection needle, the simplest and cheapest of all the accessories, is the single most useful one in controlling active bleeding. It is usually used to inject epinephrine solution (1/10 000–1/20 000 in 1–2 mL aliquots up to 10 mL or more) into and/or around a definite or probable bleeding site[26] but others have injected sclerosants such as ethanolamine (3.3% solution, 2–8 mL).[27] Once the needle has been inserted and the injection started, the needle is slowly withdrawn until resistance to injection pressure is felt and swelling or bleb formation is seen (Fig. 13.3). If in doubt, several injections can be made to surround the visible vessel or suspected bleeding point, preferably continuing until bleeding stops. The bonus of injection is that precise localization is not critical; the negative is that theoretically the effects could be short-lived, although in practice rebleeding is uncommon once controlled. Efficacy of epinephrine injection is probably due to a combination of physical compression (coaptation) and vessel contraction. There is effectively no hazard in epinephrine injection, since the portal circulation ensures no systemic or cardiac effects and intraperitoneal or extramural injection has no consequence. There is little data on the use of other agents (sodium tetradecyl sulphate, absolute alcohol). By analogy with experience in the upper gastrointestinal tract, they are likely to be more hazardous but only marginally more effective; so they are generally not advisable, except possibly in highly specific circumstances such as hemangiomas or angiodysplasias,[27] especially the raised 'blue rubber blebs' of childhood capillary hemangiomas.

Polypectomy snare (and electrosurgical unit (ESU)). The apparatus for polypectomy can equally be useful for hemorrhage control, particularly when the cause of bleeding is a polyp or cancer, or a delayed (secondary) post-polypectomy bleed, which can occur up to 12 to 14 days later, and from the site of even the smallest polyp. When the polyp (or its remnant) is stalked, the *snare* has the obvious advantage of applying strangulation (coaptive) pressure to occlude the feeding vessels, so both stopping bleeding and the heat dissipating effect of blood flow, while the tissue electrocoagulates and the plexus of vessels is hemocoagulated and sealed off (Fig. 13.4). When targeting a small bleeding point after snaring a sessile polyp, the tip of the nearly-closed snare wire can be used for local electrocoagulation (Fig. 13.5). Only a very low power setting (10 W, coagulating current) should be used, and great care taken not to risk perforation by point contact with the snare tip end-on to the surface. In most cases where there is little or no residual stalk, epinephrine injection is both the easiest and most effective option (Fig 13.3).

The *hot biopsy forceps* (or other monopolar contact probes) can target a smaller area than the snare, but has the disadvantage that, as the current flow spreads unpredictably into a wider area below the contact point, there is potential for perforation if too much heat is applied, especially in the thin-walled proximal colon. Perforations have occurred using hot biopsy forceps[28,29] and they must be used with caution, only if the mucosa will tent up and with current applied only until there is barely visible electrocoagulation at the apex ('Mount Fuji effect') (Fig. 13.6). Used in this way, and in the absence of the more predictable and sophisticated devices described below, they have been successfully employed in electrocoagulation of bleeding lesions including angiodysplasia.[30]

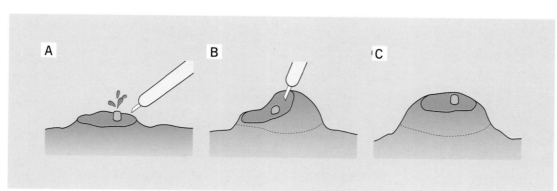

Fig. 13.3 Injection sclerotherapy of bleeding site. (**A**) Injector needle with 1:10 000 dilution of epinephrine. (**B**) Injection of 2–4 mL of solution immediately adjacent to bleeding site. (**C**) Site of polypectomy following injection of several mL of solution around bleeding site.

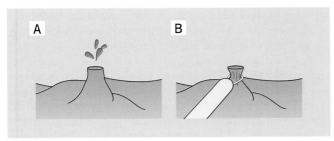

Fig. 13.4 Use of snare loop in 'co-aptation' pressure of bleeding point. (A) Polyp. stalk bleeding post-resection. (B) Residual pedicle recaptured with snare and held tightly with coaptive pressure for 5 minutes.

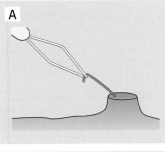

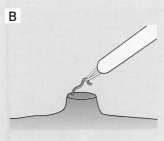

Fig. 13.5 Use of snare loop to control immediate post-polypectomy bleed. (A) Blood vessel avulsed from head of polyp during polypectomy. This only occurs with pedunculated polyps of ≤1cm diameter. The vessel is fixed by the coagulum to the snare tip. (B) Tension on vessel released. (C) The snare tip is barely protruded (about 1–2 mm) and pushed into the stalk. Additional coagulation current is given to damage the residual vessel in the stalk. The snare is then pulled free.

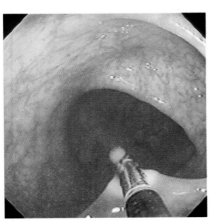

Fig. 13.6 Safe use of hot biopsy forceps – the 'Mount Fuji' effect. Very limited electrocoagulation results in whitening only of the apex of the elevated 'mountain' of tissue.

Bipolar electrocoagulation (BICAP, ACM Endoscopy; Gold probe, Microvasive) probes avoid the hazards of monopolar current spread by allowing current flow *only* through tissue in contact with the closely spaced electrodes at the tip of the probe. This means that there is no likelihood of perforation of deeper tissues, providing that low power (10–20 W) and short duration (1 second) pulses are used until there is satisfactory hemostasis or visible electrocoagulation. The system has the advantages that the probe can safely make contact at any angle, allows coaptive pressure to compress underlying vessels, can be used to 'paint' the surface of larger areas, and has a useful, inbuilt, waterjet system. The ESU employed must be designed for bipolar use (no patient plate) and there is a tendency for the probe to 'stick' to the tissue being coagulated.

Argon plasma coagulation (APC) (Erbe) is a more recent means of targeting (monopolar) current onto the mucosal surface through a plastic catheter which conducts the current from an in-built electrode through ionized argon gas flow (0.8–2 L/min) onto the tissue surface.[31] A dedicated ESU must be used, but is much cheaper than a laser. The argon gas delivery system is fully incorporated, flow being automatically activated when the electrocoagulation pedal is depressed. Care is needed to avoid overdistention of the patient by aspiration at intervals (preferably use a 3.2 mm channel colonoscope for easy deflation). The APC system has the advantage of not requiring tissue contact or precise targeting (the current will even arc sideways from the catheter to the nearest point of tissue contact) (Fig. 13.7). APC is inherently safe and tissue damage theoretically restricted to a depth of around 2–3 mm because desiccated tissue cuts off current flow, stopping further damage. In practice, there is some risk in the proximal colon, with reported peritonism and gas escape in a few cases.[32]

Laser photocoagulation (Nd:YAG) has, after initial enthusiasm and reported efficacy,[33] been substantially replaced by use of the argon plasma coagulator, which is both cheaper and safer (for patient and operator) but with similar ease of use and non-contact characteristics. The Nd:YAG laser results, invisibly, in potential deep tissue damage and so is particularly hazardous for use for bleeding lesions in the proximal colon or ulcerated areas such as sessile polypectomy sites for which the APC system is ideal and inherently safe.

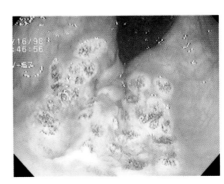

Fig. 13.7 Argon plasma coagulator effects on localized irradiation telangiectasis.

The *heater probe* (Olympus) is an ingenious microprocessor-controlled device which allows precise heating of a small volume of tissue below the point of contact with the probe, which is Teflon-coated to reduce tissue-stick problems. Its use is similar, and similarly easy to that of the bipolar electrode (BICAP, Gold), and it also has an in-built irrigation facility. Heat application is pre-dialled on its generator (typically 10–15 J). While ideal for applying coaptive pressure and heat to a point bleeding source, it is less effective than the argon plasma coagulator for 'painting' larger areas and requires accurate targeting.

The *Endoclip* or *clip-fixing device* (Olympus) is a small, stainless-steel clip with sharp, self-retaining jaws (Fig. 13.8) originally fabricated for control of bleeding peptic ulcers. It is passed through the colonoscope channel on a spiral wire introducer, targeted onto the bleeding point or visible vessel, closed tight, then released from its hook and the introducer withdrawn. Placement of the device is slightly fiddly on first acquaintance or if it is rarely used, but becomes easier with practice (which can be undertaken outside the patient). The clip, or clips, will slough off a few days later and be passed in the stools, often after successful control of bleeding.[34]

The *Endoloop* or 'detachable snare' (Olympus) is a tightenable nylon loop similar in application and introducer design to the clipping device. The loop is effectively a strangulation ligature which is perfect for placement around a polyp stalk, whether at the time of polypectomy or if there is post-polypectomy bleeding from a projecting residue of stalk.[34,35] Unfortunately, the tissue necrosis following snaring frequently means that any stalk has sloughed off, resulting in the bleed but also leaving nothing on which to close the loop.[36]

Banding devices (Wilson–Cook, Bard), primarily intended for control of esophageal varices, have also been successfully applied to flexible endoscopic management of hemorrhoids. The endoscope is retroverted in the rectum, the endoscopist suctions the vascular area into a transparent cup pre-placed onto the tip before introduction, then pulls a loop to release a tightly constricting rubber band. There are reports of direct band application onto small bleeding sites in the colon, such as Dieulafoy arteriolar lesions[37] or post-polypectomy sites.[34,38,39] A similar approach is possible using smaller versions of the Endoloop device inserted and opened within a transparent suction cap pre-placed onto the tip of the instrument.

Formaldehyde solution, applied topically (4%) with a saturated gauze or diluted as an enema, has been reported as a rapid and successful means of treating the multiple superficial telangiectases of 'irradiation proctitis', either alone or in combination with laser photocoagulation. Others have found this approach ineffective and likely to cause stricturing (Jensen D., personal communication, 1999), as well as painful at the anorectal area both immediately and subsequent to application.

Fibrin glue, applied in its two-part components down a two-channel catheter, has similarly been described in the upper gastrointestinal tract, but has not found advocates for colonic use.

COMPLICATIONS AND THEIR MANAGEMENT

Post-polypectomy bleeding is, after anorectal causes, the commonest presentation to the endoscopist (Fig. 13.9), principally because the patient knows the relevant telephone number and will make direct contact, but also because it occurs after around 1 to 2% of polypectomies.[40,41] *Immediate bleeding* can usually be anticipated from the large size of the polyp or its broad stalk and a wise endoscopist has appropriate measures ready for immediate action. If there is residual stalk, this can be rapidly grabbed and re-strangulated for 5 to 10 minutes using the snare loop already in position. If releasing the snare loop still results in rebleeding, it is possible, in the distal colon at least, to pass a pediatric endoscope up alongside the first one – allowing basal epinephrine injection before the strangulating snare-loop is re-released – and rapid placement of a clip or Endoloop if necessary.[34,40] Ordinarily, these measures are managed conventionally with the first instrument, opening and rapidly withdrawing the snare once the appropriate therapeutic device is ready for action. Basal injection of 3–10 mL 1/10 000 epinephrine solution is the easiest and quickest remedy, unless the bleeding point is small and it is felt justified to try snare-tip electrocoagulation first

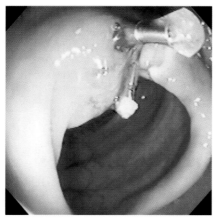

Fig. 13.8 Clips placed to control post-polypectomy bleeding site.

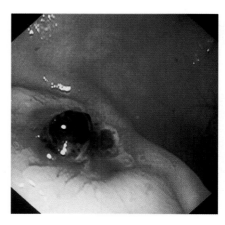

Fig. 13.9 Post-polypectomy bleeding site at 10 days.

(Figs. 13.3 to 13.5). *Delayed bleeds post-polypectomy* will usually stop spontaneously but, once the patient presents to the endoscopy facility and if the site is likely to be in the distal colon, unprepared flexible sigmoidoscopy and epinephrine injection, clipping, or banding is highly likely to be effective.[34,38] It has usually been thought preferable not to repeat electrocoagulation, mainly for safety reasons in an already damaged colon, but the availability of the argon plasma coagulator changes the situation and allows safe local re-coagulation (after epinephrine injection) as a 'belt and braces' approach.

Diverticular bleeding is the commonest cause of major colonic bleeding in most series, with 20 to 56% occurrence.[6–8] Patients with bleeding are characteristically elderly (a mean of 75 to 77 years in representative series),[5,8] so incidental diverticular disease will be a common occurrence, even if not always causative of bleeding. Minor bleeding can be caused by local mucosal traumatization with characteristic 'red folds', whereas typically a bleed from an individual diverticulum is profuse since it arises from damage to the arterial 'vasa recta' around the mouths of the diverticular sacs. Diverticular muscle hypertrophy narrows the distal colon, preparation is less effective, and there is a tendency for clot adherence in the diverticula. Colonoscopy is therefore often extremely tedious, primarily because of the difficulty of insertion but compounded by the near impossibility of getting good views when every diverticulum is blood-filled and under suspicion. It has been shown that waterjetting adherent clots does not increase the risk of rebleeding,[4] so a power washer is an invaluable accessory, preferably activated by foot switch or one of the endoscope buttons.

Therapeutically, there have been reports of 'successful' epinephrine injection, clipping, or coagulation of a visible vessel at the margin of a previously bleeding diverticulum.[26,42,43] However, diverticular bleeding seems usually to have stopped spontaneously by the time that the colonoscopy starts (or finishes), leaving the endoscopist uncertain whether the labor has been worthwhile. Rebleeding is said to occur in 25% of cases.[11] In the 'worst case', where active diverticular bleeding continues but the site cannot be localized or successfully targeted, the endoscopist can defer to angiography for selective embolization[44] or advise the surgeon which localized part of the colon requires resection.

Angiodysplasia (Fig. 13.10), although only found in 3 to 5% of patients with minor bleeding or anemia,[30] is more frequently found (11 to 30%) in series selected for severe and active bleeding.[5,8] These patients may present with anemia in up to 25% of series, iron-deficiency anemia in 10 to 15% as well as with frank bleeding, which is only acute in 15%.[45] Angiodysplasias certainly represent the single most rewarding diagnosis of all for the colonoscopist, since the appearance is definitive without histology and treatment rapid, effective, relatively safe, and usually curative. There is a 5% delayed hemorrhage rate, some patients will re-present after a long interval for 're-do', and only a minority will come to surgery (those with numerous angiodysplasias, so presumptively with other lesions inaccessible

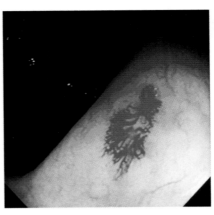

Fig. 13.10
Angiodysplasia.

proximally or in blind spots).[5] The endoscopist should remember that angiodysplasias *can* occur in the distal colon, although two-thirds are in the cecum and ascending colon, but be especially aware that they are characteristically multiple (mean 7 in Jensen's series, range 1–48).[5,45] The practical consequence of this is that the endoscopist should avoid over-rapid targeting and therapy of the first lesion seen, but rather complete a careful survey of the segment *before* therapy, in case resultant bleeding should obscure other lesions. A further corollary is that, if there are several lesions, the most dependent should be targeted first, leaving the remainder visible for treatment above the 'red sea' that can (temporarily) result. Twenty percent of 716 angiodysplasias in Jensen's series were of 1 cm diameter or greater; in these, it is desirable to target around the margin of the lesion first, so as to cause maximal surface damage before attacking the central zone where the feeding arteriole(s) is/are more likely to be. On this basis, too, it is sometimes possible to spot the 'high-flow' and high-risk smaller lesions, leaving them last in the therapy sequence, or to see superficial ulceration on the surface of the miscreant most likely to have been the cause of the presenting bleed.

Inflammatory bowel disease is one of the more likely bleeding presentations to the endoscopist, representing 15% of all causes in one series[10] but merits great caution before considering endoscopic therapy. Although some patients with longstanding Crohn's disease may have a thickened colon, it should be generally assumed that any ulcerated area is likely to be thinned, and so is hazardous for any therapeutic approach other than injection, clipping, or judicious use of the APC device. Any action taken by the endoscopist is at best a temporary measure in the hope or expectation that pharmacologic measures can save the patient from resection. Ischemic colitis is a self-limiting phenomenon of small-vessel 'shut-down'. It may present with the characteristic history of sudden onset abdominal pain and fresh bleeding but sometimes is inferred by the presence of ulceration in the 'watershed' vascular area around the splenic flexure or distally; no therapeutic action is required of the endoscopist.

Irradiation telangiectasia (Fig 13.11) is commonly misnamed as 'irradiation colitis' or 'proctitis', but is characteristically simply the scarred and vascular aftermath

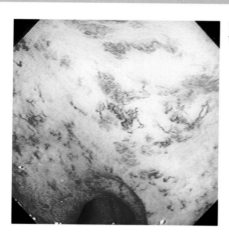

Fig. 13.11 Irradiation telangiectasia.

several years later. The worst-affected part varies according to the original 'field' of irradiation therapy, but the commonest site of bleeding is the rectum since it is usually both the most vascular area and most liable to trauma. Simple measures such as hormonal therapy have usually been tried but failed before the patient presents to the endoscopist, so there is pressure for therapy. It is highly desirable that attempted treatment should be by a non-contact modality, for which the argon plasma coagulator, laser, or formaldehyde approach is ideal.[46] Formaldehyde application alone has been found successful by some,[47] although not by others. However great the patience of the endoscopist, bleeding usually continues intermittently and several sessions of therapy and some months' time are likely to be needed before the denuded surface regenerates sufficiently.

Other causes include tumors, solitary rectal ulcer syndrome from straining, 'solitary ulcer' in the cecum or ascending colon (thought to be ischemic in origin), NSAID-induced ulceration (also typically in the proximal colon), and more extensive hemangiomas. Meckel's diverticulum, which can cause major red bleeding, is inaccessible to the endoscopist 1 m up the ileum. In children, juvenile polyps are the commonest cause of major bleeding, sometimes only occurring when the polyp twists and auto-amputates, leaving little for the endoscopist to see or do.

COST-EFFECTIVENESS OF COLONOSCOPY IN ACUTE AND SEVERE BLEEDING EPISODES

The cost-effectiveness of outpatient colonoscopy in the 'ordinary' patient having an elective procedure on a 'walk-in/walk-out' basis cannot be questioned, as no other procedure allows the same degree of diagnostic accuracy and therapeutic efficacy and safety. Until recently, the situation for patients hospitalized with acute or severe bleeding was less clear. This is attributable perhaps to the relative rarity of major colonic bleeding (as well as a paucity of referrals for emergency colonoscopy from the emergency teams); most endoscopists have been timorous to offer a colonic service comparable to that routinely in place for 'upper gastrointestinal bleeders'. However, it is now becoming clear that colonoscopy has more to offer than either isotope scanning or angiography in such patients, while the morbidity and 5 to 11% mortality of emergency surgery is unacceptable without trying the safer alternative of colonoscopy.[5,9] Nevertheless, patients with unrelenting massive (usually diverticular) bleeding may be beyond endoscopic therapy, and the endoscopist's role is simply to guide the surgeon in planning resection.

CONCLUSION

Colonoscopy is the undoubted 'gold standard' diagnostic procedure for patients with lower intestinal bleeding, especially once the proctologist has excluded anorectal lesions that are the commonest cause. Since 80 to 95% of even massive bleeds will stop spontaneously, the judgment on the 'success' of endoscopic therapy should be circumspect. Timing of colonoscopy also requires judgment. A delayed examination after full preparation will clearly be more accurate. Combining diagnostic excellence with the impressive results being achieved with newer therapeutic modalities (bipolar as well as monopolar electrocoagulation and the argon plasma coagulator), colonoscopy now generally takes precedence in the clinical 'pecking order' over adjunctive – sometimes highly valuable – techniques such as isotope scintigraphy or selective angiography. The colonoscopist is now in the front line, providing a high percentage of satisfactory and cost-effective outcomes, even in many patients with severe acute bleeding episodes. In massive exsanguination, the hope may often only be to assist the surgeon peroperatively to localize the problem and its resection, but thereby to reduce mortality. The range of therapeutic options in this 'new frontier' area of endoscopic practice is constantly changing, however, and it can be confidently expected that new therapies will emerge and results improve still further.

CHECKLIST OF PRACTICE POINTS

1. Most cases of lower GI bleeding will cease spontaneously. However, it may not be possible to predict which will stop and which will require intervention. All patients who have severe acute bleeding should be approached as if it will not stop spontaneously.
2. Injection with dilute (1:10 000) epinephrine solution is rapidly effective and inexpensive. This option should be considered when there is a point-source of bleeding.
3. In general, bleeding from diffuse areas, as in inflammatory bowel disease or ischemia, is not amenable to endoscopic therapy.
4. Blood is a cathartic and the presence of residual stool is rarely a problem with the patient who presents with acute severe rectal bleeding. However, the presence of blood is a hindrance to the successful performance of colonoscopy. A large-volume electrolyte preparation is effective for cleansing the colon of blood.
5. The frequency of bowel movements is the best parameter to assess ongoing bleeding. A decrease in the frequency of bloody motions indicates that the rate of bleeding is diminishing.
6. The approach to the patient should be:
   A. Assessment as to stability and site of bleeding.
   B. Resuscitation.
   C. If ongoing bleeding after colonoscopic polypectomy, perform urgent colonoscopy without any preparation.
   D. If ongoing severe bleeding of unknown etiology, perform upper GI endoscopy to rule out an upper source. Prep the patient with electrolyte solution. Perform colonoscopy urgently. Treat with epinephrine injection or any of the available thermal sources.
   E. If bleeding has stopped, prep the patient with electrolyte solution and perform colonoscopy when the bowel is clean.
   F. Use angiography with the capability of infusion therapy if bleeding is torrential.
   G. 'On table lavage' and preoperative colonoscopy is the final effective option for massive hemorrhage.
   H. Blind resection has an unacceptable mortality rate.

REFERENCES

1. Rossini FP, Ferrari A. Emergency colonoscopy. Acta Endoscopica 1976; 6:165–167.
2. Nuesch HJ, Kobler E, Jenny S, et al. Emergency colonoscopy. Endoscopy 1976; 6:161–163.
3. Jensen DM, Machicado GA. Diagnosis and treatment of severe hematochezia. The role of urgent colonoscopy after purge. Gastroenterology 1988; 95:1569–1574.
4. Jensen DM. Current management of severe lower gastrointestinal bleeding. Gastrointest Endosc 1995; 11:171–173.
5. Jensen DM, Machicado GA. Colonoscopy for diagnosis and treatment of severe lower gastrointestinal bleeding. Gastrointest Endosc Clin North Am 1997; 7:477–498.
6. Kok KY, Kum CK, Goh PM. Colonoscopic evaluation of severe hematochezia in an Oriental population. Endoscopy 1998; 8:675–680.
7. Wilcox CM, Clark WS. Causes and outcome of upper and lower gastrointestinal bleeding: the Grady Hospital experience. South Med J 1999; 92:44–50.
8. Chaudry V, Hyser MJ, Gracias VH, et al. Colonoscopy: the initial test for acute lower gastrointestinal bleeding. Am Surg 1998; 64:723–728.
9. Wagner HE, Stain SC, Gilg MGP. Systematic assessment of massive bleeding of the lower part of the gastrointestinal tract. Surg Gynecol Obstet 1999; 175:445–449.
10. Jaramillo E, Slezak P. Comparison between double-contrast barium enema and colonoscopy to investigate lower gastrointestinal bleeding. Gastrointest Radiol 1992; 17:81–83.
11. Vernava AM, Moore BA, Longo WE, et al. Lower gastrointestinal bleeding. Dis Colon Rectum 1997; 40:846–858.
12. Billingham RP. The conundrum of lower gastrointestinal bleeding. Surg Clin North Am 1997; 77:241–252.
13. Zuckerman GR, Prakash C. Acute lower intestinal bleeding: Part 1: Clinical presentation and diagnosis. Gastrointest Endosc 1998; 48:606–616.
14. Schrock TR. Colonoscopic diagnosis and treatment of lower gastrointestinal bleeding. Surg Clin North Am 1989; 69:1309–1325.
15. American Society for Gastrointestinal Endoscopy Guidelines: The role of endoscopy in the patient with lower gastrointestinal bleeding. Gastrointest Endosc 1998; 48:685–688.
16. Wang CY, Won CW, Shieh MJ. Aggressive colonoscopic approaches to lower intestinal bleeding. Gastroenterol J 1991; 26(Suppl 3):125–128.
17. Davis GR, Santa-Ana CA. Development of a lavage solution with minimal water and electrolyte absorption and secretion. Gastroenterology 1979; 78:991–995.
18. Campbell WB, Rhodes M, Kettlewell MG. Colonoscopy following intraoperative lavage in the management of severe colonic bleeding. Ann R Coll Surg Engl 1985; 67:219–222.
19. Scott HJ, Lane IF, Glynn MJ. Colonic hemorrhage – a technique for rapid intra-operative bowel preparation and colonoscopy. Br J Surg 1986; 73:390–391.
20. Cussons PD, Berry AR. Comparison of the value of emergency mesenteric angiography and intraoperative colonoscopy with

antegrade colonic irrigation in massive rectal haemorrhage. J R Coll Surg Edinb 1989; 34:91–93.

21. Browder W, Cerise EJ, Litwin MS. Impact of emergency angiography in massive lower gastrointestinal bleeding. Ann Surg 1986; 204:530–535.

22. Dill JE. Vasopressin in postpolypectomy bleeding. Gastrointest Endosc 1987; 33:399.

23. Adrain AL, Krevsky B. Endoscopy in patients with gastrointestinal bleeding of obscure origin. Dig Dis 1996; 14:345–355.

24. Vakil N, Huilgol V, Khan I. Effect of push enteroscopy on transfusion requirements and quality of life in patients with unexplained gastrointestinal bleeding. Am J Gastroenterol 1997; 92:425–428.

25. Setya V, Singer JA, Minken SL. Subtotal colectomy as a last resort for unrelenting, unlocalised lower gastrointestinal haemorrhage: experience with 12 cases. Am Surg 1992; 58:295–299.

26. Kim YI, Marcon NE. Injection therapy for colonic diverticular bleeding. A case study. J Clin Gastroenterol 1993; 17:46–48.

27. Bemvenuti GA, Julich MM. Ethanolamine injection for sclerotherapy of angiodysplasia of the colon. Endoscopy 1998; 30:564–569.

28. Dyer WS, Quigley EMM, Noel SM, et al. Case report: Major colonic haemorrhage following electrocoagulating (hot) biopsy of diminutive colonic polyps: relationship to colonic location and low-dose aspirin therapy. Gastrointest Endosc 1991; 37:361–364.

29. Williams CB. Small polyps – the virtues and dangers of hot biopsy. Gastrointest Endosc 1991; 37:394–395.

30. Danesh BJZ, Spiliadis C, Williams CB, et al. Angiodysplasia – an uncommon cause of colonic bleeding; colonoscopic evaluation of 1050 patients with rectal bleeding and anaemia. Int J Colorect Dis 1987; 2:218–222.

31. Conio M, Gostout CJ. Argon plasma coagulation (APC) in gastroenterology; experimental and clinical experiences – commentary. Gastrointest Endosc 1998; 48:109–110.

32. Hoyer N, Thouet R, Zellweger U. Massive pneumoperitoneum after endoscopic argon plasma coagulation. Endoscopy 1998; 30:S44–45.

33. Mathus-Vliegen EMH. Laser treatment of intestinal vascular abnormalities. Int J Colorect Dis 1989; 4:20–25.

34. Pfaffenbach B, Adamek RJ, Wegener M. Endoscopic band ligation for treatment of post-polypectomy bleeding. Z Gastroenterol 1996; 34:241–242.

35. Pontecorvo C, Pesce G. The 'safety snare' – a ligature placing snare to prevent haemorrhage after transection of large pedunculated polyps. Endoscopy 1986; 18:55–56.

36. Richter JM, Christensen MR, Kaplan LM. Effectiveness of current technology in the diagnosis and management of lower gastrointestinal hemorrhage. Gastrointest Endosc 1999; 41:93–98.

37. Gadetatter M, Wetscher G, Crookes PF, et al. Dieulafoy's disease of the large and small bowel. J Clin Gastroenterol 1998; 27:169–172.

38. Slivka A, Parsons WG, Carr-Locke DL. Endoscopic band ligation for treatment of post-polypectomy haemorrhage. Gastrointest Endosc 1994; 40:230–232.

39. Smith RE, Doull J. Treatment of post-colonoscopy bleeding site by endoscopic band ligation. Gastrointest Endosc 1994; 40:499–503.

40. Rex DK, Lewis BS, Waye JD. Colonoscopy and endoscopic therapy for delayed post-polypectomy hemorrhage. Gastrointest Endosc 1992; 38:127–129.

41. Waye JD, Kahn O, Auerbach ME. Complications of colonoscopy and flexible sigmoidoscopy. Gastroenterol Clin North Am 1996; 6:343–377.

42. Ramirez FC, Johnson DA, Zierer ST, et al. Successful endoscopic hemostasis of bleeding colonic diverticula with epinephrine injection. Gastrointest Endosc 1996; 43:167–170.

43. Savides TJ, Jensen DM. Colonoscopic hemostasis for recurrent diverticular hemorrhage associated with a visible vessel: a report of three cases. Gastrointest Endosc 1994; 40:70–73.

44. Guy GE, Shetty PC, Sharma RP, et al. Acute lower gastrointestinal hemorrhage: treatment by superselective embolization with polyvinyl alcohol particles. Am J Roentgenol 1992; 159:521–526.

45. Harford WV. Gastrointestinal angiodysplasia: clinical features. Endoscopy 1988; 20:144–148.

46. Chapuis PH, Bokey E, Galt E, et al. The development of a treatment protocol for patients with chronic radiation-induced rectal bleeding. Aust N Z J Surg 1996; 66:680–685.

47. Roche B, Chauterns R, Marti M. Application of formaldehyde for treatment of haemorrhagic radiation-induced proctitis. World J Surg 1996; 20:1094–1095.

14.
PROCTOLOGIC INTERVENTION

JOHN HARTLEY

PETER LEE

INTRODUCTION

This chapter will discuss the ambulatory endoscopic management of hemorrhoids, including the most recent technique developed in this field which is stapled hemorrhoidectomy, before summarizing the continued development of techniques for transanal excision of rectal neoplasms. Finally, the techniques available for the endoscopic palliation of rectal malignancy will be reviewed.

AMBULATORY ENDOSCOPICE MANAGEMENT OF HEMORRHOIDS

Now considered to be disordered anal cushions,[1] hemorrhoids continue to be one of the commonest medical problems of Western civilization; no age group is excluded but it seems likely that half of all people over the age of 50 years have some degree of hemorrhoidal formation.[2] Although perhaps mundane when compared to other more sophisticated treatment modalities described in this book, the endoscopic management of hemorrhoids remains an important part of the practice of both medical and surgical proctology.

INDICATIONS

Symptoms are the indication for the treatment of hemorrhoids; invasive treatment of symptomatic hemorrhoids is unnecessary. The common presenting features which demand outpatient endoscopic treatment are those of bright red rectal bleeding, anal discomfort, prolapse, mucus or fecal-mucus leakage, and pruritus ani. Perhaps 90% of all symptomatic patients can be treated on an ambulant outpatient basis with only a relatively small number now progressing to formal excisional hemorrhoidectomy.[3] Although some have attempted to relate choice of out-patient treatment to quantifiable

parameters – e.g. anal pressure measurements – most decisions as to the appropriate choice of treatment are made on clinical assessment alone, and it is inevitable therefore that the choice of treatment remains variable and subject to individual physician assessment, preference, and experience.

The appropriate modality of treatment is based on the presenting degree of hemorrhoids as classified by Goligher (Table 14.1).[5]

EQUIPMENT

Because the diagnosis of hemorrhoids is often made at the initial consultation and treatment instituted immediately, it is essential that the equipment necessary for each favored mode of treatment should be immediately available. This demands that the proctologist has a comprehensive, well-organized equipment cart at the side of the examination couch, within hand's reach (Figs 14.1 and 14.2). A suggested list of contents is:

— Disposable sigmoidoscopes
— Proctoscopes – small, large
— Appropriate light source – either fiberoptic or movable direct
— Disposable hemorrhoidal syringes
— Sclerosant fluid
— Bivalve speculum
— Long dissecting forceps
— Cotton balls/gauze squares/tissues
— Topical epinephrine
— Banding gun, rubber bands, loader and grasper
— Infrared coagulator
— Gloves
— Lubricating jelly
— Long cleansing pledgets.

It is recommended that because of transmissible disease and current health regulations regarding sterilization as much as possible of this equipment be totally *disposable*.

Classification and treatment of hemorrhoids		
Classification of hemorrhoids	Definition	Treatment
First degree	Small hemorrhoids projecting slightly into the anal canal when the veins are congested at defecation	Dietary control/injection/infrared coagulation
Second degree	Large swelling protruding into the anal canal and descending toward the anal orifice on straining but returning to the anal canal spontaneously when straining ceases	Small: injection/infrared coagulation Large: banding
Third degree	The pile masses prolapse readily at defacation and remain prolapsed until digitally replaced	No significant external component: banding *Large external component: hemorrhoidectomy

* The external components of the internal hemorrhoid are the skin tags and large, thickened anal cushions which are usually the accompaniment of long-standing hemorrhoids. Internal hemorrhoids which are permanently prolapsed – Goligher's so-called fourth-degree hemorrhoids – are not included in the outpatient regimen as they are considered more suitable for formal excisional hemorrhoidectomy.

Table 14.1 Classification and treatment of hemorrhoids

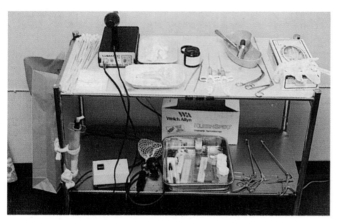

Fig. 14.1 Equipment cart for treatment of hemorrhoids.

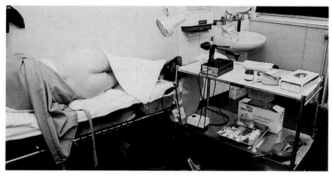

Fig. 14.2 Equipment cart, patient position, and lighting.

PATIENT PREPARATION

It is not necessary for the patient routinely to undergo any preoperative bowel preparation for the outpatient management of hemorrhoids. Indeed, such preparation may adversely affect the initial endoscopic examination by removing traces of blood or masking a mild proctitis. It is accepted that on the rare occasion when fecal loading or loose bowel contents makes treatment difficult that rectal evacuation with enemas or suppositories may be necessary with subsequent re-examination and treatment.

PROCEDURES

Injection sclerotherapy

The patient is placed in the left lateral position with the buttocks elevated on a small cushion. Other positions, such as the knee–elbow position, are also possible. Full anorectal examination is completed. A 3.5 mm diameter proctoscope (Fig. 14.3) is inserted and the main hemorrhoidal complexes identified (Fig. 14.4). Five to 10 mL of sclerosant fluid (phenol BP 5% w/v in almond oil BP 1973 or equivalent sclerosant) is prepared in a disposable hemorrhoidal syringe and a long bevelled needle is attached, either straight or angled according to preference (Fig. 14.5). The needle is inserted into the apex or the proximal aspect of the pile mass in a submucus position and 3–5 mL of sclerosant fluid injected (Figs 14.6 and 14.7). Initially, it is advisable to draw back on the syringe to avoid direct venous injection; if the needle is situated too deep, no visible weal will accompany the injection; if too superficial, the mucosa will become white; in each case, the needle should be repositioned as necessary.

After the initial injection, usually of the right anterior or left lateral hemorrhoid, better access to the remaining hemorrhoids may be obtained by placing a small cotton pledget over the previous injection site; this may also serve to control leakage of the sclerosant to some extent. It is usual to inject three sites for the initial course of treatment (right anterior, right posterior, and left lateral) using a total of approximately 10 mL of sclerosant fluid. Re-examination at 6 weeks is suggested when re-injection may occasionally be necessary for continued symptoms. If the injections have been placed correctly in the submucus position, each subsequent set of injections becomes progressively more difficult because of the consequent fibrosis and care must be taken not to inject intramucosally.

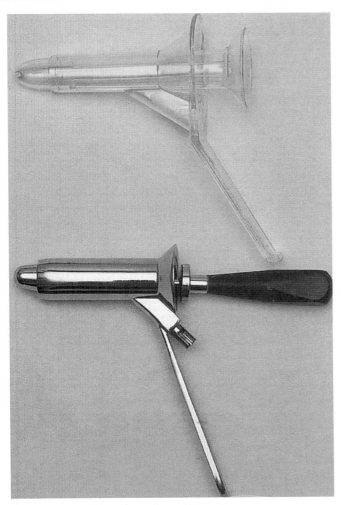

Fig. 14.3 Disposable and non-disposable proctoscopes.

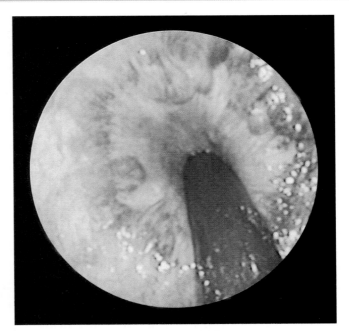

Fig. 14.4 Internal view of the hemorrhoidal ring.

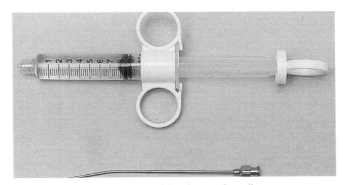

Fig. 14.5 Disposable hemorrhoidal syringe and needle.

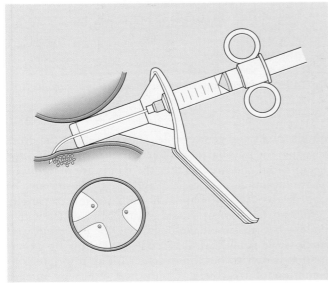

Fig. 14.6 Injection of sclerosant fluids at apex of hemorrhoid mass.

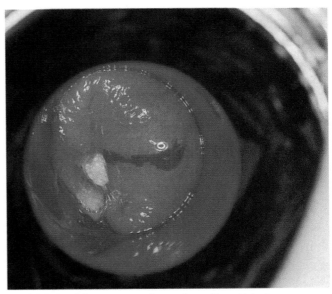

Fig. 14.7 'Cystic' appearance of correctly positioned injection.

Complications and their management

The commonest complications are:

— transient anorectal discomfort
— small amounts of rectal bleeding.

The patient may complain of mild discomfort during the injection procedure; if the procedure is painful, then the injection is in the incorrect place, either too deep or too superficial. It is not uncommon for the patient to complain of faintness or dizziness after the procedure. This usually subsides rapidly. Small amounts of bright red bleeding may occur from the injection site in the first 24 hours post-injection and the patient should be warned of this and also of the possibility of an aching discomfort within the rectum – best alleviated by warm bathing and simple analgesics. Rectal bleeding and pain at a later stage (2 to 3 weeks) may be evidence of a post-injection ulcer, a rare occurrence usually caused by injection of too large a volume of oil. This will settle down on conservative management with local steroid/anesthetic foams and laxatives if necessary. Submucus abscess formation, hematuria (caused by too deep an injection of the right anterior hemorrhoid penetrating the prostatic capsule), fibrous stricture formation, and paraffinoma have all been recorded but are extremely rare.[6]

Rubber banding

The patient position and proctoscope insertion are identical to those for injection sclerotherapy. It is helpful to have available at least two preloaded banding guns of the Barrons or McIveny type (Fig. 14.8). The conventional hemorrhoidal grasping instrument provided with the guns is in practice too short and it is more convenient to use a short biopsy forceps. Two hands are necessary for the procedure so it is helpful to have a nurse or assistant to hold the proctoscope in place; however, it is quite satisfactory to ask the patient to hold the proctoscope with the right hand. The banding gun is loaded with two rubber bands using the plastic conical attachment supplied. The grasping instrument is then placed through the barrel of the gun and the pile mass grasped at its most

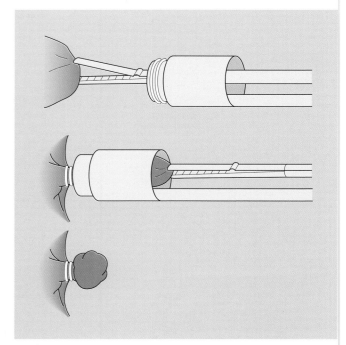

Fig. 14.9 Technique of hemorrhoidal banding.

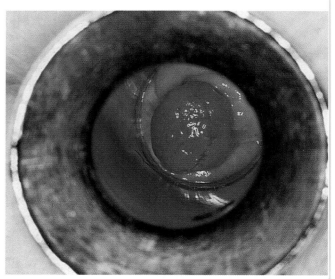

Fig. 14.10 Immediate post-banding appearance of hemorrhoids.

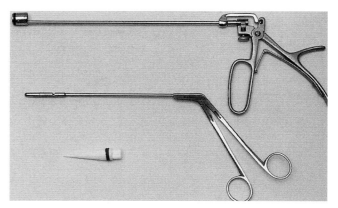

Fig. 14.8 Barron banding gun, applicator, and grasping forceps.

mobile point and gently pulled into the end of the proctoscope; the gun barrel is then slid over the positioned hemorrhoid and fired so that the bands are placed well above the anoderm (Figs 14.9 and 14.10). Positioning of one or two sets of bands at each session is usually sufficient. The patient should always be provided with a patient information leaflet regarding the procedure and its possible complications (see Box). Follow-up examination is carried out at 6 weeks with appropriate continuation of treatment if indicated either by further banding or by injections.

Complications and their management

The common complications are:

— initial post-banding discomfort
— severe immediate post-banding discomfort
— light rectal bleeding for 4 to 5 days after the pile
   sloughs off.

Less common, but more important complications are:

— significant secondary rectal hemorrhage
— urinary retention
— late severe intrarectal pain and sepsis.

The complication rate following rubber band ligation
is low. If the patient complains of severe pain immediately
post-banding, then the bands have been placed too low and
should be removed immediately. This is not easy but is best
accomplished by re-inserting the proctoscope, steadying
the bands with a long straight artery forceps, and cutting
the bands through with a 15 or 11 gauge scalpel mounted
on a long handle. Approximately 5% of patients will complain of minor complications[7] which include intrarectal discomfort, minor bleeding, early slippage of the bands and,
less commonly, prolapsed thrombosed hemorrhoids, minor
urinary difficulties, and rarely priapism. The complication
rate appears to be related to the number of hemorrhoids
banded at each session.

More severe complications will occur in approximately
2 to 3% of cases,[7,8] the most frequent of which is significant
rectal bleeding requiring hospitalization, transfusion, and
oversewing of the bleeding point under general anesthesia.
This usually occurs around 10 days after the banding procedure with a frequency of approximately 1 in 600 banding procedure-s. Severe persistent intrarectal pain must
always be regarded seriously because of the rare development of life-threatening pelvic sepsis.[9] The pain may indicate the development of complicated thrombosis
progressing to an abscess, fistula, or ulcer. The patient
should be examined under general anesthesia, the bands
removed, and treatment with intravenous antibiotics
instituted. Urinary catheterization may be required if
appropriate.

Infrared coagulation

Infrared coagulation was introduced for the treatment of
first- and second-degree hemorrhoids by Neiger[10] as an
alternative to injection sclerotherapy or banding. An
infrared delivery system specifically designed for the treatment of hemorrhoids is required (Fig. 14.11) (Infrarot
Koagulator, MBB-AT). The system delivers infrared radiation from a 14 V halogen bulb via a focused photocon-
ductor to a polymer-coated non-tissue-adhesive cap
(Fig. 14.11). A timing device and power adjuster allow a
measured amount of radiation to be delivered to the hemorrhoidal site producing a well-defined 3 mm white disc of

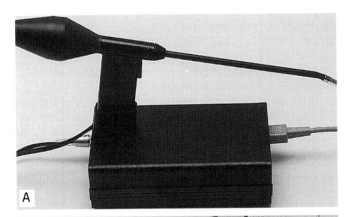

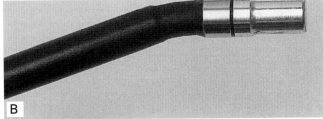

Fig. 14.11 (A) Infrared coagulator system; (B) polymer-coated
non-tissue-adhesive cap.

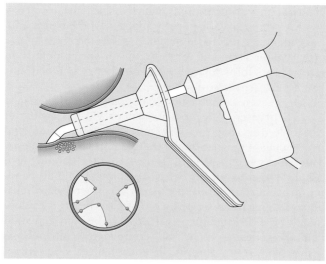

Fig. 14.12 Positioning of infrared coagulation sites.

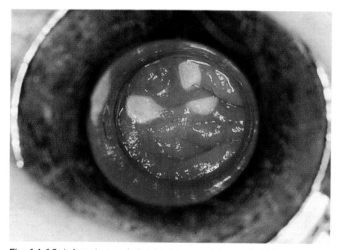

Fig. 14.13 Infrared coagulation burns around hemorrhoidal mass.

coagulated tissue extending through the full thickness of the mucosa for some 3 mm.

The patient and proctoscope position are as previously described. The coagulator tip is placed flat on the mucosa at the apex of the pile in the position similar to that used for injection sclerotherapy. The infrared coagulator is applied for a fixed 1-second period. The procedure is repeated for a total of three applications at each pile mass in the positions as shown in Figures 14.12 and 14.13. After repeated use, the copolymer tip may become burned through and is easily replaced. Sterilization procedures for the instrument should be adhered to in accordance with manufacturer's instructions.

Complications

The advantage of infrared coagulation would seem to be that it is almost complication-free.[8,11] A slight warmth is felt by the patient at the time of the coagulation; significant post-treatment pain is minimal although slight rectal bleeding may occur usually at 10 to 14 days after the treatment.

Cryosurgery

A liquid nitrogen probe (freezing to −196°C) (Fig. 14.14) or a nitrous oxide probe (KeyMed) (freezing to −89°C) is required, capable of producing a visible ice ball of sufficient size to encompass the hemorrhoidal mass.

The procedure can be carried out with anesthesia, under perineal block, or under general anesthesia depending on the fitness of the patient, the size of the hemorrhoidal mass, and the degree of external component.[12–14] Contact of the ice ball with the skin component of a hemorrhoidal plexus produces severe pain and will dictate the form of anesthesia required.

The patient is placed in the left lateral position and the internal hemorrhoidal plexus visualized using a split proctoscope of the Clifton type or a Hill Ferguson-type retractor; some prefer to use a plastic vaginal-type speculum because of cold conduction via a metal instrument. The flattened side of the probe (Fig. 14.14) is covered with water-soluble jelly and placed along the long axis of the hemorrhoidal mass. If the probe is conical, then the tip is covered with jelly and positioned at the center of the hemorrhoid. The freezing process is then applied until the ice ball envelops the pile – this is seen as a slowly advancing white plaque. The freezing time is usually of approximately 2 minutes duration. The probe is then reheated and removed when it will lift off without adhesion or trauma. The process is then repeated at the other primary hemorrhoidal sites, usually dealing with three sites at one session. Protagonists of the method would advise that a similar procedure can be used to freeze and destroy any accompanying skin tags.

The patient is warned that local swelling may occur and that a watery discharge will commence a few hours after the procedure. They are provided with absorbent pads to wear over the perineal region, advised to bathe at least daily, and change the pads as and when necessary. The patient is reviewed at 6 weeks and further cryo-destruction applied as necessary.

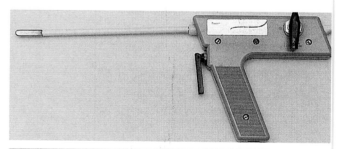

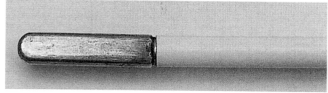

Fig. 14.14 Cryosurgical hemorrhoid probe.

Complications

The following complications have been recorded:

— pain
— local swelling and edema
— watery discharge
— hemorrhage
— urinary difficulties
— fecal impaction.

The degree of pain experienced is probably related to whether or not anoderm or skin tags have been involved in the freezing process; if the probe is applied to the internal plexus only then only discomfort is experienced.[15] Local swelling and edema occur in the first 24 hours after the procedure and a watery discharge may start within a few hours. The degree of discharge varies from series to recorded series and may be profuse on the first 3 to 4 days; the liquid nitrogen probe, which causes more tissue necrosis, may be responsible for this being more of a problem.[14] Hemorrhage does not seem to be a significant complication of cryohemorrhoidectomy[13] although Oh[16] did report two such incidents in his initial series of 100 cases. Urinary difficulties have been reported as has fecal impaction.[17]

Laser hemorrhoidectomy

The controlled tissue destruction achieved by the application of laser energy, together with the easy accessibility of hemorrhoids to the laser beam, would seem to offer advantages for this mode of treatment, perhaps somewhat driven by patient demand for sophisticated 'high tech' treatment. Although used in Japan[18] and apparently widely available on an outpatient basis in the USA,[19] there is little yet available in the way of controlled clinical trials on which to base an evaluation, especially in its use for hemorrhoids on an outpatient basis. The Nd:YAG laser (Fig. 14.15), the carbon dioxide laser (Fig. 14.16), or a combination of both have been used in non-contact mode using a 'brushing' technique for the internal component of hemorrhoids. It is suggested that this internal component is better photocoagulated by the Nd:YAG laser producing a relatively painless fibrosis and shrinkage, while the external component is better vaporized by the deformed beam of the CO_2 laser, the latter producing a more superficial injury because of energy absorption within the cells.[18]

The patient is placed in the lithotomy position and each pile mass displayed using a dull bivalve speculum. The internal hemorrhoid is photocoagulated with the Nd:YAG

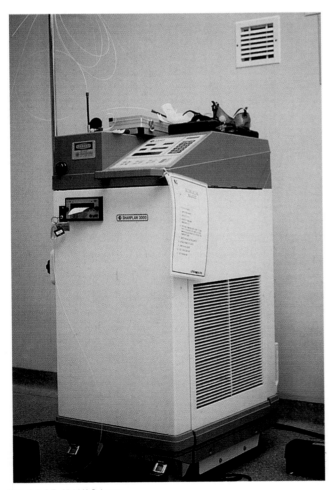

Fig. 14.15 Nd:YAG laser.

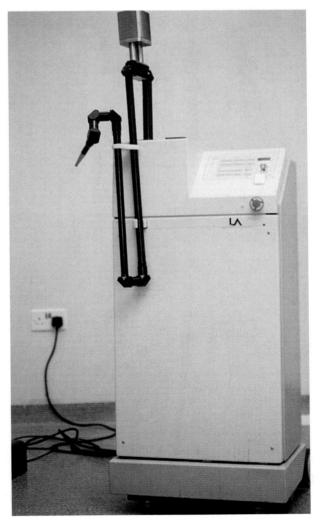

Fig. 14.16 Carbon dioxide laser.

laser from apex to base in a criss-cross, brushing motion in a non-contact manner. The power of the laser is set at 25 W with a 0.6 second pulse time, using a 3 mm diameter spot size by holding the fiber tip approximately 2 cm away from the hemorrhoidal mass. The brushing process is repeated until the hemorrhoid base becomes gray, shrunken, and flat (Fig. 14.17). The external component is then vaporized using the CO_2 laser using a non-focused, non-contact beam, the energy being applied until the tissue becomes shrunken and white (Fig. 14.18).

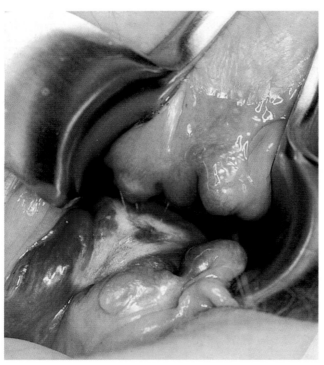

Fig. 14.17 Nd:YAG laser effect on internal hemorrhoidal component.

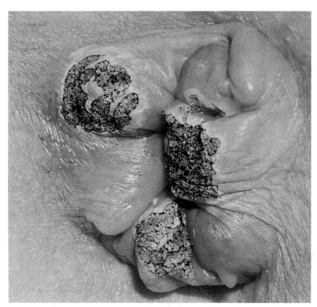

Fig. 14.18 Carbon dioxide laser effect on external component of hemorrhoid.

Complications and their management

The following complications can occur:

— local swelling and edema
— watery discharge
— pain
— formation of skin tags
— residual hemorrhoidal tissue with persistent bleeding and discomfort.

The above complications have responded to the use of frequent warm bathing, simple oral analgesia, and local foam anesthetic (Proctofoam HC). Our experience so far indicates a greater discomfort, delay in healing, and poorer cosmetic and symptomatic end result when compared to standard ligation and excision.

Stapled hemorrhoidectomy

The technique of stapled hemorrhoidectomy as described by Longo is a new method for the control of hemorrhoidal disease which has been widely undertaken in Southern Europe but has yet to be embraced elsewhere.[20] The technique centers upon the use of the circular end-to-end anastomosis (CEEA) stapler to excise a ring of mucosa above the dentate line in order to reduce the prolapsing component of the hemorrhoidal cushions, reduce the blood supply to the hemorrhoidal complex, and act as a point of fixation. The procedure is commonly undertaken under caudal anesthesia. The hemorrhoidal cushions are grasped with tissue forceps and prolapsed in order to display the dentate line. A stout pursestring suture is inserted 2–3 cm above the dentate line, the gun is then inserted in the open position, closed, and then fired. In this way, a ring of mucosa is excised above the dentate line. This draws up the external component of the hemorrhoidal complex into the anal canal, as well as excising the blood supply to these complexes and leaves a circumferential staple line above the dentate line (Fig. 14.19). This staple line is checked for hemostasis and an adsorbable hemostatic plug inserted.

Because all intervention is undertaken above the dentate line, this procedure has the potential to be pain-free and has therefore generated much excitement amongst coloproctologists in Europe. The procedure is in the early

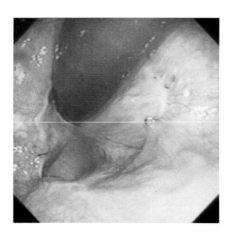

Fig. 14.19 Circumferential staple line above the dentate line following stapled hemorrhoidectomy.

stages of its clinical evaluation and should be considered unproven. However, if the technique is shown to be efficacious in terms of pain control and relief of symptoms, then it carries the potential to revolutionize the management of hemorrhoidal disease.

RESULTS

Injection sclerotherapy

Despite its wide use, there is relatively little information available regarding the long-term results of hemorrhoidal injection. Milligan[21,22] reported that at 5-year follow-up 98.3% of patients with first-degree hemorrhoids and 68% of those with second-degree hemorrhoids were asymptomatic, but that 15% and 38% respectively required injection between 1 and 3 years later. Greca et al[23] reported a 70% incidence of symptom relief in a series of mainly second-degree hemorrhoids when assessed at 1 year. Dencker et al[24] reported poor results with injection sclerotherapy with only 21% being symptom-free at 1 year, while Alexander-Williams & Crapp[25] felt it was only suitable for first-degree hemorrhoids and gave only short-term relief.

There are a limited number of trials available comparing injection to other modalities. Leicester et al[26] showed it to be less effective than infrared coagulation in non-prolapsing hemorrhoids, while Gartell et al[27] compared injection sclerotherapy to rubber banding and found the latter to be superior. Collectively the complication rate is very low and practically confined to only post-injection aching; the effects are relatively short-term and re-injection may be required. Injections are really only suitable for first- and second-degree hemorrhoids without a significant degree of prolapse.

Rubber band ligation

Several large series of rubber band ligation treatment are available. Bartizol & Slosberg[28] report on 670 patients with an incidence of pain in 4%, slight bleeding in 4% and significant bleeding in 1%. Assessment of these patients is not long-term but Steinberg et al[29] report that after a mean of 4.8 years after banding 89% of 125 patients considered themselves cured or satisfied but with only 44% completely symptom-free. Wrobleski et al,[30] Geharny & Weakley et al[31] and Lau et al[32] with much larger series report patients to be symptom-free or symptomatically improved in 70 to 90% of cases, with the most significant complications being pain (4 to 29%) and significant bleeding (1 to 3.5%).

Infrared coagulation

There are no long-term results available for the use of infrared coagulation alone; those treatment results available are in comparative trials with other modalities and give results at a maximum of 1 year. The apparent superiority of infrared coagulation over sclerotherapy has been shown by Leicester et al[26] and Ambrose et al[33]. Infrared coagulations has been extensively compared to rubber band ligation: Leicester et al[11] showed it to compare favorably with rubber band ligation in most prolapsing hemor-

rhoids. Keighley[8] in a series of 255 patients reported that infrared coagulation was almost as effective as rubber band ligation in first- and second-degree hemorrhoids and was associated with few complications. His results were reported at 4-month follow-up and showed that repeat treatment was necessary more often in the infrared coagulation group.

Templeton et al,[34] reviewing a series of patients with first- and second-degree hemorrhoids at between 3 months and 1 year, showed a satisfactory symptomatic result in 85% of a series of 66 patients treated with infrared coagulation compared to a 92% satisfactory result with 71 patients treated with rubber band ligation. They comment that the incidence of side effects was much greater with the rubber band group (especially discomfort) and that the number of treatments did not significantly differ between the two. Ambrose et al[35] in a similar series of 286 patients with first-and second-degree hemorrhoids again showed no difference in the symptomatic outcome assessed at 1 year, and confirmed a greater incidence of pain and bleeding with the rubber band group but showed that more treatment sessions were required with infrared coagulation.

Overall, it would appear that for first- and second-degree hemorrhoids, infrared coagulation is superior to injection sclerotherapy and as good as rubber band ligation, with more minor side effects but increased frequency of treatment being required.

Cryosurgery

Cryosurgery for the treatment of hemorrhoids was first reported in the later 1960s and since then many series have been reviewed.[36,37] In Wilson's[37] series of 100 patients, again treated as inpatients but without general anesthesia, 94 were found to be satisfactory at 3 months, 4 of them progressing to formal hemorrhoidectomy. In all cases, discharge was reported in the first few post-treatment days; 1 patient complained of pain in the first 5 days and 2 of pain later on. Kaufman's[38] series of 100 patients was said to have an 89% success rate at 2 months. Twenty percent complained of internal pain, 13% of edema, and 10% of post-treatment bleeding. Oh[39] has reported a series of 1000 cases and felt that pain and prolonged discharge were disadvantages of the treatment. Traynor & Carter[40] similarly reported profuse discharge in over two-thirds of patients and was disappointed with its effect on external skin tags. Overall, it would appear that banding or infrared coagulation have marked advantages over cryotherapy without the necessity for local or general anesthetic and with many fewer accompanying side effects. This opinion would be borne out by our own experiences and compounded by the relatively infrequent usage of this technique in current proctoscopic practice worldwide.

Laser

Leff[41] has reported a series of 170 patients who underwent laser hemorrhoidectomy on an outpatient basis using the CO_2 laser; some 10% of them required a subsequent stay of over 24 hours; 75% of the patients healed without problems. Urinary problems and fecal impaction were complications occurring in 14% and 6% respectively. Three of the patients suffered significant postoperative rectal bleeding when compared to a hemorrhoidectomy also performed on an outpatient basis; the postoperative pain appeared little different. Sanker & Joffe[42] have reported less pain and quicker return to work using the Nd:YAG laser.

It seems possible that the Nd:YAG laser treatment of internal hemorrhoids driven by patient demand will produce satisfactory results but there is no available data as yet to back this up. There always remain the disadvantages of expensive equipment, special training, and possibility of complications related to the laser energy itself, all of which will mitigate against its use instead of injections, infrared coagulation, or banding.

Stapled hemorrhoidectomy

To date there are no peer-reviewed publications concerning this technique. However, a variety of conference proceedings have appeared.[20,43,44] These, in the main, detail case series and report minimal postoperative pain, a low incidence of complications, and good symptoms control up to several months follow-up. A randomized trial undertaken within our own institution of stapled hemorrhoidectomy versus the standard Milligan–Morgan type procedure has shown the former procedure to be safe and well tolerated and to carry significant advantages in terms

of pain control and early return to normal activity.[45] There is as yet, however, insufficient clinical follow-up to determine the utility of the procedure for control of the hemorrhoidal complex.

Thus, at present, the role of stapled hemorrhoidectomy is unclear. It appears likely to be superior to conventional hemorrhoidectomy with regard to pain control and recovery time, and if it is shown to be comparable to standard techniques in terms of control of hemorrhoids, then one might anticipate a paradigm shift in the indications for surgical hemorrhoidectomy.

TRANSANAL ENDOSCOPIC MICROSURGERY

Villous or adenomatous polyps of the lower third of the rectum have been variously treated by prolapse and excision, snare removal via the operating endoscope,[46] and elevation and excision using a variety of per anal retractors.[47] Those lesions lying above the lower third, i.e. 6 cm from the anal verge, have proved much more difficult to treat adequately because of problems of access, and have traditionally been treated with either a low anterior resection or a local operative approach such as the Localio abdominosacral[48] or the York–Mason transphincteric approach.[49]

A modified endoscopic approach called transanal endoscopic microsurgery (TEM) offers an alternative resection technique for selected adenomas, villous adenomas, and perhaps some locally confined carcinomas lying 6–20 cm from the anal verge.[50] Larger lesions in the lower third of the rectum are probably still better treated as outlined above because of difficulties in positioning the TEM endoscope and maintaining gas flow. Lesions above this level suitable for removal may be localized or circumferential polyps and may be resected either submucosally or with a full thickness of the rectal wall, always remembering that the larger the lesions, the higher the incidence of frank malignant change within them. The design of the instruments, the development of the technique, and much of the presented data must be attributed to Buess et al in Germany.[51]

EQUIPMENT

A specially designed operating endoscope is available (Richard Wolf GMBH) (Fig. 14.20), incorporating a constant-flow CO_2 gas system to promote rectal distention, irrigation and suction, and an operating endpiece (Fig. 14.21) through which cutting diathermy and suture can be performed using a variety of specially designed instruments (Fig. 14.22). The development of a multipurpose cutting instrument which has suction, irrigation, and monopolar coagulation has aided in the ease of dissection and hemostasis. Three-dimensional vision of the operating field is obtained via a binocular lens system with a separate assistant side-channel which, if required,

---

CHECKLIST OF PRACTICE POINTS

1. Have all the necessary instruments, prepared and in working order, within easy reach.
2. Carry out a full anorectal examination with proctoscopy at its conclusion so that the hemorrhoids can be treated immediately if indicated.
3. Use injection sclerotherapy for first-degree and small second-degree hemorrhoids.
4. Inject a maximum of three sites at each session using not more than 3–5 mL at each site.
5. Pain accompanying the injection means it is in the wrong position.
6. Infrared coagulation can be used in preference to sclerotherapy if the instrument is available.
7. Rubber band ligation is the preferred treatment for internal hemorrhoids with significant prolapse.
8. Band one or two sites per session.
9. Remove the bands immediately if pain is experienced.
10. Always provide the patient with a full information sheet.
11. Cryosurgery would not seem to have any advantage over the other simpler procedures.
12. Laser treatment of hemorrhoids remains under review.

---

one of the capped operating ports has given much better access and allowed much more extensive controlled tumor destruction.

A single non-contact fiber with red guide light is used with an initial setting of 10 W at continuous mode. The laser is activated and moved over a limited area of the tumor in a brush-stroke pattern until the tumor is coagulated, first black and then white. It is often possible to then gently break off the coagulated tumor, control any bleeding with the laser, and then laser debulk the tumor further. Care must be taken when approaching the rectal wall not to perforate the tumor by too deep tissue destruction. As a working rule, always undercoagulate and repeat in 3 to 4 weeks' time if necessary. A good suction device is necessary alongside the laser fiber to remove the smoke. We have found it helpful to have the fiber held in a long slender metal suction probe with the laser tip protruding some 2–3 cm from the holding probe. This facilitates control.

Depending on the size and firmness of the tumor, increasing power wattage may be necessary, increasing by a factor of 10 W up to a maximum of 50 or 60 W. At the end of the procedure, a careful check is made for hemostasis. We routinely keep patients under observation for 24 hours in case of postoperative bleeding and because of their generally poor physical status.

Complications
Immediate

1. *Bleeding*. This is usually minor and controlled by further laser beam application. If from larger vessels, it may be better controlled by a standard diathermy probe using the long, round-tipped variety.
2. *Perforation*. This is best avoided by repeated laser tumor destruction. If intraperitoneal perforation occurs, then open excision of the tumor with all the attendant risk would have to be considered.
3. *Urine retention*. As with any pelvic procedure, this has occurred and necessitates short-term catheterization. It has not been our practice to catheterize patients routinely perioperatively.

Late

1. *Failure of treatment*. It has been accepted in some cases that local palliation has been unsuccessful in terms of symptom relief and anterior resection or abdominoperineal excision has been carried out. Unfortunately, in a significant number of cases, the anticipated complications of major surgery in the unfit elderly patient have then occurred.
2. *Fistulation* of an incompletely controlled tumor into the bladder or vagina has occurred following palliative treatment and necessitates reversion to more radical and less appropriate resectional procedures.

Urologic resectoscope
A standard 24 or 27 Fr urologic resectoscope is used together with 1.5% glycine delivery system. The anal plug can be adapted from a Lord's plastic dilator, as described above. The operation is performed under a general anesthetic with antibiotic prophylaxis and crossmatching. The resectoscope sheath with obturator is positioned in the anal plug and inserted into the anal canal. The obturator is removed and the resectoscope inserted and the glycine flow commenced. The tumor resection is carried out in exactly the same manner as for a prostatic tumor starting at the proximal margin of the tumor and working distally. If excessive bleeding occurs, then this can be controlled with the ball electrode or tamponaded by use of a 24 Fr Foley catheter placed through the anus and inflated with 30–50 mL of water. Again we have found it safer to carry out several repeated resections over a period of weeks rather than to risk perforation.

As our experience of laser has been more extensive, we have tended to use this method by choice, but the urologic resectoscope has the advantage of being much cheaper and more widely available and the necessary experience has often been obtained with previous urologic resections.

Complications In our small series, bleeding has been the most frequent complication and this has been controlled as described above. Urinary retention has occurred and we routinely catheterize the patient for 48 hours postoperatively. Larger reported series by Berry et al[55] and Wetherall et al[56] list disseminated intravascular coagulation, septicemia, intraperitoneal perforation, and rectovaginal fistulae as further complications.

These complications should be treated as appropriate, with open surgery being necessary in the last two cases.

CHECKLIST OF PRACTICE POINTS

1. Resectional removal rather than local palliation of the tumor mass remains the palliative treatment of choice if the patient's condition or prognosis permits it.
2. Careful preoperative assessment and medical treatment of this generally unfit group of patients should be carried out.
3. The risks and complications of the procedure and the necessity for repeated treatment sessions should be pointed out to the patients and their relatives.
4. The mode of palliation should be chosen appropriate to the size of tumor, degree of narrowing, the instruments available, and the preferred experience of the operator.
5. Repeated limited attempts at tumor destruction are preferred to the more risky 'over' resection or debulking.
6. Patients are best observed for 24 hours postoperatively.
7. Endoanal brachytherapy has been found to be helpful following the debulking or dilating palliation in many cases.

Dilation of stenosing lesions

This may be achievable by coagulation, laser, or resectoscope if the lumen is sufficient to allow instrument access. On infrequent occasions we have found that the safest method of widening of the tumor lumen over a defined length can be achieved by heat destruction using the BICAP heater probes. It is sometimes possible then to increase the tumor destruction by a second procedure with laser.

The procedure is carried out under general anesthesia. The tumor is viewed through the operating endoscope and the remaining lumen size estimated. The appropriate size of tumor probe is chosen, inspected, and tested by smearing with lubricating jelly and activating the probe at setting 3 with a 1-second duration. The jelly must be observed to boil. As the tumor is usually circumferential, the 360° probe is used of a size which will comfortably and gently pass into the tumor lumen. The probe is then activated for 2-second periods at setting 8 and repeated for 5 to 10 times until the tumor can be seen to coagulate. If necessary the probe can then be moved in a cephalad direction and the process repeated to widen the more proximal lumen. In the esophagus, the probe is often best placed with the use of guidewire under radiologic control but we have not found this necessary in the rectum. Rather than using increasing diameter probes at the same occasion, we have found it better to repeat the process at 3 to 4 weeks and often a wider lumen probe or the laser can be used.

Stenting of stenosing rectal lesions

An alternative for the palliation of both bulky exfoliative and stenosing malignant rectal lesions is to introduce a stent in a manner analogous to techniques more commonly used in the esophagus and biliary tree. The recent development of self-expanding metal mesh stents specifically designed for use in the colon and rectum have further facilitated this (Wallstent, Boston Scientific, St Albans, Herts, UK; Memotherm Enteral Stent, Bard, Letchworth, Herts, UK). The stent may be used in combination with laser therapy either prior to stent insertion to debulk tumor or widen the lumen or later to unblock the stent for tumor overgrowth.

The patient should have full bowel preparation if this is possible and receive prophylactic antibiotics. If necessary the procedure may be performed under intravenous sedation. A contrast enema is performed to delineate the stricture and, under fluoroscopic control, a flexible guidewire is passed across the lesion. A self-expanding stent is then passed across the guidewire and maneuvered into the correct position under radiologic control.

Complications associated with the procedure are perforation, stent displacement, and stent blockage. The latter problem has been managed by additional laser therapy or stent replacement. As a means of palliation, published data have been promising.[57,58]

Stenting for obstructed left-sided/rectosigmoid neoplasm

The use of expanding metal stents identical to those above has been introduced into the treatment of obstructed left-sided neoplasm as a means of temporary decompression

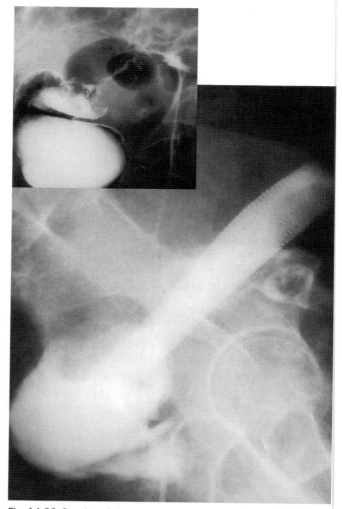

Fig. 14.30 Stenting of obstructing rectal carcinoma. Expandable metal stent in position through rectal neoplasm.

prior to definitive surgery.[59,60] This development has been driven by the recognized high mortality associated with the acutely obstructed colon, together with the attractive possibility of immediate resection and anastomosis rather than temporary 'defunctioning' surgery.

The stent is placed either by the procedure described above with contrast enema assessment and guidewire insertion of the stent or by the placement of the stent under colonoscopic control (Fig. 14.30).

Stent perforation is clearly a potential concern of this procedure, but appears to be sufficiently infrequent to justify further studies of this technique. Investigation by a randomized trial of stenting versus immediate surgery for obstructed left-sided colonic and rectosigmoid obstructions is imperative, but as yet not available.

ANAL FISSURE

Non-inflammatory-bowel-disease-related anal fissure is the second most commonly occurring benign pathology in practical proctology. It is related to an area of relative ischemia in the anal canal. It occurs equally in males and

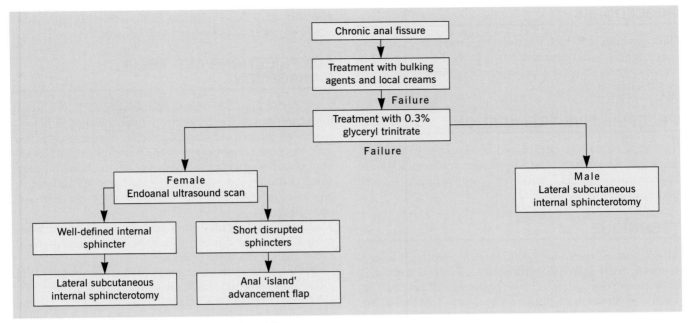

Fig. 14.31 Suggested treatment protocol for chronic anal fissure.

females, and more commonly posteriorly than anteriorly. Presenting typically with severe pain on and after defecation accompanied by bright red rectal bleeding, it is frequently, although not always, associated with an episode of either diarrhea or constipation with straining. Some 40% of fissures are acute and shallow and will heal spontaneously or with the use of bulking agents and local anesthetic creams. The classic chronic fissure is deeper, has fibrotic margins, often shows the internal sphincter as a white band in its base, and is accompanied by an external skin tag and a hypertrophic papilla at its apex.

Some recent reports[61] have detailed the success of glyceryl trinitrate paste in the healing of both acute and chronic fissure. Failure of conservative management necessitates surgical intervention (see Fig. 14.31).

ANAL ADVANCEMENT FLAP

This operation should be performed in the female patient with chronic anal fissure who, on endoanal ultrasound scanning, is shown to have either a short internal sphincter or any degree of external or internal sphincter disruption.

CHECKLIST OF PRACTICE POINTS

1. Use conservative management initially.
2. If conservative management fails, use lateral, internal sphincterotomy in the male (open technique).
3. Always perform an endoanal ultrasound scan of the anal sphincter in the female.
4. Use advancement flap technique if sphincters are short or disrupted.

BENIGN RECTAL STRICTURE

ETIOLOGY

The majority of benign rectal strictures are due to post-surgery anastomotic strictures, inflammatory bowel disease, and post-radiotherapy changes. The rare causes of rectal stricture should be remembered. This section primarily involves the management of anastomotic stricture, which occurs after some 8% of all anterior resections of the rectum. The incidence is higher in those anastomoses which have leaked, in those which have had a covering stoma in place, and probably in those performed by a double staple technique.

DIAGNOSIS

The stricture should be defined as such only if it is symptomatic and not on purely physical characteristics alone. Its position, length, and degree should *always* be defined, if necessary with a combination of examination under anesthesia, direct endoscopy with a rigid or a flexible sigmoidoscope, and by barium radiology. Local or recurrent disease *must* be excluded by direct or needle biopsy, cytology brushing, and MRI scanning.

CHECKLIST OF PRACTICE POINTS

1. Exclude malignant recurrence.
2. Do not treat unless symptomatic.
3. Define the length and configuration of the stricture.

PROCEDURES

Balloon dilation, which distends the narrow segment with incremental radial pressure has now replaced the use of finger or metal bougie dilation in the treatment of benign rectal stricture.

PREOPERATIVE PREPARATION

The patient should receive full mechanical bowel preparation. The use of broad-spectrum antibiotics should be considered. Light sedation is appropriate for the procedure.

TECHNIQUE

The patient is placed in the left lateral position. The rectum is initially opacified with water-soluble contrast and then air introduced to achieve double-contrast visualization over the entire length of the stricture. At this point, a straight 6 Fr catheter is introduced per rectum across the stricture with the aid of a 0.035 inch angiographic, J-tipped guidewire. If the anatomy is more complex, C-arm fluoroscopy can help to clarify the situation. In addition, tight or more complex strictures can be controlled using hydrophilic-angled guidewires (Turomo Corporation, Tokyo, Japan). The initial guidewire is exchanged for a stiffer guidewire such as Amplatz wire. A 2–3 cm balloon (Boston Scientific, Watertown, Ma., USA) is placed across the stricture under fluoroscopic guidance. Subsequent, gentle dilation is then undertaken and abolition of the balloon waisting is clearly visualized as the stricture opens up. Some gastroenterologists would prefer to place the balloon or the guidewire across the stricture under direct vision using a flexible sigmoidoscope together with fluoroscopic control.[63]

COMPLICATIONS AND THEIR MANAGEMENT

1. **Perforation** This may occur in up to 2% of cases.[63] Initial conservative management with continued antibiotic cover and intravenous fluid should be instituted, together with frequent reassessment of the patient's general condition and, in particular, the presence of the signs of generalized peritonitis. Development of the latter will necessitate operative intervention with drainage and fecal diversion and a stoma.

2. **Stenosis.** This may occur and require repeat dilations; the use of further dilation should be based on symptoms rather than endoscopic finding.

3. **Failed dilation.** Laser stricturoplasty, ureterotome or ERCP papillotomy knife,[64] urological resectoscope,[65] staple cutter,[66] Endo GIA stapler,[67] and a circular stapling instrument[68] have all been used to widen relatively short anastomotic strictures. Re-resection and an anastomosis or a loop stoma may have to be considered in the long-term failure.

CHECKLIST OF PRACTICE POINTS

1. Do not treat a stricture unless symptomatic.
2. Balloon dilation under radiological control is the initial treatment of choice.
3. Only use other stricture-relieving techniques if balloon dilation fails and if the stricture is short.

REFERENCES

1. Thomson WH. The nature of haemorrhoids. Br J Surg 1975; 62:542–552.

2. Goligher J. Surgery of the anus, rectum and colon. 5th ed. London: Baillière Tindall; 1984:98.

3. Anonymous. Outpatient treatment of haemorrhoids. BMJ 1975; 2:651.

4. Keighley MR, Buchmann P, Minervini S, et al. Prospective trials of minor surgical procedures and high-fibre diet for haemorrhoids. BMJ 1979; 2:967–969.

5. Goligher J. Surgery of the anus, rectum and colon. 5th ed. London: Baillière Tindall; 1984:101.

6. Goligher J. Surgery of the anus, rectum and colon. 5th ed. London: Baillière Tindall; 1984:112.

7. Bat L, Melzer E, Koler M, et al. Complications of rubber band ligation of symptomatic internal haemorrhoids. Dis Colon Rectum 1993; 36:287–290.

8. Keighley MR. Randomized trial to compare photocoagulation with rubber band ligation for treatment of haemorrhoids. Coloproctology 1982; 4:132–134.

9. Russell TR, Donohue JH. Haemorrhoidal banding: a warning. Dis Colon Rectum 1985; 28:291–293.

10. Neiger A. Haemorrhoids in everyday practice. Proctology 1979; 2:22–28.

11. Leicester RJ, Nicholls RJ, Mann CV. Infrared coagulation: a new treatment for haemorrhoids. Dis Colon Rectum 1981; 24:602–605.

12. Williams KL, Haq IU, Elem B. Cryodestruction of haemorrhoids. BMJ 1973; 1:666–668.

13. Kaufman HD. Outpatient treatment of haemorrhoids by cryotherapy. Br J Surg 1976; 63:462–463.

14. Wilson MC, Schofield P. Cryosurgical haemorrhoidectomy. Br J Surg 1976; 63:497–498.

15. Macleod JH. In defense of cryotherapy for hemorrhoids. A modified method. Dis Colon Rectum 1982; 25:332–335.

16. Oh C. The role of cryosurgery in management of anorectal disease: cryohemorrhoidectomy evaluated. Dis Colon Rectum 1975; 18:289–291.

17. O'Connor JJ. Cryohemorrhoidectomy: indications and complications. Dis Colon Rectum 1976; 19:41–43.

18. Wang JY, Chang-Chien CR, Chen JS, et al. The role of lasers in hemorrhoidectomy. Dis Colon Rectum 1991; 34:78–82.

19. Leff EI. Hemorrhoidectomy – laser vs nonlaser: outpatient surgical experience. Dis Colon Rectum 1992; 35:743–746.

20. Longo A.Treatment of hemorrhoids disease by reduction of mucosa and hemorrhoidal prolapse with a circular suturing device: a new procedure. Proceedings of the 6th World Congress of Endoscopic Surgery. Rome, Italy 3–6 June 1998.

21. Milligan ET. Haemorrhoids. BMJ 1939; 2:412.

22. Milligan ET. The treatment of haemorrhoids in recruits. Med Press Circ 1943; 210:84–85.

23. Greca F, Hares MM, Nevah J. A randomized trial to compare rubber band ligation with phenol injection for treatment of haemorrhoids. Br J Surg 1981; 68:250–252.

24. Dencker H, Hjorth N, Norryd C. Comparison of results obtained with different methods of treatment of internal haemorrhoids. Acta Chir Scan 1973; 139:742–745.

25. Alexander-Williams J, Crapp AR. Conservative management of haemorrhoids. Clin Gastroenterol 1975; 4:595–618.

26. Leicester RJ, Nicholls RJ, Chir M. Infrared coagulation: a new treatment for haemorrhoids. Dis Colon Rectum 1981; 24:602–605.

27. Gartell PC, Sheridan RJ, McGinn FP. Out-patient treatment of haemorrhoids: a randomized clinical trial to compare rubber band ligation with phenol injection. Br J Surg 1985; 72:478–479.

28. Bartizol J, Slosberg P. An alternative to haemorrhoidectomy. Arch Surg 1963; 105:563.

29. Steinberg DM, Liegois H, Alexander-Williams J. Long-term review of the results of rubber band ligation of haemorrhoids. Br J Surg 1975; 62:144–146.

30. Wrobleski DE, Corman ML, Veidenheimer MC. Long-term evaluation of rubber band ligation in haemorrhoidal disease. Dis Colon Rectum 1980; 23:478–482.

31. Geharny RA, Weakley FL. Internal haemorrhoidectomy by elastic ligation. Dis Colon Rectum 1974; 17:347–353.

32. Lau WY, Chow HP, Poon GP. Rubber band ligation of three primary haemorrhoids in a single session. A safe and effective procedure. Dis Colon Rectum 1982; 25:336–339.

33. Ambrose NS, Morris D, Alexander-Williams J. A randomized trial of photocoagulation or injection sclerotherapy for the treatment of first- and second-degree haemorrhoids. Dis Colon Rectum 1985; 28:238–240.

34. Templeton JL, Spence RA, Kennedy TL. Comparison of infrared coagulation and rubber band ligation for first and second degree haemorrhoids: a randomized prospective clinical trial. BMJ 1983; 286:1387–1389.

35. Ambrose NS, Hares MM, Alexander-Williams J. Prospective randomized comparison of photocoagulation and rubber band ligation in treatment of haemorrhoids. BMJ 1983; 286:1389–1391.

36. Williams KL, Haq IU, Elem B. Cryodestruction of haemorrhoids. Br Med J 1973; 1:666–668.

37. Wilson MC, Schofield P. Cryosurgical haemorrhoidectomy. Br J Surg 1976; 63:497–498.

38. Kaufman HD. Outpatient treatment of haemorrhoids by cryotherapy. Br J Surg 1976; 63:462–463.

39. Oh C. One thousand cryohaemorrhoidectomies: an overview. Dis Colon Rectum 1981; 24:613–617.

40. Traynor OJ, Carter AE. Cryotherapy for advanced haemorrhoids: a prospective evaluation with 2 year follow-up. Br J Surg 1984; 71:287–289.

41. Leff EI. Hemorrhoidectomy – laser vs nonlaser: outpatient surgical experience. Dis Colon Rectum 1992; 35:743–746.

42. Sankar MY, Joffe SN. Laser surgery in colonic and anorectal lesions. Surg Clin North Am 1988; 68:1447–1469.

43. Pescatori M, Favetta U, Dedola S, et al. Transanal stapled excision of rectal mucosal prolapse. Techniques Coloproctol 1997; 1:96–98.

44. Milito G, Cortese F, Casciani CU. Surgical treatment of mucosal prolapse and haemorrhoids by stapler. Proceedings of the 6th World Congress of Endoscopic Surgery. Rome, Italy 3–6 June 1998.

45. Mehigan BJ, Hartley JE, Monson JRT 1999 (unpublished data).

46. Goligher J. Surgery of the anus, rectum and colon. 5th ed. London: Baillière Tindall; 1984:378–380.

47. Parks AG. A technique for excising extensive villous papillomatous change in the lower rectum. Proc R Soc Med 1968; 61:441–442.

48. Localio SA, Baron B. Abdomino-trans-sacral resection and anastomosis for mid-rectal cancer. Ann Surg 1973; 178:540–546.

49. Mason AY. Transphincteric exposure of the rectum. Ann R Coll Surg Engl 1972; 51:320.

50. Saclarides TJ, Smith L, Ko St. Transanal endoscopic microsurgery. Dis Colon Rectum 1992; 35:1183–1191.

51. Buess G, Mentges B, Manncke K, et al. Technique and results of transanal endoscopic microsurgery in early rectal cancer. Am J Surg 1992; 163:63–70.

52. Steele RJ, Hershman MJ, Mortenson NJ, et al. Transanal endoscopic microsurgery – initial experience from three centres in the United Kingdom. Br J Surg 1996; 83:207–210.

53. Smith LE, Ko ST, Saclarides T, et al. Transanal endoscopic microsurgery. Initial registry results. Dis Colon Rectum 1996; 39:S79–84.

54. Courtney SP, Nankivell C, Davidson CM. Endoscopic transanal resection of rectal lesions: facilitation by adaptation of Lord's dilator. J R Coll Surg Edinb 1991; 36:249–250.

55. Berry AR, Souter RG, Campbell WB. Endoscopic transanal resection of rectal tumours – a preliminary report of its use. Br J Surg 1990; 77:134–137.

56. Wetherall AP, Williams NM, Kelly MJ. Endoscopic transanal resection in the management of patients with sessile rectal adenomas, anastomotic stricture and rectal cancer. Br J Surg 1993; 80:788–793.

57. Tack J, Gevers AM, Rutgeerts P. Self expandable metallic stents in the palliation of rectosigmoid carcinoma: a follow up study. Gastrointest Endosc 1998; 3:267–271.

58. Dohmoto M, Hunerbein M, Schlag PM. Application of rectal stents for palliation of obstructing rectosigmoid cancer. Surg Endosc 1997; 11:758–761.

59. Soonawalla Z, Thakur K, Boorman P, et al. Use of self expanding metallic stents in the management of obstruction of the sigmoid colon. AJR Am J Roentgenol 171; 633:6.

60. Tefero E, Fernandez-Lobato R, Mainar A, et al. Initial results of a new procedure for treatment of malignant obstruction of the left colon. Dis Colon Rectum 1997; 40:432–436.

61. Lund J, Scholefield J. A randomised prospective double blind placebo controlled trial of glyceryl trinitrate ointment in the treatment of anal fissure. Lancet 1997; 349:11–14.

62. Banerjee AK, Walters TK, Wilkins R, et al. Wire guided balloon coloplasty – a new treatment for colorectal strictures. J R Soc Med 1991; 84:136–139.

63. Johansson C. Endoscope dilation of rectal strictures. Dis Colon Rectum 1996; 39:423–428.

64. Accordi F, Sogno O, Carniato S, et al. Endoscopic treatment of stenosis following stapler anastomosis. Dis Colon Rectum 1987; 30:647–649.

65. Kelly M. Use of urological resectoscope in benign and malignant lesions. J R Soc Med 1989; 82:588–590.

66. Shimada S, Matsuda M, et al. A new device for the treatment of coloproctostomic stricture after double stapling anastomosis. Ann Surg 1996; 224:603–608.

67. Pagni S, McLaughlin C. Simple technique for the treatment of strictured colorectal anastomosis. Dis Colon Rectum 1995; 38:433–434.

68. Ovnae A, Peiser J, Avinoah E, et al. A new approach to rectal anastomotic stricture. Dis Colon Rectum 1989; 32:351–353.

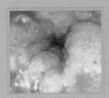

15.

ENDOSONOGRAPHY-GUIDED INTERVENTIONS

MANOOP S. BHUTANI

INTRODUCTION

Endosonographic imaging can be performed with radial or linear array echoendoscopes. The radial instruments provide a 360° circular scan, which is perpendicular to the long axis of the echoendoscope. This provides excellent anatomic orientation and thus radial echoendoscopes are the most widely used instruments for endoscopic ultrasound (EUS) imaging. However, because of the perpendicular scan of a radial echoendoscope, a needle passed through the biopsy channel of the instrument is seen merely as an echogenic dot. Although EUS-guided intervention has been performed under radial EUS guidance, because of the technical difficulties of performing intervention with needles that cannot be imaged or monitored along their length, EUS-guided intervention is mostly performed using linear array endosonography. In linear array endosonography, the echoendoscope scans parallel to the long axis of the echoendoscope. Thus needles can be seen on the ultrasonic screen and real-time EUS-guided intervention performed.

There are a variety of indications for EUS-guided intervention. As more widespread use of EUS is developing, there are increasingly greater indications for interventional usage (Table 15.1). Because of the possibility of hemorrhage when advancing a needle deeply into bodily tissues, coagulopathy is a contraindication as is the inability to use drugs for conscious sedation. The procedure should not be performed when the information derived from this investigation will not alter clinical management (Table 15.2).

EQUIPMENT

Linear array echoendoscopes
FG32UA, FG36UX, FG38UX (Pentax Corp.®, Orangeburg, NY) (Fig. 15.1)
These instruments have a curved linear array transducer with 60° oblique endoscopic view. Pulse and color Doppler are available.

Indications for EUS-guided intervention

- EUS-guided fine needle aspiration of lymph nodes
- EUS-guided pancreatic fine needle aspiration
- EUS-guided fine needle aspiration of submucosal gastrointestinal lesions
- EUS-guided fine needle aspiration of other lesions
  - —Adrenal gland
  - —Peri-rectal masses
  - —Liver lesions
  - —Prominent gastric and rectal folds
- EUS-guided pancreatic pseudocyst drainage
- EUS-guided celiac plexus neurolysis
- EUS-guided botulinum toxin injection for achalasia
- EUS-guided cholangiopancreatography
- EUS-guided paracentesis/thoracentesis

Table 15.1 Indications for EUS-guided intervention

Contraindications for EUS-guided intervention

- Coagulopathy
- Severe co-morbid conditions preventing conscious sedation
- When the information obtained will not alter clinical management (e.g. histologically proven primary tumor with known distant metastases)

Table 15.2 Contraindications for EUS-guided intervention

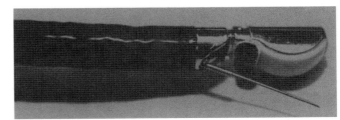

Fig. 15.1 Example of a linear array echoendoscope (Pentax FG32UA; Pentax Corp.®, Orangeburg, NY).

GF-UC30P (Olympus Corp.®. Melville, NY)
This is a curved linear array echoendoscope with oblique optics (45°). Color Doppler is available on this instrument as well.

Operating characteristics of linear array echoendoscopes		
	Olympus GFUC 30P	Pentax FG32UA, FG36UX FG38UX
Optics	45° oblique	60° oblique
Biopsy channel	2.8 mm	2.0, 2.4, 3.2 mm
Elevator	+	+
Length	1255 mm	1250 mm
Ultrasound display mode	B-mode M-mode Color Doppler	B-mode Color Doppler
Scanning direction	Convex linear	Convex linear
Frequency	7.5 MHz	5.0 MHz, 7.5 MHz
Scanning range	180°	100°

Table 15.3 Operating characteristics of linear array echoendoscopes. (Adapted from Bhutani MS. Interventional endoscopic ultrasound. In: Bhutani MS, Tandon RK, eds. Advances in gastrointestinal endoscopy. New Delhi: JayPee Brothers Medical Publishers; 1999 (in press).)

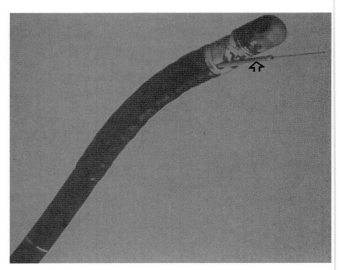

Fig. 15.3 Mechanical sector scanning echoendoscope (GF-UMP, Olympus Corp.®, Melville, NY) with NA-10J-1 needle (Olympus Corp.®) passed through the biopsy channel of the instrument. Arrow points to protective sheath around the needle.

Table 15.3 is a comparison of the operating characteristics of Pentax and Olympus linear array echoendoscopes.

PEF-703FA (Toshiba Corp.®, Tokyo, Japan) (Fig. 15.2)

This echoendoscope is different from the instruments described above as it has forward viewing optics. Color Doppler is available. The instrument has two biopsy channels, one is for standard endoscopic biopsy and the other is for EUS-guided interventional procedures.

Mechanical sector scanning echoendoscope

A mechanical sector scanning echoendoscope is also available (GF-UMP, Olympus Corp., Melville, NY) that allows EUS-guided intervention (Fig. 15.3). This instrument uses a rotating mirror to orient a radial image along the shaft of the echoendoscope, allowing visualization of a needle along its length. Even though intervention is feasible under EUS guidance with this instrument, the general sense among EUS practitioners is that this instrument is more

difficult to use than linear array instruments. The advantage of this echoendoscope is that it uses the same console as a radial echoendoscope (Olympus Corp.) and thus avoids the purchase of a separate console for EUS-guided intervention.

Needle devices for interventional endoscopic ultrasound

GIP Medi-Globe needle system (Grassau, Germany, Tempe, AZ)

This device consists of a steel needle with a stylet, covered with a metal spiral sheath and connected to a biopsy handle with a piston. The needle is 170 cm long and 22 gauge. The tip of the needle is sandblasted to improve ultrasonic visualization. The piston on the biopsy handle is used to push the needle into the target organ or lesion during EUS-guided interventions (Fig. 15.4). This device

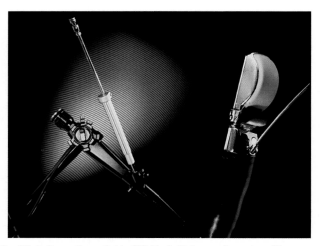

Fig. 15.4 Currently available GIP-Medi-Globe needle system (Grassau Germany; Tempe, AZ, USA) inserted through a linear echoendoscope (Pentax FG32UA).

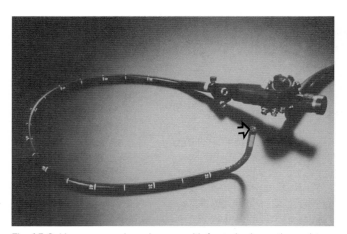

Fig. 15.2 Linear array echoendoscope with front-viewing optics and two biopsy channels (Toshiba PEF-703FA; Toshiba Corp.®, Tokyo, Japan).

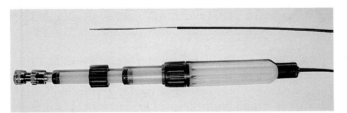

Fig. 15.5 Single use, Sonotip needle system for EUS-guided FNA (GIP-Medi-Globe).

is designed for Pentax linear array echoendoscopes. A single use needle system (Sonotip) will soon be released by this manufacturer (Fig. 15.5) to replace the currently available system.

Olympus NA-10J-1 needle (Olympus Corp.)

This needle system is used with Olympus linear array (GF-UC30P) and mechanical sector scanning (GF-UMP) echoendoscopes. The needle is 22 gauge and it is covered with a 145 cm metal spiral coil sheath. The tip of the needle is dimpled to improve ultrasonic visualization. The needle can be advanced up to 65 mm beyond the spiral sheath. The length of the spiral sheath beyond the echoendoscope can be adjusted as well in this device.

EUSN-1 Echotip ultrasound needle (Wilson–Cook, Winston-Salem, NC)

This is a 22-gauge needle designed for use with the Pentax linear array echoendoscopes but can also be used with the Olympus echoendoscopes. The needle is covered with a metallically reinforced outer catheter, which is 5.5 Fr and 140 cm long. The needle can be connected to a 10 mL syringe that has a self-sustaining vacuum lock (Fig. 15.6A). The needle can be advanced up to 8 cm beyond the echoendoscope and a movable guard is present to adjust the maximum distance of needle advancement beyond the echoendoscope based on the size of the target lesion (Fig. 15.6B).

PATIENT PREPARATION

Patient preparation in general is similar to any other therapeutic endoscopy:

- Patient fasting for 6 to 8 hours
- Informed consent
- Discontinuation of aspirin or other non-steroidal anti-inflammatory drugs for 5 to 7 days prior to the procedure date
- Platelet count, prothrombin time, international normalized ratio and partial thromboplastin time should be checked on the day of the procedure or a few days before.

PROCEDURE

Endoscopic ultrasound-guided fine needle aspiration

The majority of EUS-guided fine needle aspiration (FNA) procedures are performed with linear array echoendoscopes. However, a large number of centers have both radial and linear echoendoscopes. In such centers, most endosonographers prefer to perform diagnostic imaging with a radial echoendoscope because of its easier anatomic orientation. If a lesion is seen during radial EUS and histology is considered clinically necessary and the lesion is suitable for EUS-guided FNA, the radial echoendoscope is withdrawn and a linear echoendoscope inserted into the gastrointestinal tract lumen to image the target lesion in preparation for FNA. Alternatively, at many centers where only linear echoendoscopes are available or when another imaging modality (e.g. CT scan) has already shown an unequivocal lesion suitable for EUS-guided FNA, linear EUS instruments are inserted into the gastrointestinal tract lumen without prior imaging. Both practices (radial followed by linear EUS imaging or linear imaging alone) are

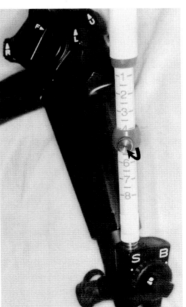

Fig. 15.6B The EUS N$_1$ Echotip needle has an adjustable guard (arrow) to limit the maximum protrusion of the needle beyond the echoendoscope.

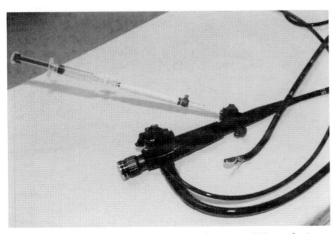

Fig. 15.6A EUS N$_1$ Echotip ultrasound needle system (Wilson–Cook, Winston-Salem, NC, USA) inserted through a linear echoendoscope.

acceptable and the method selected depends on the factors discussed above.

Once the linear echoendoscope is inserted into the upper or lower gastrointestinal tract lumen and the target lesion (e.g. pancreatic mass, lymph node, submucosal lesion) is imaged, the control knobs are adjusted to bring the lesion in close proximity to the tip of the echoendoscope. The FNA assembly is then inserted into the biopsy channel of the echoendoscope and positioned such that the outer sheath projects beyond the tip of the echoendoscope. This can usually be seen as a thick echogenic line at the periphery of the lesion. In addition, the ultrasonic image of the sheath provides the endosonographer with a fairly good estimate of the projected needle path. Some needle devices have an adjustable sheath with a guard that can be set to a specific distance before the needle is advanced beyond the sheath (Olympus NA-10J-1). Once the sheath is properly locked in, a re-adjustment of the ultrasonic image is accomplished by moving or rotating the echoendoscope to get an optimal position for puncture. Generally at this point, the endosonographer removes the right hand from the shaft of the echoendoscope and has an assistant stabilize the echoendoscope shaft. The optimal image for endosonographic-guided puncture often requires a clockwise or anti-clockwise torque of the shaft. Thus, before switching the shaft grasp to the assistant, it is important that the operator alerts the assistant to the direction of torque so that the optimal image for needle puncture can be stabilized.

The stylet is withdrawn about 10 mm and the needle is then slowly advanced into the middle of the target lesion (e.g. pancreatic mass, lymph node) under ultrasonic guidance. The stylet is then pushed all the way into the needle. The stylet is removed and suction is applied with a syringe. Continuous suction with a 10 mL syringe tends to provide the best cellular yield when compared to intermittent suction or larger syringe sizes. The endosonographer then moves the needle back and forth within the lesion for 30 to 60 seconds while monitoring the needle movement on the ultrasonic screen. Care should be taken to avoid overshooting the needle during its movement beyond the outer margin of the lesion. This is important since large blood vessels are frequently present around pancreatic masses and lymph nodes and it is desirable to prevent accidental needle stick of such vessels with the potential for bleeding complications. Once the needle has been moved to and fro within the lesion for 30 to 60 seconds, the syringe is disconnected. The whole needle/catheter assembly is withdrawn and the aspirated material is expressed onto a glass slide using an air flush with a syringe. The stylet is then re-inserted and another pass is made.

EUS-guided FNA is preferably performed in the presence of an attending cytopathologist or at least a cytology technician who can perform some rapid stains and microscopy of the aspirated material. Successive passes are made until malignant cells are seen or benign cells are harvested with acceptable cellularity for a reasonable cytopathologic interpretation. If a cytologist or cytopatho-

logist cannot be present, multiple passes (3–5) should be performed to maximize the cytologic yield.

Endoscopic ultrasound-guided lymph node fine needle aspiration

Various echo features have been used to predict malignant invasion of lymph nodes during EUS imaging.[1,2] However, echo features have the limitation of lack of standardized criteria, interobserver variability, and overlap between echo features of malignant and benign lymph nodes.[3] EUS-guided FNA is thus an important modality for determination of malignant invasion in lymph nodes in gastrointestinal malignancies, pulmonary malignancies, and mediastinal lymphadenopathy of unknown origin (Figs 15.7 to 15.9). Bhutani et al[3] subjected 22 patients with

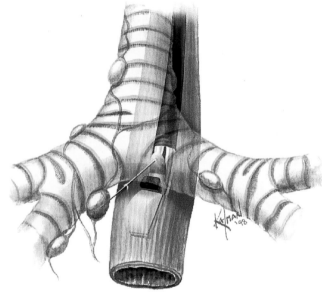

Fig. 15.7 Representation of the technique of EUS-guided transesophageal fine needle aspiration of a mediastinal lymph node. (Reproduced with permission from Bhutani MS. Interventional endoscopic ultrasonography: state of the art. Endoscopy 2000; in press.)

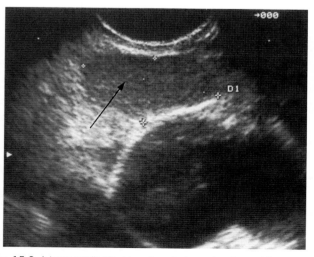

Fig. 15.8 A large mediastinal lymph node (arrow) as imaged by a linear array echoendoscope in the esophagus.

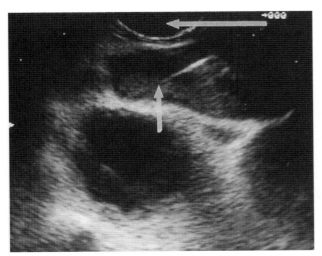

Fig. 15.9 EUS-guided FNA of a large mediastinal lymph node in the aortopulmonary window. Short arrow: needle tip within the lymph node. Long arrow: transducer within the esophagus.

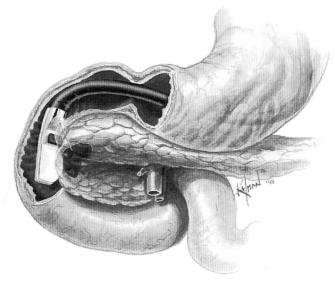

Fig. 15.10 Representation of the technique of EUS-guided transduodenal fine needle aspiration of a pancreatic head mass with a linear array echoendoscope. (Reproduced with permission from Bhutani MS. Interventional endoscopic ultrasonography: state of the art. Endoscopy 2000; in press.)

esophageal, pancreatic and lung cancer to EUS-guided FNA of lymph nodes located in the subcarinal, aortopulmonary window, para-aortic area, para-esophageal area, celiac axis, and peripancreatic area. Cytopathologic examination of the needle aspirates revealed malignant cells in 16 cases and these patients were thus not considered suitable for surgery with a curative intent. Another series of EUS-guided lymph node FNA in patients with gastrointestinal malignancies has shown a sensitivity of 80% and specificity of 94% for detecting malignant lymph node invasion.[4] EUS-guided lymph node FNA is also becoming an important modality for sampling mediastinal lymph nodes for staging patients with known, non-small cell, lung carcinoma and in the work-up of mediastinal lymphadenopathy of unknown cause. In the presence of lymph nodes on CT scan in the subcarinal, aortopulmonary window, or in the para-esophageal locations, a positive EUS-guided transesophageal FNA for malignancy can avert more invasive procedures such as a mediastinoscopy or thoracotomy.[5-7]

Endoscopic ultrasound-guided fine needle aspiration of the pancreas

EUS is extremely useful for the detection and staging of pancreatic masses.[8-10] In addition, EUS-guided transduodenal or transgastric FNA can also provide a tissue diagnosis (Figs 15.10 and 15.11). Pancreatic tumors by EUS are imaged as focal, irregular, hypoechoic areas. At institutions where both radial and linear echoendoscopes are available, radial instruments are generally used to detect, image, and stage a mass and then a linear array echoendoscope is inserted to perform EUS-guided FNA. However, some endosonographers prefer to image as well as perform EUS-guided FNA with a linear array echoendoscope. This is an acceptable approach. A study comparing radial and linear EUS instruments revealed a comparable accuracy for imaging and staging pancreatic carcinoma.[11] Sensitivity and specificity of EUS-guided pancreatic FNA

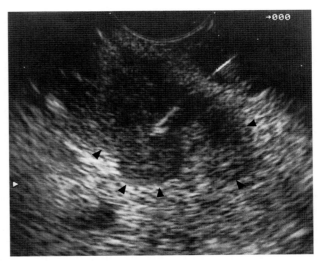

Fig. 15.11 Hypoechoic pancreatic mass imaged by linear EUS (within arrow heads) and punctured by EUS-guided FNA with the needle seen in the mass.

for detection of cancer range from 64 to 90% and 85 to 100% respectively.[12-15]

EUS-guided pancreatic FNA is useful for tissue diagnosis of pancreatic masses that appear to be unresectable by EUS or other imaging modalities. If an adenocarcinoma is found, the patient can then be considered for chemotherapy or radiation therapy protocols. Other pancreatic tumors may include small cell carcinoma, lymphoma, or neuroendocrine tumors; a diagnostic EUS-guided FNA in these cases will lead to appropriate therapy. In patients with a potentially resectable pancreatic mass, a negative EUS-guided FNA will not rule out the presence of a neoplasm (because of low negative predictive value of EUS-guided pancreatic FNA). Thus, a surgical exploration may be undertaken anyway. Theoretically, seeding of malignant cells would be a concern in resectable pancreatic body/tail lesions. However, in pancreatic head lesions, the needle track would be included in the surgical specimen in resectable lesions. Thus, in potentially resectable pancreatic lesions, EUS-guided FNA should be undertaken if tissue-based, preoperative, neo-adjuvant chemotherapy or radiation is being considered or if the information obtained is going to assist in clinical decision-making on a case-to-case basis.[12]

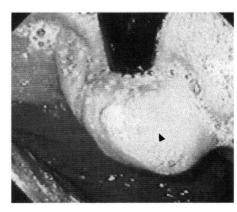

Fig. 15.12A Submucosal gastric mass at the cardia (retroflexed view) seen during regular endoscopy (arrow head).

Endoscopic ultrasound-guided fine needle aspiration of submucosal lesions

Once EUS determines that a submucosal compression of the gastrointestinal tract lumen is due to an intramural lesion arising deeper to the mucosa, EUS-guided FNA could be used as an adjunct to achieve diagnostic information. Certain submucosal lesions have a classic appearance on EUS. These include a lipoma (homogenous, echogenic lesion arising from the submucosa), submucosal cyst (anechoic lesion in the submucosa), and a myogenic tumor (hypoechoic lesion arising from the muscularis propria). However, many other submucosal lesions seen on EUS imaging may have a diagnostic overlap.[16–18] A hypoechoic lesion arising in the submucosa has a broad differential diagnosis including pancreatic rest, granular cell tumor, carcinoid tumor, metastasis, lymphoma, neurilemmoma, or a myogenic tumor superficial to the muscularis propria. Such submucosal lesions can be punctured during routine endoscopy with a fine needle even without using EUS.[19] However, with EUS-guided FNA, it can be ensured that the needle is actually within a lesion instead of being superficial or deeper to it (Fig. 15.12A–C).[20] The overall accuracy of EUS-guided FNA for diagnosis of submucosal lesions is generally lower than EUS-guided pancreatic or lymph node FNA. This is probably because many of the intramural submucosal lesions are benign and are the result of overgrowth of normal elements (e.g. neural, myogenic, adipose) and thus individual cells on a needle aspirate may appear normal in morphology. Differentiation between a benign leiomyoma and a malignant leiomyosarcoma also cannot be reliably made during EUS-guided FNA. Larger bore needles that provide a core sample for histology have been developed to increase the accuracy of EUS-guided puncture of submucosal lesions.[21,22]

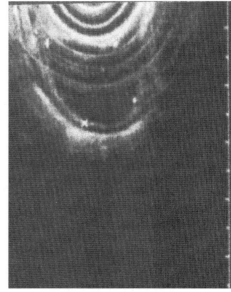

Fig. 15.12B Radial EUS imaging reveals the submucosal mass at the cardia to be a hypoechoic lesion arising within the submucosa. Note the intact muscularis propria underneath the lesion.

Endoscopic ultrasound-guided fine needle aspiration of other lesions

An important indication for endosonography is the further work up of prominent gastric folds seen during endoscopy. When the muscularis propria or muscularis propria and the submucosa are thickened, the likelihood of an infiltrating gastric carcinoma (linitis plastica) or lymphoma is very high. If standard endoscopic biopsies are non-diagnostic, a full thickness surgical biopsy is usually recommended in these patients. Prior to proceeding with an open surgical or a laparoscopic biopsy, linear EUS-guided FNA of the deeper layers of the gastric wall can be attempted to help

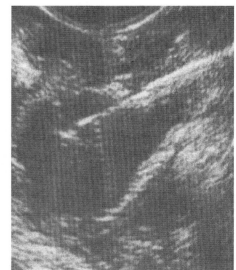

Fig. 15.12C Using linear EUS (magnified view), the hypoechoic submucosal mass in Figure 15.12A and B is punctured to perform EUS-guided FNA.

obtain a clinical diagnosis.[23] Similarly, EUS-guided FNA of deeper layers of the rectal wall[24] can be performed in rectal linitis plastica (Fig. 15.13A and B). Perirectal masses can also be sampled with EUS-guided FNA.[25] Such lesions may include adenocarcinoma, cervical carcinoma, and lym-

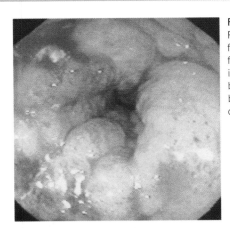

Fig. 15.13A Prominent, indurated, friable rectal folds on flexible sigmoidoscopy in a patient with rectal bleeding. Endoscopic biopsies were non-diagnostic.

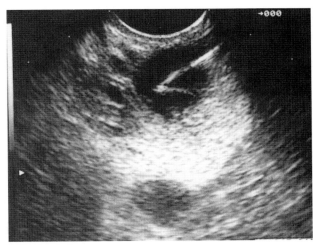

Fig. 15.14 Pancreatic pseudocyst imaged as an anechoic well-defined lesion with a linear array echoendoscope. A needle is inserted through the gastric wall into the pseudocyst under linear EUS guidance.

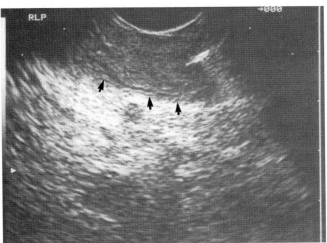

Fig. 15.13B Linear EUS of the rectal wall in Figure 15.13A, revealing significant thickening of the rectal wall (arrows) with loss of five layer echo-pattern consistent with rectal linitis plastica. Note the needle within the deeper rectal wall inserted under linear EUS guidance. Cytology revealed rectal linitis plastica secondary to an infiltrating prostate carcinoma.

phoma. Other lesions sampled during EUS-guided FNA with limited data include left adrenal masses.[23,26,27]

Endoscopic ultrasound-guided pancreatic pseudocyst drainage

Endoscopic drainage of pseudocysts is a minimally invasive approach employed instead of a surgical drainage in selected patients. Endoscopic drainage of a pseudocyst involves creation of a cystogastrostomy or a cystoduodenostomy when an endoscopically visible luminal bulge is present. EUS-guided pseudocyst drainage can be particularly helpful when submucosal compression of the gastrointestinal lumen is absent or minimal. In addition, color Doppler can help to avoid major vessels or varices. EUS can readily measure the distance between the cyst wall and the gastrointestinal tract lumen, with a distance of >10 mm considered to be a contraindication to endoscopic cyst drainage.

When EUS is used for endoscopic pseudocyst drainage, an option is to image the pseudocyst by a radial echoendoscope or miniprobe and study the suitability for endoscopic drainage such as its distance from the gut wall of <10 mm, if it is unilocular and if there are no interposed varices. In these situations, EUS is followed by endoscopic cyst drainage in the usual fashion.[28,29] The other option is real-time EUS-guided pseudocyst puncture for endoscopic drainage. Antibiotics are given before and after the procedure to minimize the chances of infection. Linear array endosonography is performed in the usual fashion. Once the cyst is imaged by EUS as a localized anechoic area and considered suitable for endoscopic drainage (e.g. within 10 mm of the gastrointestinal tract lumen, no major blood vessels by Doppler in the projected needle path, homogeneous, unilocular cyst), EUS-guided transgastrointestinal puncture is performed (Fig. 15.14). This is usually performed by the same needles that are used for EUS-guided FNA. Although the initial report on this technique used diathermy with a needle-knife to achieve this goal,[30] the same group of authors subsequently reported that diathermy may not be necessary in this approach.[31] After the cyst is punctured, cyst fluid is aspirated for biochemical and cytological markers. The options after this procedure are:[31]

1. to insert a guidewire through the needle into the cyst and insert a stent or nasocystic catheter through the linear echoendoscope
2. to insert a guidewire into the cyst and exchange the echoendoscope with a duodenoscope, then insert a 10 Fr stent after dilation of the tract
3. complete aspiration of cyst contents and follow-up of the patient; if the cyst recurs, then resort to continuous drainage by percutaneous or endoscopic route.

Endoscopic ultrasound-guided celiac nerve block

In patients with upper abdominal malignancies such as pancreatic cancer or chronic pancreatitis, celiac nerve block has been performed under CT guidance via a posterior percutaneous approach for alleviation of pain.[32] Celiac nerve block can now also be performed under real-time EUS. The celiac ganglion is not visible during EUS guidance but the celiac ganglion has a consistent relationship to the celiac artery take-off from the aorta which is generally well visualized during EUS. EUS-guided celiac neurolysis is performed under conscious sedation similar to other EUS procedures.[33] While imaging with a linear array echoendoscope, the celiac artery is imaged as it emanates from the aorta. One of the needle systems used for EUS-guided FNA is primed for EUS-guided celiac neurolysis by removing the stylet and flushing the needle with saline. The needle system is passed through the biopsy channel.

While imaging the aorta and the celiac artery take-off, the echoendoscope is rotated clockwise or anti-clockwise in a way that the celiac artery is no longer seen but the aorta is still visualized. The needle is then advanced under EUS guidance into the peri-aortic space at this point. The needle is flushed with 1 mL of saline and then 25% preservative-free bupivacaine is injected followed by 10 mL of 98% dehydrated absolute alcohol (Figs 15.15 and 15.16). The needle is then withdrawn and the same process repeated on the other side of the celiac artery. If there is difficulty in rotating to either side while keeping the aorta in view, a single injection could also be performed around the celiac artery.

Normal saline is infused intravenously during and after the procedure to prevent hypotension from neural blockade and sedation. Bupivacaine and steroids have been injected by some authors during EUS-guided nerve block in chronic pancreatitis.[34] The results of celiac nerve block in pancreatic cancer have been good with significant improvement in pain scores in up to 88% of patients.[33–35] The results of celiac block in patients with chronic pancreatitis have been less favorable both with EUS-guided anterior approach and CT-guided posterior approach.[36]

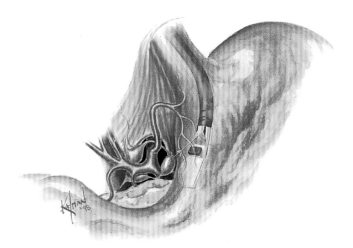

Fig. 15.15 Representation of the technique of EUS-guided celiac nerve block. (Reproduced with permission from Bhutani MS. Interventional endoscopic ultrasonography: state of the art. Endoscopy 2000; in press.)

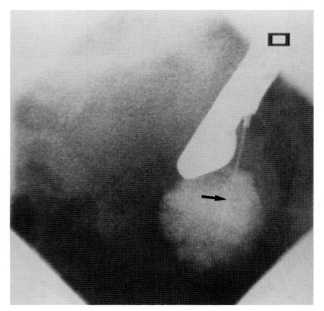

Fig. 15.16 Fluoroscopic image of EUS-guided celiac nerve block after adding a small amount of radiographic contrast to bupivacaine and alcohol or steroids. Fluoroscopy is generally not needed as long as an aspiration test is performed to ensure that there is no blood return and the needle is not within a vascular structure. Arrow indicates the needle.

Endoscopic ultrasound-guided botulinum toxin injection for achalasia

Recently, botulinum toxin injection into the lower esophageal sphincter with a sclerotherapy needle (during regular endoscopy) has been reported in achalasia and it has become an acceptable treatment for achalasia in patients who are not candidates for surgical myotomy or balloon dilation.[37–39] Even though an immediate response to injection of botulinum toxin into the lower esophageal sphincter was seen in 90% of patients, 42% of patients had to be re-treated with botulinum toxin.[37,38] We have postulated that in patients who do not respond to injection of botulinum toxin with a standard sclerotherapy needle, the needle may be either superficial to or beyond the lower esophageal sphincter. In some cases the needle may be only partly into the sphincter. The lower esophageal sphincter is visualized as a hypoechoic band above the gastro-esophageal junction as the muscularis propria (4th EUS layer) by radial and linear echoendoscopy. Using a linear echoendoscope after the lower esophageal sphincter has been visualized (Fig. 15.17A), an EUS-guided FNA needle can be inserted into the sphincter (Fig. 15.17B). Twenty units of botulinum toxin is injected under real-time EUS guidance. The echoendoscope is rotated and the procedure repeated in four quadrants. Initial data on the EUS-guided botulinum toxin injection reveal that this approach may help to decrease the relapse rate and improve the initial response rate when this toxin is used for achalasia.[40–42] Comparative trials with and without EUS are needed.

Endoscopic ultrasound-guided paracentesis

Frequently during EUS imaging, a small amount of ascites is seen around tumors (e.g. gastric, pancreatobiliary,

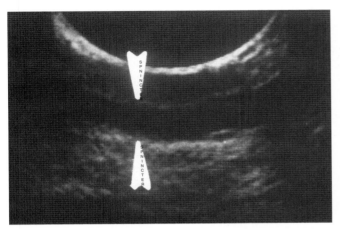

Fig. 15.17A Linear EUS examination above the gastroesophageal junction in a patient with achalasia revealing the lower esophageal sphincter as a hypoechoic layer (between arrows).

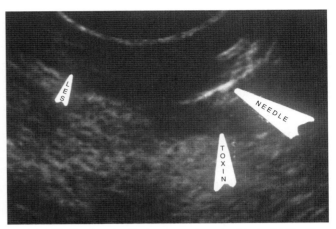

Fig. 15.17B After imaging the lower esophageal sphincter (LES) with a linear echoendoscope, a needle is inserted under EUS guidance within the LES, and botulinum toxin is injected which can be observed as an enlarging anechoic zone around the needle in real-time.

rectal). This is typically imaged as an anechoic triangular area. Many patients with this minimal amount of ascites on EUS do not have clinically detectable ascites and imaging studies such as transabdominal ultrasound or CT scan may also be negative for ascites. This minimal ascites can be malignant ascites or a reactive phenomenon. In a manner similar to EUS-guided transgastrointestinal FNA, a needle can be inserted under EUS guidance into the ascites and the fluid aspirated for cytological examination.[43–45] This should only be done if the needle can be passed into the ascites without traversing the primary tumor and if a malignant cytology in the aspirated fluid will help in clinical decision-making regarding therapy.

Endoscopic ultrasound-guided cholangiopancreatography

The distal bile duct and the pancreatic duct are visualized during EUS. Using linear EUS, the bile duct or the pancreatic duct can be punctured with a needle in locations where these ducts are in close proximity to the gastrointestinal tract lumen (Fig. 15.18). EUS-guided cholangiopancreatography has thus been performed by injecting contrast after entering the bile duct or the pancreatic duct under

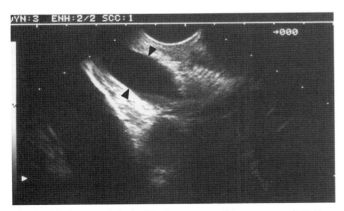

Fig. 15.18 Common bile duct (between arrows) is seen very close to the linear array transducer during transduodenal imaging.

EUS guidance in patients with unsuccessful ERCP.[46–48] With the development of magnetic resonance cholangiopancreatography (MRCP), the utility for the EUS-guided approach may be limited but this accomplishment may act as a stepping stone for other innovative developments such as the creation of a biliary-enteric anastomosis to bypass unresectable biliary obstruction.

COMPLICATIONS AND THEIR MANAGEMENT

Diagnostic EUS without intervention is a safe test in experienced hands. Although EUS procedures take longer than diagnostic endoscopy and require a greater amount of sedatives, the rate of minor complications such as changes in blood pressure, pulse rate, and oxygen desaturation is the same.[49] A large multicenter study of 37 915 upper EUS examinations revealed an overall major complication rate of 0.05%.[50] These included esophageal perforation, pharyngeal perforation, duodenal perforation, and bleeding. Esophageal perforation primarily occurred in patients who underwent dilation of a stenotic esophageal tumor just prior to passing an echoendoscope. This appears to be the situation with the highest risk of complications in diagnostic EUS and should be avoided unless the information obtained is going to have a major clinical impact.

Complications during interventional endosonography

EUS-guided FNA has an overall complication rate of 1.1%.[51] The complications attributable to the FNA aspect of EUS included hemorrhage, infection, and pancreatitis. When cystic lesions in the pancreas or elsewhere are punctured under EUS guidance, the risk of infectious complications has been reported to be as high as 14% in some studies with the complication rate for solid lesions being only 0.5%.[51] Similarly in another study, cystic masses had a complication rate of 19% compared to

0.06% for solid masses.[52] Because of the risk of infection, when a cystic lesion is punctured during EUS, prophylactic antibiotics should be given before and after the procedure. In addition, the entire cyst fluid should be aspirated to minimize the chance of infection. Needless to say, the clinical necessity of the information obtained should be kept in mind before deciding to puncture a cystic lesion or mass during EUS. There is a small risk (less than 2%) of pancreatitis from EUS-guided pancreatic FNA.[53,54] A study has also documented a post-pancreatic FNA rise in serum lipase.[55] Although no patients in that series had clinical pancreatitis, when a patient presents with idiopathic acute pancreatitis and a referral is made for EUS to look for an occult pancreatic tumor, it is my preference to wait for 4 to 6 weeks prior to performing EUS with possible FNA. This allows the pancreatic inflammation to 'cool down' and to lessen the chance of EUS-guided FNA making the already existing pancreatitis worse. In addition, pancreatic inflammation can mask pancreatic tumors or focal inflammation can masquerade as a pancreatic tumor on imaging by EUS.

The risk of hemorrhage during EUS-guided FNA can be minimized by ensuring the absence of significant coagulopathy and paying close attention to the vascular structures around the lesion that is being sampled. EUS-guided FNA with a radial scanner has been reported and because of its inability to monitor the depth of a needle during EUS, there has been a higher risk of bleeding complications during EUS-guided pancreatic FNA with a radial echoendoscope when compared to a linear echoendoscope.[53] Thus, EUS-guided intervention should preferably be performed with a linear echoendoscope or a mechanical sector scanning echoendoscope because these instruments allow monitoring of the depth of insertion of a needle.

EUS-guided celiac nerve block has also been reported to have some unique complications. Patients undergoing this procedure have had minor complications which are transient postural hypotension and diarrhea.[33,34] Intravenous saline should thus be infused during and after EUS-guided celiac nerve block to minimize the chances of developing postural hypotension which is usually transitory. Postural hypotension and diarrhea are a result of the autonomic nerve blockade from the procedure. Two major complications have been reported during EUS-guided celiac nerve block. A pseudoaneurysm and a retroperitoneal bleed have been reported after EUS-guided celiac block using ethanol.[36] Another patient in whom steroids were used instead of ethanol developed a peripancreatic abscess.[36] This patient was on a proton pump inhibitor and the authors postulated that this might

have resulted in bacterial overgrowth in the stomach. Thus, one may choose to give antibiotics during celiac nerve block with steroids or alcohol. Some may suggest that antibiotics may not be necessary if alcohol is used because of its bactericidal effects. Clearly more data are needed.

No major complications have been reported with EUS-guided botulinum toxin injection for achalasia. Minor complications include transient chest pain (8%) and gastroesophageal reflux (4%) but these have also been reported with non-EUS-guided botulinum toxin injection for achalasia.[39]

CONCLUSIONS

EUS-guided interventions open an exciting phase of possibilities. This is technology in evolution. However, interventional EUS and EUS-guided FNA have already become clinically useful and accepted modalities. Further developments in this area are expected to continue and with rapid developments in non-invasive imaging techniques such as virtual endoscopy, MRCP, helical CT, and MRI, the greatest utility of EUS in the future may be in its ability to perform endosonography-guided interventions.[56]

CHECKLIST OF PRACTICE POINTS

1. Avoid using radial echoendoscope for interventional EUS (especially for pancreatic lesions).
2. Ensure the absence of significant coagulopathy before EUS-guided intervention.
3. Do not traverse the primary tumor when a lymph node or ascitic fluid is being sampled during EUS.
4. Use antibiotics before and after the procedure if a cystic lesion is to be punctured during EUS-guided FNA.
5. Have a cytologist present to assess the adequacy of specimen during EUS-guided FNA. If a cytologist is not present, perform multiple passes. Save some material for flow cytometry studies if a lymphoma is suspected.
6. Stop acid-suppressive medicines for a few days prior to EUS-guided celiac block.

REFERENCES

1. Catalano MF, Sivak MV Jr, Rice T, et al. Endoscopic features predictive of lymph node metastases. Gastrointest Endosc 1994; 40:442–446.

2. Grimm H, Hamper K, Binmoeller KR, et al. Enlarged lymph nodes: malignant or not? Endoscopy 1992; 24(Suppl 1):320–333.

3. Bhutani MS, Hawes RH, Hoffman BJ. A comparison of the accuracy of echo features during endoscopic ultrasound (EUS) and EUS-guided fine-needle aspiration for diagnosis of malignant lymph node invasion. Gastrointest Endosc 1997; 45:474–479.

4. Harada N, Wiersema M, Wiersema L. Endosonography guided fine-needle aspiration biopsy (EUS FNA) in the evaluation of lymphadenopathy: staging accuracy of EUS FNA versus EUS alone (abstract). Gastrointest Endosc 1997; 45:AB31.

5. Bhutani M, Hoffman B, Reed C, et al. Lymph node staging of esophageal and non-small cell lung cancer by endoscopic ultrasound guided fine-needle aspiration cytology (abstract). Gastrointest Endosc 1995; 41:299.

6. Bhutani MS. Pros and cons of transesophageal endoscopic ultrasound guided access to the mediastinum in patients with lung cancer. Adv Gastroenterol Hepatol Clin Nutr 1998; 3:59–62.

7. Gress FG, Savides TJ, Sandler A, et al. Endoscopic ultrasonography, fine-needle aspiration biopsy guided by endoscopic ultrasonography, and computed tomography in the preoperative staging of non-small-cell lung cancer: a comparison study. Ann Intern Med 1997; 127:604–612.

8. Yasuda K, Tanaka Y, Fujimoto S, et al. Use of endoscopic ultrasound in small pancreatic cancer. Scand J Gastroenterol 1984 (Suppl 102); 19:9–17.

9. Bhutani M, Hoffman B, van Velse A, et al. Is CT scan really the gold standard for the diagnosis of pancreatic masses? (abstract). Am J Gastroenterol 1995; 90:1598.

10. Rösch T, Braig C, Gain T, et al. Staging of pancreatic and ampullary carcinoma by endoscopic ultrasonography. Comparison with conventional sonography, computed tomography, and angiography. Gastroenterology 1992; 102:188–199.

11. Gress F, Savides T, Cummings O, et al. Radial scanning and linear array endosonography for staging pancreatic cancer: a prospective randomized comparison. Gastrointest Endosc 1997; 45:138–142.

12. Bhutani MS, Hawes RH, Baron PL, et al. Endoscopic ultrasound guided fine needle aspiration of malignant pancreatic lesions. Endoscopy 1997; 29:854–858.

13. Chang KJ, Wiersema M, Giovannini M, et al. Multi-center collaborative study on endoscopic ultrasound (EUS) guided fine needle aspiration (FNA) of the pancreas (abstract). Gastrointest Endosc 1996; 43:417.

14. Gress F, Hawes R, Ikenberry S, et al. A prospective evaluation of EUS-guided fine needle aspiration (FNA) biopsy for diagnosing pancreatic masses (PM) with comparison to CT and ERCP cytology (abstract). Gastrointest Endosc 1996; 43:422.

15. Nguyen P, Chang RJ. Endoscopic ultrasound (EUS) and EUS guided fine needle aspiration (FNA) in predicting survival in pancreatic cancer patients (abstract). Gastrointest Endosc 1996; 43:427.

16. Rösch T. Endoscopic ultrasonography in upper gastrointestinal submucosal tumors: a literature review. Gastrointest Endosc Clin North Am 1995; 5:609–614.

17. Caletti GC, Zani L, Bolondi L, et al. Endoscopic ultrasonography in the diagnosis of gastric submucosal tumor. Gastrointest Endosc 1989; 35:413–418.

18. Yasuda K, Nakajima M, Yoshida S, et al. The diagnosis of submucosal tumors of the stomach by endoscopic ultrasonography. Gastrointest Endosc 1989; 35:10–15.

19. Benya RV, Metz DC, Hijazi YM, et al. Fine needle aspiration cytology of submucosal nodules in patients with Zollinger–Ellison syndrome. Am J Gastroenterol 1993; 88:258–265.

20. Harada N, Kouzu T, Isono K. Fine needle aspiration biopsy of a submucosal tumor of the stomach using endoscopic ultrasonography. Dig Endosc 1993; 5:417.

21. Caletti GC, Brocchi E, Ferrari A, et al. Guillotine needle biopsy as a supplement to endosonography in the diagnosis of gastric submucosal tumors. Endoscopy 1991; 23:251–254.

22. Harada N, Kouzu T, Arima M, et al. Endoscopic ultrasound-guided histologic needle biopsy: preliminary results using a newly developed endoscopic ultrasound transducer. Gastrointest Endosc 1996; 44:327–330.

23. Giovannini M, Seitz JF, Monges G, et al. Fine-needle aspiration cytology guided by endoscopic ultrasonography: results in 141 patients. Endoscopy 1995; 27:171–177.

24. Bhutani MS. EUS and EUS-guided fine needle aspiration for the diagnosis of rectal linitis plastica secondary to prostate carcinoma. Gastrointest Endosc 1999; 50:117–119.

25. Hoffman B, Bhutani M, Aabakken L, et al. Endoscopic ultrasound-guided fine needle aspiration in the evaluation of extrarectal pelvic masses (abstract). Gastrointest Endosc 1996; 43:423.

26. Wegener M, Adamek RJ, Wedmann B, et al. Endosonographically guided fine-needle aspiration puncture of paraesophagogastric mass lesions: preliminary results. Endoscopy 1994; 26:586–591.

27. Chang KJ, Erickson RA, Nguyen P. Endoscopic ultrasound (EUS) and EUS-guided fine-needle aspiration of the left adrenal gland. Gastrointest Endosc 1996; 44:568–572.

28. Savides TJ, Gress F, Sherman S, et al. Ultrasound catheter probe assisted endoscopic cystogastrostomy. Gastrointest Endosc 1995; 41:145–148.

29. Chan AT, Heller SJ, Van Dam J, et al. Endoscopic cystogastrostomy: role of endoscopic ultrasonography. Am J Gastroenterol 1996; 91:1622–1625.

30. Grimm H, Binmoeller KF, Soehendra N. Endosonography guided drainage of a pancreatic pseudocyst. Gastrointest Endosc 1992; 38:170–171.

31. Binmoeller KF. Endosonographic pseudocyst puncture and drainage. In: Bhutani MS, ed. Interventional endoscopic ultrasonography. Harwood Academic Publishers, Amsterdam 1999 (in press).

32. Brown DL, Bulley CK, Quiel EL. Neurolytic celiac plexus block for pancreatic cancer pain. Anesth Analg 1987; 66:869–873.

33. Wiersema MJ, Wiersema LM. Endosonography-guided celiac plexus neurolysis. Gastrointest Endosc 1996; 44:656–662.

34. Harada N, Wiersema MJ, Wiersema LM. Endosonography-guided celiac plexus neurolysis. Gastrointest Endosc Clin North Am 1997; 7:237–245.

35. Harada N, Wiersema M, Wiersema L. Endosonography guided celiac plexus neurolysis (EUS CPN) for abdominal pain:

comparison of results in patients with chronic pancreatitis versus malignant disease (abstract). Gastrointest Endosc 1997; 45:AB30.

36. Gress F, Ciaccia D, Kiel J, et al. Endoscopic ultrasound (EUS) guided celiac plexus block (CB) for management of pain due to chronic pancreatitis (CP): a large single center experience (abstract). Gastrointest Endosc 1997; 45:AB173.

37. Pasricha PJ, Ravich WJ, Hendrix TR, et al. Treatment of achalasia with intersphincteric injection of botulinum toxin: a pilot trial. Ann Intern Med 1994; 121:590–591.

38. Pasricha PJ, Ravich WJ, Hendrix TR, et al. Intersphincteric botulinum toxin for the treatment of achalasia. N Engl J Med 1995; 332:774–778.

39. Bhutani MS. Gastrointestinal uses of botulinum toxin. Am J Gastroenterol 1997; 92:929–933.

40. Hoffman BJ, Bhutani MS, Knapple WL, et al. Treatment de l'achalasie par injection de toxine botulinique sous controle echoendoscopique. (Treatment of achalasia by injection of botulinum toxin under endoscopic ultrasound guidance.) Acta Endosc 1995; 25:485–490.

41. Hoffman BJ, Knapple W, Bhutani MS, et al. EUS-guided injection of botulinum toxin for achalasia (abstract). Gastrointest Endosc 1996; 43:424.

42. Hoffman BJ, Knapple W, Bhutani MS, et al. Treatment of achalasia by injection of botulinum toxin under endoscopic ultrasound guidance. Gastrointest Endosc 1997; 45:77–79.

43. Chang K, Albers CG, Ashby K. Endoscopic ultrasound (EUS)-guided fine-needle aspiration (FNA) of pleural and ascitic effusions in cancer staging. Am J Gastroenterol 1994; 89:1635.

44. Chang KJ, Albers CG, Nguyen P. Endoscopic ultrasound-guided fine needle aspiration of pleural and ascitic fluid. Am J Gastroenterol 1995; 90:148–150.

45. Nguyen P, Rezvani A, Chang K. Endoscopic ultrasound (EUS) and EUS-guided fine needle aspiration (FNA) of abdominal fluid (abstract). Gastrointest Endosc 1997; 45:AB176.

46. Koito K, Nagakawa T, Murashima Y, et al. Endoscopic ultrasonographic-guided punctured pancreatic ductography: an initial and successful trial. Abdom Imaging 1995; 20:222–224.

47. Wiersema MJ, Sandusky D, Carr R, et al. Endosonography-guided cholangiopancreatography. Gastrointest Endosc 1996; 43:102–106.

48. Gress F, Ikenberry S, Sherman S, et al. Endoscopic ultrasound-directed pancreatography. Gastrointest Endosc 1996; 44:736–739.

49. Kallimanis G, Gupta PK, Kankaria AG, et al. Complications of endoscopic ultrasonography using conscious sedation at a university hospital. Gastrointest Endosc 1994; 40:P27.

50. Rosch T, Dittler HJ, Fockens P, et al. Major complications of endoscopic ultrasonography: results of a survey of 42,105 cases. Gastrointest Endosc 1993; 39:341.

51. Wiersema MJ, Vilmann P, Giovannini M, et al. Endosonography guided fine needle aspiration biopsy: diagnostic accuracy and complication assessment. Gastroenterology 1997; 112:1087–1095.

52. Catalano MF, Hoffman B, Wassef W, et al. Endoscopic ultrasound guided fine needle aspiration of gastrointestinal tract lesions: multicenter practice guidelines (abstract). Gastrointest Endosc 1997; 45.

53. Gress FG, Hawes RH, Savides TJ, et al. Endoscopic ultrasound guided fine needle aspiration biopsy using linear array and radial scanning endosonography. Gastrointest Endosc 1997; 45:243–250.

54. Giovannini M, Monges G, Bernardini D, et al. Diagnostic and therapeutic value of the endoscopic ultrasound guided biopsy: results in 453 patients. Endoscopy 1997; 29:E3.

55. Gress F, Ikenberry S, Ciaccia D, et al. Is pancreatitis a complication of endoscopic ultrasound guided fine needle aspiration of the pancreas? Gastrointest Endosc 1997; 45:174.

56. Bhutani MS, ed. Interventional endoscopic ultrasonography. Harwood Academic Publishers, Amsterdam.

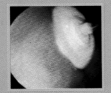

16.
GASTROSTOMY AND ENTEROSTOMY

E.M.H. MATHUS-VLIEGEN

Since 1980, two major non-surgical procedures for insertion of gastrostomy tubes have become available, one using percutaneous radiologic and another using percutaneous endoscopic techniques. Neither requires general anesthesia.

Whichever technique is used, it is of vital importance to exclude any interposed organ between the anterior gastric and anterior abdominal walls and to achieve apposition of the stomach to the anterior parietal peritoneum. During the percutaneous radiologic technique, ultrasonography or CT scan is used to exclude interposed organs such as liver or colon. This can also be confirmed during the procedure, after insufflation of the stomach, by anterior–posterior and lateral (biplanar) fluoroscopy. In the endoscopic procedure, an attempt is made to avoid interposed organs by abdominal wall transillumination by the bright light from the endoscope shining through the stomach and observed on the skin of the abdomen. Sufficient gastric distention by air insufflation is needed to displace the colon downward and liver and spleen laterally (Fig. 16.1). This also apposes the anterior gastric and anterior abdominal walls. In the radiologic technique, distention of the stomach can be obtained by air insufflation through a nasogastric tube, sometimes provided with an inflatable occluding balloon at the level of the gastric cardia, via the percutaneous needle after puncture of the hollow viscus, or by swallowing effervescent granules. In the endoscopic procedure, endoscopic insufflation distends the stomach and effects adequate apposition of the gastric and anterior abdominal walls.

Both methods also differ with respect to the gastric puncture and the gastrostomy placement but, more importantly, the subsequent fixation is different.

Under fluoroscopic or ultrasound guidance, the stomach is punctured transabdominally and a gastrostomy tube is placed either directly into the stomach (percutaneous radiologic gastrostomy) or subsequently manipulated through the pylorus into the duodenum and beyond the duodenojejunal junction (percutaneous radiologic gastrojejunostomy).[1–3] In neither of the two radiologic procedures is the anterior gastric wall closely apposed to the anterior abdominal wall. However, in the first proce-

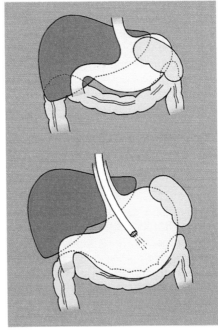

Fig. 16.1
Displacement of the colon downward and the liver and spleen laterally by gastric air distention through a nasogastric tube (radiology) or an endoscope (endoscopy).

dure, the (pigtail) shape of the catheter will prevent it from being dislodged during intragastric feeding and the inflammatory reaction will seal off both holes in the gastric and abdominal walls. In the second procedure, the long path of the catheter through the stomach and duodenum and the delivery of food in the jejunum will protect against catheter displacement and intraperitoneal leakage of fluids. In children, an antegrade radiologic approach combines features of the radiologic and endoscopic procedure.[4] After the percutaneous puncture of the stomach and the insertion of a guidewire through the needle, the guidewire is grasped and pulled out of the mouth by a Dotter intravascular sheath and retrieval basket, which is inserted orally up to the level of the body of the stomach. Over the guidewire, a gastrostomy tube is passed antegradely through the mouth as with the endoscopic (Sacks–Vine) method. The inner retention disc provides inner fixation of the anterior gastric wall to the skin. In ultrasound-guided percutaneous gastrostomy and jejunostomy, Cope anchors or T-shape anchoring devices can be used for the fixation of viscera to skin.[5]

In the endoscopic method, the stomach is punctured under endoscopic view with a sheathed needle via the abdominal wall. After removal of the needle, a string or loop wire (Ponsky–Gauderer, pull-(on)-string method) or a guidewire (Sacks–Vine, push-over-wire method; Russell, introducer or poke method) is advanced through the sheath into the stomach.[6–8] The three methods differ with respect to the means of introduction of the gastrostomy tube. In the Ponsky–Gauderer[6] and Sacks–Vine techniques,[7] the string/loop wire or the guidewire is grasped with a biopsy forceps or polypectomy snare. Withdrawal of the endoscope will bring the string/loop wire or the guidewire out of the mouth. Fixed at the string/loop wire or passed over the guidewire, the gastrostomy tube is positioned via the mouth and the esophagus into the stomach, finally piercing the abdominal wall. In the Russell method,[8] the immediate transabdominal gastric puncture and gastrostomy positioning are almost analogous to the percutaneous radiologic technique but under endoscopic control. In contrast to most of the radiologic procedures, in all three endoscopic methods the gastric wall is fixed to the abdominal wall by an inner retention disc, an inflated balloon, or a mushroom-like tip at the end of the catheter and by an outer retention disc, sleeve, or clipping device.

INDICATIONS

A gastrostomy is indicated when enteral feeding is anticipated for a period of more than 1 month. In that case, a non-surgical gastrostomy should be performed without any attempt at inserting a feeding tube. However, individuals with rapidly progressive disease are better served with nasogastric and nasojejunal tubes.[9–12] This consideration together with reports of a considerably high 30-day mortality (cited in the literature as between 6% and 33%, own series 6.7%[13]) resulted in a decision-making algorithm for gastrostomy placement.[14,15] This algorithm categorizes patients clinically into groups of anorexia–cachexia, permanent vegetative state, or dysphagia patients with or without symptoms and then considers the benefits defined as positive effects on physiological parameters such as nutritional status and effects on quality of life. In the decision process, prognostic markers of early mortality and raised complication risks should be taken into account, i.e. old age, male sex, low albumin, the presence of diabetes mellitus, multiorgan failure, or oropharyngeal aspiration and the indications for a gastrostomy. Central nervous system disease and non-cancer illnesses carry the best prognosis.[16–21]

Indications for a gastrostomy

The indications can be subdivided into three main categories:[22–28]

1. Nutrition in patients with:
   — reversible disease with potential for recovery (Guillain–Barré polyneuritis, cerebrovascular accident, failure to thrive in children with Crohn's disease or cystic fibrosis)
   — incurable disease with potential for extended survival (amyotrophic lateral sclerosis, head and neck cancer)
   — terminal or seriously debilitating disease (malignancy, trauma, brain damage)
   Here, frequent tube removal, long-term necessity for enteral feeding and hospital discharge to home care or step-down care are the common factors.
2. Gastric decompression in patients with similar conditions to those in group 1, with:
   — reversible disease with potential for recovery (decompensated gastric atony)
   — incurable disease with potential for extended survival (intestinal pseudo-obstruction and total parenteral nutrition)
   — terminal or severely debilitating disease (malignancy, aerophagia in brain-damaged patients).[29]

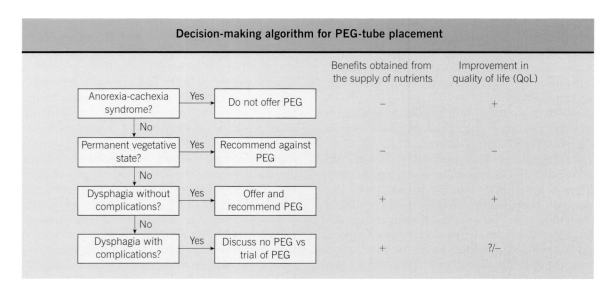

Decision-making algorithm for PEG-tube placement

			Benefits obtained from the supply of nutrients	Improvement in quality of life (QoL)
Anorexia-cachexia syndrome?	Yes →	Do not offer PEG	−	+
↓ No				
Permanent vegetative state?	Yes →	Recommend against PEG	−	−
↓ No				
Dysphagia without complications?	Yes →	Offer and recommend PEG	+	+
↓ No				
Dysphagia with complications?	Yes →	Discuss no PEG vs trial of PEG	+	?/−

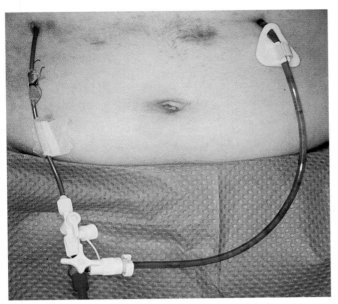

Fig. 16.2 Recirculation of bile recovered from external drainage into the stomach via a gastrostomy in a young patient after bile duct transection during laparoscopic cholecystectomy.

3. Bypass in patients with similar characteristics of group 1 patients, in whom biliary recirculation after bile duct trauma or complete bile duct obstruction is needed; the bile recovered from external drainage is deviated through the gastrostomy back into the gastrointestinal tract (Fig. 16.2). Occasionally, a gastrostomy is used to fasten the stomach in recurrent gastric volvulus or to enable transgastric instrumentation. In the literature, most reports feature patients with neurological disease, ear, nose, and throat problems, and respiratory illnesses as the candidates for gastrostomy feeding.

Indications for a gastrojejunostomy or jejunostomy

The conversion of a gastrostomy into a gastrojejunostomy or direct placement of a jejunostomy[25,30–34] is indicated for:

1. feeding purposes in patients with severe gastroesophageal reflux, food regurgitation, gastric dysmotility states or (impending) pulmonary aspiration
2. gastric decompression/gastric bypass together with jejunal feeding in patients on assisted ventilation or maxillomandibular fixation after facial trauma with a need to keep the stomach empty and in patients with gastroparesis (the critically ill, burns, neurosurgery, diabetic gastroparesis).

Occasionally, a gastrojejunostomy is used for the intrajejunal administration of medications, e.g. in therapy-resistant Parkinson's disease.

CONTRAINDICATIONS

Contraindications are related to the gastrostomy procedure itself or to the subsequent fistulous track formation.[22,25] They may be evident beforehand, or may only become so at the time of the initial endoscopy.[29,35,36]

Absolute and relative contraindications related to the gastrostomy procedure

The gastrostomy procedure itself is absolutely contraindicated in the presence of interposed organs (liver, colon), gastric mucosal abnormalities at the site of the puncture (ulcer, varices, congestive gastropathy, angiodysplasias, watermelon stomach), and severe coagulation disturbances in so far as they cannot be corrected. Until recently, absent transillumination (adiposity, abnormal anatomy after surgery, body deformity in cerebral palsy) always precluded the procedure. With certain precautions the procedure can be safely carried out.[37,38]

In the presence of a completely obstructing ear, nose, and throat process or esophageal cancer, when an endoscope cannot be introduced, only the radiologic or surgical approach is feasible. The Russell (introducer) method is preferred when gastric intubation is only feasible by pediatric endoscope or after dilation in cases of more severe degrees of obstruction, and certainly when an esophagotracheal fistula is present. The method is preferable to the peroral route in the presence of upper aerodigestive cancer as implantation metastases in the gastrostomy opening have been reported.[39] This also holds true for patients with severe oropharyngeal infection and probably also for patients with methicillin-resistant *Staphylococcus aureus* (MRSA), and AIDS, where the retrograde insertion by mouth may facilitate the dispersal and translocation of pathogens. Furthermore, the Russell method is preferred in patients with esophageal varices without evidence of gastric varices or ascites.

Some of the former absolute contraindications, such as esophageal fistula, esophageal obstruction, and esophageal varices, are now considered to be relative ones, provided the Russell method is used.

Other relative contraindications are prior abdominal surgery, as the procedure will be less successful (i.e. Billroth II resection), and prior intra-abdominal sepsis or peritonitis, where the procedure will be more prone to complications because of adhesions, interposed organs, and abnormal anatomy.[40,41]

Absolute and relative contraindications related to the cutaneous track formation

Low albumin levels (≤25 g/L) and the inability to appose the gastric and anterior abdominal walls (ascites) impede formation of a safe fistulous skin track.

Because of the risk of contamination, the procedure is contraindicated in peritoneal dialysis and where peritoneovenous shunts are inserted. In peritoneovenous shunts, there is an extra risk of air embolism. Notwithstanding the initial reservations in view of the risk of infection, the potential for shunt malfunction and neurological decompensation, percutaneous gastrostomies have been performed in more than 60 cases with ventriculoperitoneal shunts, both in adults and children.[40–43] It can be safely done, if the area of the shunt is avoided and is even preferred over surgery by some because of a reduced risk of adhesion formation and a larger remaining peritoneal surface. In portal hypertension with ascites, diffuse peritoneal metastases, immunosuppression, or corticosteroid treatment, a mature fistulous track may fail to develop or may only develop after a protracted period. A gastrostomy may be contraindicated unless precautions for a safe and prolonged fixation, for instance by T-anchors, are provided.

EQUIPMENT

Equipment for placement of a percutaneous endoscopic gastrostomy (PEG)

The endoscopic part of the procedure requires the normal equipment for endoscopy. As videoendoscopes are increasingly used, one should be aware that it is more difficult to produce transillumination since the instrument does not provide the same amount of light in the interior of the stomach.[37] In the presence of esophageal stenosis, a small-caliber endoscope is required and, if dilation is necessary, a guidewire and dilating bougies should be available. Additional equipment which should be available:

- a biopsy- or saw-toothed forceps (Ponsky–Gauderer) or a polypectomy snare (Ponsky–Gauderer; Sacks–Vine; Russell) according to the method used
- skin dressing materials
- metric tape measure
- plastic siphon bag
- sedative medications for intravenous use
- 1 g of a first- (cefazolin) or second-generation (cefoxitin/mefoxin) cephalosporin.

The sterile-draped table for the positioning of the gastrostomy tube should include:

- povidone-iodine
- local anesthesia, lidocaine 1% or bupivacaine 0.25–0.5% with or without epinephrine
- syringe and needle (21 gauge (0.8 mm diameter) and 5.0 mm in length) for local skin infiltration
- sterile drapes, sterile gauzes
- sterile clamps, sterile scissors, and surgical scalpel
- provisions, depending upon method used:
  1. Ponsky–Gauderer and Sacks–Vine method (Fig. 16.3)
     — a puncture needle with Teflon outer sheath
     — a cotton string or metal loop wire and a gastrostomy tube with a loop of cotton or metal material at the tapered end (Ponsky–Gauderer)
     — a guidewire and a gastrostomy tube with an open tapered end (Sacks–Vine)
     — in either method, a retention disc or propeller-like bumper at the opposite site of the gastrostomy tube
     — an abdominal retention disc or clipping device
     — a feeding system adaptor to be pushed or screwed onto the gastrostomy tube.
  2. Russell method (Fig. 16.4)
     — a puncture needle
     — a guidewire
     — a tapering introducer which can pass over a guidewire with a peel-away sheath around it; if a tapering introducer is not available, several dilators and a peel-away sheath
     — a gastrostomy tube (Foley bag balloon catheter; replacement balloon gastrostomy tube; Friction-Lock Malecot Russell gastrostomy catheter, Cook)

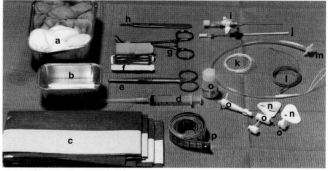

Fig. 16.3 Sterile draped table for the positioning of the Ponsky–Gauderer or Sacks–Vine gastrostomy tube: (a) povidone-iodine swabs; (b) lidocaine 1% local infiltration anesthesia; (c) sterile drapes; (d) syringe and needle for skin infiltration anesthesia; (e) sterile scissors; (f) catgut or nylon sutures; (g) sterile clamp; (h) surgical scalpel; (i) puncture needle with (j) Teflon outer sheath; (k) cotton string or (l) metal wire; (m) gastrostomy tube with retention disc at the one end and tapered at the other end, with (Ponsky–Gauderer) or without (Sacks–Vine) a loop; (n) abdominal retention disc or clipping device; (o) feeding system adaptor; (p) metric tape measure.

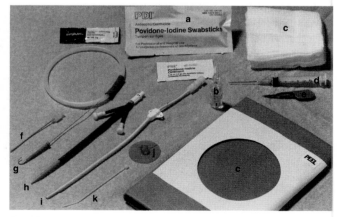

Fig. 16.4 Sterile draped table for the positioning of the Russell gastrostomy tube: (a) povidone-iodine swabs; (b) lidocaine 1% for local anesthesia; (c) sterile drapes and gauzes; (d) syringe and needle for local skin infiltration anesthesia; (e) small scalpel; (f) puncture needle; (g) J-tipped guidewire; (h) peel-away sheath (black) mounted on a tapering 16 Fr dilator (grey); (i) Malecot gastrostomy catheter; (j) abdominal retention disc; (k) fixation for retention disc.

— syringe filled with water for use with the balloon catheter

— an abdominal retention disc

— optional: two sets of 2 T-shaped anchoring devices (Brown/Mueller T-fastener set, Ross Laboratories; Cope suture anchors, Cook; Dennison anchors, Dennison Manufacturing; Meditech; Moss anchors, Moss).

Ready-to-use sets are available as well (*Ponsky–Gauderer/Sacks–Vine type*: Bard Interventional Products; Biosearch Medical Products; Corpak Medsystems; Fresenius; Medical Innovations; Mill–Rose; Novartis; Ross Laboratories; Wilson–Cook; *Russell type*: Cook; Microvasive; Moss; Ross Laboratories).

Equipment for the conversion of a gastrostomy into a gastroduodenostomy (jejunal tube through a gastrostomy; JETPEG or PEG/J)

In addition to the equipment needed for the positioning of a gastrostomy tube the following should be available:

- a biopsy or saw-toothed forceps
- catgut or nylon suture material
- a guidewire or a glidewire with a 12 Fr, 40 cm biliary catheter (Meditech)
- a separate intestinal feeding tube of appropriate size, small enough to be introduced via the gastrostomy opening. Some intestinal tubes are supplied with a grip-tip or silk thread at the tip to facilitate grasping with the forceps (Fig. 16.5). Coiled and Tungsten weighted tips are designed to

prevent early displacement. If simultaneous gastric decompression is required, enough space for drainage should be left between the gastrostomy opening and the intestinal feeding tube (Bard Interventional Products; Biosearch Medical Products; Corpak Medsystems; Fresenius; Medical Innovations; Novartis; Ross Laboratories; Wilson–Cook).

Equipment for placement of a percutaneous endoscopic jejunostomy (PEJ)

With the exception of a push enteroscope or a 1.60 m long endoscope and an extra-long cotton string, the same equipment as used in the Ponsky–Gauderer technique is required.

Equipment for placement of a gastric button

Sets for placement of gastric buttons through an already existing gastrocutaneous track are ready to use and should contain:

- viscous 2% lidocaine or lubricating jelly
- a gastrocutaneous track-measuring device
- the button (Figs 16.6 and 16.7), which consists of four parts:
    1. a small outer retention disc with a feeding port and feeding port cap; in balloon-tipped buttons, it also contains a balloon inflation port with a built-in valve
    2. a gastrostomy tube to bridge the distance between skin level and gastric inner wall via the gastrocutaneous track
    3. a mushroom- or dome-shaped tip which can be straightened with an obturator, or an inflatable balloon tip
    4. a one-way, antireflux valve, which can only be opened by clipping the feeding catheter at the time of the administration of food in balloon-tip buttons. In mushroom- or dome-shaped

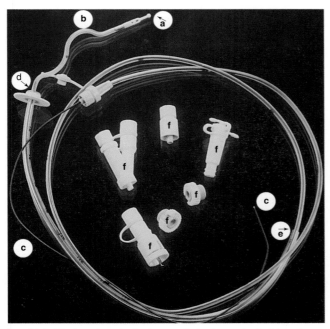

Fig. 16.5 The long intestinal tube supplied with a grip-tip (a) and a coiled end (b) which unfolds after removal of the guidewire (c). Both ends of the gastrostomy tube (d,e), where the intestinal tube enters and exits the gastrostomy tube, are shown. When cut to an appropriate length, the adaptors, (f) screwed onto the gastrostomy and jejunal tube catheter, either allow feeding or decompression and feeding.

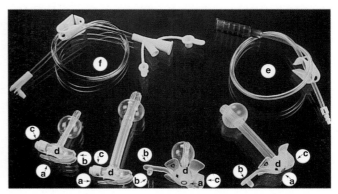

Fig. 16.6 Balloon-tipped buttons. The external end of the shaft is equipped with a feeding port (a), a snap-on plug (b) to prevent gastrocutaneous reflux, a balloon inflation port (c) with a built-in valve to prevent the escape of balloon contents. In the external part of the shaft, a one-way, antireflux valve is designed to prevent leakage of gastric contents (d). Both extremes of shaft length and diameter are shown. Tubes for bolus feeding (e) or continuous administration of food (f) are plugged onto the feeding port.

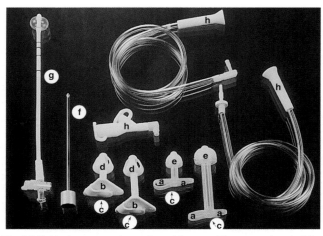

Fig. 16.7 Mushroom- or dome-shaped buttons. The external end of the shaft is equipped with retention flaps (a) or retention disc (b) to prevent internal migration. It contains the feeding port and feeding port cap (c). Different lengths and sizes of the shaft are shown. At the internal end of the shaft, the mushroom (d) or dome (e) of the button contains a one-way, antireflux valve to prevent leakage of gastric contents. To stretch the mushroom or dome an obturator (f) has to be introduced into the shaft. A balloon-tipped measuring device (g) with outer markings is provided to estimate the required button size. (h) Tubes for feeding.

buttons, the valve is at the opposite site near the mushroom or the dome and opens by the flow of feeding
(*Balloon-tipped buttons*: Bard Interventional Products; Biosearch Medical Products; Corpak Medsystems; Medical Innovations; *mushroom- or dome-shaped buttons*: Bard Interventional Products; Ross Laboratories; Surgitek)

- a water-filled syringe for use with a balloon-tipped button; an obturator to elongate the mushroom- or dome-shaped buttons.

Should intrajejunal feeding with or without gastric decompression become necessary in a patient with a gas-

tric button, a gastrojejunal button is available (Bard Interventional Products; Medical Innovations) (Fig. 16.8). Also, a gastrostomy tube can be converted into a button by cutting the gastrostomy tube at skin level (Bard Interventional Products). A device that contains a one-way, antireflux valve is positioned into the tube and an appliance containing two retention flaps and a feeding port cap is mounted over this device (Fig. 16.9).

Equipment for placement of a one-step gastric button

A gastric button placed as a one-step procedure requires the equipment and sterile-draped table as used for the positioning of a gastrostomy tube. The ready-to-use set (Bard Interventional Products, Surgitek) (Fig. 16.10) should contain:

- a puncture needle
- a guidewire
- a measuring device
- an assembly containing the appropriate length one-step-button
- a set of disc spacers
- a specially designed tube to allow gastric decompression.

Equipment for gastrostomy removal and/or replacement

Foley bag balloon catheters or replacement balloon gastrostomy tubes, where the balloon can be emptied, and gastrostomy tubes with a collapsible internal retention disc (Bard Interventional Products; Biosearch Medical Products; Corpak Medsystems; Friction-Lock Malecot Russell gastrostomy, Cook; Medical Innovations; Ross Laboratories;

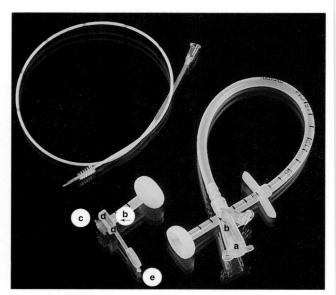

Fig. 16.9 The conversion of an existing gastrostomy tube into a button. The original gastrostomy tube (a) is cut off at the 3 cm marking (b). A yellow device containing a one-way, antireflux valve is positioned into the tube (c) and an appliance with two retention flaps (d) and the feeding port cap (e) is mounted onto this device. Also, a brush to clean the gastrostomy tube or button is shown.

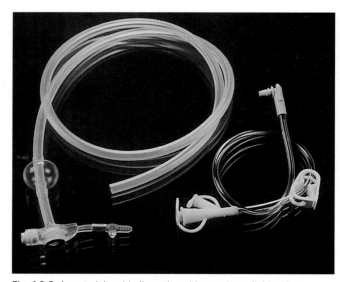

Fig. 16.8 A gastrojejunal balloon-tipped button is available when intrajejunal feeding is necessary.

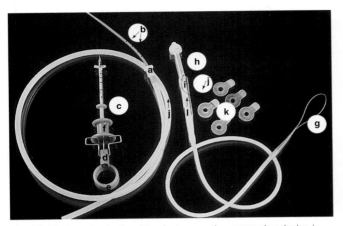

Fig. 16.10 One-step button. The first-generation measuring device is introduced over the guidewire through the mouth until the internal bolster (a) rests against the gastric wall. The markings on the outside (blue part, b) denote the required size (1.7 cm, 2.4 cm, 3.4 cm, and 4.4 cm) of the button. The recent redesigned measurement device: a sheathed needle (c) to puncture the stomach, after removal of the needle (d), allowing the introduction of a guidewire. By squeezing the other handle parts (e,f), the distal part of the sheath folds up to a star-shaped end. After pulling the star-shaped end against the gastric wall, the markings on the outside denote the required size. The plastic catheter contains a dilating tip and looped wire at the one end (g) and the enshrouded button (h) with a red colored guide strip (i) that incorporates a silk suture (j) to tear and peel away the shroud at the other end. Disc spaces (k) that can be positioned on the shaft are provided to better appose both gastric and abdominal walls.

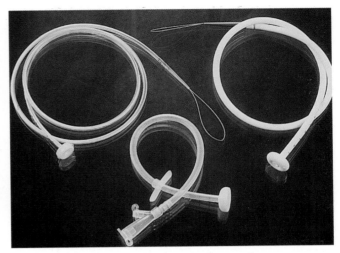

Fig. 16.11 Gastrostomy tubes with collapsible internal retention disc that do not require endoscopic removal but can be extracted by gently pulling on the shaft.

Wilson–Cook; Fig. 16.11) do not require endoscopic removal. If there is a rigid internal retention disc, endoscopic removal requires:

- an endoscope
- a polypectomy snare
- scissors
- occasionally, a long suture.

To carry out replacement, a ready-to-use gastrostomy or gastric button should be available. Otherwise, a choice of one of the many replacement balloon gastrostomy tubes should be made (Bard Interventional Products; Corpac Medsystems; Medical Innovations; Moss; Novartis; Sandoz Nutrition Biosystems; Sherwood; Ross Laboratories).

PATIENT PREPARATION

Regardless of the method, patients should be fasting and the skin of the left upper quadrant of the abdomen should be shaved and cleaned. Local pharyngeal anesthesia is obtained by spraying with lidocaine 1%. An IV cannula is inserted when midazolam and/or antibiotics are administered. Opinions differ on the issue of antibiotic prophylaxis and oral hygienic measures, mainly with reference to gastrostomy placement via the oral route.[44–50] Most sources report the administration of 1 g IV first-generation cefalosporin (cefazolin) 30 minutes before the procedure.[44,45] This may be repeated twice thereafter, every 6 to

8 hours. In patients already on antibiotics, cefazolin prophylaxis is not indicated.[45] There are reports that a more broad-spectrum antibiotic and a more prolonged duration of administration may be significant factors determining the risk of infection, stemming not only from the oral route, but also from the skin and the water in the water bottle of the endoscope.[44,46,47] It is important to note that a second-generation cefalosporin, i.e. cefoxitin, did not demonstrate any benefit of antibiotic prophylaxis.[48,49] Third-generation cefalosporins may be preferred to cover more adequately the throat-harboring bacteria such as *Haemophilus* and *Neisseria*. Few authors follow the suggestion of vigorous dental hygiene and of extensive rinsing, gargling, and scrubbing of mouth and teeth with povidone-iodine. Similarly, the advised discontinuation of H$_2$-receptor antagonists at least 24 hours beforehand and the administration of four doses of 1 g neomycin in hypochlorhydric patients[50] is not common practice.

PROCEDURE

Procedure of gastrostomy (PEG) placement

In all three methods of endoscopic gastrostomy placement, endoscopic inspection as far as the duodenum with the patient in the left lateral position is of paramount importance. Abnormal findings may preclude tube placement in 5% of patients or may dictate the conversion of a gastrostomy into a gastroduodenostomy or jejunostomy procedure in another 5%.[29,35,36]

The gastric fluid is aspirated and the patient is turned to the supine position. The stomach is then inflated to displace neighboring organs laterally and downward and to appose the gastric and anterior abdominal walls (Fig. 16.1). Room lights are dimmed and bright red transillumination should be visible in the left upper quadrant of the abdomen (Fig. 16.12). Interposed organs are visible, as are large veins present in the abdominal wall. In children, the transverse

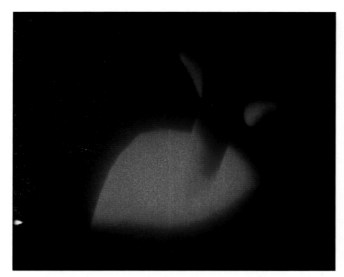

Fig. 16.12 The bright red transillumination of the gastric and abdominal wall in the left upper quadrant of the abdomen. Interposed organs and large veins in the abdominal wall are absent.

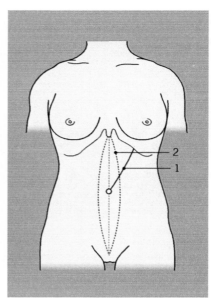

Fig. 16.13 Puncture site located on the line between the umbilicus and the midclavicular line at the left inferior costal margin, at the junction of the middle and outer one-third (1). Adjustment by endoscopy often results in a somewhat higher puncture site (2).

colon can lie across the lower part of the stomach. During transillumination, a dark shadow may be seen running transversally, usually across the lower third of the illuminated stomach, which represents the greater omentum and the transverse colon.[51]

A line is drawn between the umbilicus and the left inferior costal margin at the midclavicular line (Fig. 16.13). The site of the puncture should be at the junction of the middle third and the outer third.[6] Together with the help of maximally intense transillumination and the internally visible indentation of the finger palpating the outer abdominal wall (Fig. 16.14), the optimal endoscopic site, along the anterior wall of the stomach and opposite the incisura, is determined. Often, the puncture site determined according to the line between the umbilicus and costal margin has to be adjusted and is usually situated higher up in the epigastrium and just left of the rectus muscle. Ideally, puncture should be directed between, and not on top of, the gastric rugae, as elongation of these rugae in advance of the penetrating cannula may impede the passage of the needle into the stomach or may increase the risk of puncture through the stomach into the posterior gastric wall (Fig. 16.15).[23] The introduction of the trochar needle in short, controlled jabs prevents the stomach from being pushed away.[51]

Failure to identify the stomach in the usual position, or a less desirable puncture site despite an adequate start of the procedure, may result from overinflation of the stomach, which displaces the antrum to the left and downwards. In children, excessive insufflation causes the small bowel to push stomach and colon cranially. The stomach rotates upward on its transverse axis, pulling the colon with it and thereby increasing the risk of colonic puncture.[42,51]

As soon as the puncture site is selected, the lights are switched on, the skin is prepared with povidone-iodine and sterile drapes applied. After local skin infiltration with lidocaine 1%, the needle with the lidocaine-filled syringe is introduced perpendicularly into the stomach while aspir-

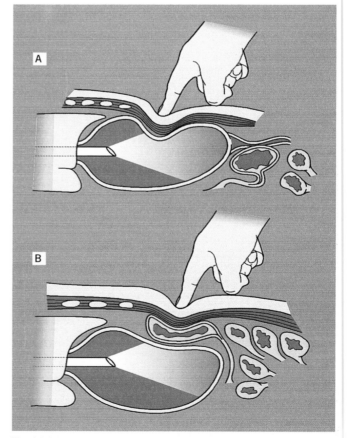

Fig. 16.14 (A) Palpation of the stomach by the finger is seen as a sharp and clearly visible indentation through the endoscope. (B) In a case of interpositioned bowel loops, no sharp indentation and only referred motion are seen.

ating. Care should be taken not to puncture the endoscope. This maneuver, the so-called 'double-check' or 'safe track' is used to check the safe gastrocutaneous puncture track

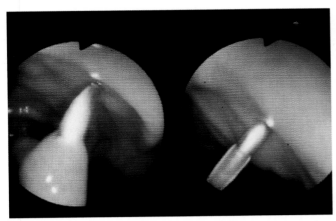

Fig. 16.15 Elongation of a gastric rugal fold when the puncture site is on top of a fold and when the selected puncture site is situated too far toward the greater curvature. This may prevent entry of the needle or further attempts at pushing may result in puncture of the posterior gastric wall.

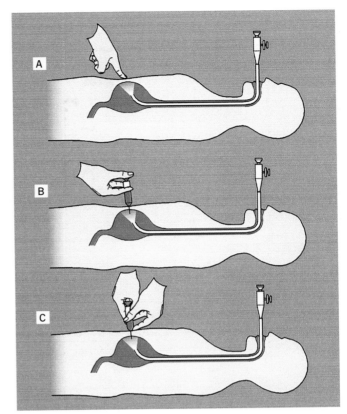

Fig. 16.16 Initial steps similar in all three endoscopic gastrostomy tube placements. (**A**) Determination of the optimal puncture site by combined maximal transillumination and indentation of the palpating finger; (**B**) local infiltration anesthesia of the skin; (**C**) 'double-check' or 'safe-track' maneuver, consisting of observing for air return in the aspirating needle and visualization of the needle in the stomach.

(Fig. 16.16). Tracks are safe in the presence of simultaneous air return in the aspirating syringe and endoscopic visualization of the intragastric needle.[52] In the presence of air bubbles upon aspiration, while the needle is not visualized, another hollow viscus (esophagus, gastric cardia or fundus, duodenum, or even colon) has probably been punctured. Sometimes, the endoscopist has difficulty in locating the needle. The injection of fluid and the visible jet may help the endoscopist locate the puncture site. When still in doubt, methylene blue may be added to the syringe fluid for proper visualization in difficult cases, such as severe body deformity in cerebral palsy.

With the scalpel, an incision 1.5 times wider than the diameter of the selected gastrostomy tube is made through the skin layer. The stomach is reinflated and a sheathed needle is then thrust across the apposed abdominal and gastric walls, again controlled by the endoscopist. As soon as the proper position of both needle and sheath has been confirmed, the needle is removed. Continued insufflation is of paramount importance to prevent gastric collapse and dislocation of the sheath from the stomach into the abdominal cavity. A trick to prevent dislodgement is to introduce a polypectomy snare and to tighten the snare around the sheath. Some sets (Fresenius) have sheaths, provided with a one-way valve which closes after needle removal to prevent the escape of air. A special device is provided to open the valve upon the introduction of the string or wire.

Ponsky–Gauderer (pull-(on)-string) method

In this method,[6,22,41] a cotton string (or metal loop wire) is inserted via the cannula into the stomach (Fig. 16.17). If a snare was used to hold the cannula, the string can be grasped by loosening the snare and allowing it to slip down over the string. Then, the snare is retightened. The string can also be grasped by a biopsy or saw-toothed forceps. With the snare or forceps tightly closed, the endoscope is removed, pulling the string with it and finally leaving the string projecting from the patient's mouth. The string may

be lost upon premature opening of the snare or forceps or may slip out upon withdrawal of the endoscope. To prevent this, the string can be pulled completely through the instrumentation channel, until it appears at the upper end of the endoscope. By opening the snare or the forceps, the string is freed. The endoscope is removed, leaving the string in the patient's mouth.

The gastrostomy tube is supplied with a loop at the tapered end which is tied to the string at the mouth. Where a loop wire is used instead of a cotton string, the loop on the gastrostomy tube can be interlooped with the end which protrudes from the mouth. By careful pulling at the abdominal end of the string (or metal loop wire), the gastrostomy tube passes from the mouth into the esophagus and the stomach and finally emerges through the abdominal wall. The tapered end dilates the tiny puncture wound in the abdominal wall while traversing it. This should be the only part during tube passage where some resistance is met. The gastrostomy tube is extracted until the round or propeller-like retention disc reaches the gastric wall and prevents further withdrawal of the gastrostomy tube.

Repeat endoscopy will confirm the full introduction of the tube and the proper positioning of the inner retention disc, and should exclude blanching of the gastric mucosa, indicative of excessive compression and traction

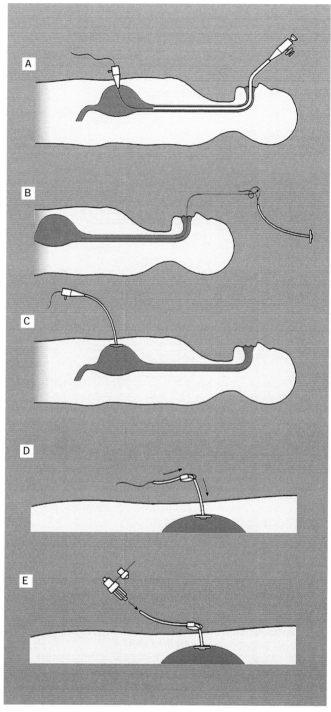

Fig. 16.17 Gastrostomy tube placement according to the Ponsky–Gauderer and Sacks–Vine methods. (**A**) Gastric puncture with a sheathed needle and introduction of a string or metal wire through the sheath after removal of the needle. While grasping the string or the metal wire, the endoscope is removed; (**B**) with the Ponsky–Gauderer method, the loop of the gastrostomy tube is knotted at the string projecting from the mouth and by pulling at the abdominal end of the string, the gastrostomy tube passes through the esophagus and stomach and finally pierces the abdominal wall. In the Sacks–Vine method, the gastrostomy tube is pushed over the metal wire projecting from the mouth into the esophagus and stomach and through the abdominal wall; (**C**) the retention disc of the gastrostomy tube is apposed against the gastric wall; (**D**) the outer retention disc and (**E**) the feeding adaptor are put in place.

(Fig. 16.18). The retention disc should rotate freely when the tube is rotated. Alternatively, endoscopists can rely upon the markings on the outer surface of the tube or on the length of the outer remaining tube, to ascertain the entire introduction of the gastrostomy tube.[53] Also, pulling on the tube itself elevates the abdomen along the contours of the inner retention disc (Fig. 16.19). Moreover, by palpating the abdomen around the tube with a V-shape formed by the index and middle fingers, the internal bumper can often be detected and when finger palpation is considered satisfactory, sufficient looseness is obtained by allowing the tube to slide back 1.5–2.0 cm through the abdominal wall track. This reduces the necessity for a second passage of an endoscope to cases with insufficient satisfactory finger palpation and to morbidly obese patients.[54] After cutting the gastrostomy tube at the desired length, the outer retention disc or clipping device designed for fixation is placed so as to ensure close approximation of both walls to allow proper track formation. Finally, the feeding adaptor is pushed or screwed onto the gastrostomy tube.

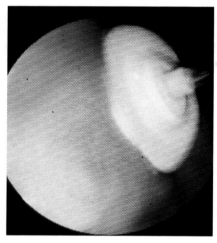

Fig. 16.18 Endoscopic confirmation of proper positioning of the gastrostomy tube without blanching of the underlying gastric mucosa.

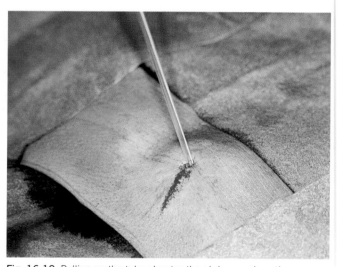

Fig. 16.19 Pulling on the tube elevates the abdomen along the contours of the inner retention disc and allows palpation of the disc. When this sign is present, a second control endoscopy is unnecessary.

Sacks–Vine (push-over-wire) method

This procedure is very similar to the pull-(on)-string technique, but uses a very long, firm gastrostomy tube with a tapered end which can be passed over a guidewire.[7,24,55] The patient is prepared as described above. The endoscope is passed and the correct site chosen by abdominal wall transillumination and finger pressure, and confirmed by the 'double-check' or 'safe-track' control (Fig. 16.16). After skin incision and needle puncture, a flexible guidewire is passed through the sheath. A snare is tightened around the wire and the endoscope, and snare and wire are withdrawn (Fig 16.17). After opening the snare, the wire lies free in the patient's mouth. The gastrostomy tube is then loaded onto the wire with the tapered end first and pushed over the guidewire down the esophagus, into the stomach and through the abdominal wall. As with the pull-(on)-string method, a control endoscopy can be performed to assess the adequate introduction of the entire gastrostomy tube and the appropriate positioning of the inner retention disc. In most instances, it is only necessary to measure the outer gastrostomy tube length and confirm the proper location of the retention disc against the gastric wall by a slight pull on the tube. The gastrostomy tube should be shortened to the appropriate length, the outer retention disc properly fixed, and the feeding port mounted on the tube. In both methods, with the introduction via the oral route, gel or neosporin ointment may be used for lubrication of the gastrostomy tube.

Russell (introducer or poke) method

For this procedure,[8,22,24,56] the patient is prepared as described for the two other methods of percutaneous endoscopic gastrostomy. The endoscope is introduced and the appropriate site for puncture identified. A small skin incision is made and a needle is thrust into the stomach (Fig 16.20). A flexible J-wire guide is passed through the lumen of the needle and the needle is removed. All steps are controlled by endoscopy. Next, the inner dilator (or introducer) and the outer peel-away sheath are threaded as one unit over the guidewire. Using a rotary clockwise–counterclockwise motion, the dilator and sheath are introduced into the stomach, where both have to be visualized by the endoscopist.

During the procedure, the path of the guidewire has to be followed when inserting the dilator and sheath; they must follow the same insertion angle as the original needle. If not, the wire may kink or buckle into the peritoneum and placement may be either difficult or unsuccessful, or otherwise, the dilator and sheath may not penetrate the gastric lumen and they may tunnel subserosally in the gastric wall. During the critical step of dilator insertion over the guidewire, the stomach must be kept fully inflated. Three measures are available when difficulties arise. The wire can be caught with a snare (introduced via the endoscope) and kept taut by the nurse at the outer end. Also, the endoscope can be used to stabilize the gastric wall.[8,57] An alternative technique is to anchor the gastric and abdominal walls by means of T-shaped anchoring devices (Fig. 16.21).[5,58,59] These are mounted in a needle. After

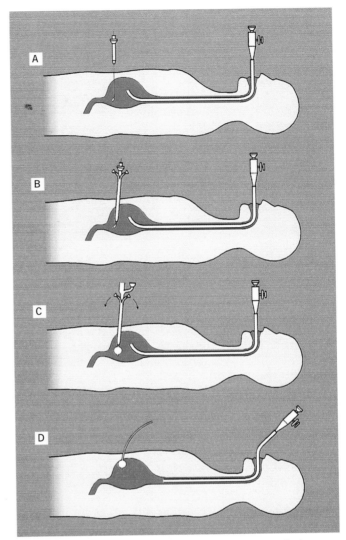

Fig. 16.20 Gastrostomy tube positioning by the Russell method. (A) Gastric puncture with a needle and introduction of a flexible J-wire into the stomach via the lumen of the needle; (B) removal of the needle and insertion of the inner dilator and outer peel-away sheath over the guidewire; (C) after dilation, the inner dilator and J-wire are removed and a Foley bag balloon catheter is introduced into the stomach through the peel-away sheath, which is peeled off after balloon filling; (D) the final positioning of the balloon gastrostomy tube, controlled by endoscopy before removal of the endoscope.

transabdominal gastric puncture with the needle, the T-anchor can be pulled out of the needle: it assumes the T-shape by unfolding. Usually, four T-anchors are placed in a four-square surrounding the guidewire and knotted two-by-two together at skin level.

Once the introducer and its sheath are well inside the gastric lumen, the introducer is removed and a Foley bag balloon, a replacement balloon gastrostomy tube, or a Malecot catheter is introduced through the sheath into the stomach. Under endoscopic view, the balloon is filled with the indicated volume, but fluid (water) is used instead of air to prevent premature dangerous deflation. Where a Malecot catheter is used, the mushroom tip is stretched over an inner probe so that the bulbous end is markedly

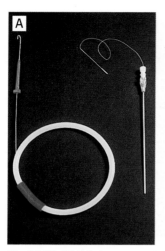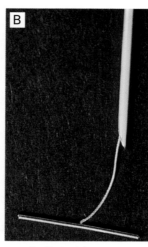

Fig. 16.21 (A) T-fastener, mounted in a needle. To the left, the wire needed to expel the T-fastener from the needle; (B) the T-fastener assuming its T-shape as it is expelled from the needle.

deformed into a straight line. Once the end is inserted into the stomach through the sheath, the inner probe is pulled back which allows the mushroom tip to unfold. The peel-away sheath is torn off and peeled away. The gastrostomy tube is placed in the sleeve of the outer retention disc and fixed at the skin with appropriate tension. After a final inspection, the endoscope is withdrawn.

Gastrostomy tubes in children

The correct site for puncture is more critical in the child as the stomach is small and the distance between esophagogastric junction and pylorus relatively short.[22,60,61] Also, the procedure is somewhat more difficult as during needle puncture (in order to avoid scope damage) the endoscope has to be withdrawn from the puncture site. The endoscope will therefore be at the esophagogastric junction, where peristalsis and respiratory movements are present. For these reasons, in small children the procedure is done under general anesthesia. The inner retention disc should be cut down or small V-shaped cuts made in three places (in a 'Mercedes-Benz sign'). In children younger than 12 months of age, the inner retention disc should be 1.5 cm or less in order to pass the cricopharyngeal area.[4] A second pass of the endoscope is more often required, especially when finger palpation is unsatisfactory. Measurement of the length of the outer remaining tube is less reliable. The inner retention disc may be stuck in the esophagus behind the cardia and the small difference in distance may go unrecognized.

Choice of method

Both methods of oral placement of gastrostomy tubes (Ponsky–Gauderer and Sacks–Vine) are comparable[62] and technically easier[57] but not as fast[63] as the Russell (introducer) method. Furthermore, both oral methods have the advantage of creating a small abdominal wall defect with less risk of leakage and easier conversion into a gastrojunostomy. The disadvantages of the Ponsky–Gauderer

(pull-(on)-string) method are string rupture, difficult introduction of the string into the needle when moistened, and mechanical laceration of hypopharynx, cricopharyngeus or the gastroesophageal junction. The Sacks–Vine (push-over-wire) method circumvents these disadvantages. However, contamination with oral flora is possible with both methods.

The Russell (introducer) method is free of the risk of oral bacterial contamination of the puncture site and is therefore preferred in oral candidiasis, in MRSA and in AIDS patients. Also, the direct abdominal puncture is advantageous in severe esophageal obstruction and esophagotracheal fistulae. Here the disadvantages are a more difficult conversion into a gastrojejunostomy, a larger abdominal wall defect with more chance of leakage, displacement of the anterior gastric wall without piercing it, and difficult apposition and fixation of both gastric and abdominal walls. Also, the loss of gastric insufflation and the resultant pneumoperitoneum during tract dilation should be taken into account when T-fasteners are not used. In that case, premature balloon deflation or removal may be life-threatening.

When looking at complications, complications are more frequent and more severe in the Russell and Sacks–Vine method.[55,64] In children, the Ponsky–Gauderer technique is preferred to the Sacks–Vine method, because of the rather large catheter with a stiff tube segment in the latter. It is also preferred to the Russell technique, in which the stomach can be pushed away during insertion or the balloon catheter may deflate prematurely.[42]

Post-procedure actions

After the procedure, wound care is given. The gastrostomy tube length is measured and a gastric siphon bag is connected. Nil by mouth and an analgesic suppository in case of wound pain are advised. In the absence of fever, abnormal bowel sounds, and gross evidence of pneumoperitoneum such as the disappearance of liver dullness, oral intake is resumed the next morning. The IV line and the gastric siphon are disconnected. Enteral feeding is given by bolus feeding (200 mL every 2 hours) for the rest of the day. Before and after each feed, the tube is flushed with 20 mL water. The patient can be discharged the same day, if feeding is well tolerated. At home, feeding is gradually augmented over 5 days (200 mL every 2 hours seven times daily; 250 mL every 3 hours six times daily; 300 mL every 3 hours five times daily; 400 mL every 4 hours four times daily, and finally 500 mL every 4 hours four times daily). In the hospital, 24-hour continuous administration is usually preferred. This is started at 20 mL/h for the first 8 hours. If tube feeding is well tolerated, a stepwise increase with 20 mL/h is planned every 8 hours up to 100 mL/h. The patient is instructed to measure the length of the outer tubing daily and to contact the hospital in case of a change in length of more than 1 cm. Bathing is not allowed for the first 7 days. Handling of the tube, particularly close to the point of insertion, should be minimized.

At the outpatient appointment, 1 week later, the skin dressing is removed and the wound is inspected. The for-

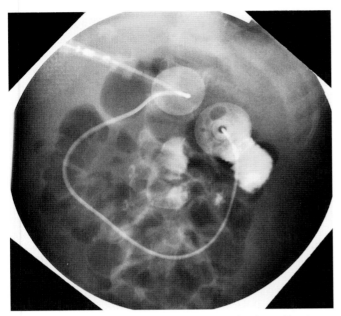

Fig. 16.22 Complete obstruction at the duodenojejunal transition by a gastrostomy catheter in an infant because of insufficient care and control of the outer remaining tube length. The remaining outer part is indicated (arrows).

mation of the fistulous track can be seen by tenting up the tube: a smooth, rose-colored moistened layer is visible around the tube, which slides easily in- and outward without resistance. When adequate fistula formation has occurred, the outer retention disc is loosened about 0.5–1 cm and fixed again. Bathing and swimming are now allowed, and daily measurement of the tube length is no longer necessary. Most gastrostomy tubes have centimeter markings, which allow estimation of the outer tube length. In children, however, careful inspection of the remaining tube length is indicated. Owing to a shorter distance between the retention disc located in the antrum and the pyloric channel, gastric outlet obstruction by migration of the inner retention disc may occur in children after a change of only a few centimeters of extra tube length (Fig. 16.22).[22] When nylon T-fasteners are used, they are cut at skin level to release the T ends after 3 weeks and they pass uneventfully in the stools.[5]

Patients are instructed to return immediately and at least within 24 hours in case of accidental removal of the gastrostomy tube or tube rupture to prevent fistula closure.

Procedure of gastrojejunostomy (JETPEG or PEG/J) placement

A gastrostomy can be converted into a gastrojejunostomy (jejunal tube through a gastrostomy; JETPEG or PEG/J) either during the procedure of gastrostomy positioning in both oral methods or in the case of the Russell (introducer) method, when T-anchors have been used, after at least 1 week after the track has been fully formed.[25]

Most of the intestinal tubes have a silk thread or a grip-tip at the end; else, a suture should be knotted at the tip (Fig. 16.5).

The intestinal tube is introduced into the stomach via the gastrostomy tube opening and maneuvered under endoscopic view toward the antrum until it lies in front of the pyloric channel. Redundant loop formation should be avoided. Here the thread or grip-tip is grasped by a biopsy or saw-toothed forceps. Upon introduction of the endoscope into the small intestine, the intestinal tube will follow. When the desired level is reached, the thread or grip-tip should be released. The endoscope should be carefully removed in order not to displace the intestinal tube. This can be prevented to some extent by stiffening the intestinal tube with a guidewire. More helpful is to wedge the tube in between the opened forceps and intestinal wall upon withdrawal of the endoscope. This requires a coordinated outward withdrawal of the endoscope and a synchronous insertion of an equivalent length of the shaft of the forceps. The stepwise motion is repeated until the endoscope is removed from the duodenum. Two recent modifications using an over-the-wire technique or using a steerable glidewire have been reported.[65,66] In both techniques, the wire is inserted inside the stomach via the gastrostomy opening, grasped with the forceps, and guided into the third part of the duodenum by the endoscope. In the over-the-wire technique, the guidewire is straightened and held tight at both ends. The jejunostomy tube is guided over the wire into the duodenum under direct vision. As soon as the tube reaches the end of the guidewire, the forceps is released and the tip of the jejunal tube is passing distally. Slow withdrawal of the endoscope is used to verify that a large loop of the enteral tube is not left in the stomach.

In the glidewire method, loop formation is prevented by advancing a 12 Fr, 40 cm straight biliary catheter over the wetted glidewire. Again, the glidewire is guided into the third part of the duodenum by the endoscope. Once the glidewire is in place, the forceps is released. The glidewire is then advanced slowly and gently for 10–15 cm, followed by the biliary catheter. Also, a torque device can be attached to the glidewire to enable advancement of the glidewire by a continuous forward clockwise motion of the torque device. Upon encountering resistance, the assembly has to be withdrawn partially and the maneuver repeated. The advancement is visualized by endoscopy. Upon reaching the desired distance, the biliary catheter (and torque device) are removed and the jejunostomy tube is passed over the glidewire in a twisting motion.

The intestinal tube is used for feeding, and, if necessary, gastric decompression or gastric suction can be applied via the gastrostomy tube.

Procedure of jejunostomy (PEJ) placement

Direct percutaneous endoscopic jejunostomy (DPEJ or PEJ) placement requires the introduction of a long (1.60 m) endoscope distal to the ligament of Treitz into the jejunum,[67] until the transilluminated light, concentrated in a small 2–3 cm diameter area, is seen clearly on the abdominal wall. Pressure applied with the finger tip should give a discrete indentation. After skin preparation and infiltration anesthesia and after an incision is made, the sheathed needle is introduced with a swift stab, instead of a slow push, into the jejunum. Once the sheathed needle is in view in the jejunum, the needle is removed, the string inserted, grasped by the biopsy forceps and pulled out of the patient's mouth by the endoscope. The internal retention disc of the gastrostomy tube has to be reduced to 2 cm in diameter to avoid jejunal obstruction or ulceration. The cotton loop of the gastrostomy tube is knotted at the string and carefully pulled through until resistance is met. Before outer fixation of the tube, a second endoscopy should confirm the proper position of the tube. It is essential to proceed quickly after identification of the site of puncture because bowel peristalsis may cause a loss of the transilluminated position and may interfere with the insertion of the sheathed needle.

Procedure of gastric button placement

Gastric buttons permit a psychologically and socially normal and acceptable life (Figs 16.6 to 16.9). Before the placement of a button is considered, a mature fistulous gastrocutaneous track must be present, which can resist some external forces without separation of the adherent abdominal and gastric wall layers. This applies especially for obturator-type buttons which carry a higher risk of gastrostomy tract disruption and gastric separation.[68] It may take 4 weeks for perpendicularly piercing short tracks (up to 2.7 cm) and 8 weeks for obliquely running long (2.7–4.3 cm) tracks.[69] In children, a 3-month interval is advised and an even longer period in the presence of malnutrition or use of steroids.[70,71] If an earlier replacement is needed, a balloon-tipped button is preferred. In case approximation of the gastric to the abdominal wall was not accomplished initially,[72] the formation of thin-walled fibrous tracks precludes the safe positioning of a gastric button.

First, the gastrostomy tube has to be removed and the length of the track between skin and stomach has to be measured. The original rigid stoma-measuring device occasionally became falsely engaged in the abdominal wall fascia and failed to identify the true tract length, so the use of the old gastrostomy tube and the measurement of the inner retention disc to skin length was strongly recommended.[68,70,71] The currently used small balloon-catheter-type measuring device is able to more adequately identify longer tracts: it is introduced into the tract and inflated when lying free in the stomach (Fig. 16.7). When pulled against the gastric wall the centimeter markings at the outside indicate the required length and size of the button. When the mushroom- or dome-shaped button is used, an obturator is needed to straighten the dome of the button. Under constant stretch, the button is thrust through the existing gastrocutaneous track into the stomach. When the obturator is removed, the button assumes its preformed mushroom or dome shape. Where a button with a balloon is used, the button is introduced into the stomach and is filled with the appropriate amount of water. After insertion, the button should have some to-and-fro play indicating that the head of the device is in the stomach rather than in the track.[70] When in doubt, radiographic or endoscopic control should follow.[68]

Also, an existing gastrostomy tube can be converted into a button. The tube is cut off at skin level and a one-way, antireflux valve-containing device is positioned into the gastrostomy tube. An appliance with two retention flaps and a feeding port plug is mounted onto this device (Fig. 16.9). Gastrojejunal buttons require subsequent endoscopy to position the feeding tube into the jejunum (Fig. 16.8).

Procedure of one-step button placement

Up to the insertion of the guidewire, the method is analogous to the Sacks–Vine (push-over-wire) gastrostomy technique. Over the guidewire, a measuring device with markings to denote 1.7 cm, 2.4 cm, 3.4 cm, and 4.4 cm is advanced with the dilator tip pushing the needle out until the internal bolster rests against the gastric wall (Fig. 16.10). The marking on the outside denotes the required size of the button. By pulling it back over the wire, the measuring device is removed through the mouth, leaving the guidewire in place. The appropriate length one-step button consisting of a plastic catheter enshrouding an 18 or 24 Fr button at the one end and a dilating tip on the other end is pulled through or advanced over the wire. Once the dilator comes through the abdominal wall, it is carefully pulled out until the shroud covering the external components of the button and the red colored guide strip that incorporates a silk suture, become visible (Fig. 16.23). By pulling the suture upward, the strip is torn and the shroud peeled away. The wings of the button are released. Disc spacers can be added to the shaft when the apposition of gastric and abdominal walls seems to be too loose. The lingering controversy over the safety of the procedure[73–76] (twice instrument passage, inadequate button sizing, difficult pull through the abdominal wall, impossible gastric decompression) has recently resulted in two improvements: an adaptor that violates the continent internal valve to

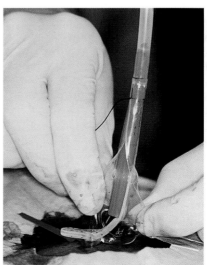

Fig. 16.23 The dilator part of the plastic catheter enshrouding the button has been carefully pulled out. The shroud covering the external components of the button is peeled away by pulling at the silk suture on the red colored guide strip. One of the two wings of the button is released; the other one has yet to be detached from the catheter.

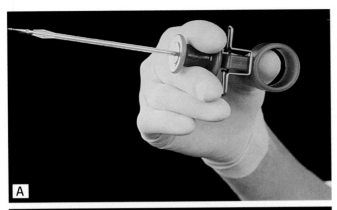

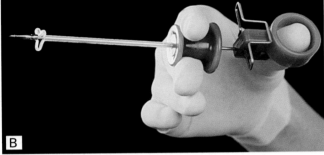

Fig. 16.24 (A) The measuring device as held during the puncture and (B) the star-shaped end that is formed by pulling apart the two handle components as soon as the needle has entered the stomach. After pulling this end against the gastric wall, markings at the outside indicate the required button size.

enable postinsertion gastric decompression and a redesign of the measurement device (Fig. 16.10).[77] It consists of a 14 Fr intussuscepting sheathed needle, that – like the Russell (introducer) method – punctures the stomach and after needle removal allows the introduction of a guide-wire (Fig. 16.24). By pulling at an outer handle, the distal part of the sheath folds up to a star-shaped end. By pulling this end against the gastric wall, the markings at the outside indicate the required button size.

Procedure of gastrostomy tube removal and/or replacement

For removal or replacement, a Foley bag balloon catheter or replacement balloon gastrostomy tube can be emptied and removed. In the presence of a collapsible internal retention disc, gentle traction outward via the fistulous track is advised (Fig. 16.11). However, where there is a rigid internal retention disc, two different approaches are feasible: removal via endoscopy or per vias naturales.[78–80] At endoscopy, the retention disc or mushroom tip can be grasped with an opened snare in such a way that, on closing the snare, the tube is caught just behind the disc. Care should be taken not to include a knuckle of mucosa. If the tube is freely movable in the track, the tube is cut as close as possible to skin level. Withdrawal of the endoscope results in removal of the gastrostomy tube remnant, caught in the snare, usually without the need for an overtube. Should the gastrostomy tube be replaced, or if there is some doubt as to

whether the retention disc will pass the cardia and the esophagus freely, it is a handy trick to stitch a long suture in the tube remnant at skin level. After removal of the endoscope and the gastrostomy tube, the string remains at the mouth and allows replacement of the tube through the original track by pulling at the abdominal part of the string, as in the initial procedure. Moreover, if the gastrostomy tube obstructs or hooks in the cardia or esophagus and oral removal seems impossible, it can be pulled back into the stomach.[80] If transintestinal passage is considered safe, the string has to be cut and no further attempt should be taken to extract it orally. In young (<6 years) and small children (<20 kg) and in the presence of motility disturbances or abnormal anatomy, endoscopic removal is required.[81] Whenever free intestinal passage of the disc is considered to be safe,[78,80] an unimpeded to-and-fro movement of the tube inside the gastrocutaneous track and an easy rotation of the retention disc should exclude gastric submucosal migration. The tube should then be cut as close as possible to the internal retention disc and pushed into the stomach. Spontaneous passage has proved to be a safe procedure, but a few cases of intestinal obstruction from the disc being lodged in the small bowel have been reported. After removal, the cutaneous track will be obliterated uneventfully in the next 24 to 72 hours.

COMPLICATIONS

Accurate information regarding the incidence of gastrostomy complications is difficult to obtain.[22,24,82,83] Sources in the literature include a number of large retrospective series and there are only limited prospective data. Also, there is no uniform reporting system and the often debilitated state of the patient interferes with the differentiation between the procedure-related complications or disease-related events. Moreover, insertion-related complications are not always clearly separated from mechanical in-use complications. The same holds true for the distinction between early and late complications.[22,24] The duration of follow-up seems to be the main determinant factor in the specific complications.

A recent meta-analysis of the literature on gastrostomies included 10 radiologic, 48 endoscopic, and 11 surgical reports with a minimum number of 15 patients.[84] Especially in the endoscopic literature, many small series from inexperienced centers were reviewed. Therefore, it was not surprising that rates of successful tube placement were higher for radiologic gastrostomy than for the endoscopic procedure and procedure-related mortality and major complications occurred less frequently after radiologic gastrostomies (Table 16.1). Wound-related major problems and aspiration occurred significantly more frequently in endoscopic procedures (3.3% vs 0.8% and 2.1% vs 0.6%, respectively) and peritonitis was more frequent in radiologic procedures (1.3% vs 0.5%). A literature search of detailed articles reporting on 100 patients[21,55,59,64,85–96] or more showed a comparable

Meta-analysis covering data for 5752 patients in detailed articles of at least 15 treated patients	Surgical gastrostomy	Radiologic gastrostomy	Endoscopic gastrostomy	Radiology vs endoscopy (P value)
No. of series	11	9	48	
No. of patients	721	837	4149	
Success rate (%)	100	99.2	95.7	<0.001
Procedure-related mortality (%)	2.5	0.3	0.5	<0.001
30-day mortality (%)	16.2	15.4	14.7	
Total complications (%)	29.0	13.3	15.4	
Major (%)	19.9	5.9	9.4	<0.001
Minor (%)	9.0	7.8	5.9	
Tube-related complications (%)	NR	12.1	16.0	<0.03

NR = not reported.

Table 16.1 Meta-analysis covering data for 5752 patients in detailed articles of at least 15 treated patients

success rate, procedure-related and 30-day mortality rates for the radiologic and endoscopic procedure, with lower rates of complications in the radiologic procedure (Table 16.2). To some extent, this can be explained by the fact that patients in whom preprocedural assessment with ultrasound demonstrated the impossibility of the procedure are not included in the analysis while this problem is only detected in the course of the procedure itself during an attempt at endoscopic gastrostomy.[99] Also, the follow-up is different: the only long-term follow-up studies[13,16,18,97–102] come from gastroenterologists with, as can be expected, higher rates of complications, mainly of infectious origin and tube-related problems (Tables 16.3 and 16.4).

Results of percutaneous gastrostomy procedures in detailed studies with more than 100 treated patients with short-term follow-up

		N	Success rate	Mortality % Procedure-related	30-day	Morbidity % Total	Major	Minor
Endoscopy*								
Ponsky 1985[85]	P–G	307	100	0.3	NR	5.9	NR	NR
Stern 1986[86]	P–G	100	100	1.0	7.0	4.0	NR	NR
Larsson 1987[87]	P–G	314	95	1.0	15.9	16.3	3.3	13.0
Sangster 1988[88]	P–G	155	100	0	NR	9.8	3.2	6.4
Gibson 1992[21]	P–G	349	96	0.3	NR	11.1	NR	NR
Bussone 1992[89]	P–G	101	99	3.0	14.0	12.0	5.0	7.0
Foutch 1988[55]	S–V	120	96	0.8	4.1	16.8	4.4	12.4
Miller 1989[90]	R	316	96	0.6	16.7	6.0	2.2	3.8
Saunders 1991[91]	R	140	97	0	NR	5.0	NR	NR
Petersen 1997[64]	R	135	100	5.1	17.7	41.3	12.5	28.8
Overall no. of patients		2037	1983	19	153	236	49	121
% patients			95.7	0.9	14.1	11.6	4.3	10.6
Radiology								
Ho 1988[92]		133	100	1.5	7.5	5.3	4.5	0.8
Halkier 1989[93]		252	99	0.8	14.2	6.0	1.6	4.4
O'Keeffe 1989[94]		100	99	0	15.0	15.0	0	15.0
Saïni 1990[59]		125	99	0	11.0	11.1	1.6	9.5
Hicks 1990[95]		158	100	1.9	26.0	18.0	6.0	12.0
Bell 1995[96]		474	95	0.4	17.1	4.2	1.3	2.9
Overall no. of patients		1242	1215	9	181	95	28	67
% patients			97.8	0.7	14.6	7.6	2.3	5.4

*P–G = Ponsky–Gauderer (pull-(on)-string) method; S–V = Sacks–Vine (push-over-wire) method; R = Russell (introducer) method; NR = not reported.

Table 16.2 Results of percutaneous gastrostomy procedures in detailed studies with more than 100 treated patients with short-term follow-up

Results of percutaneous endoscopic gastrostomy procedures in detailed studies with more than 100 treated patients with data on prolonged follow-up

		N	Success rate	Mortality % Procedure-related	30-day	Morbidity % Total	Major	Minor
Taylor 1992[16]*	P–G	97	94	0	22.6	69.6	27.2	42.4
Grant 1993[41]	P–G	595	99	0.2	NR	8.9	1.3	7.6
Wenk 1994[97]	P–G	180	98	1.1	NR	11.6	3.3	8.3
Raha 1994[98]	P–G	161	99	0.6	19.9	12.4	0.6	11.8
Meier 1994[99]	P–G	165	99	0.6	NR	13.3	3.0	10.3
Gossner 1995[100]*	P–G	1182	NR	0.5	NR	33.0	1.0	32.0
Del Piano 1995[101]	P–G	259	98	0	10.0	10.3	1.2	9.1
de Ledinghen 1995[18]	P–G	140	99	2.1	10.0	15.9	3.6	12.3
Mathus-Vliegen 1999[13]*	P–G	286	94	1.0	6.7	65.6	17.5	48.1
Horton 1991[102]	S–V	224	100	0	8.2	32.2	7.6	24.6
Overall no. of patients		3289	2067	17	120	866	129	737
% patients			98.1	0.5	11.1	26.3	3.9	22.4

*Detailed studies with longest follow-up; P–G = Ponsky–Gauderer (pull-(on)-string) method; S–V = Sacks–Vine (push-over-wire) method; NR = not reported.

Table 16.3 Results of percutaneous endoscopic gastrostomy procedures in detailed studies with more than 100 treated patients with data on prolonged follow-up

Table 16.4 Prevalence of complications in short-term radiologic and endoscopic gastrostomy studies and in prolonged endoscopic gastrostomy follow-up

Prevalence of complications in short-term radiologic and endoscopic gastrostomy studies and in prolonged endoscopic gastrostomy follow-up

	Radiologic PG/PGJ procedure-related short-term	Endoscopic PEG procedure-related short-term	Endoscopic PEG prolonged follow-up
No. of patients	1242	2037	3289
Peritonitis/peritonism	29 (2.3%)	24 (1.2%)	58 (1.8%)
GI perforation	0	7 (0.3%)	5 (0.2%)
GI ulceration/hemorrhage	8 (0.6%)	8 (0.4%)	24 (0.7%)
Aspiration (pneumonia)	10 (0.8%)	22 (1.1%)	22 (0.7%)
Pneumoperitoneum	2 (0.2%)	1 (0.04%)	9 (0.3%)
Infection deep and superficial	24 (1.9%)	68 (3.3%)	285 (8.7%)
Wound hematoma/bleed	0	3 (0.1%)	45 (1.4%)
Stoma leakage	12 (1.0%)	22 (1.1%)	46 (1.4%)
Catheter erosion/buried bumper	2 (0.2%)	5 (0.2%)	7 (0.2%)
Gastrocolonic fistula	0	3 (0.1%)	1 (0.03%)
Tube-related problems	NR	26 (1.3%)	263 (8.0%)

GI = gastrointestinal; NR = not reported; PEG = percutaneous endoscopic gastrostomy; PG/PGJ = percutaneous gastrostomy/percutaneous gastrojejunostomy.

MANAGEMENT OF COMPLICATIONS

Unsuccessful placement

Transillumination is necessary to avoid puncturing neighboring organs such as the colon. In cases of absent or inadequate transillumination, ultrasonography can be used first to rule out interposed organs. The alternative is to continue with the procedure and to perform the 'double-check' or 'safe-track' technique by slowly advancing a syringe, partially filled with fluid and with the barrel of the syringe pulled back to create negative pressure.[52] When air is aspirated before the needle appears in the gas-tric lumen, an interposed air-containing hollow viscus is very likely. If this is not the case and when there is a direct and prominent indentation on external finger pressure and not only referred motion, the procedure can be safely completed.[37,38]

Usually, the positioning of a gastrostomy will fail in an unduly high horizontal location of the stomach obscured by the costal margin and liver and in subjects with severe spine deformities (e.g. in brain-damaged children). The only solution, i.e. oblique puncturing in a cephalad direction, is only acceptable under endoscopic and fluoroscopic control with anterior–posterior and lateral (biplanar) beam exposure. Another option is to proceed with a combined surgical and endoscopic procedure. A small subcostal horizontal incision is made to expose a small area of the stomach. Transillumination with the endoscope can be helpful. The stomach is punctured with the sheathed needle by the surgeon and the procedure completed as with the Ponsky–Gauderer method. Other possibilities are a radiologic procedure or a laparoscopic gastrostomy or jejunostomy.

Complicated placement

In cases of insufficient insufflation or substantial escape of air via the puncture site, the stomach may move back into the abdomen, thus leaving the needle behind in the peritoneal cavity. Termination of the procedure, insertion of a nasogastric tube for gastric decompression and siphoning, or needle decompression paracentesis in cases of severe pneumoperitoneum (and eventually surgery) is one option (Fig. 16.25). The other and more preferable option is to repeat the whole procedure immediately.[56] This also holds true for the Russell (introducer) procedure in the unlikely event that the stomach has been punctured by the introducer, and the outer peel-away sheath cannot be introduced into the stomach. A considerable pneumoperitoneum has to be expected and, when necessary, should be evacuated by needle paracentesis. The stomach should be kept empty after the procedure by nasogastric and gastrostomy drainage, and feeding should be postponed until the opening has sealed.

Tube displacement/tube dislodgement

In the first 7 to 10 days, only appropriate close approximation of the gastric and abdominal walls will result in sealing and in the formation of a gastrocutaneous fistulous track. In these early days, dislodgement of the tube from the stomach or even complete removal may occa-sionally result in an uneventful pneumoperitoneum, but usually will cause severe peritonitis owing to intraperitoneal leakage of gastric contents or intraperitoneal tube feeding both of which are surgical emergencies. A collapsed balloon or unfolded Malecot catheter may be responsible for tube dislodgement but also pressure necrosis and ulceration caused by excessive tension on both retention discs. Also, repeated pulling on the tube by a confused patient will result in an opening in the gastric wall which is wider than the diameter of the feeding tube and will cause a loss of the usual apposition of gastric and anterior abdominal walls.[103] Sometimes, the tube is expelled entirely by the patient.

Later in the follow-up, tube dislodgement or complete removal requires only tube exchange. This is easy when a replacement tube is substituted immediately or within the first 24 hours. Thereafter, the gastrostomy tube fistula may have closed. To avoid a false route, the introduction of a guidewire through a narrow and closing track into the stomach under fluoroscopy is advised. Difficulty in either probing the complete track or in the rotatory motion and to-and-fro movement of the gastrostomy tube is a warning sign that the retention disc has ulcerated submucosally or even into the abdominal wall layers, the so-called 'buried bumper' (Fig. 16.26). Occasionally, the retention disc which is partially extruded into the stomach's submucosal tissues can be pushed back or grasped with a biopsy forceps and pulled back into the lumen under endoscopic view. If repositioning into the gastric lumen is not successful and the retention

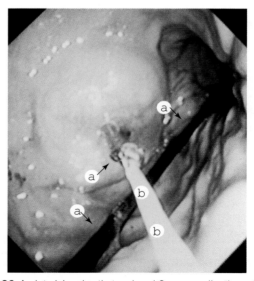

Fig. 16.26 An intrajejunal catheter placed 3 years earlier through the opening of a gastrostomy tube was clogged and required exchange. Resistance was met when pulling at the jejunal catheter. At endoscopy, both the internal retention disc of the gastrostomy catheter and the exit site of the intrajejunal tube were covered by gastric mucosa. The intrajejunal tube (a) was cut with the help of a pair of scissors introduced through the instrumentation channel of the endoscope and a wire (b) was introduced through the gastrostomy opening. The wire was grasped and a new gastrostomy tube was placed; after a skin excision, the old one was expelled driven by the new gastrostomy catheter.

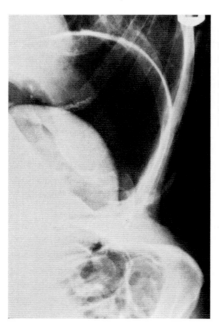

Fig. 16.25 Massive pneumoperitoneum after successful resuscitation of a patient in cardiac and ventilatory arrest during gastrostomy placement. Reabsorption of the inflated air took 5 weeks.

disc is only superficially covered by a layer of gastric mucosa, penetration into the more superficial layers of the abdominal wall and towards the skin can be afforded by a weight fixed at the distal part of the external tube. If at subsequent endoscopy neither the retention disc nor any trace of its exit from the stomach is visible, surgical incision of the skin and the deeper layers alongside the tube is needed for removal.

If probing of the gastrocutaneous track is unsuccessful and a new tube is still needed, the picture at endoscopy is decisive.[104,105] Sometimes, the retention disc is no longer visible but an excavated ulceration with converging folds is present, in the center of which the tube opening can be seen. In that case, the introduction of a guidewire from the outside will be successful. Where the retention disc is totally embedded in the soft tissues outside the abdominal wall, the gastrostomy tube is cut at skin level and a long Seldinger needle introduced into the stomach via the lumen of the tube under endoscopic view. Through that same needle, a string is introduced into the stomach and the needle removed. As with the initial introduction, the endoscopist grasps the guidewire or the string and brings it out of the mouth by withdrawing the endoscope. Then the embedded internal retention disc is partially exposed by the surgeon by blunt dissection and a new gastrostomy tube introduced over the guidewire or knotted at the string. By advancing the tube over the wire, or by pulling at the string, the partially extruded tube remnant will be removed and simultaneously a new tube is positioned. Regardless of the method used, a repeat endoscopy should confirm the proper position of the new inner retention disc.

Measures to prevent the above-mentioned buried bumper syndrome are simple:

1. avoid excessive traction at the time of insertion and a too tight skin disc thereafter
2. loosen the skin disc for a distance of 1–2 cm after the formation of the fistulous tract and adjust the disc after weight gain
3. advise against inadvertent pulling or manipulation of the tube; multiple gauze pads beneath the external bumper may pull on the internal bumper causing pressure necrosis of the mucosal surface.[106]

Tube dislodgement and removal are notoriously frequent with the Foley bag balloon catheter because of acid corrosion of the balloon material. Either a more acid-resistant replacement balloon gastrostomy tube or a mushroom- or dome-shaped gastric button may be preferred.

Tube blockage

Blockage usually results from protein-enriched formulae or medications administered through the tube and from insufficient tube care. The size of the gastrostomy tube is important; 9 Fr-sized tubes clog notoriously frequently when compared to 15 Fr tubes, whereas no difference in clogging rate is observed between 12 and 20 Fr-sized tubes.[13,108] The considerable number of silicone tube failures from obstruction related to fungus colonies lends support to the recommendation for use of polyurethane materials.[107] Flushing with carbonated fluids, acetylcysteine, elase, and chymotrypsin may assist in clearing the obstruction. Probing the tube with a flexible wire should be attempted before the decision to exchange the tube. Before this procedure, the proper position of the tube should be ascertained by a free rotation and in-and-out movement because obstructed flow may also be a result of partial submucosal tube dislodgement.[104] The especially high rate of catheter failure of the 9 Fr-sized jejunal tubes in gastrojejunostomy, mainly owing to blockage, accounts for the rather pessimistic view regarding its benefit.[109–112]

Tube leakage

Some leakage of fluid is sometimes inevitable with high abdominal pressure (severe coughing), but is innocuous. Significant leakage of tube feeding and gastric contents causing peristomal excoriation of the skin should be a reason to evaluate the gastric emptying.[83] Sometimes, gentle traction on the gastrostomy resolves the leak but too much pressure may lead to necrosis and worsening of the leak. Removal of the tube for several days may allow the stoma to approximate the tube more closely. Occasionally, the tube must be removed and a new site selected for a repeat gastrostomy placement. The excoriated skin can be treated by topical application of aldegrate/magnesium (hydr)oxide or sucralfate. Tube feeding may leak from the gastrostomy site where there is partial submucosal extrusion of the tube.[104] Ascitic fluid leakage is highly problematic. Therefore, it is a relative contraindication when deciding whether to place a gastrostomy.

Wound infection/necrotizing fasciitis

At wound inspection, erythema and induration should be distinguished from exudate. Peristomal erythema needs only adequate wound care with hydrogen peroxide and povidone-iodine ointment. Topical application of an antibiotic ointment (erythromycin or tetracycline) will help when a slight inflammation or some purulent discharge is present. In more severe inflammation, such as manifest infiltration or even abscess formation, systemic antibiotic treatment or surgical drainage has to be considered. Persisting pain after 2 to 3 days is an early sign of infection and should lead to an investigation by ultrasound. Necrotizing fasciitis is an infrequent complication which should be recognized early, within 24 hours, and which requires aggressive and emergency treatment because of the high mortality.[50] Surgical debridement, antibiotic treatment, or hyperbaric oxygen are some of the proposed therapeutic measurements. Unfavorable and predisposing conditions such as diabetes, atherosclerosis, malnutrition, immunosuppression, corticosteroids, and adiposity should be noted. Incorrectly small incisions of the skin, inappropriate antibiotic treatment, and impaired gastric mucosal blood flow because of forceful traction also play a role.

Aspiration pneumonia

Aspiration is the most frequent complication of the procedure. It may also develop later and its cause should be precisely defined whether by oropharyngeal secretion, gastroesophageal acid reflux, or reflux of food.[30,83] In the last case, two alternatives are available: one is adjusting the feeding volume and rate by continuous drip feeding instead of bolus feeding,[32] with evaluation of gastric residuals and elevation of the head. The other option is a conversion of a gastrostomy into a gastrojejunostomy.[31–33,65,66,111–113] Whether jejunal feeding offers advantage over gastric feeding in those high-risk patients is still an unresolved controversy. To be of benefit, at least two conditions should be fulfilled: the placement of the feeding tube far beyond the ligament of Treitz and the simultaneous decompression of the stomach with rerouting the gastric contents into the jejunum if needed.[31,65,66,113,114] Another unresolved question is whether a gastrostomy influences the lower esophageal sphincter and causes or aggravates gastroesophageal reflux. This is important, especially in brain-damaged children, where the necessity of a fundoplication in addition to a gastrostomy is debated. As of now, the issue is elegantly solved by Gauderer, who advises a 4- to 6-week trial period of nasogastric tube feeding.[42,115] If this period passes uneventfully, a gastrostomy is indicated; if there are problems with reflux, a combined gastrostomy and antireflux surgery seem indicated.

Pneumoperitoneum

With more sophisticated diagnostic methods, a benign pneumoperitoneum, not requiring medical intervention, is increasingly found.[23,116] The air will be absorbed over the following days. Exceptionally, massive amounts of air in the absence of signs of peritonitis can be removed by needle paracentesis (Fig. 16.24). In true peritonitis, caused by perforation or tube feeding leakage, surgery is necessary.

Gastric ulceration and gastric bleeding

Pressure necrosis because of traction or inappropriate handling and pulling at the tube may result in gastric ulceration and gastric bleeding underneath the fixation disc. Removal of the tube is then indicated. The initially reported high incidence of ulceration and bleeding in percutaneous endoscopic gastrojejunostomies (10/43, 23%)[109,110] is striking and only partially explained by alkaline reflux or by a high frequency (12%) of peptic ulcer disease at initial endoscopy in patients with no previous history.[35,36] It is no longer reported in later studies that describe intrajejunal feeding together with gastric decompression.[113,114]

Esophageal laceration and gastric perforation

The posterior larynx can be damaged by endoscopy or by the pull through of the internal retention disc, especially in children, where a gastrostomy tube size of maximally 15 Fr is advised under the age of 2 or below a body weight of 10 kg.[30,83] A longitudinal tear in the esophagus is caused if the guidewire is hooked near its tip, which shreds the esophagus longitudinally during extraction. The use of plastic-coated wires or completely pulling the wire through the instrumentation channel before removing the endoscope circumvents this problem.

Early gastric perforation may result from failed positioning after needle puncture. In the presence of a tight stricture in the esophagogastric region, the retention disc may strip off the mucosa when the gastrostomy tube is pulled through the narrowed area.[87] This also holds true for esophagotracheal fistulas. When it occurs, surgery is indicated.

Gastrocolic fistula

Most of the fistulae described were discovered in children and only late in the history during an unsuccessful exchange procedure. The replacement tube then only entered the colon without entering the tract towards the stomach. Subsequent feeding resulted in diarrhea or feculent vomiting. Removal of the tube is indicated with spontaneous closure of the track and a renewed successful endoscopic insertion thereafter. Elevation of the head of the bed to displace the colon toward the pelvis may help to prevent the complication.

Rare complications

In rare cases, transhepatic placement had no untoward effects. Duodenal obstruction by a partially deflated balloon catheter and jejunal obstruction and retrograde jejunoduodenal intussusception owing to the migration of the inner retention disc have been reported (Fig. 16.23). Deflation of the balloon or slight pulling at the feeding catheter will often result in successful repositioning into the stomach. Occasionally, operation is necessary. This also holds true for the occasional obstruction from bumper discs migrating through the small bowel after being cut and released at the time of tube exchange or removal.

CONCLUSION

Percutaneous endoscopic gastrostomy is becoming a routinely performed procedure, easy and fast in most circumstances and only problematic in some patients with Billroth II resection, brain damage, and amyotrophic lateral sclerosis. It is well accepted by the patient. Dislocation and blockage occur less often than in nasoenteric tubes, nasopharyngeal irritation is absent, and the lower esophageal sphincter function is less compromised.

However, for those patients who need intrajejunal feeding over prolonged periods, radiologic placement may be technically superior to endoscopic placement as the endoscopic method requires first a (fast and easy) gastrostomy procedure, followed by a rather difficult, tedious and time-consuming positioning of an intestinal tube with, because of its small size, a high rate of catheter failure in prolonged follow-up. On the other hand, only the endoscopic techniques provide the possibility of simultaneous gastric decompression and intrajejunal feeding.

CHECKLIST OF PRACTICE POINTS

1. Evaluate the indication and estimated duration of enteral feeding by tube.
2. Pay attention to the desired gut level of food administration.
3. Decide whether a nasogastric tube or a gastrostomy is more appropriate.
4. Decide upon the method for gastrostomy either via the oral or transabdominal route.
5. Consider also the conversion into a gastrojejunostomy, the need for a direct jejunostomy, or the placement of a gastric button, now or in the near future.
6. Check the feasibility of transabdominal illumination where a videoendoscope is used.
7. Seek the presence of transillumination, finger indentation, and the 'safe track' (visualization of needle and air bubbles) maneuver.
8. Use adequate insufflation to displace neighboring organs and to appose gastric and abdominal walls.
9. When inexperienced or in doubt, check adequate positioning and apposition of the gastrostomy tube by a second endoscopy.
10. Give special attention to proper apposition of gastric and abdominal wall layers and to proper fixation of both inner and outer retention discs.
11. Explain to the patient the importance of the daily measurement of the remaining tube length in the first week to avoid premature displacement. Emphasize the importance of checking this regularly thereafter to avoid intestinal migration.
12. See the patient as early as possible, and at the outside within 24 hours, whenever the tube slips out.
13. Ascertain the presence of a mature gastrocutaneous track before embarking on the placement of a gastrostomy button.

REFERENCES

1. Wills JS, Oglesby JT. Percutaneous gastrostomy. Radiology 1983; 149:449–453.

2. Ho CS. Percutaneous gastrostomy for jejunal feeding. Radiology 1983; 149:595–596.

3. Yeung EJ, Ho CS. Percutaneous radiologic gastrostomy. Baillieres Clin Gastroenterol 1992; 6:297–317.

4. Towbin RB, Ball WS Jr, Bissett GS. Percutaneous gastrostomy and percutaneous gastrostomy in children: antegrade approach. Radiology 1988; 168:473–476.

5. Brown AS, Mueller PR, Ferrucci JT Jr. Controlled percutaneous gastrostomy: nylon T-fastener for fixation of the anterior gastric wall. Radiology 1986; 158:543–545.

6. Gauderer MWL, Ponsky JL, Inzant RRJ. Gastrostomy without laparotomy: a percutaneous endoscopic technique. J Pediatr Surg 1980; 15:872–875.

7. Sacks BA, Vine HS, Palestrant AM, et al. A nonoperative technique for establishment of a gastrostomy in the dog. Invest Radiol 1983; 18:485–487.

8. Russell TR, Brotman M, Norris F. Percutaneous gastrostomy: a new simplified and costeffective technique. Am J Surg 1984; 148:132–137.

9. Park RHR, Allison MC, Lang J, et al. Randomised comparison of percutaneous endoscopic gastrostomy and nasogastric tube feeding in patients with persisting neurological dysphagia. BMJ 1992; 304:1406–1409.

10. Wicks C, Gimson A, Vlavianos P, et al. Assessment of the percutaneous endoscopic gastrostomy feeding tube as part of an integrated approach to enteral feeding. Gut 1992; 33:613–616.

11. Editorial. Percutaneous endoscopic gastrostomy: the end of the line for nasogastric feeding? BMJ 1992; 304:1395–1396.

12. Norton B, Homer-Ward M, Donnelly MT, et al. A randomised prospective comparison of percutaneous endoscopic gastrostomy and nasogastric tube feeding after acute dysphagic stroke. BMJ 1996; 312:13–16.

13. Mathus-Vliegen EMH, Koning H. Percutaneous endoscopic gastrostomy and gastrojejunostomy: a critical reappraisal of patient selection, tube function and the feasibility of nutritional support during extended follow-up. Gastrointest Endosc 1999; 50:746–754.

14. Rabeneck L, Wray NP, Petersen NJ. Long-term outcomes of patients receiving percutaneous endoscopic gastrostomy tubes. J Gen Intern Med 1996; 11:287–293.

15. Rabeneck L, McCullough LB, Wray NP. Ethically justified, clinically comprehensive guidelines for percutaneous endoscopic gastrostomy tube placement. Lancet 1997; 349:496–498.

16. Taylor CA, Larson DE, Baillard DJ, et al. Predictors of outcome after percutaneous endoscopic gastrostomy: a community-based study. Mayo Clin Proc 1992; 67:1042–1049.

17. Kaw M, Sekas G. Long-term follow-up of consequences of percutaneous endoscopic gastrostomy (PEG) tubes in nursing home patients. Dig Dis Sci 1994; 29:738–743.

18. de Ledinghen V, Beau P, Labat J, et al. Compared effects of enteral nutrition by percutaneous endoscopic gastrostomy in cancer and in non-cancer patients: a long-term study. Clin Nutr 1995; 14:17–32.

19. Marin OE, Glassman MS, Schoen BT, et al. Safety and efficacy of percutaneous endoscopic gastrostomy in children. Am J Gastroenterol 1994; 89:357–361.

20. Friedenberg F, Jensen G, Gujral N, et al. Serum albumin is predictive of 30-day survival after percutaneous endoscopic gastrostomy. JPEN 1997; 21:72–74.

21. Gibson SE, Wenig BL, Watkins JL. Complications of percutaneous endoscopic gastrostomy in head and neck cancer patients. Ann Otol Rhinol Laryngol 1992; 101:46–50.

22. Ponsky JL, Gauderer MWL. Percutaneous endoscopic gastrostomy: indications, limitations, techniques, and results. World J Surg 1989; 13:165–170.

23. Mamel JJ. Percutaneous endoscopic gastrostomy. Am J Gastroenterol 1989; 84:703–710.

24. Moran BJ, Taylor MB, Johnson CD. Percutaneous endoscopic gastrostomy. Br J Surg 1990; 77:858–862.

25. Railey DJ, Calleja GA, Barkin JS. Percutaneous endoscopic jejunostomy: indications, techniques and evaluation. Gastrointest Endosc Clin North Am 1992; 2:223–230.

26. Stellato JA. Expanded applications of percutaneous gastroscopy. Gastrointest Endosc Clin North Am 1992; 2:249–257.

27. Boyle JT. Nutritional management of the developmentally disabled child. Pediatr Surg Int 1991; 6:76–81.

28. Goretsky MJ, Johnson N, Farrell M, et al. Alternative techniques of feeding gastrostomy in children: a critical analysis. J Am Coll Surg 1996; 182:233–240.

29. Campagnutta E, Cannizzaro R, Gallo A, et al. Palliative treatment of upper intestinal obstruction by gynecological malignancy: the usefulness of percutaneous endoscopic gastrostomy. Gynecol Oncol 1996; 62:103–105.

30. Baskin WN. Advances in enteral nutrition techniques. Am J Gastroenterol 1992; 87:1547–1553.

31. Lewis BS. Perform PEJ, not PED. Gastrointest Endosc 1990; 36:311–313.

32. Coben RM, Weintraub H, DiMarino AJ, et al. Gastroesophageal reflux during gastrostomy feeding. Gastroenterology 1994; 106:13–18.

33. Patel PH, Thomas E. Risk factors for pneumonia after percutaneous endoscopic gastrostomy. J Clin Gastroenterol 1990; 12:389–392.

34. Cogen R, Weinryb J, Pomerantz C, et al. Complications of jejunostomy tube feeding in nursing facility patients. Am J Gastroenterol 1991; 86:1610–1613.

35. Scott JS, Edelman DS, Unger SW. Percutaneous endoscopic gastrostomy: a mandate for complete diagnostic upper endoscopy. Am Surg 1989; 55:85–87.

36. Wolfsen HC, Kozarek RA, Ball TJ, et al. Value of diagnostic upper endoscopy preceding percutaneous gastrostomy. Am J Gastroenterol 1990; 85:249–251.

37. Ponsky JL. Transilluminating percutaneous endoscopic gastrostomy. Endoscopy 1998; 30:656.

38. Stewart JAD, Hagan P. Failure to transilluminate the stomach is not an absolute contraindication to PEG insertion. Endoscopy 1998; 30:621–622.

39. van Erpecum KJ, van Akkersdijk WL, Wárlám-Rodenhuis CC, et al. Metastasis of hypopharyngeal carcinoma in the gastrostomy tract after placement of a percutaneous endoscopic gastrostomy catheter. Endoscopy 1995; 27:124–127.

40. Stellato TA, Gauderer MWL, Ponsky JL. Percutaneous endoscopic gastrostomy following previous abdominal surgery. Ann Surg 1984; 200:46–50.

41. Grant JP. Percutaneous endoscopic gastrostomy. Initial placement by single endoscopic technique and long-term follow-up. Ann Surg 1993; 217:168–174.

42. Gauderer MWL. Percutaneous endoscopic gastrostomy: a 10-year experience with 220 children. J Pediatr Surg 1991; 26:288–294.

43. Graham SM, Flowers JL, Scott TS, et al. Safety of percutaneous endoscopic gastrostomy in patients with a ventriculoperitoneal shunt. Neurosurgery 1993; 32:932–934.

44. Raskin JB, Rams H, Garrido J, et al. A prospective study on the source of the infectious complications associated with percutaneous endoscopic gastrostomy. Gastrointest Endosc 1986; 32:150 (A47).

45. Jain NK, Larson DE, Schroeder KW, et al. Antibiotic prophylaxis for percutaneous endoscopic gastrostomy. Ann Intern Med 1987; 107:824–828.

46. Akkersdijk WL, van Bergeijk JD, van Egmond T, et al. Percutaneous endoscopic gastrostomy (PEG): comparison of push and pull methods and evaluation of antibiotic prophylaxis. Endoscopy 1995; 27:313–316.

47. Sturgis TM, Yancy W, Cole JC, et al. Antibiotic prophylaxis in percutaneous endoscopic gastrostomy. Am J Gastroenterol 1996; 91:2301–2304.

48. Jonas SK, Neimark S, Panwalker AP. Effect of antibiotic prophylaxis in percutaneous endoscopic gastrostomy. Am J Gastroenterol 1985; 80:438–441.

49. Kozarek RA, Ball TJ, Patterson DJ. Prophylactic antibiotics in percutaneous endoscopic gastrostomy (PEG): need or nuisance. Gastrointest Endosc 1986; 32:147–148 (A36).

50. Greif JM, Rayland JJ, Ochsner MG, et al. Fatal necrotizing fasciitis complicating percutaneous endoscopic gastrostomy. Gastrointest Endosc 1986; 32:292–294.

51. Beasly SW, Catton-Smith AG, Davidson PM. How to avoid complications during percutaneous endoscopic gastrostomy. J Pediatr Surg 1995; 30:671–673.

52. Foutch PG, Talbert GA, Waring JP, et al. Percutaneous endoscopic gastrostomy in patients with prior abdominal surgery: virtues of the safe tract. Am J Gastroenterol 1988; 83:248–251.

53. Aisenberg J, Cohen L, Lewis BS. Marked endoscopic gastrostomy tubes permit one-pass Ponsky-technique. Gastrointest Endosc 1991; 37:552–553.

54. Sartori S, Trevisani L, Nielsen I, et al. Percutaneous endoscopic gastrostomy placement using the pull-through or push-through techniques: is the second pass of the gastroscope necessary? Endoscopy 1996; 28:686–688.

55. Foutch PG, Woods GA, Talbert GA, et al. A critical analysis of the Sacks–Vine gastrostomy tube: a review of 120 consecutive procedures. Am J Gastroenterol 1988; 83:252–255.

56. Miller RE, Winkler WP, Kotler DP. The Russell percutaneous endoscopic gastrostomy: key technical steps. Gastrointest Endosc 1988; 34:339–342.

57. Kozarek RA, Ball TJ, Ryan JA Jr. When push comes to shove: a comparison between two methods of percutaneous endoscopic gastrostomy. Am J Gastroenterol 1986; 81:642–646.

58. Wu TK, Welch HF. New method of percutaneous gastrostomy using anchoring devices. Am J Surg 1987; 153:230–232.

59. Saïni S, Mueller PR, Gaa J, et al. Percutaneous gastrostomy with gastropexy: experience in 125 patients. AJR Am J Roentgenol 1990; 154:1003–1006.

60. Gauderer MWL, Stellato TA. Percutaneous endoscopic gastrostomy in children: the technique in detail. Pediatr Surg Int 1991; 6:82–87.

61. Coughlin JP, Gauderer MWL, Stellato TA. Percutaneous endoscopic gastrostomy in children under 1 yr of age: indications, complications and outcome. Pediatr Surg Int 1991; 6:88–91.

62. Hogan RB, Demarro DC, Hamilton JK, et al. Percutaneous endoscopic gastrostomy: to push or to pull: a prospective randomized trial. Gastrointest Endosc 1986; 32:253–258.

63. Deitel M, To T, Spratt E, et al. Percutaneous endoscopic gastrostomy (PEG) by the 'pull' and 'push' methods. Gastrointest Endosc 1987; 33:147.

64. Petersen TI, Kruse A. Complications of percutaneous endoscopic gastrostomy. Eur J Surg 1997; 163:351–356.

65. Duckworth PF, Kirby DP, McHenry L, et al. Percutaneous endoscopic gastrojejunostomy made easy: a new over-the-wire technique. Gastrointest Endosc 1994; 40:350–353.

66. Parasher VK, Abramowicz CJ, Bell C, et al. Successful placement of percutaneous gastrojejunostomy using steerable glidewire – a modified controlled push technique. Gastrointest Endosc 1995; 41:52–55.

67. Shike M, Latkany L, Gerdes H, et al. Direct percutaneous endoscopic jejunostomies for enteral feeding. Nutr Clin Pract 1996; 12:S38–S42.

68. Romero R, Martinez FL, Robinson SYJ, et al. Complicated PEG-to-skin level gastrostomy conversions: analysis of risk factors for tract disruption. Gastrointest Endosc 1996; 44:230–234.

69. Foutch PG, Talbert EA, Gaines JA, et al. The gastrostomy button: a prospective assessment of safety, success, and spectrum of use. Gastrointest Endosc 1989; 35:41–44.

70. Gauderer MWL, Olsen MM, Stellato TA, et al. Feeding gastrostomy button: experience and recommendations. J Pediatr Surg 1988; 23:24–28.

71. Gauderer MWL, Stellato TA, Wade DC. Complications related to gastrostomy button placement. Gastrointest Endosc 1993; 39:467.

72. Chung RS, Schertzer M. Pathogenesis of complications of percutaneous endoscopic gastrostomy. A lesson in surgical principles. Am Surg 1990; 56:134–137.

73. Ferguson DR, Harig JM, Kozarek RA, et al. Placement of a feeding button ('one-step button') as the initial procedure. Am J Gastroenterol 1997; 88:501–504.

74. Marion MT, Zweng TN, Strodell WE. One-stage gastrostomy button: an assessment. Endoscopy 1994; 26:666–670.

75. Treem WR, Etienne NL, Hyams JC. Percutaneous endoscopic placement of the 'button' gastrostomy tube as the initial procedure in infants and children. J Pediatr Gastroenterol Nutr 1993; 17:382–386.

76. Kozarek RA, Payne M, Barkin J, et al. Prospective multicenter evaluation of an initially placed button gastrostomy. Gastrointest Endosc 1995; 41:105–108.

77. Strodell WG. Technique for placement of one-stage gastrostomy button. Gastrointest Endosc 1996; 43:629.

78. Korula J, Harma C. A simple and inexpensive method of removal and replacement of gastrostomy tubes. JAMA 1991; 265:1426–1428.

79. Ponsky JL. Percutaneous endoscopic gastrostomy: techniques of removal and replacement. Gastrointest Endosc Clin North Am 1992; 2:215–229.

80. Dye KR, Pattison CP, Dye NV. Percutaneous endoscopic gastrostomy: technical modifications for improved results. South Med J 1986; 79:24–27.

81. Yaseen M, Steele MI, Grunow JE. Non-endoscopic removal of percutaneous endoscopic gastrostomy tubes: morbidity and mortality in children. Gastrointest Endosc 1996; 44:235–238.

82. Foutch PG. Complications of percutaneous endoscopic gastrostomy and jejunostomy: recognition, prevention and treatment. Gastrointest Endosc Clin North Am 1992; 2:231–248.

83. Schapiro GD, Edmundowicz SA. Complications of percutaneous endoscopic gastrostomy. Gastrointest Endosc Clin North Am 1996; 6:409–422.

84. Wollman B, D'Agostino H, Walus-Wigle JR, et al. Radiologic, endoscopic, and surgical gastrostomy: an institutional evaluation and meta-analysis of the literature. Radiology 1995; 197:699–704.

85. Ponsky JL, Gauderer MWL, Stellato TA, et al. Percutaneous approach to enteral alimentation. Am J Surg 1985; 149:102–105.

86. Stern JS. Comparison of percutaneous endoscopic gastrostomy with surgical gastrostomy at a community hospital. Am J Gastroenterol 1986; 81:1171–1173.

87. Larsson DE, Burton DD, Schroeder KW, et al. Percutaneous endoscopic gastrostomy. Indications, success, complications, and mortality in 314 consecutive patients. Gastroenterology 1987; 93:48–52.

88. Sangster W, Cuddington BD, Backulis BL. Percutaneous endoscopic gastrostomy. Am J Surg 1988; 155:677–679.

89. Bussone M, Lalo M, Piette F, et al. The value of percutaneous endoscopic gastrostomy in assisted feeding in malnutritioned elderly patients based on 101 consecutive cases in patients over the age of 70 years. Ann Chir 1992; 46:59–66.

90. Miller RE, Castlemain B, Lacqua FJ, et al. Percutaneous endoscopic gastrostomy. Results in 316 patients and review of the literature. Surg Endosc 1989; 3:186–190.

91. Saunders JR, Brown MS, Hirata RM, et al. Percutaneous endoscopic gastrostomy in patients with head and neck malignancies. Am J Surg 1991; 162:381–383.

92. Ho CS, Yee ACN, McPherson R. Complications of surgical and percutaneous non-endoscopic gastrostomy: review of 233 patients. Gastroenterology 1988; 95:1206–1210.

93. Halkier BK, Ho CS, Yee ACN. Percutaneous feeding gastrostomy with the Seldinger technique: review of 252 patients. Radiology 1989; 171:359–362.

94. O'Keeffe F, Carrasco CH, Charnsangayej C, et al. Percutaneous drainage and feeding gastrostomies in 100 patients. Radiology 1989; 172:341–343.

95. Hicks ME, Surrat RS, Picus D, et al. Fluoroscopically guided percutaneous gastrostomy and gastroenterostomy: analysis of 158 consecutive cases. AJR Am J Roentgenol 1990; 154:725–728.

96. Bell SD, Carmody EA, Yeung EY, et al. Percutaneous gastrostomy and gastrojejunostomy: additional experience in 519 procedures. Radiology 1995; 194:817–820.

97. Wenk A, Krauss EC, Markreiter M, et al. Komplikationen der perkutanen endoskopischen kontrollierten Gastrostomie (PEG) – Erfahrungsbericht über 180 Patienten. Verdauungskrankheiten 1994; 12:61–66.

98. Raha SK, Woodhouse K. The use of percutaneous endoscopic gastrostomy (PEG) in 161 consecutive elderly patients. Age Ageing 1994; 23:162–163.

99. Meier R, Bauerfeind P, Gyr K. Die perkutane endoskopische Gastrostomie in der Langzeiternährung. Schweiz Med Wochenschr 1994; 124:655–659.

100. Gossner L, Ludwig J, Hahn EG, et al. Risiken der perkutanen endoskopischen Gastrostomie. Dtsch Med Wochenschr 1995; 120:1768–1772.

101. Del Piano M, Montino F, Occhipinti P, et al. La gastrostomie percutanée endoscopique: techniques et expérience personelles. Acta Endosc 1995; 25:239–246.

102. Horton WL, Colwell DL, Burton DT. Experience with percutaneous endoscopic gastrostomy in a community hospital. Am J Gastroenterol 1991; 86:168–170.

103. Haslam D, Hughes S, Harrison RP. Peritoneal leakage of gastric contents, a rare complication of percutaneous endoscopic gastrostomy. J Parenter Enteral Nutr 1996; 20:433–434.

104. Fay DE, Luther R, Gruber M. A single procedure endoscopic technique for replacing partially extruded percutaneous endoscopic gastrostomy tubes. Gastrointest Endosc 1990; 36:298–300.

105. Shallman RW, Norfleet RG, Hardache JM. Percutaneous endoscopic gastrostomy feeding tube migration and impaction in the abdominal wall. Gastrointest Endosc 1988; 34:367–368.

106. Heximer B. Pressure necrosis: implications and interventions for PEG tubes. Nutr Clin Pract 1997; 12:256–258.

107. Iber FL, Lwak A, Patel M. Importance of fungus colonization in failure of silicone rubber percutaneous gastrostomy tubes (PEGs). Dig Dis Sci 1996; 41:226–231.

108. Duncan HD, Bray MJ, Kapadia SA, et al. Prospective randomized comparison of two different sized percutaneous endoscopically placed gastrostomy tubes. Clin Nutr 1996; 15:317–320.

109. Kaplan DS, Murthy UK, Linscheer WC. Percutaneous endoscopic jejunostomy: long-term follow-up of 23 patients. Gastrointest Endosc 1989; 35:403–406.

110. DiSario JA, Foutch PG, Sanowski RA. Poor results with percutaneous endoscopic jejunostomy. Gastrointest Endosc 1990; 36:257–260.

111. Wolfsen HC, Kozarek RA, Ball TJ, et al. Tube dysfunction following percutaneous gastrostomy and jejunostomy. Gastrointest Endosc 1990; 36:261–263.

112. Henderson JM, Strodel WE, Gilensky NH. Limitations of percutaneous endoscopic jejunostomy. J Parenter Enteral Nutr 1993; 17:546–550.

113. DeLegge M, Duckworth PF, McHenry L, et al. Percutaneous endoscopic gastrojejunostomy: a dual center safety and efficacy trial. J Parenter Enteral Nutr 1995; 19:239–243.

114. DeLegge M, Patrick P, Gibbs R. Percutaneous endoscopic gastrojejunostomy with a tapered tip, nonweighted jejunal feeding tube: improved placement success. Am J Gastroenterol 1996; 91:1130–1134.

115. Gauderer MWL. An updated experience with percutaneous endoscopic gastrostomy in children. Gastroenterol Endosc Clin North Am 1992; 2:195–205.

116. Gottfried EB, Plumser AB, Clair MR. Pneumoperitoneum following percutaneous endoscopic gastrostomy: a prospective study. Gastrointest Endosc 1986; 32:397–399.

Abdominal pain
  chronic pancreatitis, 188, 189
  intestinal bleeding and, 236
Abscesses
  EUS-guided celiac nerve block, 274
  liver, after sphincterotomy, 142
  stents, 51–52
Absolute alcohol
  celiac nerve block, 272
  sclerotherapy, esophageal varices, 5, 19
Absorption coefficients, photodynamic therapy, 105
Achalasia
  dilation procedures, 34, 35
  dilators, 31
  EUS-guided botulinum toxin injection, 272, 274
Acid corrosion, Foley bag balloon catheter, gastrostomy, 295
Acid suppression
  esophageal varices therapy, 19
  EUS-guided celiac block and, 274
  gastrostomy and, 283
  peptic ulcer bleeding, 9
Active bleeding, peptic ulcers, 3
Acute bleeding per rectum, 235
Adenomas
  argon plasma coagulation, 91
  colon, 218
  laser therapy, 78, 82–83
    results, 81
  papilla of Vater, 130
    obstruction, 139, 187
  transanal endoscopic microsurgery, 254
  see also Polypectomy
Adherent clots, 3, 65–66
Adjuvant therapy, esophageal varices, 21
Admission to hospital, sphincterotomy, 134
Adrenaline, see Epinephrine injection
Aerobilia, 141
Age
  peptic ulcer bleeding, 1
  stenting for cholelithiasis, 160
Aggregates, photosensitizers, 102
Air
  bubbles mistaken for stones, 152
  colon polypectomy
    aspiration, 220, 221, 225
    free in peritoneum, 227–228
  insufflation for gastrostomy, 277, 283, 285
Airway compression, stenting and, 40, 44
Alanine aminotransferase, photodynamic therapy and, 106
Albumin, serum levels, gastrostomy, 279
Alcohol, see Absolute alcohol
Alkaline phosphatase, photodynamic therapy and, 106
Allergy, contrast medium, 166
Alternate-site burns, from electrocoagulation, 62
Ambulatory procedures, sphincterotomy, 134, 143
5–Aminolevulinic acid, 102–103, 108
  Barrett's esophagus, 109
  energy density for, 106
  skin phototoxicity, 111
Ampullary obstruction, 139
  see also Papilla of Vater; Sphincter of Oddi dysfunction
Amsterdam-type stents, biliary, 199
Anal advancement flap, 261
Anal fissure, 260–261
Anastomotic strictures
  esophageal, 35
  gastrointestinal, 35
  rectal, 261–262
Anchoring devices, T-shaped, Russell method, 287, 288 (Fig.)
Angiodysplasia, 241
  argon plasma coagulation, 91–96, 92
  enteroscopy, 237
  sclerotherapy, 238
Angioectasias, electrocoagulation, 72
  colonic, 68, 69
  upper gastrointestinal, 67, 69
Angiographic catheters, pancreatic duct cannulation, 177–178

Angiography, gastrointestinal bleeding, 229, 236
Angiomas, laser therapy, 79
Angled stenoses, stenting, 44
Anorexia-cachexia syndrome, gastrostomy and, 278
Antegrade approach, gastrostomy, 277–278
Antibiotics
  biliary procedures, 132, 138, 168
  colon polyp marking, 227
  endoscopic mucosal resection, 126
  ERCP, 179
  esophageal varices treatment, 16, 20, 21
  EUS-guided celiac nerve block, 274
  gastrostomy, 283
  stricture dilation, 31
Anticoagulants
  intestinal bleeding, 236
  polypectomy, 213
Aortic grafts, intestinal bleeding, 236
Argon lasers, 76
Argon plasma coagulation, 62, 87–100
  colon bleeding, 239, 241
  colon lesions, 214, 221
  equipment, 88–89
  peptic ulcer hemorrhage, 6
  procedure, 89–90
  technique, 98
  troubleshooting, 90 (Box)
Arteries, peptic ulcer bleeding, 1, 3, 4 (Table)
  electrocoagulation, 64
Ascites, 272–273
  gastrostomy and, 295
Aspartate aminotransferase, photodynamic therapy and, 106
Aspirating catheters, pancreatic duct, 182
Aspiration pneumonia, gastrostomy, 296
Aspirin
  colonoscopy and, 213
  endosonography, 267
Automatic regulation, electrosurgical generators, 61–62
Automatic stone-tissue discrimination systems, 137, 151, 158, 167–168, 171

Babyscopes
  bile duct cannulation, 149
  pancreatoscopy, 179
  shockwave lithotripsy, 155
  transpapillary stone removal, 148–149
Bacteremia, esophageal varices therapy, 19–20
Bacteria, bile content after sphincterotomy, 141
Balloon catheters, biliary stone extraction, 131–132
Balloon dilation, 30–31
  benign rectal strictures, 262
  biliary stenting, 201, 204
  papilla of Vater, 131, 142, 143 (Fig.)
Balloons
  photodynamic therapy, 104–105
  transpapillary stone removal, 149, 152
'Balloon-tomes', transpapillary stone removal, 149
Band ligation, see Ligation; Rubber banding, hemorrhoids
Barbs, pancreatic duct stents, 182
Barium enemas
  polyp localization, 226
  see also Enemas, soluble contrast medium
Barrett's esophagus
  argon plasma coagulation, 95 (Fig.)
    recurrence, 96
  bipolar electrocoagulation, 59, 71–72
  carcinoma, 71
    lymph node metastases, 106
    photodynamic diagnosis, 107 (Fig.)
  endoscopic mucosal resection, 118
  photodynamic therapy, 106, 109–110
Barron banding equipment, 248 (Fig.)
Baskets
  cable fracture, 155
  with mechanical lithotripsy systems, 150
  pancreatic duct, 178
  transpapillary stone removal, 149, 151
    problems, 154–155
  see also Dormia baskets

Baylor Bleeding Score, 9
'Benign' pneumoperitoneum, 227–228
Benign rectal strictures, 261–262
BICAP probes
  hemostasis probe, 63
    colon polyps, 214
    colonic bleeding, 239
    peptic ulcer, 66
  thermal coagulation, 6
  tumor probes, 72
    esophageal tumors, 70–71
    rectal carcinoma palliation, 257–258
    for strictures, 260
Bifurcation strictures
  biliary stenting, 204
    cholangitis after, 209
  malignant, 207–208
Bile acids, sphincterotomy on, 141
Bile ducts
  photodynamic therapy, 106
  see also Common bile duct; Cystic duct; Intrahepatic radicles
Biliary catheters, intestinal tube placement, 289
Biliary decompression, 189
Biliary drainage, 139–140
Biliary obstruction, 47 (Fig.)
  see also Choledocholithiasis
Biliary pancreatitis, 130, 183–184
  sphincterotomy, 138–139
Biliary peritonitis, percutaneous transhepatic cholangioscopy, 173
Biliary recirculation, via gastrostomy, 279
Biliary reflux, after sphincterotomy, 141
Bilirubin, serum levels, photodynamic therapy and, 106
Billroth-II gastrectomy
  choledocholithiasis, 136
  sphincterotomy, 131, 133, 134, 136
Biophysics, electrocoagulation, 59–62
Biopsies
  staging for photodynamic therapy, 107
  see also Endoscopic mucosal resection; Fine needle aspiration
Biopsy forceps, bipolar, 63
  see also 'Hot biopsy' forceps
Bipolar electrocoagulation, 62, 63
  colonic bleeding, 239
  peptic ulcer, 64–67
Bipolar hemostasis probes, power density, 60
BLEND mode, 61
  colon polypectomy, 216
Blockage, see Occlusion
Blood
  coagulation
    sclerosants, 20
    see also Anticoagulants; Coagulopathy
  transport of photosensitizers, 102
Blood transfusion, intestinal bleeding, 236
BML systems, Olympus
  results, 157
  stone impaction, 154
Botulinum toxin injection, 272, 274
Bougienage, see Dilation procedures
Bougies
  biliary stenting, 201
  percutaneous transhepatic cholangioscopy, 166, 169, 172
  see also Savary–Gilliard dilators
Bowel preparation, see Cleansing regimens
Brachytherapy
  esophageal tumors, 82
  rectal carcinoma palliation, 259
Braun enteroenterostomy, sphincterotomy results, 136
Bronchoscopy, see Tracheobronchial system
Bupivacaine, celiac nerve block, 272
'Buried bumper', gastrostomy, 294–295
Burns
  colon polypectomy, 219
    prevention, 221
  from electrocoagulation, 62
  transmural, 228
Buttons
  gastrojejunal, 282, 290
  see also Gastric buttons
Butyl-cyanoacrylate, esophageal varices, 15, 17

Cachexia, gastrostomy and, 278
Calculi
    pancreatic duct, 181
        chronic pancreatitis, 189–190
        strictures, 140–141
    see also Choledocholithiasis
Calibrated integrating sphere, photodynamic
        therapy monitoring, 105
Capacitive coupling, electrocoagulation, 62
Caps, endoscopic mucosal resection, 119–120
Carbon dioxide, colon insufflation, 213
Carbon dioxide laser, hemorrhoids, 251, 252
Carcinogenesis, sphincterotomy, 141
Carcinoma
    ampullary, 139
    Barrett's esophagus, 71
        lymph node metastases, 106
        photodynamic diagnosis, 107 (Fig.)
    gastrostomy, 279
    see also Tumors; named sites
Cardiac function, esophageal varices therapy, 20
Carpet polyps, colon, 217, 225
Catheters
    biliary stenting, 200–201, 202–203
    percutaneous transhepatic cholangioscopy, 166
    see also specific types
Caustic strictures, 35
Cecostomy-tube colonic lavage, 236
Cefazolin, gastrostomy, 283
Cefoxitin, gastrostomy, 283
Celiac nerve block, 271–272
    complications, 274
Center for Ulcer Research and Education
        Hemostasis Research Group,
        electrocoagulation guidelines, 67, 68
        (Table)
Cervical esophagus
    laser therapy, 77
    strictures, electrocoagulation, 71
    tumors, argon plasma coagulation, 95 (Fig.)
Chiba needle, 166, 168–169
Children
    gastric buttons, 290
    gastrostomy, 288
        antegrade approach, 277–278
        gastro-oesophageal reflux, 296
        post-procedure care, 289
Chlorins, 102
Cholangiopancreatography
    EUS-guided, 273
    see also Endoscopic retrograde
        choledochopancreatography
Cholangioscopes, percutaneous transhepatic,
        166, 170
Cholangioscopy, 137
    vs fluoroscopy, biliary lithotripsy, 158
Cholangitis, 130, 138
    from biliary stenting, 209
    percutaneous transhepatic cholangioscopy,
        172–173
    after sphincterotomy, 142
        prevention, 135
    sphincterotomy for, 138
Cholecystectomy, 129–130
    functional effects, 141
    after sphincterotomy, 142
    transpapillary stone removal after, 147
Cholecystitis, from biliary stenting, 209, 210
Cholecystokinin, microlithiasis diagnosis, 185
Choledochoceles, 187
Choledochoduodenostomy (fistulotomy),
        133–134
Choledocholithiasis
    misdiagnosis, 152–154
    missed stones, 153–154
    percutaneous transhepatic stone removal,
        165–176
        results, 173–174
    recurrent pancreatitis, 185
    sphincterotomy, 129–130
        residual stones, 142
        results, 136–138
    stone size, 157
        stenting on, 159
    transpapillary management, 147–163
    see also Biliary pancreatitis

Cholestasis, 189
Cholesterol
    crystal formation after sphincterotomy, 141
    stone types, 154
Chromoendoscopy, 107
    colonic polypectomy, 217
    endoscopic mucosal resection, 120, 122
    indigocarmine solution, 118, 120
    iodine-dye method, 117–118, 120
Circular end-to-end anastomosis stapler,
        hemorrhoidectomy, 252
Cirrhosis, 13–14
Clamshell polyps, colon, 217, 224
    submucosal saline, 220
Cleansing regimens
    colonoscopy, 213
        for bleeding, 236
    electrocoagulation, 62
    hemorrhoids and, 246
    rectal carcinoma palliation, 258
Clips
    colon polypectomy, 215, 226
    fixing device (Endoclip), 240
    peptic ulcer hemorrhage, 7
Clogging, see Occlusion
Closure sensation, snares, 215, 216
Clots, adherent, 3, 65–66
COAG mode
    colon polypectomy, 216
    electrocoagulation, 61
Coagulation
    infrared, hemorrhoids, 249–250, 253
    see also Electrocoagulation
Coagulation zones, argon plasma coagulation, 88
Coagulopathy
    colonoscopy, 213
    ERCP, 179
    percutaneous transhepatic cholangioscopy, 166
    transpapillary stone removal, 148
Coaptive coagulation, 6, 62, 64–65
'Cold biopsy' forceps, colon polypectomy, 218
Collapsible internal disks, gastrostomy tubes, 282,
        283 (Fig.)
Collaterals, esophageal varices, 20
Colon
    bleeding
        emergency electrocoagulation, 64
        see also Gastrointestinal bleeding, lower
    carcinoma
        in adenomas, 82–83
        argon plasma coagulation, 95 (Fig.)
        early detection, 118–119
        electrocoagulation, 68 (Table)
        at polypectomy, 220
            tracking risk, 220
        stenting, 260
        see also Rectosigmoid tumors
    electrocoagulation, 68
    laser therapy
        angiomas, 79
        perforation, 79
    stenting, 39, 44, 46
        results, 54–56
    see also Angiodysplasia
Colonoscopes, 214
    for bleeding, 237
    rotation for polypectomy, 222
Colonoscopy
    for hemorrhage, 235–244
    polypectomy, 213–233
        polyp size, 217, 225
Colorectal stenoses, 35
    malignant, laser therapy, 82
Combination therapy, peptic ulcer bleeding, 8
Combustible gases, see Explosion
Common bile duct
    decompression, 189
    laparoscopy, 130
    sphincterotomy, 186
        see also Sphincterotomy, ampulla of Vater
    see also Choledocholithiasis; Strictures;
        Transpapillary stone removal
Congestive gastropathy, 14, 20
Consent
    expandable stent procedures, 44
    transanal endoscopic microsurgery, 256

Contact quality monitors, electrocoagulation, 62
Contact thermal methods, for peptic ulcer
        hemorrhage, 6–7
Contrast media
    allergy, 166
    dilation procedures, 31
    ERCP, 179
    injection, transpapillary stone removal, 151,
        153
    lipiodol, with butyl-cyanoacrylate, 17
    stenting procedures, 44
Cooling media, laser therapy, 76
Cost-effectiveness, colonoscopy for bleeding, 242
Coumarin-green lasers, lithotripsy, 158
Covered stents, esophagus, results, 53–54
Creatinine, photodynamic therapy and, 106
Crohn's disease
    bleeding, 241
    duodenal stenoses, 35
    ileocolonic stenoses, 35
    laser therapy, 81–82, 83
Cryosurgery, hemorrhoids, 250–251, 253
CUT mode, 61
    colon polypectomy, 216
Cylindrical diffusers, photodynamic therapy, 104
Cystic duct, biliary stenting, 205
Cystoenterostomy, pancreatic pseudocysts,
        190–191, 271
Cysts
    EUS-guided puncture, complications,
        273–274
    submucosal, 270
Cytology, see Fine needle aspiration
Cytology brushes
    biliary stenting, 203
    pancreatic duct, 178
Cytology catheters, pancreatic duct, 178

Daughter endoscopes, see Babyscopes
Debulking
    before argon plasma coagulation, 96
    rectal carcinoma palliation, 258–259
Decompression
    common bile duct, 189
    one-step gastric button procedure, 290–291
    stomach, 278
Decompression tubes, with laser therapy,
        malignant tumors, 78
Defibrillators, implanted, electrocoagulation and,
        62, 72
Detachable snare loops
    colonic bleeding, 240
    colonic polypectomy, 214–215
        hemostasis, 228
Dextrose, injection therapy, 5
Diathermy snare excision, adenomas, ampullary
        obstruction, 187
Diet, esophageal stenting, 46
Dieulafoy's lesions
    argon plasma coagulation, 92, 93 (Fig.)
        hemorrhage from, 97
    electrocoagulation, 67, 72
Dihematoporphyrin ether/ester, 102
Dilating catheters, see Bougies
Dilation procedures, 29–37
    common bile duct strictures, 204
    pancreatic duct strictures, 181
    papilla of Vater, 131, 142
    for stenting, 44
    tumors, results, 52
Diode lasers, photodynamic therapy, 103
Direct current hemorrhoid probe, 69
Discharge (watery), cryohemorrhoidectomy, 251,
        253
Disposable sphincterotomes, 131
Distension, for gastrostomy, 277, 283, 285
Divergence, laser beams, 76
Diverticula
    colon, hemorrhage, 68, 69, 241
    juxtapapillary, sphincterotomy, 134, 157
Dormia baskets
    biliary stent retrieval, 205, 206
    biliary stone extraction, 131–132
    lithotripsy, 136–137
Dosimetry, photodynamic therapy, 105–106
Double duct sign, pancreas, 180

'Double-check' ('safe track') maneuver, gastrostomy puncture, 284–285
Down-hill varices, 13
Dry hemostasis probes, 63
  peptic ulcer, 64
Duodenoscopes
  side-viewing, 130
  stenting, 46
  for transpapillary stone removal, 148–149
Duodenum
  endoscopic mucosal resection, results, 123–124
  peptic ulcer, laser therapy and, 75, 79
  perforation, 210
  stenoses, 35, 47 (Fig.)
Duration, electrocoagulation, 60–61
Duty cycles, electrocoagulation, 61
Dye lasers
  lithotripsy, 156
    pulsed flashlamp, 151, 158, 167–168
  photodynamic therapy, 103, 108
Dye marking, colonic polyps, 226
Dysmotility, esophageal varices treatment, 20
Dysphagia, gastrostomy, 278
Dysplasia
  argon plasma coagulation, 96
  Barrett's esophagus, 71, 109, 110
  photodynamic therapy, 106

Echoendoscopes, 265–266
Eder–Puestow guidewires, 31
Eder–Puestow metal olives, 29–30
Electric field strength, argon plasma coagulation, 88
Electrocoagulation, 59–74
  biophysics, 59–62
  equipment, 63
  hazards, 62–63
Electrodes, argon plasma coagulation, 89
Electrohydraulic lithotripsy, choledocholithiasis, 137, 150, 155–156, 167
  extracorporeal, 151
  results, 158
Electrohydrothermal probes, 64
Electromagnetic extracorporeal lithotripsy, choledocholithiasis, 151
Electromagnetic fields, inductive sensing, colonoscope position, 226
Electron spin conversion, photosensitizers, 101
Electronic devices, implanted, electrocoagulation and, 62, 72
Electroshockwave lithotripsy (ESWL)
  choledocholithiasis, 137, 150, 155–156
  pancreatic duct stones, 141
Electrosurgical units, see Generators
Elevation, carcinoma of colon, at polypectomy, 220
Elevator bridges, biliary stenting, 203
Emergency electrocoagulation, colonic bleeding, 64
Emergency endoscopy, gastrointestinal bleeding
  lower, 235, 236
  upper, 1–2, 64
  varices, 15
Emphysema, intestinal, after argon plasma coagulation, 94, 97
EMR tube procedure, endoscopic mucosal resection, 119
Endoclip, colon bleeding, 240
Endoloop, see Detachable snare loops
Endoprostheses, see Stenting
Endoscopic mucosal resection, 117–127
  colon carcinoma, 118–119
  procedure, 119–122
  results, 123–124
Endoscopic retrograde choledochopancreatography, 177–197
  complications, 181–183
  see also Cholangiopancreatography, EUS-guided
Endosonography, 265–276
  choledocholithiasis, 183–184
  complications, 273–274
  pancreatitis, 185
  pseudocyst drainage, 191
  staging for photodynamic therapy, 108

Endotracheal intubation, gastrointestinal bleeding, 2
Enemas
  electrocoagulation and, 62
  soluble contrast medium, 228
    polyp localization, 226
  see also Barium enemas
Energy
  electrocoagulation, 60
  photodynamic therapy, 103
Energy density, photodynamic therapy, 106
Enteral feeding, gastrostomy, 278, 288
Enteral Wallstents, 46
Enteroenterostomy (Braun), sphincterotomy results, 136
Enteroscopy, gastrointestinal bleeding, 236–237
Epigastric access, percutaneous transhepatic cholangioscopy, 168
Epinephrine injection, 4–5, 8
  bleeding ulcers, 66, 79
  colon
    bleeding, 238, 240–241
    polypectomy, 219, 229
  in endoscopic mucosal resection technique, 120
Equipment carts, hemorrhoid management, 245, 246 (Fig.)
Erlangen basket system, 150
Erosions, laser therapy, 79
Eska–Buess stents, 40
Esophacoils, 42
  malplacement, 50–51
  non-esophageal use, 46
  perforation from, 50 (Fig.)
  rectosigmoid tumors, 48 (Fig.)
Esophagus
  benign stenoses, 34–35
  carcinoma
    argon plasma coagulation, 93 (Fig.), 95 (Fig.)
    early detection, 117–118
    electrocoagulation, 70–71
    photodynamic therapy, 110
    stenting, 40
  endoscopic mucosal resection, results, 123
  intramural saline, 125
  laceration, gastrostomy procedures, 296
  paving, 56
  photodynamic therapy, 105
  stenting, 44–46
    benign stenoses, 39
    perforation, 46
    results, 52–54
    tumors, 35, 40, 82
  transection, vs sclerotherapy, 21
  varices, 13–27
  see also Cervical esophagus
ESWL, see Electroshockwave lithotripsy
Ethanolamine, sclerotherapy
  esophageal varices, 15, 17, 19
  peptic ulcer, 5
EUSN-1 Echotip ultrasound needle, 267
Excoriation, gastrostomy, 295
Expandable stents, 41–43
  benign strictures and, 54
  esophagus, 46
  procedure, 43–46
  vs rigid stents, 39
  see also Self-expanding metal stents
Experience of operators
  dilation procedures, 34
  sphincterotomy, 136
Explosion
  argon plasma coagulation, 89–90
  electrocoagulation, 62
  laser therapy, 79
Extended polyps, colon, 217
Extracorporeal shock wave lithotripsy
  biliary tract, 151, 156, 167
  pancreatic duct, 181
  sepsis, 190
Eyes, after photodynamic therapy, 112

Familial adenomatous polyposis (FAP syndrome), argon plasma coagulation, 95 (Fig.), 97
Famotidine, 9

Fibrin sealant
  colonic bleeding, 240
  esophageal varices, 15
  fistulae, 80
    argon plasma coagulation before, 97
  peptic ulcer, 5–6, 8–9
Fibrosis, tissue resistance, 60
Field strength, argon plasma coagulation, 88
Fine needle aspiration
  EUS-guided, 267–271
    complications, 273, 274
  needles for, botulinum toxin injection, 272
First pass effect, 4
Fistula prostheses, Wilson-Cook, 40
Fistulae
  argon plasma coagulation, before fibrin sealant, 97
  esophageal stenting, results, 53 (Table)
  gastrostomy, 289
    abnormal, 296
    measurement, 290
  from laser therapy, 79–80
  rectal carcinoma palliation, 259
  for transhepatic stone removal, 169
    postprocedure care, 172
Fistulotomy (choledochoduodenostomy), 133–134
Flattening, mucosal folds, photodynamic therapy, 105
Fluorescence, photosensitizers, 101
Fluoroscopy
  vs cholangioscopy, biliary lithotripsy, 158
  colonoscope position, 226
  dilation procedures, 31, 34, 44
  gastrostomy, 277
  shockwave lithotripsy, 155
  transpapillary stone removal, 148, 153–154
Foley bag balloon catheter, acid corrosion, 295
Food impaction, 51
Foreign bodies, removal from biliary tree, 138
Formaldehyde solution, for colonic bleeding, 240, 242
Forrest classification, peptic ulcers, 3, 4 (Table)
Foscan, see Metatetra(hydroxyphenyl)chlorin
Four-barb stents, pancreatic duct, 182
Fracture, basket cables, 155
'Freddy', see Frequency-doubled neodymium: yttrium aluminum garnet lasers
Free air, after colon polypectomy, 227–228
Frequency-doubled neodymium: yttrium aluminum garnet lasers, 76
  lithotripsy, 151, 158–159
Fresenius set, gastrostomy, 285
Frimberger stent coupling device, 204
Fulguration, 61
  colon polypectomy, 218, 220, 221

Gallbladder, after sphincterotomy, 141, 142
Gallstone pancreatitis, see Biliary pancreatitis
Gas
  free after colon polypectomy, 227–228
  see also Explosion
Gastrectomy, see Billroth-II gastrectomy
Gastric buttons
  equipment, 281–282
  procedures, 290–291
Gastric decompression, 278
Gastric lavage, 2
Gastric outlet obstruction, malignant, stenting, 39, 44, 54
Gastric stasis, 31
Gastrocolic fistulae, gastrostomy, 296
Gastroduodenostomy, conversion of gastrostomy, equipment, 281
Gastro-esophageal reflux
  esophageal varices treatment, 20
  gastrostomy, 296
  stenosis above stents, 52
  valved stents, 42
  see also Peptic stenoses
Gastrointestinal bleeding
  electrocoagulation, 64–69
  lower, 235–244
  upper
    non-variceal, 1–11
    see also Peptic ulcer
  variceal, 13–27

Gastrojejunal buttons, 282, 290
Gastrojejunostomy
    blockage, 295
    indications, 279, 296
    ulcers, 296
    see also Roux-en-Y gastrojejunostomy
Gastropathy, 14, 20
Gastroplasty
    endoscopy of ampulla of Vater, 148
    stenoses, 35
Gastroscopes, colon polypectomy, 224
Gastroscopy, lower gastrointestinal bleeding, 236
Gastrostomy, 277–300
    complications, 291–296
    conversion to button, 282, 290
    equipment, 280–283
    failure of placement, 293–294
    post-procedure care, 288–289
    procedure, 283–285
    removal/replacement
        equipment, 282–283
        procedure, 291
    tube displacement, 294–295
Geenen–Hogan classification, sphincter of Oddi
    dyskinesia, 139
General anaesthesia, stricture dilation, 31
Generators, electrosurgical, 60, 63
    automatic regulation, 61–62
    colonic polypectomy, 213, 216–217
    sphincterotomy, 131
GF-UC30P echoendoscope (Olympus), 265, 266
    (Table)
GIP Medi-Globe needle system, endosonography,
    266–267
Glasgow criteria (modified), acute pancreatitis,
    184 (Table)
Glidewire method, intestinal tube placement, 289
Glyceryl trinitrate paste, anal fissure, 261
Glycylpressin, esophageal varices treatment, 16
Gold probes, 63, 65, 66
    colonic bleeding, 239
    thermal coagulation, 6
'Grasping and snaring', endoscopic mucosal
    resection, 119
Green lasers, lithotripsy, 158
Grounding pads, electrocoagulation, 62
Guidewires
    benign rectal strictures, 262
    biliary stenting, 201, 202, 203
        positioning, 205
    dilation procedures, 31–32
    gastrostomy, Sacks–Vine method, 287
    intestinal tube placement, 289
    for olives, 29–30
    pancreatic duct cannulation, 177–178
    percutaneous transhepatic stone removal, 166,
        169
    sphincterotomy, 131, 134
        hemorrhage control, 135
    stenting procedures, 44

H₂ receptor antagonists, see Acid suppression
Handles, outside-the-scope mechanical
    lithotriptors, 149
Healing, endoscopic mucosal resection, 123
Heart, esophageal varices therapy, 20
Heat
    electrocoagulation, 59–60
    laser therapy, 76
Heat sink effect, electrocoagulation, 61
Heater probes, 7, 63
    colon bleeding, 240
    colon polyps, 214
    peptic ulcer, 66
Helium-neon pilot lasers, 76
Hematoma, esophageal varices, 19
Hematoporphyrin derivative, 101, 102
    strictures, 111
Hemobilia, 172, 173
Hemoclips, 7, 8 (Fig.)
Hemodynamics, esophageal varices therapy, 20
Hemorrhage
    banding of hemorrhoids, 249
    colon polypectomy, 228–229
    EUS-guided fine needle aspiration, 274
    gastrostomy, 296

from laser therapy, 79
    percutaneous transhepatic cholangioscopy, 172
    rectal carcinoma palliation, 259
    retroperitoneal, EUS-guided celiac nerve block,
        274
    sphincterotomy, ampulla of Vater, 132, 135
    ulcers from esophageal varices therapy, 19
    see also Gastrointestinal bleeding
Hemorrhoid probe, multipolar, 63
Hemorrhoids, 245–254
    bleeding, 236
    classification, 246 (Table)
    electrocoagulation, 69
Hemostasis
    argon plasma coagulation, 91–96
    colonic polypectomy, 217, 225, 228–229,
        240–241
    electrocoagulation, 61, 64
    at endoscopic mucosal resection, 121, 125
    laser therapy, 75, 78–79, 83
    results, 82
Hemostasis probes, 63
    bipolar, power density, 60
Heparin, polypectomy, 213
Hepaticojejunostomy, transhepatic approach, 174
Hepatolithiasis, see Intrahepatic radicles, stone
    removal
High-brightness lamps, photodynamic therapy,
    104
Histopathology
    endoscopic mucosal resection, 122
    see also Fine needle aspiration
History-taking, intestinal bleeding, 236
Holmium lasers, lithotripsy, 150–151, 159
Home-made stents, 40
Hospital admission, sphincterotomy, 134
'Hot biopsy' forceps
    colon angioectasias and, 68
    colon polypectomy, 214, 218
        hemostasis, 229
        precautions, 229
    colonic bleeding, 238
Huibregtse catheter, 200–201
Human thrombin, peptic ulcer injection therapy, 5
Hydatid disease, removal of parasites, 138
Hydrophilic guidewires
    biliary stenting, 201
    percutaneous transhepatic stone removal, 169
Hydroxyl radicals, photodynamic therapy, 102
Hypertensive gastropathy, 14, 20

Idiopathic acute recurrent pancreatitis, 185
Ileocolonic stenoses, 35
Impaction, biliary calculi, 154
Implanted electronic devices, electrocoagulation
    and, 62, 72
India ink, colonic polyps, 226–227
Indigocarmine solution, carcinoma detection, 118,
    120
Indocyanine green, colonic polyps, 226
Inductive sensing, colonoscope position, 226
Inflammatory bowel disease
    bleeding, 241
    see also Crohn's disease
Inflammatory polyps, after argon plasma
    coagulation, 97
Inflatable balloons, see Balloons
Information sheet, hemorrhoid banding, 249
Infrared coagulation, hemorrhoids, 249–250, 253
'Injection and snaring', endoscopic mucosal
    resection, 119
'Injection, pre-cutting and snaring', endoscopic
    mucosal resection, 119
Injection therapy
    peptic ulcer bleeding, 4–6
    see also Sclerotherapy
Injection-Gold probe, 65
    thermal coagulation, 6
    see also Gold probes
Injector needles
    botulinum toxin for achalasia, 272
    colonic bleeding, 238
    colonic polypectomy, 213–214, 219–220
Instrument channels, position, 218
Insufflation for gastrostomy, 277, 283, 285
Insulation failure, electrocoagulation, 62

Integrated fiber detectors, photodynamic therapy
    monitoring, 105
Intelligent laser lithotripsy, 137, 151, 158,
    167–168, 171
Intensive care, transpapillary stone removal, 148
Intermittent current, electrocoagulation, 61
International classification, chronic pancreatitis,
    180 (Table)
Intersystem crossover, photosensitizers, 101
Intestinal bleeding, 235–244
Intestinal emphysema, after argon plasma
    coagulation, 94, 97
Intestinal obstruction, gastrostomy tubes, 296
Intestinal tubes, see Jejunal tubes
Intraductal secretin test, chronic pancreatitis, 188
Intrahepatic radicles, stone removal
    transhepatic, 168, 170, 173–174
    transpapillary, 152
Intramural saline
    argon plasma coagulation, 95
    colon
        argon plasma coagulation, 92
        laser therapy, 79
        polypectomy, 219–220
    endoscopic mucosal resection, 117, 119, 122
        experimental study, 124–125
        technique, 120
Intra-operative colonoscopy, 226
    gastrointestinal bleeding, 229
Intravariceal injection, 16
Intravenous access, esophageal varices treatment,
    16
Introducer method, see Russell method
Intussusception, gastrostomy tubes, 296
Iodine-dye method, carcinoma of esophagus,
    117–118, 120
Irradiation telangiectasias, see Radiation-induced
    telangiectasias
Irrigation
    adherent clots, 66
    colonic bleeding, 237
        diverticular disease, 241
    shockwave lithotripsy, 155, 171
    stomach, 2
Ischemia, abdominal pain and intestinal bleeding,
    236
Ischemic colitis, bleeding, 241
Isolated generator outputs, electrocoagulation, 62
Isosorbide dinitrate, papilla of Vater dilation, 142
Isotope scanning, lower gastrointestinal bleeding,
    236

Jag guidewire, biliary stenting, 201
Jejunal tubes, 281, 289
    aspiration pneumonia, 296
    blockage, 295
Jejunostomy
    equipment, 281
    procedure, 289–290
JETPEG, see Gastrojejunostomy
Juvenile polyps, 242
Juxtapapillary diverticula, sphincterotomy, 134,
    157

Kasugai classification, chronic pancreatitis, 179
KeyMed–Atkinson prostheses, 40
Kidneys, function, photodynamic therapy, 106
KTP lasers, photodynamic therapy, 103, 104

Lamps, high-brightness, photodynamic therapy,
    104
Laparoscopy
    biliary system, 129–130, 147, 148
    colonic surgery, 225
    for post-polypectomy perforation, 228
Larynx, laceration, gastrostomy procedures, 296
Laser light, photodynamic therapy, 101
    sources, 103
Laser lithotripsy, 137, 150–151, 167–168
    vs extracorporeal shock wave lithotripsy, 159
    results, 158–159
    transhepatic approach, 170–171
Laser therapy, 75–85
    vs argon plasma coagulation, 89 (Fig.), 97
    colonic bleeding, 239
    damage to metal stents, 97

esophageal tumors, *vs* electrocoagulation, 70, 71
hemorrhoids, 251–252, 253–254
for peptic ulcer hemorrhage, 6, 66
puncture of pseudocysts, 191
rectal carcinoma palliation, 258–259
Leakage, gastrostomy, 295
Left hepatic duct, guidewire insertion, 205
Leiomyomas, 270
Leukopenia, 106
Life support, gastrointestinal bleeding, 2
'Lift and cut', endoscopic mucosal resection, 119
Ligation
endoscopic mucosal resection procedure, 119
esophageal varices, 14
complications, 19
devices, 15
vs sclerotherapy, 21–22
technique, 17–18
hemorrhoids, 240
vs electrocoagulation, 69
post-polypectomy bleeding, 229
Light application systems, photodynamic therapy, 104–105
Light guides, laser therapy, 76
Light sources, photodynamic therapy, 103–104
Linear array echoendoscopes, 265–266
fine needle aspiration, 267–268, 269
Linitis plastica, EUS-guided fine needle aspiration, 270
Lipiodol, with butyl-cyanoacrylate, 17
Lipomas, submucosal, 270
Lipoproteins, photosensitizers, 102
Liquid hemostasis probes, 63
peptic ulcer, 64
Liquid nitrogen, cryosurgery of hemorrhoids, 250
Lithotripsy
choledocholithiasis, 136–137, 149–150
difficulties, 154–155
results, 157–158
systems, 167–168
transhepatic approach, 170–171, 174
pancreatic, sepsis, 190
Liver
abscess, after sphincterotomy, 142
cirrhosis, 13–14
epinephrine metabolism, 4
function
5–aminolevulinic acid, 111
photodynamic therapy, 106
porphyrins, 106
see also Intrahepatic radicles, stone removal
Loops, nylon, colonic polypectomy, 214
Lord's anal dilator, rectal carcinoma palliation, 258, 259
Low molecular weight heparin, polypectomy and, 213
Lower esophageal sphincter, botulinum toxin injection, 272, 273 (Fig.)
Lymph nodes
EUS-guided fine needle aspiration, 268–269
metastases, stomach carcinoma, 106, 118
Lymphoma, stomach, EUS-guided fine needle aspiration, 270

Magnetic fields, inductive sensing, colonoscope position, 226
Magnifying colonoscopes, chromoendoscopy, 217
Major papilla sphincterotomy, pancreatic duct, 180–181
Makuuchi tube, endoscopic mucosal resection, 119
Malecot catheter, Russell gastrostomy method, 287–288
Mallory-Weiss tears
electrocoagulation, 67, 69
epinephrine and, 4
laser therapy, 79
Malplacement, stents, 50–51
Mannitol, 62, 213
Manometry, pancreatic duct, complications, 182
Marble-type polyps, colon, 217
Marking
colonic polyps, 226
snares, colonic polypectomy, 215–216
see also Chromoendoscopy

Massive necrosis, acute pancreatitis, 187–188
Measurement, gastrostomy tracts, 290
Measuring devices, one-step gastric button procedure, 290, 291
Mechanical lithotripsy, 136–137, 149–150, 154–155
results, 157–158
Mechanical methods, for peptic ulcer hemorrhage, 7
Mechanical sector scanning echoendoscope, 266
Meckel's diverticulum, 242
Mediastinal lymph nodes, fine needle aspiration, 268–269
Medication pumps, electrocoagulation and, 62
Medi-Globe needle system (GIP), endosonography, 266–267
Medoc-Celestin tubes, 40–41
Memory catheters, sphincterotomes, 131
Mesenteric veins, thrombosis, sclerosants, 20
Mesothelioma, photodynamic therapy, 103
Metal clips, for peptic ulcer hemorrhage, 7
Metal olives, 29–30
Metal stents
biliary drainage, 139–140
damage
argon plasma coagulation, 97
electrocoagulation, 69–70
laser therapy, 97
electrocoagulation and, 69–70
see also Self-expanding metal stents
Metaplasia, Barrett's esophagus, 71
Metastases, *see* Lymph nodes
Metatetra(hydroxyphenyl)chlorin, 102, 108
carcinoma of stomach, 110
energy density for, 106
squamous esophagus, 102
Methylene blue
Barrett's esophagus, 107
colon polypectomy, 217
gastrostomy puncture, 285
Methyl-terbutyl-ether, 138
Microlens, photodynamic therapy of stomach, 105
Microlithiasis, pancreatitis, 185
Microsurgery, transanal endoscopic, 254–257
Midazolam, esophageal varices treatment, 16
Migration
biliary stents, 206
pancreatic duct stents, 182
Z stents, 51
Minibaskets, pancreatic duct, 178
Minimally invasive biliary surgery, 130
Miniscopes, *see* Babyscopes
Minisnare, colon polypectomy, 218, 223–224
Minisphincterotomes, 178
Minor papilla
pre-cannulation excision, 181
sphincterotomy, 181, 186–187
Modified Glasgow criteria, acute pancreatitis, 184 (Table)
Monoaspartyl chlorin e6, 102
Monochromators, photodynamic therapy monitoring, 105
Monolith lithotriptor, 149–150, 157
Monopolar electrocoagulation, 59, 62, 63, 64
'Mother–baby' systems
cholangioscopy, 137, 149
shockwave lithotripsy, 155
transpapillary stone removal, 148–149
'Mount Fuji' effect, 238, 239 (Fig.)
Mountain-type polyps, colon, 217
MTHPC, *see* Metatetra(hydroxyphenyl)chlorin
Mucosal carcinoma, resection, 118
Mucosal clips, colon polypectomy, 215, 226
Mucosal folds, flattening, photodynamic therapy, 105
Mucosal resection, colon carcinoma, 118–119
Mucosectomy, simple suction technique, 119
Multiligators, esophageal varices, 16 (Fig.)
Multipolar electrocoagulation, *see* Bipolar electrocoagulation
Multipolar hemorrhoid probe, 63
Multipolar hemostasis probes, 63
Multipolar tumor probe, 63
Myogenic tumors, submucosal, 270

NA-10J-1 needle (Olympus), endosonography, 267
Nasogastric tube feeding, trial of (Gauderer), 296
Nasopancreatic catheters, 178
for pseudocysts, 190
Nausea, 5–aminolevulinic acid, 111
Necrosis
massive, acute pancreatitis, 187–188
stomach, peptic ulcer sclerotherapy, 5
Necrotizing fasciitis, gastrostomy, 295
Needle systems, endosonography, 266–267
Needle-knife sphincterotomes, 130 (Fig.), 131
pancreatic duct, 180–181
Needles
botulinum toxin injection of lower esophageal sphincter, 272
colonic polyp marking, 227
hemostasis probes, 63, 66
injection therapy, 4
esophageal varices, 15
peptic ulcer, 4
percutaneous transhepatic cholangioscopy, 166
Needle-tip catheters, papilla cannulation, 177
Neodymium: yttrium aluminum garnet lasers, 76
colonic bleeding, 239
frequency-doubled, 76
lithotripsy, 151, 158–159
hemorrhoids, 251–252, 254
peptic ulcer hemorrhage, 6
rectal carcinoma palliation, 257
see also KTP lasers
Neomycin, gastrostomy and, 283
Nimura-type bougies, percutaneous transhepatic cholangioscopy, 166
Nitrates
glyceryl trinitrate paste, anal fissure, 261
papilla of Vater dilation, 142
Nitrogen, liquid, cryosurgery of hemorrhoids, 250
Nitrous oxide, cryosurgery of hemorrhoids, 250
Non-contact thermal methods, for peptic ulcer hemorrhage, 6
Non-ionic contrast media, ERCP, 179
'Non-lifting sign', carcinoma of colon, 220
Non-steroidal anti-inflammatory drugs
colon ulcers, 242
endosonography, 267
intestinal bleeding, 236
Nuclear medicine, lower gastrointestinal bleeding, 236
Nylon loops, colonic polypectomy, 214

Oasis system, biliary stenting, 203
Obstructive cholangitis, sphincterotomy for, 138
Obstructive pancreatitis, chronic, 140–141
Occlusion
biliary stents, 206, 209–210
gastrostomy tubes, 295
pancreatic duct stents, 183
Octreotide, esophageal varices treatment, 16
Olives, 29–30
Olympus
BML systems
results, 157
stone impaction, 154
cholangioscopes, percutaneous transhepatic, 166 (Table)
GF-UC30P echoendoscope, 265, 266 (Table)
NA-10J-1 needle, endosonography, 267
triple layer lithotriptor, 150
video-chip baby cholangioscope, 149
Omeprazole, ulcers from esophageal varices therapy, 21
One-step gastric button
equipment, 282, 283 (Fig.)
procedure, 290–291
Operating endoscopes, transanal endoscopic microsurgery, 254–255, 258–259
Operators
dilation procedures, 34
sphincterotomy, 136
Oral hygiene, 283
Outpatients, sphincterotomy, 134, 143
'Outside-the-scope' mechanical lithotriptors, 149, 154, 157
Overdistension, photodynamic therapy, 105

Overgrowth, stents
 argon plasma coagulation, 97
 biliary, 210
 electrocoagulation, 70
 photodynamic therapy, 106
Overholt balloons, photodynamic therapy,
  104–105
'Over-the-wire' balloon dilators, 30, 33
 achalasia, 34
'Over-the-wire' intestinal tube placement, 289
Overtubes
 Esophacoil retrieval, 51
 esophageal varices ligation, 15
 gastric lavage, 2
Oxygen, photodynamic therapy, 101–102
Oxygen therapy, explosion, argon plasma
  coagulation, 90

Pacemakers, electrocoagulation and, 62
Pain
 hemorrhoids
  banding, 249
  cryosurgery, 251
 see also Abdominal pain
Pancreas
 benign diseases, 177–197
 carcinoma, 191
  celiac nerve block, 272
  duct stenting, 207
 EUS-guided fine needle aspiration, 269–270
 tumors, 187
 see also Pseudocysts
Pancreas divisum, 130, 136, 141, 186–187,
  207
Pancreatic duct
 diameters, 179
 strictures, 140–141, 180, 181, 187, 189
 see also Stenting, pancreatic duct
Pancreatic sphincter
 sphincterotomy, 134, 136, 140
 see also Minor papilla
Pancreatitis
 acute, 183–188
  with massive necrosis, 187–188
 biliary, 130, 183–184
  sphincterotomy, 138–139
 bipolar vs monopolar sphincterotomy, 63
 chronic, 179, 188–191
  celiac nerve block, 272
  obstructive, 140–141
  stenting, 140, 207
 duodenal stenoses, 35
 after ERCP, 181–182
 after interventional endosonography, 274
 after percutaneous transhepatic cholangioscopy,
  173
 post-traumatic, 191
 after sphincterotomy, 134–135
Pancreatography, 179
 pancreatic duct rupture, 191
Pancreatoscopy, 179
Papilla of Vater
 ampullary obstruction, 139
 cannulation, 202
 tumors, 130
 see also Transpapillary drainage
Papillectomy, 134
Papillotomy, 130
Paracentesis, EUS-guided, 272–273
Parasites, removal, 138
Paravariceal injection, 16
Patient, see Positioning of patient
Patient information sheet, hemorrhoid banding,
  249
Patulous orifice, transpapillary stone removal, 154
Pauldrach basket system, transpapillary stone
  removal, 150
Paving, esophagus, 56
Pediatric duodenoscopes, for transpapillary stone
  removal, 148
Pediatrics, see Children
Pedunculated polyps, colon, 217, 218
PEF-703FA echoendoscope, Toshiba, 266
PEG-electrolyte purge regimen, 236
PEG/J, see Gastrojejunostomy
Pelvic sepsis, hemorrhoid banding, 249

Penetration depth, photodynamic therapy, 105
Pentax cholangioscopes, percutaneous
  transhepatic, 166 (Table)
Pentax echoendoscopes, 265, 266 (Table)
Peptic stenoses
 esophagus, 34–35
 pylorus, 35
Peptic ulcer, 1
 assessment, 3–4
 duodenum, laser therapy and, 75, 79
 electrocoagulation, 64–67, 72
 laser therapy, 78–79, 83
  results, 82
Percutaneous transhepatic cholangiography, 136
Percutaneous transhepatic cholangioscopy, 137
Percutaneous transhepatic stone removal,
  165–176
 results, 173–174
Perforation
 after argon plasma coagulation, 96
 argon plasma coagulation for, 93 (Fig.)
 balloon dilation, 33, 34
 bile ducts, 209
 colon polypectomy, 219, 227–228
 duodenum, 210
 endoscopic mucosal resection, 117, 123
  mechanism studies, 124–125
 endosonography, 273
 esophageal varices, 19
 gastrostomy, 296
 laser therapy, 79
 peptic ulcer electrocoagulation, 65
 rectum
  benign stricture dilation, 262
  carcinoma palliation, 259
 retroperitoneal, sphincterotomy, 135
 stenting, 46, 50
Peristalsis, esophageal varices treatment, 20
Peritoneal dialysis, gastrostomy and, 279
Peritoneovenous shunts, gastrostomy and,
  279–280
Peritonitis
 benign rectal stricture dilation, 262
 biliary, percutaneous transhepatic
   cholangioscopy, 173
 esophageal varices treatment, 20
 gastrostomy displacement, 294
 post-polypectomy, 228
Permanent vegetative state, gastrostomy and, 278
Pharmacologic dilation of ampulla, 142
Phenol, hemorrhoids, 246
Phospho-soda preparation, colon cleansing
  regimen, 213
Photobiological equivalence, 104
Photodynamic diagnosis, 107
Photodynamic therapy, 101–115
Photofrin (porfimer sodium), 102, 108
Photosensitivity, after photodynamic therapy, 112
Photosensitizers, 101–103
Piecemeal polypectomy, colon, 216, 220–221,
  224
Piezo-electric extracorporeal lithotripsy,
  choledocholithiasis, 151
Pigtail catheters
 gastrostomy, 277–278
 percutaneous transhepatic stone removal, 166,
  169
Pigtail stents, biliary, 199
Plastic expandable stents, 43
 biliary drainage, 139–140
 see also Teflon stents
Platelet count
 for percutaneous transhepatic cholangioscopy,
  166
 for transpapillary stone removal, 148
Plug technique, fibrin sealant injection therapy,
  5–6
Pneumonia, aspiration, gastrostomy, 296
Pneumoperitoneum
 'benign', 227–228
 gastrostomy, 294, 296
  Russell method, 288, 294
Poke method, see Russell method
Polidocanol, sclerotherapy
 esophageal varices, 17, 19
 peptic ulcer, 5, 6, 8

Polydiagnost cholangioscope, percutaneous
  transhepatic, 166 (Table)
Polyethylene glycol, bowel cleansing, 213, 217
Polyp traps, 223
Polypectomy
 colonoscopy, 213–233
  polyp size, 217, 225
 electrocoagulation, 71 (Fig.)
  instruments, 63
  post-operative, 71
 hemorrhage, 68, 69, 240–241
 laser therapy, 82, 83
  post-operative, 78
 transanal microsurgery, 254–257
Polyps
 familial adenomatous polyposis, argon plasma
   coagulation, 95 (Fig.), 97
 see also Adenomas
Polyurethane, vs silicones, gastrostomy tubes, 295
Polyvinyl dilators
 technique, 32–33
 see also Savary–Gilliard dilators
Polyvinyl stents, 40
Ponsky–Gauderer method, gastrostomy, 278
 choice, 288
 equipment, 280
 procedure, 285–286
Popcorn effect, laser therapy, 76
Porfimer sodium, 102, 108
Porphyria, 106
Porphyrins, tissue distribution, 102
Portacaval shunting, vs sclerotherapy, 21
Portal hypertension, 13
 reduction after sclerotherapy, 21
 see also Congestive gastropathy
Portal vein, thrombosis, sclerosants, 20
Portocaval shunting, see Transjugular intrahepatic
   portosystemic shunting
Positioning of patient
 colonoscopy
  bleeding, 237
  polypectomy, 223
 gastrointestinal bleeding, 2
Post-polypectomy coagulation syndrome, 228
Post-traumatic pancreatitis, 191
Postural hypotension, EUS-guided celiac nerve
  block, 274
Potassium iodide, iodine-dye method, carcinoma
  of esophagus, 117–118, 120
Povidone-iodine, oral hygiene, 283
Power, power density
 argon plasma coagulation, limits, 98 (Table)
 electrocoagulation, 60, 63, 72
 photodynamic therapy, 105
Pre-cannulation excision of minor papilla, 181
Precut sphincterotomy, 130 (Fig.), 131, 133,
  157
Pregnancy, stenting in choledocholithiasis, 151
Pre-looping, endoscopic mucosal resection, 121
Premalignant lesions
 argon plasma coagulation, 96
 photodynamic therapy, 96
 see also Barrett's esophagus
Pressure necrosis, stents, 51–52
Primary sclerosing cholangitis, stenting, 140, 207
Proctitis, radiation, strictures after argon plasma
  coagulation, 96
Proctology, 245–264
 see also Rectosigmoid tumors; Rectum
Proctoscopes, 247 (Fig.)
Proctoscopy, for bleeding, 236
Prograde stone removal, transhepatic approach,
  169–170
Prophylaxis, esophageal variceal bleeding, 22
Propofol
 esophageal varices treatment, 16
 stricture dilation, 31
Propranolol, esophageal varices, 21
Prostheses, see Stenting
Prothrombin time
 for percutaneous transhepatic cholangioscopy,
  166
 for transpapillary stone removal, 148
Proton pump inhibitors, 9
Protoporphyrin IX, 103
 skin phototoxicity, 111

Pseudoaneurysm, EUS-guided celiac nerve block, 274
Pseudocysts, pancreas, 130, 141, 190–191
  ERCP, complications, 182
  EUS-guided drainage, 271, 273
Pull-string method, see Ponsky–Gauderer method
Pull-type sphincterotomes, 130 (Fig.)
Pulmonary circulation, sclerosants, 20
Pulsed flashlamp dye lasers, lithotripsy, 151, 158, 167–168
Puncture sites, gastrostomy, 284
'Push' enteroscopes, 237
Pusher tubes, stenting, 41
  biliary, 203
Push-over-wire method, see Sacks–Vine method
Push-type sphincterotomes, 130 (Fig.), 131
Pylorus
  peptic stenoses, 35
  stenting, 46
  see also Gastric outlet obstruction

Radial echoendoscopes, 265
  fine needle aspiration, 267, 269
    hemorrhage, 274
Radiation proctitis, strictures after argon plasma coagulation, 96
Radiation-induced telangiectasias
  colon, 241–242
  electrocoagulation, 68, 69
Radiofrequency current, electrocoagulation, 59–60
Radiologic gastrostomy, 277–278
  results, 291–292
Radionuclide scanning, lower gastrointestinal bleeding, 236
Ranitidine
  vs proton pump inhibitors, 9
  ulcers from esophageal varices therapy, 21
Ranson criteria, acute pancreatitis, 184 (Table)
Rapid-start, electrosurgical generators, 131
Reactive oxygen products, photodynamic therapy, 102
Rectosigmoid tumors, 48 (Fig.)
  electrocoagulation, 71
  stenting, 260
    results, 55–56
Rectum, 245–264
  benign strictures, 261–262
  carcinoma, 49 (Fig.)
    argon plasma coagulation, 92 (Fig.)
    endoscopic palliation, 257–260
  EUS-guided fine needle aspiration, 270–271
  gastroscopes, polypectomy, 224
  intramural saline, 125
  laser therapy, 77
Recurrence
  bleeding, argon plasma coagulation, 94
  esophageal tumors, after laser therapy, 82
  esophageal varices, 18
    bleeding, 21
  peptic ulcer bleeding, 9
    laser therapy, 79
Recurrent pancreatitis, acute, 184–185
Red folds, diverticular disease, 241
Red-out, 2
Renal function, photodynamic therapy, 106
Rendez-vous technique, sphincterotomy, 134, 165
Repeat treatment
  colon polypectomy, 224–225
  esophageal varices treatment, 18–19
  hemorrhoids, sclerotherapy, 246
  malignant tumors, laser therapy, 77
  peptic ulcer bleeding, 8–9
Repositioning
  balloon dilation, 44
  stents, esophagus, 45–46
Rescue devices, 'outside-the-scope' mechanical lithotriptors, 149, 154, 157
Resistance of tissue, electrocoagulation, 60, 61
Respiratory arrest, sedation, 179
Respiratory function, sclerosants, 20
Respiratory tract, see Tracheobronchial system
Restenosis, after sphincterotomy, 142
Resuscitation, gastrointestinal bleeding, 2
Retention discs, 'buried bumper', gastrostomy, 294–295

Retrieval
  Esophacoils, malplacement, 50–51
  stents, 46
    biliary, 205–206
Retroperitoneal hemorrhage, EUS-guided celiac nerve block, 274
Retroperitoneal perforation, sphincterotomy, 135
Retroversion, see U-turn maneuver
Re-use, sphincterotomes, 131
Rhodamine laser lithotripsy, choledocholithiasis, 137, 151, 158, 167–168
Rigid stents
  esophagus, 44–46
    results, 53
    vs expandable stents, 39
Rigiflex dilators, achalasia, 31
Risk scores, esophageal varices, 14
Roll-over technique, 2
Rotation, colonoscopes
  for bleeding, 237
  for polypectomy, 222
Roux-en-Y choledochojejunostomy, transpapillary stone removal, 148
Roux-en-Y gastrojejunostomy, sphincterotomy results, 136
Rubber banding, hemorrhoids, 248–249
  band removal, 249
  results, 253
Rugae, gastrostomy puncture, 284, 285 (Fig.)
Rupture (post-traumatic pancreatitis), 191
Russell method, gastrostomy, 278, 279
  choice, 288
  equipment, 280–281
  pneumoperitoneum, 288, 294
  procedure, 287–288

Sacks–Vine method, gastrostomy, 278
  choice, 288
  equipment, 280
  procedure, 286 (Fig.), 287
'Safe track' maneuver, gastrostomy puncture, 284–285
Safety sphincterotomes, 131
Saline, see Intramural saline
Sapphire tips, laser therapy, 76
Savary–Gilliard dilators, 30
  photodynamic therapy, 104
  tumors, 35
Scarring, tissue resistance, 60
Schatzki rings, 35
Sclerosants
  colonic bleeding, 238
  esophageal varices, 15
  peptic ulcer, 5, 8–9, 66
  systemic effects, 20
Sclerotherapy
  esophageal varices, 14
    with banding, 19
    results, 21–22
    technique, 16–17
  hemorrhoids, 246–248, 253
  see also Injector needles
Second look endoscopy, peptic ulcer bleeding, 8–9
Secretin test, chronic pancreatitis, 188
Sector scanning echoendoscope, 266
Sedation
  biliary stenting, 202
  ERCP, 179
  esophageal varices treatment, 16
  photodynamic therapy, 107
  stricture dilation, 31
Self-expanding metal stents
  biliary, 200, 204, 206, 208, 210
  rectal stenosing lesions, 260
Sepsis
  pancreatic lithotripsy, 190
  pelvis, hemorrhoid banding, 249
Septostomy, Zenker's diverticulum, argon plasma coagulation, 97
Serositis, 228
Sessile polyps
  colon, 217, 218, 220–221, 224
    bleeding after resection, 229
  rectum, 257
Sheaths
  echoendoscopes, 268

gastrostomy placement, 285
percutaneous transhepatic cholangioscopy, 169
Shockwave lithotripsy, see Electroshockwave lithotripsy; Laser lithotripsy
Shortening, stents, 46
Shunts (peritoneovenous), gastrostomy and, 279–280
Side viewing endoscopes, 130
  biliary stenting, 199
  gastrointestinal bleeding, 2
Silicone oil, 17, 33
Silicone prostheses, esophageal tumors, vs electrocoagulation, 70
Silicones, vs polyurethane, gastrostomy tubes, 295
Simple suction technique, mucosectomy, 119
Single-shot duration limits, argon plasma coagulation, 98 (Table)
Singlet photosensitizers, 101
Site localization
  colonic polyps, 225–227
  see also Puncture sites, gastrostomy
Skin
  excoriation, gastrostomy, 295
  phototoxicity, 102, 103, 111
Smart laser lithotripsy, 137, 151, 167–168, 171
Smoke
  argon plasma coagulation and, 97
  rectal carcinoma palliation, 259
Snares
  colonic bleeding, 238
  colonic polypectomy, 215–216
  endoscopic mucosal resection, 119, 121
  gastrostomy placement, 285
  gastrostomy tube removal, 291
  pancreatic duct, 178
  see also Detachable snare loops
Sodium phosphate, colon cleansing regimen, 213
Sodium tetradecyl sulfate, sclerotherapy
  esophageal varices, 15, 17
  peptic ulcer, 5
Soehendra ('outside-the-scope') mechanical lithotriptors, 149, 154, 157
Solitary ulcer, colon, 242
Soluble contrast medium enemas, 228
  polyp localization, 226
Somatostatin, after sphincterotomy, 135
Song stents, see Z stents
Sonotip needle system (GIP), 267
Sorbitol, 62
Space irradiance, photodynamic therapy, 105
Sphincter of Oddi dysfunction, 185–186
  sphincterotomy, 139
Sphincteroplasty, 186
Sphincterotomes, 63, 130–131
  pancreatic duct, 178
  power density, 60
Sphincterotomy
  ampulla of Vater, 129–146
    assessment for stone removal, 154
    biliary stenting and, 202
    complications, 134–136, 141–142, 208–209
    hemorrhage, 132, 135
    for microlithiasis, 185
    precut, 130 (Fig.), 131, 133, 157
    procedure, 132–134
    results, 136–141
    for sphincter dysfunction, 185–186
  anal fissure, 261
  colon, hemorrhage, 68, 69
  pancreatic duct, 180–181
Spiral Z and ZA-stents, biliary, 200
Splanchnic veins, thrombosis, sclerosants, 20
Splenorenal shunts, esophageal varices therapy, 20
Split proctoscopes, 250
Squamous cell carcinoma, lymph node metastases, 106
Squamous esophagus, photodynamic therapy, 110
Staging procedures, for photodynamic therapy, 107–108
Stapled hemorrhoidectomy, 252–253, 254
Stent coupling device (Frimberger), 204

Stent retrievers, 201, 202 (Fig.)
  biliary stents, 206
Stenting, 39–58
  ampullary strictures, 139–140
  biliary, 199–212
    choledocholithiasis, 136, 151, 159–160
    common bile duct decompression, 189
    complications, 208–210
  contraindications, 39–40
  esophageal tumors, 35, 40, 82
  pancreatic duct, 182, 192, 207
    changes after, 183
    complications, 182–183
    minor papilla, 186–187
    pain relief, 189
    pseudocysts, 190
    at sphincterotomy, 180
  rectal stenosing lesions, 260
  sphincterotomes for, 130
  tumor ingrowth, 47 (Fig.), 51, 69–70, 97, 106
    argon plasma coagulation, 97
    biliary, 210
    electrocoagulation, 69–70
    photodynamic therapy, 106
Stents
  delivery systems, 46
  pancreatic duct, 178
  see also specific types
Steroids
  at celiac nerve block, 272
  with laser therapy, malignant tumors, 78
Stigmata of hemorrhage, peptic ulcer, 3
Stomach
  carcinoma
    early detection, 118
    EUS-guided fine needle aspiration, 270
    photodynamic therapy, 106, 111
  decompression, 278
  distension, gastrostomy, 277
  endoscopic mucosal resection, results, 123
  intramural saline, 125
  lavage, 2
  muscularis propria thickening, EUS-guided fine
    needle aspiration, 270
  necrosis, peptic ulcer sclerotherapy, 5
  photodynamic therapy, 105
  stasis, 31
    see also Gastric outlet obstruction
  stenoses, 35
  varices, 14
Stones, see Calculi; Choledocholithiasis
Stone-tissue discrimination systems, 137, 151,
    158, 167–168, 171
Strictures
  benign, rectum, 261–262
  biliary, stenting, 204–205, 206–208
  common bile duct
    chronic pancreatitis, 189
    stenting, 204
    transhepatic stone removal, 174
    transpapillary stone removal, 152
  dilation, see Dilation procedures
  after endoscopic mucosal resection, 123
  esophageal varices therapy, 19
  impeding endoscopy, 148
  laser therapy, 75, 78, 83
    results, 81–82
  malignant, 83
    argon plasma coagulation, 91
    dilation, 35, 52
    electrocoagulation, 70–71
  pancreatic duct, 141–141, 180, 181, 187,
    189
  after photodynamic therapy, 105, 111
  rectal carcinoma palliation, 260
Stridor, stenting and, 40, 44
Strings
  gastrostomy tube replacement, 291
  Ponsky–Gauderer method, 285
'Strip biopsy', endoscopic mucosal resection, 119
Subcapsular hematoma, percutaneous
    transhepatic cholangioscopy, 172
Submucosal carcinoma, resection, 118
Submucosal lesions, EUS-guided fine needle
    aspiration, 270

Submucosal saline, see Intramural saline
Suction, rectal carcinoma palliation, 259
Sump syndrome, 130, 138
Superoxide anions, photodynamic therapy, 102
Surface area, photodynamic therapy, 105
Surgery
  biliary pancreatitis, 184
  colonic polyps, 225
  intestinal bleeding, 237
  massive pancreatic necrosis, 188
  pancreatic pain, 188
  recurrent peptic ulcer bleeding, 9
Surgical anastomoses, see Anastomotic strictures
Surgical emphysema, after argon plasma
    coagulation, 94, 97
Surveillance (second look endoscopy, peptic ulcer
    bleeding), 8–9
Sutures
  biliary stone formation, 153
  transanal endoscopic microsurgery, 256
Systemic effects, sclerosants, 20

T-anchors, Russell method, 287, 288 (Fig.)
'Tannenbaum' stents, biliary, 199–200
Teflon stents, biliary, 199–200
Telangiectasias, radiation-induced, 68, 69,
    241–242
'Ten rules of APC', 98
Terumo guidewire, 201
T-fasteners, Russell method, 287, 288 (Fig.)
Therapeutic splitting, minimally invasive biliary
    surgery, 130
Thermal methods, for peptic ulcer hemorrhage,
    6–7, 9
Three-layer stents, biliary, 199–200
Thrombin, peptic ulcer injection therapy, 5
Thrombocytopenia, 106
Thrombogenic substances, peptic ulcer injection
    therapy, 5
Thrombosis, distant, sclerosants, 20
'Through-the-scope' balloon dilators, 30–31, 33,
    36, 44
'Through-the-scope' mechanical lithotriptors,
    149–150, 154, 157
Time duration, electrocoagulation, 60–61
Tin etiopurpurin, 102
TIPS, see Transjugular intrahepatic portosystemic
    shunting
Tissue distribution, porphyrins, 102
Tissue resistance, electrocoagulation, 60, 61
Torquable guidewires, biliary stenting, 201
Torque
  colonoscope positioning, 222–223
  echoendoscopes, 268
Torque devices, glidewire intestinal tube
    placement, 289
Toshiba PEF-703FA echoendoscope, 266
Tracer guidewire, biliary stenting, 201
Tracheobronchial system
  argon plasma coagulation, 92
  explosion, 90
  fistulae from laser therapy, 80
Tracking risk, carcinoma of colon at polypectomy,
    220
Transabdominal ultrasonography, biliary
    pancreatitis, 183
Transanal endoscopic microsurgery, 254–257
Transfusion, intestinal bleeding, 236
Transhepatic cholangioscopy, 137
Transillumination
  gastrostomy, 279, 283–284
  videoscopes and, 280
Transjugular intrahepatic portosystemic shunting,
    14
  vs sclerotherapy, 22
Transmural burn, 228
Transpapillary drainage, 190
Transpapillary stone removal, 147–163
  difficulties, 154–156
  procedure, 151–156
  results, 157–160
Transplantation of liver, esophageal varices, 22
Trauma, pancreatitis, 191
Treatment time calculation, photodynamic therapy,
    105
Triple layer lithotriptor, Olympus, 150

Triplet photosensitizers, 101
TTS ('through-the-scope') balloon dilators, 30–31,
    33, 36, 44
Tube feeding, trial of (Gauderer), 296
Tumor probe, multipolar, 63
Tumors
  ampulla of Vater, 130, 187
  argon plasma coagulation, 91, 96
  dilation
    duodenum, 35
    esophagus, 35
    results, 52
  electrocoagulation, 69–71, 72
  laser therapy, 75, 77–78, 82–83
    results, 80–81
  mistaken for stones, 152
  pancreas, 187
  photodynamic therapy, 106
  stenting, 39
  see also Carcinoma; Stenting, tumor ingrowth;
      Strictures, malignant; specific sites
Tuohy–Borst valve, irrigation for shockwave
    lithotripsy, 155
Twin-channel endoscopes, gastrointestinal
    bleeding, 2
Two-barb stents, pancreatic duct, 182
Two-channel endoscopes, colon polypectomy,
    225
Tygon tubing, stents from, 40

U-turn maneuver, colonoscopy
  bleeding, 237
  polypectomy, 225
Ulcers
  endoscopic mucosal resection, 123
    hemostasis, 125
  esophageal varices therapy, 19
    management, 21
  gastrostomy, 296
  hemorrhoid sclerotherapy, 248
  see also Peptic ulcer
Ultraflex stents, 41–42
  biliary Diamond stents, 200
  esophagus, results, 53–54
  non-esophageal use, 46
  rectal carcinoma, 49 (Fig.), 50 (Fig.)
Ultraslim cholangioscope
  ERCP, 179
  percutaneous transhepatic, 167
Ultrasonography
  transabdominal, biliary pancreatitis, 183
  see also Endosonography
Uni-Dwell needle, 166, 169
Urine retention, rectal carcinoma palliation, 259
Urologic resectoscopes, rectal carcinoma
    palliation, 258, 259
Ursodeoxycholic acid
  for microlithiasis, 185
  with stenting, 159–160
U-turn maneuver, colonoscopy
  bleeding, 237
  polypectomy, 225

Vaporization defects, laser therapy, 76
Variable rigidity guidewire, biliary stenting, 201
Varices
  laser therapy and, 75
  upper gastrointestinal bleeding, 13–27
  see also Ligation
Vasopressin
  angiography, gastrointestinal bleeding, 236
  sclerosants and, blood coagulation, 20
Vasopressors, esophageal varices, 16, 21
Vegetative state, gastrostomy and, 278
Ventilation, esophageal varices treatment, 16
Ventriculoperitoneal shunts, gastrostomy and,
    280
Video-chip baby cholangioscope, Olympus, 149
Videoscopes
  colonic chromoendoscopy, 217
  percutaneous transhepatic cholangioscopy,
    167
  transillumination and, 280
Villous adenomas
  laser therapy, results, 81
  transanal endoscopic microsurgery, 254

Wallstents, 41, 47 (Fig.), 50 (Fig.)
  biliary, 200, 204
  Enteral Wallstents, 46
  esophagus, results, 52 (Table), 53
  tumor ingrowth, 51
Water, injection therapy, 5
Water-jet systems, laser therapy, 76, 79, 82
Watermelon stomach
  argon plasma coagulation, 93 (Fig.), 96
  electrocoagulation, 67, 69
Water-pik device, 2

Wavelengths, phototherapy, 102
  monitoring, 105
Webs, esophagus, 35
Wilson-Cook stents, 40
'Windsock' stents, 42
Wire-guided systems, transpapillary stone
  removal, 149
Wound infection, gastrostomy, 295

X-rays, colonoscope position, 226

Yamakawa-type bougies, percutaneous
  transhepatic cholangioscopy, 166, 169,
  172

Z stents, 42, 46
  esophagus, results, 52 (Table), 53
  inadequate expansion, 50 (Fig.)
  migration, 51
  see also Spiral Z and ZA-stents
Zenker's diverticulum, septostomy, argon plasma
  coagulation, 97